Renal Cell Carcinoma

Renal Cell Carcinoma

Special Issue Editor

José I. López

MDPI • Basel • Beijing • Wuhan • Barcelona • Belgrade • Manchester • Tokyo • Cluj • Tianjin

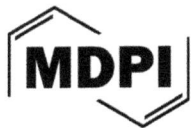

Special Issue Editor
José I. López
Cruces University Hospital
Spain

Editorial Office
MDPI
St. Alban-Anlage 66
4052 Basel, Switzerland

This is a reprint of articles from the Special Issue published online in the open access journal *Cancers* (ISSN 2072-6694) (available at: https://www.mdpi.com/journal/cancers/special_issues/RCC_cancers).

For citation purposes, cite each article independently as indicated on the article page online and as indicated below:

LastName, A.A.; LastName, B.B.; LastName, C.C. Article Title. *Journal Name* **Year**, *Article Number*, Page Range.

ISBN 978-3-03928-638-6 (Pbk)
ISBN 978-3-03928-639-3 (PDF)

Cover image courtesy of José I. López.

© 2020 by the authors. Articles in this book are Open Access and distributed under the Creative Commons Attribution (CC BY) license, which allows users to download, copy and build upon published articles, as long as the author and publisher are properly credited, which ensures maximum dissemination and a wider impact of our publications.

The book as a whole is distributed by MDPI under the terms and conditions of the Creative Commons license CC BY-NC-ND.

Contents

About the Special Issue Editor ix

Claudia Manini and José I. López
The Labyrinth of Renal Cell Carcinoma
Reprinted from: *Cancers* **2020**, *12*, 521, doi:10.3390/cancers12020521 1

Riuko Ohashi, Silvia Angori, Aashil A. Batavia, Niels J. Rupp, Yoichi Ajioka, Peter Schraml and Holger Moch
Loss of CDKN1A mRNA and Protein Expression Are Independent Predictors of Poor Outcome in Chromophobe Renal Cell Carcinoma Patients
Reprinted from: *Cancers* **2020**, *12*, 465, doi:10.3390/cancers12020465 7

Alexander Groß, Dmitry Chernyakov, Lisa Gallwitz, Nicola Bornkessel and Bayram Edemir
Deletion of Von Hippel–Lindau Interferes with Hyper Osmolality Induced Gene Expression and Induces an Unfavorable Gene Expression Pattern
Reprinted from: *Cancers* **2020**, *12*, 420, doi:10.3390/cancers12020420 21

Jochen Rutz, Sebastian Maxeiner, Saira Justin, Beatrice Bachmeier, August Bernd, Stefan Kippenberger, Nadja Zöller, Felix K.-H. Chun and Roman A. Blaheta
Low Dosed Curcumin Combined with Visible Light Exposure Inhibits Renal Cell Carcinoma Metastatic Behavior in Vitros
Reprinted from: *Cancers* **2020**, *12*, 302, doi:10.3390/cancers12020302 39

Luis Palomero, Lubomir Bodnar, Francesca Mateo, Carmen Herranz-Ors, Roderic Espín, Mar García-Varelo, Marzena Jesiotr, Gorka Ruiz de Garibay, Oriol Casanovas, José I. López and Miquel Angel Pujana
EVI1 as a Prognostic and Predictive Biomarker of Clear Cell Renal Cell Carcinoma
Reprinted from: *Cancers* **2020**, *12*, 300, doi:10.3390/cancers12020300 55

Lucia Santorelli, Giulia Capitoli, Clizia Chinello, Isabella Piga, Francesca Clerici, Vanna Denti, Andrew Smith, Angelica Grasso, Francesca Raimondo, Marco Grasso and Fulvio Magni
In-Depth Mapping of the Urinary N-Glycoproteome: Distinct Signatures of ccRCC-related Progression
Reprinted from: *Cancers* **2020**, *12*, 239, doi:10.3390/cancers12010239 67

Caroline Roelants, Catherine Pillet, Quentin Franquet, Clément Sarrazin, Nicolas Peilleron, Sofia Giacosa, Laurent Guyon, Amina Fontanell, Gaëlle Fiard, Jean-Alexandre Long, Jean-Luc Descotes, Claude Cochet and Odile Filhol
Ex-Vivo Treatment of Tumor Tissue Slices as a Predictive Preclinical Method to Evaluate Targeted Therapies for Patients with Renal Carcinoma
Reprinted from: *Cancers* **2020**, *12*, 232, doi:10.3390/cancers12010232 85

Sven Wach, Helge Taubert, Katrin Weigelt, Nora Hase, Marcel Köhn, Danny Misiak, Stefan Hüttelmaier, Christine G. Stöhr, Andreas Kahlmeyer, Florian Haller, Julio Vera, Arndt Hartmann, Bernd Wullich and Xin Lai
RNA Sequencing of Collecting Duct Renal Cell Carcinoma Suggests an Interaction between miRNA and Target Genes and a Predominance of Deregulated Solute Carrier Genes
Reprinted from: *Cancers* **2020**, *12*, 64, doi:10.3390/cancers12010064 103

Tanja Radic, Vesna Coric, Zoran Bukumiric, Marija Pljesa-Ercegovac, Tatjana Djukic, Natasa Avramovic, Marija Matic, Smiljana Mihailovic, Dejan Dragicevic, Zoran Dzamic, Tatjana Simic and Ana Savic-Radojevic
GSTO1*CC Genotype (rs4925) Predicts Shorter Survival in Clear Cell Renal Cell Carcinoma Male Patients
Reprinted from: Cancers **2019**, *11*, 2038, doi:10.3390/cancers11122038 . . . . **121**

Yong-Syuan Chen, Tung-Wei Hung, Shih-Chi Su, Chia-Liang Lin, Shun-Fa Yang, Chu-Che Lee, Chang-Fang Yeh, Yi-Hsien Hsieh and Jen-Pi Tsai
MTA2 as a Potential Biomarker and Its Involvement in Metastatic Progression of Human Renal Cancer by miR-133b Targeting MMP-9
Reprinted from: Cancers **2019**, *11*, 1851, doi:10.3390/cancers11121851 . . . . **139**

Joanna Bogusławska, Piotr Popławski, Saleh Alseekh, Marta Koblowska, Roksana Iwanicka-Nowicka, Beata Rybicka, Hanna Kędzierska, Katarzyna Głuchowska, Karolina Hanusek, Zbigniew Tański, Alisdair R. Fernie and Agnieszka Piekiełko-Witkowska
MicroRNA-Mediated Metabolic Reprograming in Renal Cancer
Reprinted from: Cancers **2019**, *11*, 1825, doi:10.3390/cancers11121825 . . . . **155**

Minsun Jung, Jeong Hoon Lee, Cheol Lee, Jeong Hwan Park, Yu Rang Park and Kyung Chul Moon
Prognostic Implication of pAMPK Immunohistochemical Staining by Subcellular Location and Its Association with SMAD Protein Expression in Clear Cell Renal Cell Carcinoma
Reprinted from: Cancers **2019**, *11*, 1602, doi:10.3390/cancers11101602 . . . . **177**

Riuko Ohashi, Peter Schraml, Silvia Angori, Aashil A. Batavia, Niels J. Rupp, Chisato Ohe, Yoshiro Otsuki, Takashi Kawasaki, Hiroshi Kobayashi, Kazuhiro Kobayashi, Tatsuhiko Miyazaki, Hiroyuki Shibuya, Hiroyuki Usuda, Hajime Umezu, Fumiyoshi Fujishima, Bungo Furusato, Mitsumasa Osakabe, Tamotsu Sugai, Naoto Kuroda, Toyonori Tsuzuki, Yoji Nagashima, Yoichi Ajioka and Holger Moch
Classic Chromophobe Renal Cell Carcinoma Incur a Larger Number of Chromosomal Losses Than Seen in the Eosinophilic Subtype
Reprinted from: Cancers **2019**, *11*, 1492, doi:10.3390/cancers11101492 . . . . **191**

Antonia Franz, Bernhard Ralla, Sabine Weickmann, Monika Jung, Hannah Rochow, Carsten Stephan, Andreas Erbersdobler, Ergin Kilic, Annika Fendler and Klaus Jung
Circular RNAs in Clear Cell Renal Cell Carcinoma: Their Microarray-Based Identification, Analytical Validation, and Potential Use in a Clinico-Genomic Model to Improve Prognostic Accuracy
Reprinted from: Cancers **2019**, *11*, 1473, doi:10.3390/cancers11101473 . . . . **205**

Mi-Ae Kang, Jongsung Lee, Sang Hoon Ha, Chang Min Lee, Kyoung Min Kim, Kyu Yun Jang and See-Hyoung Park
Interleukin4Rα (IL4Rα) and IL13Rα1 Are Associated with the Progress of Renal Cell Carcinoma through Janus Kinase 2 (JAK2)/Forkhead Box O3 (FOXO3) Pathways
Reprinted from: Cancers **2019**, *11*, 1394, doi:10.3390/cancers11091394 . . . . **229**

Ayham Al Ahmad, Vanessa Paffrath, Rosanna Clima, Jonas Felix Busch, Anja Rabien, Ergin Kilic, Sonia Villegas, Bernd Timmermann, Marcella Attimonelli, Klaus Jung and David Meierhofer
Papillary Renal Cell Carcinomas Rewire Glutathione Metabolism and Are Deficient in Both Anabolic Glucose Synthesis and Oxidative Phosphorylation
Reprinted from: Cancers **2019**, *11*, 1298, doi:10.3390/cancers11091298 . . . . **253**

Paranita Ferronika, Joost Hof, Gursah Kats-Ugurlu, Rolf H. Sijmons, Martijn M. Terpstra, Kim de Lange, Annemarie Leliveld-Kors, Helga Westers and Klaas Kok
Comprehensive Profiling of Primary and Metastatic ccRCC Reveals a High Homology of the Metastases to a Subregion of the Primary Tumour
Reprinted from: *Cancers* **2019**, *11*, 812, doi:10.3390/cancers11060812 275

Kendrick Yim, Ahmet Bindayi, Rana McKay, Reza Mehrazin, Omer A. Raheem, Charles Field, Aaron Bloch, Robert Wake, Stephen Ryan, Anthony Patterson and Ithaar H. Derweesh
Rising Serum Uric Acid Level Is Negatively Associated with Survival in Renal Cell Carcinoma
Reprinted from: *Cancers* **2019**, *11*, 536, doi:10.3390/cancers11040536 289

Tsung-Chieh Lin, Yuan-Ming Yeh, Wen-Lang Fan, Yu-Chan Chang, Wei-Ming Lin, Tse-Yen Yang and Michael Hsiao
Ghrelin Upregulates Oncogenic Aurora A to Promote Renal Cell Carcinoma Invasion
Reprinted from: *Cancers* **2019**, *11*, 303, doi:10.3390/cancers11030303 303

Iñigo Terrén, Ane Orrantia, Idoia Mikelez-Alonso, Joana Vitallé, Olatz Zenarruzabeitia and Francisco Borrego
NK Cell-Based Immunotherapy in Renal Cell Carcinoma
Reprinted from: *Cancers* **2020**, *12*, 316, doi:10.3390/cancers12020316 317

Farshid Siadat and Kiril Trpkov
ESC, ALK, HOT and LOT: Three Letter Acronyms of Emerging Renal Entities Knocking on the Door of the WHO Classification
Reprinted from: *Cancers* **2020**, *12*, 168, doi:10.3390/cancers12010168 341

Rohan Garje, Josiah An, Austin Greco, Raju Kumar Vaddepally and Yousef Zakharia
The Future of Immunotherapy-Based Combination Therapy in Metastatic Renal Cell Carcinoma
Reprinted from: *Cancers* **2020**, *12*, 143, doi:10.3390/cancers12010143 357

Véronique Debien, Jonathan Thouvenin, Véronique Lindner, Philippe Barthélémy, Hervé Lang, Ronan Flippot and Gabriel G. Malouf
Sarcomatoid Dedifferentiation in Renal Cell Carcinoma: From Novel Molecular Insights to New Clinical Opportunities
Reprinted from: *Cancers* **2020**, *12*, 99, doi:10.3390/cancers12010099 371

Reza Alaghehbandan, Delia Perez Montiel, Ana Silvia Luis and Ondrej Hes
Molecular Genetics of Renal Cell Tumors: A Practical Diagnostic Approach
Reprinted from: *Cancers* **2020**, *12*, 85, doi:10.3390/cancers12010085 383

Lucía Carril-Ajuria, María Santos, Juan María Roldán-Romero, Cristina Rodriguez-Antona and Guillermo de Velasco
Prognostic and Predictive Value of *PBRM1* in Clear Cell Renal Cell Carcinoma
Reprinted from: *Cancers* **2020**, *12*, 16, doi:10.3390/cancers12010016 407

Nicole Brighi, Alberto Farolfi, Vincenza Conteduca, Giorgia Gurioli, Stefania Gargiulo, Valentina Gallà, Giuseppe Schepisi, Cristian Lolli, Chiara Casadei and Ugo De Giorgi
The Interplay between Inflammation, Anti-Angiogenic Agents, and Immune Checkpoint Inhibitors: Perspectives for Renal Cell Cancer Treatment
Reprinted from: *Cancers* **2019**, *11*, 1935, doi:10.3390/cancers11121935 423

Javier C. Angulo and Oleg Shapiro
The Changing Therapeutic Landscape of Metastatic Renal Cancer
Reprinted from: *Cancers* **2019**, *11*, 1227, doi:10.3390/cancers11091227 447

Anna Caliò, Diego Segala, Enrico Munari, Matteo Brunelli and Guido Martignoni
MiT Family Translocation Renal Cell Carcinoma: from the Early Descriptions to the Current Knowledge
Reprinted from: *Cancers* **2019**, *11*, 1110, doi:10.3390/cancers11081110 . . . . **461**

Siarhei Kandabarau, Janna Leiz, Knut Krohn, Stefan Winter, Jens Bedke, Matthias Schwab, Elke Schaeffeler and Bayram Edemir
Hypertonicity-Affected Genes Are Differentially Expressed in Clear Cell Renal Cell Carcinoma and Correlate with Cancer-Specific Survival
Reprinted from: *Cancers* **2020**, *12*, 6, doi:10.3390/cancers12010006 . . . . **473**

Renate Pichler, Eva Compérat, Tobias Klatte, Martin Pichler, Wolfgang Loidl, Lukas Lusuardi and Manuela Schmidinger
Renal Cell Carcinoma with Sarcomatoid Features: Finally New Therapeutic Hope?
Reprinted from: *Cancers* **2019**, *11*, 422, doi:10.3390/cancers11030422 . . . . **483**

About the Special Issue Editor

José I. López is Head of Department of Pathology at the Hospital Universitario Cruces and principal investigator of the Biomarkers in Cancer Unit at the Biocruces-Bizkaia Health Research Institute. He graduated at the Faculty of Medicine, University of the Basque Country, Leioa, Spain, and trained in Pathology at the Hospital 12 de Octubre, Madrid, Spain. He received his PhD degree at the Universidad Complutense of Madrid, Spain. Dr. López has served as pathologist for more than 30 years in several hospitals in Spain, and is specialized in Uropathology, where he has published more than 170 peer-reviewed articles and reviews. Dr. López is interested in translational uropathology in general and in renal cancer in particular, and collaborates with several international research groups unveiling the genomic landscape of renal and prostate cancer. Intratumor heterogeneity, tumor sampling, tumor microenvironment, immunotherapy, and basic mechanisms of carcinogenesis are his main topics of research.

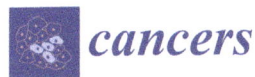

Editorial

The Labyrinth of Renal Cell Carcinoma

Claudia Manini [1] and José I. López [2,*]

1. Department of Pathology, San Giovanni Bosco Hospital, 10154 Turin, Italy; claudiamaninicm@gmail.com
2. Department of Pathology, Cruces University Hospital, Biocruces-Bizkaia Institute, University of the Basque Country, Plaza de Cruces s/n, 48903 Barakaldo, Bizkaia, Spain
* Correspondence: jilpath@gmail.com; Tel.: +34-94-600-6084

Received: 18 February 2020; Accepted: 21 February 2020; Published: 24 February 2020

Renal cell carcinoma (RCC) ranks in the top-ten list of malignancies both in males and females [1], and its frequency is increasing as a consequence of the increase in aging and obesity in Western societies [2]. Clear cell renal cell carcinoma (CCRCC) is by far the most common histological variant [3]. CCRCC has received much attention in recent years due to some new therapeutic approaches that are improving the life expectancy of many of these patients. In this way, a tumor traditionally resistant to chemo- and radiotherapy, in which only surgery and early detection had a significant prognostic impact, is becoming ultimately treatable with evident success with antiangiogenic drugs and immune checkpoint blockade, either alone or in combination [4]. However, the problem is far from being solved in many cases, due in part to intra- and inter-tumor heterogeneity [4,5].

Roughly 30% of RCCs are other than CCRCC. The list of non-CCRCC tumors grows steadily, and includes classically recognized entities and new ones which are sometimes not yet fully characterized [6]. The maze is particularly complex in the field of RCC with papillary architecture. The classical papillary renal cell carcinoma (PRCC) included types 1 and 2, but today this classification seems insufficient and is no longer recommended [7]. A recent study has identified a new subtype (type 3) with a distinct molecular signature and morphologic overlapping with types 1 and 2 [8]. As a result of this complexity, the diagnosis of PRCC is increasingly becoming a descriptive term among practical pathologists.

To make matters worse, some oncocytic/eosinophilic RCCs (other than ChRCC/oncocytoma) may display papillary, tubule-papillary or solid-papillary architectures. These cases represent a challenge even for experienced pathologists, who used to shelter their diagnoses under the descriptive term "oncocytic papillary renal cell carcinoma". This descriptive diagnosis, although not very informative, is still valid for the patient since it includes critical data such as tumor grade, necrosis, staging. However, the impression is that the term is too broad for use in daily practice.

Probably more than in any other human neoplasm, CCRCC and PRCC are hostages of the terminology's restrictions. Strictly speaking, CCRCC was the classical name given to RCC composed of clear cells and PRCC the one for RCCs architecturally arranged in the papillae, but experience has shown that some CCRCC are not composed of clear cells and some PRCC do not show papillae. Moreover, CCRCC may display a predominantly papillary architecture [9] and PRCC a prominent cytoplasmic clearance [10]. Even worse, some RCC includes different overlapping cell types and architectures, intermingled altogether in different proportions [11]. Currently, we include these cases in the "unclassified" category. The broad spectrum of morphological appearances may be quite confusing, as has been shown in a recent study [12].

Renal oncocytoma (RO) and ChRCC are the best-characterized eosinophilic renal tumors under the microscope [13]. However, a papillary architecture has been very recently described in ChRCC [14], thus favoring diagnostic confusion. The use of the term "oncocytic", applied to cells with large and deeply granular eosinophilic cytoplasm, is a mistake because, although all oncocytes are eosinophilic, not all eosinophilic cells are oncocytes. As a consequence, the terms eosinophilic and oncocytic are exchanged erroneously with some frequency. The elusive word "hybrid" is applied to those cases that seem to fall in between RO and ChRCC with very unprecise limits [13]. Some of them likely represent genomic RO [15]. Such hybrid oncocytic tumors are also observed in the so-called renal oncocytosis, a condition characterized by multifocal and bilateral oncocytic tumors [16].

Regarding molecular analyses, the issue remains incomplete when considering *VHL* gene malfunctions as the hallmark of CCRCC, and the trisomy of chromosomes 7 and 17 as the signature for PRCC. We know that a subset of CCRCC is *VHL* wild-type [17] and that PRCC may display a wide spectrum of molecular alterations [18]. Therefore, the classification of most RCCs based on molecular signatures is also imperfect and still under construction. Is there any molecular signature specifically linked to the papillary phenotype regardless of the RCC subtype? We do not know the answer to date, but we could hypothesize and, in such a case, the papillary architecture will not be a tumor-specific mark anymore, but a mere trait.

A reductionist prejudice when identifying the varied morphological subtypes of RCC is to link tumor morphology with a precise site of origin along the nephron. As far as we know, a reliable analysis linking CCRCC and PRCC to the proximal convoluted tubule is lacking, and there are no scientific reasons to deny that other elements of the nephron cannot be a potential site of origin for kidney tumors. How might the proximal convoluted tubule be the origin of two different tumors if only one cell type has been histologically described there? This question also remains unanswered, but Gu et al. [19], based on a modeling study on renal cell carcinoma in mice, have proposed that CCRCC may originate in Bowman's capsule.

The list of new renal cell neoplasms, either recognized as true entities or pending recognition, is still growing, as it has been recently reviewed [6]. Many of them may show some morphologic overlap, so strategic approaches based on immunohistochemistry have been developed trying to overcome this question [20]. The problem at this point is their correct identification in routine practice, since many of them are histologically indistinguishable and are defined only by molecular analyses [21] that are not always performed. This situation leads to the question of how many of these newly described cases are buried in pathology labs under irrecoverable descriptive diagnoses. As several of these diagnoses carry out prognostic and eventually therapeutic implications, the reversal of this situation seems an urgent task for pathologists now that personalized oncology is being increasingly implemented worldwide.

This Special Issue of *Cancers* regards the RCC labyrinth from very different perspectives, including the intimate basic mechanisms governing this disease and the clinical practice principles of their diagnoses and treatments. Thus, the interested reader will have the opportunity to discover some of the most recent findings in renal carcinogenesis and be updated with excellent reviews on new therapeutic approaches and the genetic bases of the disease.

Original articles in this issue show interesting findings with potential clinical application. Examples of the science and research presented in this Special Issue include: the influence of *VHL* deletion in the expression of an unfavorable genetic pattern in CCRCC [22]; how a low dose of curcumin inhibits RCC's metastatic behavior [23]; the predictive value of the overexpression of EVI1 in CCRCC [24]; the poor outcome of ChRCC patients who lose CDKN1A mRNA and protein expression [25]; the identification of distinct signatures of CCRCC progression through in-depth mapping of urinary *N*-glycoproteome [26]; how a preclinical evaluation method may evaluate the response to targeted therapies in patients with RCC [27]; the RNA sequencing results obtained in two examples of collecting duct renal cell carcinoma, an aggressive rare variant of RCC [28]; how *GSTO1*CC* genotype predicts shorter survival in CCRCC male patients [29]; the importance of MTA2 as a biomarker of metastatic progression in RCC [30]; the metabolic reprograming in RCC [31]; the prognostic implications of pAMPK immunostaining and its association with SMAD protein expression in CCRCC [32]; the different amount of chromosomal losses in classic ChRCC compared with the eosinophilic subtype of this neoplasm [33]; the potential influence of circular RNAs in CCRCC prognosis [34]; the association of interleukins 4Rα and 13Rα1 with the progression of RCC [35]; the glutathione metabolism in PRCC [36]; how the profiling of primary and metastatic samples of CCRCC reveals a high homology of metastases with a specific subregion of the primary tumor [37]; the interrelationship between serum uric acid levels and RCC survival [38]; and the importance of ghrelin promoting RCC invasion [39].

A total of nine reviews have also been published. Predominantly clinical reviews deal with the emerging new therapeutic landscape of metastatic renal cancer [40–43], the genetic approach to this complex disease [44–47], and the histopathological diagnostic criteria of newly appearing entities [48].

A brief report shows how hypertonicity-affected genes are differentially expressed in CCRCC correlating with cancer survival [49]. Finally, a short commentary focuses on the therapeutic possibilities of sarcomatoid RCC [50].

Funding: This research received no external funding.

Conflicts of Interest: The authors declare no conflict of interest.

References

1. Siegel, R.; Miller, K.D.; Jemal, A. Cancer statistics, 2020. *CA Cancer J. Clin.* **2020**, *70*, 7–30. [CrossRef] [PubMed]
2. Turajlic, S.; Swanton, C.; Boshoff, C. Kidney cancer: The next decade. *J. Exp. Med.* **2018**, *215*, 2477–2479. [CrossRef] [PubMed]
3. López, J.I. Renal tumors with clear cells. A review. *Pathol. Res. Pract.* **2013**, *209*, 137–146. [CrossRef] [PubMed]
4. Angulo, J.C.; Lawrie, C.H.; López, J.I. Sequential treatment of metastatic renal cancer in a complex evolving landscape. *Ann. Transl. Med.* **2019**, *7*, S272. [CrossRef] [PubMed]
5. Nunes-Xavier, C.; Angulo, J.C.; Pulido, R.; López, J.I. A critical insight into the clinical translation of PD-1/PD-L1 blockade therapying clear cell renal cell carcinoma. *Curr. Urol. Rep.* **2019**, *20*, 1. [CrossRef] [PubMed]
6. Trpkov, K.; Hes, O. New and emerging renal entities: A perspective post-WHO 2016 classification. *Histopathology* **2019**, *74*, 31–59. [CrossRef] [PubMed]
7. Akhtar, M.; Al-Bozom, I.A.; Al-Hussain, T. Papillary renal cell carcinoma (PRCC): An update. *Adv. Anat. Pathol.* **2019**, *26*, 124–132. [CrossRef]
8. Saleeb, R.M.; Brimo, F.; Farag, M.; Rompré-Brodeur, A.; Rotondo, F.; Beharry, V.; Wala, S.; Plant, P.; Downes, M.R.; Pace, K.; et al. Toward biological subtyping of papillary renal cell carcinoma with clinical implications through histologic, immunohistochemical, and molecular analysis. *Am. J. Surg. Pathol.* **2017**, *41*, 1618–1629. [CrossRef]
9. Alaghehbandan, R.; Ulamec, M.; Martinek, P.; Pivovarcikova, K.; Michalova, K.; Skenderi, F.; Hora, M.; Michal, M.; Hes, O. Papillary pattern in clear cell renal cell carcinoma: Clinicopathologic, morphologic, immunohistochemical and molecular genetic analysis of 23 cases. *Ann. Diagn. Pathol.* **2019**, *38*, 80–86. [CrossRef]
10. Klatte, T.; Said, J.W.; Seligson, D.B.; Rao, P.N.; de Martino, M.; Shuch, B.; Zomorodian, N.; Kabbinavar, F.F.; Belldegrun, A.S.; Pantuck, A.J. Pathological, immunohistochemical and cytogenetic features of papillary renal cell carcinoma with clear cell features. *J. Urol.* **2011**, *185*, 30–35. [CrossRef]
11. Michalova, K.; Steiner, P.; Alaghehbandan, R.; Trpkov, K.; Martinek, P.; Grossmann, P.; Montiel, D.P.; Sperga, M.; Straka, L.; Prochazkova, K. Papillary renal cell carcinoma with cytologic and molecular genetic features overlapping with renal cell oncocytoma: Analysis of 10 cases. *Ann. Diagn. Pathol.* **2018**, *35*, 1–6. [CrossRef] [PubMed]
12. Cai, Q.; Christie, A.; Rajaram, S.; Zhou, Q.; Araj, E.; Chintalapati, S.; Cadeddu, J.; Margulis, V.; Pedrosa, I.; Rakheja, D.; et al. Ontological analyses reveal clinically-significant clear cell renal cell carcinoma subtypes with convergent evolutionary trajectories into an aggressive type. *EBioMedicine* **2019**. [CrossRef] [PubMed]
13. Williamson, S.R.; Gadde, R.; Trpkov, K.; Hirsch, M.S.; Srigley, J.R.; Reuter, V.E.; Cheng, L.; Kunju, L.P.; Barod, R.; Rogers, C.G.; et al. Diagnostic criteria for oncocytic renal neoplasms: A survey of urologic pathologists. *Hum. Pathol.* **2017**, *63*, 149–156. [CrossRef]

14. Michalova, K.; Tretiakova, M.; Pivovarcikova, K.; Alaghehbandan, R.; Montiel, D.P.; Ulamec, M.; Osunkoya, A.; Trpkov, K.; Yuan, G.; Grossmann, P.; et al. Expanding the morphologic spectrum of chromophobe renal cell carcinoma: A study of 8 cases with papillary architecture. *Ann. Diagn. Pathol.* **2020**, *44*, 151448. [CrossRef] [PubMed]
15. Poté, N.; Vieillefond, A.; Couturier, J.; Arrufat, S.; Metzger, I.; Delongchamps, N.B.; Camparo, P.; Mège-Lechevallier, F.; Molinié, V.; Sibony, M.; et al. Hybrid oncocytic/chromophobe renal cell tumors do not display genomic features of chromophobe renal cell carcinomas. *Virchows. Arch.* **2013**, *462*, 633–638. [CrossRef] [PubMed]
16. Giunchi, F.; Fiorentino, M.; Vagnoni, V.; Capizzi, E.; Bertolo, R.; Porpiglia, F.; Vatrano, S.; Tamberi, S.; Schiavina, R.; Papotti, M.; et al. Renal oncocytosis: A clinicopathological and cytogenetic study of 42 tumours occurring in 11 patients. *Pathology* **2016**, *48*, 41–46. [CrossRef]
17. Turajlic, S.; Xu, H.; Litchfield, K.; Rowan, A.; Horswell, S.; Chambers, T.; O'Brien, T.; Lopez, J.I.; Watkins, T.B.; Nicol, D.; et al. Deterministic evolutionary trajectories influence primary tumor growth: TRACERx *Renal*. *Cell* **2018**, *173*, 595–610. [CrossRef]
18. Cancer Genome Atlas Research Network. Comprehensive molecular characterization of papillary renal cell carcinoma. *N. Eng. J. Med.* **2016**, *374*, 135–145. [CrossRef]
19. Gu, Y.-F.; Cohn, S.; Christie, A.; McKenzie, T.; Wolff, N.; Do, Q.N.; Madhuranthakam, A.J.; Pedrosa, I.; Wang, T.; Dey, A.; et al. Modeling renal cell carcinoma in mice: *Bap1* and *Pbrm1* inactivation drive tumor grade. *Cancer Discov.* **2017**, *7*, 900–917. [CrossRef]
20. Kryvenko, O.N.; Jorda, M.; Argani, P.; Epstein, J.I. Diagnostic approach to eosinophilic renal neoplasms. *Arch. Pathol. Lab. Med.* **2014**, *138*, 1531–1541. [CrossRef]
21. Beaumont, M.; Dugay, F.; Kammerer-Jacquet, S.-F.; Jaillard, S.; Cabillic, F.; Mathieu, R.; Verhoest, G.; Bensalah, K.; Rioux-Leclercq, N.; Belaud-Rotureau, M.-A. Diagnosis of uncommon renal epithelial neoplasms: Performances of fluorescence in situ hybridization. *Hum. Pathol.* **2019**, *92*, 81–90. [CrossRef] [PubMed]
22. Groß, A.; Chernyakov, D.; Gallwitz, L.; Bornkessel, N.; Edemir, B. Deletion of Von Hippel–Lindau Interferes with Hyper Osmolality Induced Gene Expression and Induces an Unfavorable Gene Expression Pattern. *Cancers* **2020**, *12*, 420. [CrossRef] [PubMed]
23. Rutz, J.; Maxeiner, S.; Justin, S.; Bachmeier, B.; Bernd, A.; Kippenberger, S.; Zöller, N.; Chun, F.; Blaheta, R. Low Dosed Curcumin Combined with Visible Light Exposure Inhibits Renal Cell Carcinoma Metastatic Behavior In Vitro. *Cancers* **2020**, *12*, 302. [CrossRef] [PubMed]
24. Palomero, L.; Bodnar, L.; Mateo, F.; Herranz-Ors, C.; Espín, R.; García-Varelo, M.; Jesiotr, M.; Ruiz de Garibay, G.; Casanovas, O.; López, J.; et al. EVI1 as a Prognostic and Predictive Biomarker of Clear Cell Renal Cell Carcinoma. *Cancers* **2020**, *12*, 300. [CrossRef]
25. Ohashi, R.; Angori, S.; Batavia, A.A.; Rupp, N.J.; Ajioka, Y.; Schraml, P.; Moch, H. Loss of CDKN1A mRNA and protein expression are independent predictors of poor outcome in chromophobe renal cell carcinoma patients. *Cancers* **2020**, *12*, 465. [CrossRef]
26. Santorelli, L.; Capitoli, G.; Chinello, C.; Piga, I.; Clerici, F.; Denti, V.; Smith, A.; Grasso, A.; Raimondo, F.; Grasso, M.; et al. In-depth mapping of the urinary *N*-glycoproteome: Distinct signatures of ccRCC-related progression. *Cancers* **2020**, *12*, 239. [CrossRef]
27. Roelants, C.; Pillet, C.; Franquet, Q.; Sarrazin, C.; Peilleron, N.; Giacosa, S.; Guyon, L.; Fontanell, A.; Fiard, G.; Long, J.-A.; et al. Ex-vivo treatment of tumor tissue slices as a predictive preclinical method to evaluate targeted therapies for patients with renal carcinoma. *Cancers* **2020**, *12*, 232. [CrossRef]
28. Wach, S.; Taubert, H.; Weigelt, K.; Hase, N.; Köhn, M.; Misiak, D.; Hüttelmaier, S.; Stöhr, C.G.; Kahlmeyer, A.; Haller, F.; et al. RNA sequencing of collecting duct renal cell carcinoma suggests an interaction between miRNA and target genes and a predominance of deregulated solute carrier genes. *Cancers* **2020**, *12*, 64. [CrossRef]
29. Radic, T.; Coric, V.; Bukumiric, Z.; Pljesa-Ercegovac, M.; Djukic, T.; Avramovic, N.; Matic, M.; Mihailovic, S.; Dragicevic, D.; Dzamic, Z.; et al. *GSTO1*CC* genotype (rs4925) predicts shorter survival in clear cell renal cell carcinoma male patients. *Cancers* **2019**, *11*, 2038. [CrossRef]

30. Chen, Y.-S.; Hung, T.-W.; Su, S.-C.; Lin, C.-L.; Yang, S.-F.; Lee, C.-C.; Yeh, C.-F.; Hsieh, Y.-H.; Tsai, J.-P. MTA2 as a potential biomarker and its involvement in metastatic progression of human renal cancer by miR-133b targeting MMP-9. *Cancers* **2019**, *11*, 1851. [CrossRef]
31. Bogusławska, J.; Popławski, P.; Alseekh, S.; Koblowska, M.; Iwanicka-Nowicka, R.; Rybicka, B.; Kędzierska, H.; Głuchowska, K.; Hanusek, K.; Tański, Z.; et al. MicroRNA-mediated metabolic reprograming in renal cancer. *Cancers* **2019**, *11*, 1825. [CrossRef] [PubMed]
32. Jung, M.; Lee, J.H.; Lee, C.; Park, J.H.; Park, Y.R.; Moon, K.C. Prognostic implication of pAMPK immunohistochemical staining by subcellular location and its association with SMAD protein expression in clear cell renal cell carcinoma. *Cancers* **2019**, *11*, 1602. [CrossRef] [PubMed]
33. Ohashi, R.; Schraml, P.; Angori, S.; Batavia, A.A.; Rupp, N.J.; Ohe, C.; Otsuki, Y.; Kawasaki, T.; Kobayashi, H.; Kobayashi, K.; et al. Classic chromophobe renal cell carcinoma incur a larger number of chromosomal losses than seen in the eosinophilic subtype. *Cancers* **2019**, *11*, 1492. [CrossRef] [PubMed]
34. Franz, A.; Ralla, B.; Weickmann, S.; Jung, M.; Rochow, H.; Stephan, C.; Erbersdobler, A.; Kilic, E.; Fendler, A.; Jung, K. Circular RNAs in clear cell renal cell carcinoma: Their microarray-based identification, analytical validation, and potential use in a clinico-genomic model to improve prognostic accuracy. *Cancers* **2019**, *11*, 1473. [CrossRef] [PubMed]
35. Kang, M.; Lee, J.; Ha, S.; Lee, C.; Kim, K.; Jang, K.; Park, S. Interleukin4Rα (IL4Rα) and IL13Rα1 Are Associated with the Progress of Renal Cell Carcinoma through Janus Kinase 2 (JAK2)/Forkhead Box O3 (FOXO3) Pathways. *Cancers* **2019**, *11*, 1394. [CrossRef] [PubMed]
36. Ahmad, A.; Paffrath, V.; Clima, R.; Busch, J.; Rabien, A.; Kilic, E.; Villegas, S.; Timmermann, B.; Attimonelli, M.; Jung, K.; et al. Papillary Renal Cell Carcinomas Rewire Glutathione Metabolism and Are Deficient in Both Anabolic Glucose Synthesis and Oxidative Phosphorylation. *Cancers* **2019**, *11*, 1298. [CrossRef]
37. Ferronika, P.; Hof, J.; Kats-Ugurlu, G.; Sijmons, R.H.; Terpstra, M.M.; de Lange, K.; Leliveld-Kors, A.; Westers, H.; Kok, K. Comprehensive profiling of primary and metastatic ccRCC reveals a high homology of the metastases to a subregion of the primary tumour. *Cancers* **2019**, *11*, 812. [CrossRef]
38. Yim, K.; Bindayi, A.; McKay, R.; Mehrazin, R.; Raheem, O.; Field, C.; Bloch, A.; Wake, R.; Ryan, S.; Patterson, A.; et al. Rising Serum Uric Acid Level Is Negatively Associated with Survival in Renal Cell Carcinoma. *Cancers* **2019**, *11*, 536. [CrossRef]
39. Lin, T.; Yeh, Y.; Fan, W.; Chang, Y.; Lin, W.; Yang, T.; Hsiao, M. Ghrelin Upregulates Oncogenic Aurora A to Promote Renal Cell Carcinoma Invasion. *Cancers* **2019**, *11*, 303. [CrossRef]
40. Terren, I.; Orrantia, A.; Mikelez-Alonso, I.; Vitallé, J.; Zenarruzabeitia, O.; Borrego, F. NK cell-based immunotherapy in renal cell carcinoma. *Cancers* **2020**, *12*, 316. [CrossRef]
41. Garje, R.; An, J.; Greco, A.; Vaddepally, R.K.; Zakharia, Y. The future of immunotherapy-based combination therapy in metastatic renal cell carcinoma. *Cancers* **2020**, *12*, 143. [CrossRef] [PubMed]
42. Brighi, N.; Farolfi, A.; Conteduca, V.; Gurioli, G.; Gargiulo, S.; Gallà, V.; Schepisi, G.; Lolli, C.; Casadei, C.; De Giorgi, U. The interplay between inflammation, anti-angiogenic agents, and immune checkpoint inhibitors: Perspectives for renal cancer treatment. *Cancers* **2019**, *11*, 1935. [CrossRef]
43. Angulo, J.C.; Shapiro, O. The changing therapeutic landscape of metastatic renal cancer. *Cancers* **2019**, *11*, 1227. [CrossRef] [PubMed]
44. Caliò, A.; Segala, D.; Munari, E.; Brunelli, M.; Martignoni, G. MiT family translocation renal cell carcinoma: From early descriptions to the current knowledge. *Cancers* **2019**, *11*, 1110. [CrossRef]
45. Alaghehbandan, R.; Perez Montiel, D.; Luis, A.S.; Hes, O. Molecular genetics of renal cell tumors: A practical diagnostic approach. *Cancers* **2020**, *12*, 85. [CrossRef]
46. Carril-Ajuria, L.; Santos, M.; Roldán-Romero, J.M.; Rodriguez-Antona, C.; de Velasco, G. Prognostic and predictive value of *PBRM1* in clear cell renal cell carcinoma. *Cancers* **2020**, *12*, 16. [CrossRef] [PubMed]
47. Debien, V.; Thouvenin, J.; Lindner, V.; Barthélémy, P.; Lang, H.; Flippot, R.; Malouf, G. Sarcomatoid Dedifferentiation in Renal Cell Carcinoma: From Novel Molecular Insights to New Clinical Opportunities. *Cancers* **2020**, *12*, 99. [CrossRef] [PubMed]
48. Siadat, F.; Trpkov, K. ESC, ALK, HOT, LOT: Three letter acronyms of emerging renal entities knocking on the door of the WHO classification. *Cancers* **2020**, *12*, 168. [CrossRef]

49. Kandabarau, S.; Leiz, J.; Krohn, K.; Winter, S.; Bedke, J.; Schwab, M.; Schaeffeler, E.; Edemir, B. Hypertonicity-Affected Genes Are Differentially Expressed in Clear Cell Renal Cell Carcinoma and Correlate with Cancer-Specific Survival. *Cancers* **2020**, *12*, 6. [CrossRef]
50. Pichler, R.; Compérat, E.; Klatte, T.; Pichler, M.; Loidl, W.; Lusuardi, L.; Schmidinger, M. Renal Cell Carcinoma with Sarcomatoid Features: Finally New Therapeutic Hope? *Cancers* **2019**, *11*, 422. [CrossRef]

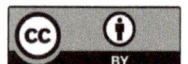

© 2020 by the authors. Licensee MDPI, Basel, Switzerland. This article is an open access article distributed under the terms and conditions of the Creative Commons Attribution (CC BY) license (http://creativecommons.org/licenses/by/4.0/).

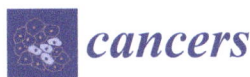

Article

Loss of CDKN1A mRNA and Protein Expression Are Independent Predictors of Poor Outcome in Chromophobe Renal Cell Carcinoma Patients

Riuko Ohashi [1,2,3], Silvia Angori [2], Aashil A. Batavia [2], Niels J. Rupp [2], Yoichi Ajioka [1,3], Peter Schraml [2,*,†] and Holger Moch [2,†]

1. Histopathology Core Facility, Faculty of Medicine, Niigata University, Niigata 951-8510, Japan; riuko@med.niigata-u.ac.jp (R.O.); ajioka@med.niigata-u.ac.jp (Y.A.)
2. Department of Pathology and Molecular Pathology, University and University Hospital Zurich, Zurich CH-8091, Switzerland; Silvia.Angori@usz.ch (S.A.); Aashil.Batavia@usz.ch (A.A.B.); niels.rupp@usz.ch (N.J.R.); holger.moch@usz.ch (H.M.)
3. Division of Molecular and Diagnostic Pathology, Graduate School of Medical and Dental Sciences, Niigata University, Niigata 951-8510, Japan
* Correspondence: Peter.Schraml@usz.ch; Tel.: +41-44-255-2114
† shared last authors.

Received: 23 November 2019; Accepted: 13 February 2020; Published: 17 February 2020

Abstract: Chromophobe renal cell carcinoma (chRCC) patients have good prognosis. Only 5%–10% patients die of metastatic disease after tumorectomy, but tumor progression cannot be predicted by histopathological parameters alone. chRCC are characterized by losses of many chromosomes, whereas gene mutations are rare. In this study, we aim at identifying genes indicating chRCC progression. A bioinformatic approach was used to correlate chromosomal loss and mRNA expression from 15287 genes from The Cancer Genome Atlas (TCGA) database. All genes in TCGA chromophobe renal cancer dataset (KICH) for which a significant correlation between chromosomal loss and mRNA expression was shown, were identified and their associations with outcome was assessed. Genome-wide DNA copy-number alterations were analyzed by Affymetrix OncoScan® CNV FFPE Microarrays in a second cohort of Swiss chRCC. In both cohorts, tumors with loss of chromosomes 2, 6, 10, 13, 17 and 21 had signs of tumor progression. There were 4654 genes located on these chromosomes, and 13 of these genes had reduced mRNA levels, which was associated with poor outcome in chRCC. Decreased CDKN1A expression at mRNA ($p = 0.02$) and protein levels ($p = 0.02$) were associated with short overall survival and were independent predictors of prognosis ($p < 0.01$ and <0.05 respectively). CDKN1A expression status is a prognostic biomarker independent of tumor stage. CDKN1A immunohistochemistry may be used to identify chRCC patients at greater risk of disease progression.

Keywords: chromophobe renal cell carcinoma; copy number loss; CDKN1A expression; patient survival; prognosis

1. Introduction

Chromophobe renal cell carcinoma (chRCC) is the third most common histological subtype of RCC and accounts for approximately 5–7% of RCC [1–3]. Although chRCC patients have better prognoses than patients with clear cell RCC (ccRCC) or papillary RCC (pRCC) [1–5], about 5–7% of patients die of metastatic disease [4,6,7]. Therefore, it is of utmost importance to identify prognostic factors, which can better predict the small patient group with clinical progression after surgical resection.

The current 2016 World Health Organization (WHO)/International Society of Urological Pathology (ISUP) grading system and the older Fuhrman grading are not recommended for chRCC [1,8], although several studies have challenged to develop a histopathological grading system for chRCC [4,6,7,9–13]. Therefore, chRCCs are currently not graded. Interestingly, only recently, it was reported that classic chRCC harbors a larger number of chromosomal losses than in the eosinophilic subtype [14], which is often accompanied by reduced expression of "CYCLOPS" (Copy-number alterations Yielding Cancer Liabilities Owing to Partial losS)" genes [15].

Recent comprehensive genomic analyses of two chRCC cohorts demonstrated a low exonic somatic mutation rate in these tumours and identified *TP53* (20–32%) and *PTEN* (6–9%) as the most frequently mutated genes [16,17]. Casuscelli et al. [7] found increased mutation rates in *TP53* (58%) and *PTEN* (24%) as well as imbalanced chromosome duplication (≥ 3 chromosomes, 25%) in chRCC patients with metastatic disease. As the prognostic relevance of these genomic alterations was analyzed separately, the combinatorial impact of these parameters remained unclear.

In this study, we aimed to identify molecular alterations associated with survival in chRCC. We analyzed the The Cancer Genome Atlas (TCGA) Kidney Chromophobe (KICH) database [16] and a Swiss chRCC cohort for chromosomal copy number variation (CNV). Next, we focused on genes, whose mRNA expression correlated with copy number (CN) loss of chromosomes 2, 6, 10, 13, 17 and 21. Reduced CDKN1A mRNA and protein expression levels were associated with poor outcome in chRCC.

2. Results

2.1. Chromosomal Loss and Patient Outcome

The loss of one copy of chromosomes 1, 2, 6, 10, 13, 17, 21 and Y occurs in the majority of chRCC cases. Since losses of chromosomes 1 and Y have been reported in benign oncocytoma [5,16,18,19], we speculated that only loss of chromosomes 2, 6, 10, 13, 17 and 21 may be associated with outcome in chRCC patients. The frequencies of loss of these chromosomes were similar in both the TCGA-KICH and the Swiss cohort. The data are summarized in Table S1. As recently described by our group [14], CN loss of chromosome 2, 6, 10, 13, 17, and 21 in single analysis is not associated with worse survival (Figure S1). In contrast, tumors without loss of chromosomes 2, 6, 10, 13, 17 and 21 had 100% survival in both, the TCGA and Swiss cohort (Figure 1).

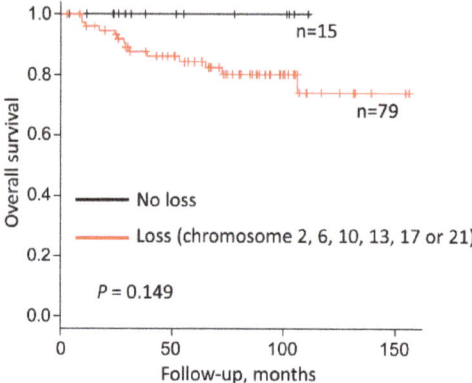

Figure 1. Combined survival analysis of chRCCs categorized by loss or no loss of chromosomes 2, 6, 10, 13, 17 and 21 (TCGA-KICH: No loss n = 12; Loss n = 52; Swiss cohort: No loss n = 3; Loss n = 27).

2.2. Identification of Genes Associated with Chromosomal Loss, Decreased Expression and Patient Survival

In search of molecular prognostic markers, we hypothesized that the expression of several genes located on chromosomes 2, 6, 10, 13, 17 and 21 is influenced by allele loss, which may affect prognosis of chRCC. The strategy to identify such genes is presented in Figure 2 and described in detail in the Materials and Methods section. The 13 candidate genes associated with chromosomal loss, decreased expression and patient survival in chRCC according to combination of UALCAN [20,21] and the Human Protein Atlas [22,23] websites are listed in Table 1 and Table S2. Scatter plots showing the correlation between CNV and mRNA expression levels of the 13 genes according to the analyzed result acquired from the Broad Institute FIREHOSE [24] website are presented in Figure S2. mRNA expression levels of the 13 genes in normal tissue and tumors with CN loss and no loss are illustrated in Figure S3. We performed also Protein–Protein Interaction Networks Functional Enrichment Analysis using the STRING database to find interactions and pathways shared between the 13 genes/proteins. The interaction network of the 13 genes is illustrated in Figure S4. We observed strong interactions between FBXW4 (F-Box and WD Repeat Domain Containing 4), FBXL15 (F-Box and Leucine Rich Repeat Protein 15) and SOCS3 (Suppressor of cytokine signaling 3) and a weaker interaction between KLF6 (Krueppel-like factor 6) and CDKN1A. According to the Reactome Pathway Database FBXW4, FBXL15 and SOCS3 are involved in ubiquitination. Interestingly, KLF6 activates CDKN1A transcription independent from TP53 and is frequently downregulated in human tumors [25].

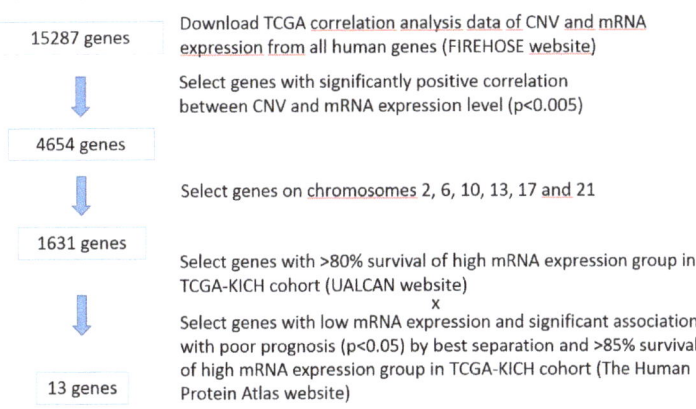

Figure 2. Strategy for identification of prognostic markers.

Table 1. Genes with a highly significant correlation between CNV and mRNA expression level, cellular localization of their proteins and their function.

Gene Name	Chromosomal Locus [1]	CNV vs mRNA Pearson's Correlation Coefficient [2]	Protein Expression [3]	Protein Function (GeneCards [4])
CDKN1A	6p21.2	R = 0.4434, p = 0.0002	nucleus	Cell cycle regulation
KLF6	10p15.2	R = 0.5474, p < 0.0001	nucleus	Transcriptional activator
FAM160B1	10q25.3	R = 0.7632, p < 0.0001	cytoplasm	unknown
PAOX	10q26.3	R = 0.6088, p < 0.0001	cytoplasm	Polyamine oxidase
PWWP2B	10q26.3	R = 0.52, p < 0.0001	cytoplasm	unknown
FBXW4	10q24.32	R = 0.4296, p = 0.0003	golgi	Ubiquitination
FBXL15	10q24.32	R = 0.4048, p = 0.0007	cytoplasm	Ubiquitination
CASKIN2	17q25.1	R = 0.4364, p = 0.0002	cytoplasm	unknown
RTN4RL1	17p13.3	R = 0.4013, p = 0.0008	secreted	Brain development
FMNL1	17q21.31	R = 0.3974. p = 0.001	cytoplasm	Regulation of cell morphology
RAB37	17q25.1	R = 0.369, p = 0.002	cytoplasm	GTPase
SOCS3	17q25.3	R = 0.3611, p = 0.003	cytoplasm	Cytokine signaling suppression
C21orf2	21q22.3	R = 0.5435, p < 0.0001	mitochondria	Regulation of cell morphology, DNA damage repair

[1] Gene, National Center for Biotechnology Information [26], [2] Data from the FIREHOSE, Broad Institute [24], [3] Data from The Human Protein Atlas [23], [4] GeneCards, The Human Gene Database [27].

2.3. CDKN1A mRNA and Protein Expression

Among these 13 genes, we focused on *CDKN1A* whose gene product acts as a cell cycle regulator being involved in genomic stability [28] for the following reasons: (i) according to the Human Protein Atlas database for several proteins (PAOX, FBXL15, RAB37, C21orf2) antibodies suitable for immunohistochemical staining are not available or unspecific; (ii) all proteins but CDKN1A are either not or only weakly expressed in renal cell carcinoma, which significantly hampers reliable TMA expression analysis.

In the TCGA-KICH cohort, tumors with high *CDKN1A* mRNA expression separated by both the best separation cutoff (p = 0.02, log rank test, Figure 3A and Table S2) and median expression (p = 0.026, Table S2) had a significantly better prognosis than tumors with low *CDKN1A* mRNA expression.

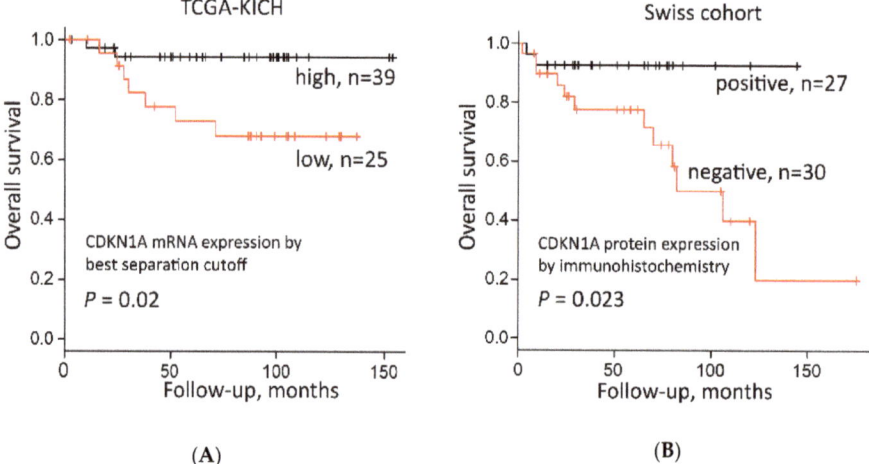

Figure 3. Survival analysis of CDKN1A expression in chRCC. (**A**) CDKN1A mRNA expression and overall survival of 64 chRCC patients in the TCGA-KICH dataset from the Human Protein Atlas [23]—best cut off was according to FPKM values (Fragments per kilo base per million mapped reads); (**B**) CDKN1A protein expression and overall survival of 57 chRCC patients from the Swiss cohort dataset.

In parallel, we examined CDKN1A protein expression in 57 Swiss chRCCs by immunohistochemistry (IHC). All normal renal cells including glomeruli, renal tubules, endothelial cells, fibroblasts, inflammatory cells were CDKN1A negative (n = 46), with the exception of a few tubules with very weak nuclear CDKN1A staining (Figure 4A). CDKN1A-positive clear cell RCC from a previous study served as positive controls (Figure 4B) [29]. A representative image of CDKN1A-positive chRCC is shown in Figure 4C and Figure S5. An amount of 30 chRCCs (52.6%) were CDKN1A negative, 27 tumors (47.4%) were CDKN1A positive (cut off ≥ 2% tumor cells). There was a significant correlation between CDKN1A negativity and shorter overall survival (Figure 3B).

Nuclear staining was weak in 19 (70.4%) tumors and 8 (29.6%) showed moderate to strong nuclear staining. The mean (range) of the H-score (described in Materials and Methods) among CDKN1A positive tumors was 16.6 (2–110) (Figure S6). Neither staining intensity nor H-score (>20) improved overall survival rate. Nuclear staining with any intensity and a cutoff of ≥2% positive tumor cells proved to be the best criteria to differentiate between CDKN1A expression status and patient outcome.

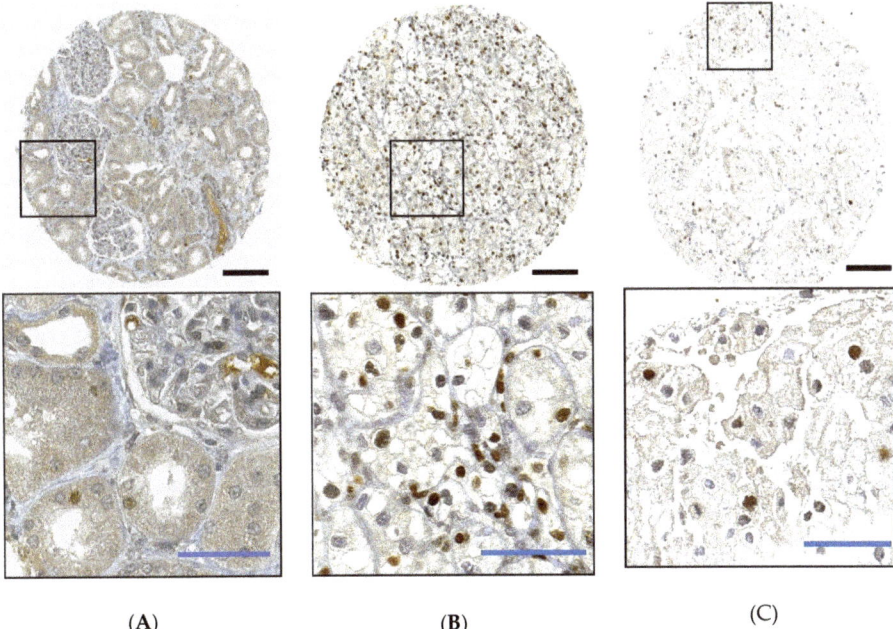

Figure 4. Immunohistochemistry of CDKN1A in the Swiss cohort. (**A**) Weak nuclear CDKN1A expression in some tubular cells in normal kidney; (**B**) strong nuclear CDKN1A expression in clear cell RCC; (**C**) strong nuclear CDKN1A expression in chRCC. Black bars: 100 μm; blue bars: 10 μm.

2.4. CDKN1A Expression, Tumor Stage, Grade and Outcome

Analysis of the TCGA and the Swiss cohort revealed no correlation between CDKN1A expression (RNA and protein) and tumor stage. Univariate Cox regression analysis showed that both T stage ($p = 0.004$) and low *CDKN1A* mRNA expression ($p = 0.001$) were significant prognostic factors in the TCGA-KICH cohort (Table 2). In the Swiss dataset, only the absence of CDKN1A protein expression by IHC was significantly associated with poor outcome ($p < 0.05$), whereas advanced pT stage did not correlate with survival by univariate Cox regression analysis. A recently published two-tiered grading system was available for the TCGA-KICH cohort [30] and included in our calculations. Univariate Cox regression analysis demonstrated strong prognostic relevance of this grading system ($p < 0.001$) (Table 2).

Table 2. Tumor stage, histological grading according to necrosis and/or sarcomatoid differentiation, CDKN1A expression separated by the best separation cutoff from FIREHOSE [24] mRNA data and overall survival in chromophobe renal cell carcinoma.

Cohort	TCGA-KICH				Swiss Patients			
Variables	Univariate		Multivariate[2]		Univariate		Multivariate	
	HR (95%CI)	*p*-value	HR (95%CI)	*p*-value	HR (95%CI)	*p*-value	HR (95%CI)	*p*-value
Tumor stage (3–4 vs 1–2)[1]	10.22 (2.12–49.29)	0.004	6.442 (1.488–37.214)	0.012	1.447 (0.398–5.264)	n.s.	1.266 (0.343–4.678)	n.s.
Grade (High vs Low)	18.03 (4.448–73.05)	<0.001	6.087 (1.374–32.266)	0.017	-	-	-	-
CDKN1A expression (Low vs High)[2,3]	22.528 (2.862–2904.443)	<0.001	12.527 (1.289–1675.059)	0.026	4.812 (1.07–21.64)	<0.05	4.741 (1.051–21.390)	<0.05

HR, hazard ratio; CI, confidence interval; n.s.: not significant; [1] TCGA-KICH: T stage, Swiss patients: pT stage; [2] Firth correction was used because of quasi-complete separation; there was no event in one of the subgroups; [3] *CDKN1A* mRNA expression in TCGA-KICH cohort and CDKN1A protein expression in Swiss cohort.

Multivariate analysis using Cox proportional hazard model revealed T stage ($p = 0.012$), grade ($p = 0.017$) and low *CDKN1A* mRNA expression ($p = 0.026$) as significant independent predictors of poor outcome in the TCGA cohort. In the Swiss dataset, only loss of CDKN1A expression ($p < 0.05$) was confirmed as a significant independent predictor of poor outcome (Table 2).

3. Discussion

In this study, we attempted to identify molecular biomarkers with prognostic value in chRCC. For this purpose, we screened TCGA-KICH data to extract genes located on frequently deleted chromosomes whose expression is associated with patient outcome. Tumor suppressor Cyclin-dependent kinase inhibitor 1A (*CDKN1A*) was among 13 genes which fulfilled these criteria. We demonstrated that decreased CDKN1A expression at the mRNA and protein levels is an independent predictor of outcome in two independent chRCC cohorts.

The tumor suppressive role of CDKN1A, also known as p21/Waf1/Cip1, has been widely accepted. Cellular stressors, such as DNA damage or UV-light, activate tumor suppressor p53, which leads to the transient expression of CDKN1A. CDKN1A inhibits cyclin-CDK1, -CDK2, and CDK4/6, which regulates cell cycle progression of G1 and S phases and mediates senescence or apoptosis [28]. Previous studies emphasize CDKN1A's important tumor suppressive role by showing that its depletion in cell line models leads to DNA damage and chromosomal instability [28,31] but also permits carcinogenesis from chronically damaged kidney epithelial cells [32].

CDKN1A, which resides in 6p21.2, is affected by the frequent loss of one chromosome 6 allele in chRCC. Analysis of TCGA-KICH data demonstrated that the loss of one *CDKN1A* allele was closely linked to lower *CDKN1A* mRNA expression levels compared to tumors that retained both *CDKN1A* alleles. Notably, the overall mRNA expression level in normal renal tissue was higher than in chRCC with *CDKN1A* loss and lower than in tumors without *CDKN1A* loss. This is consistent with the immunohistochemical CDKN1A protein expression analysis of the Swiss cohort. chRCC cells were either CDKN1A negative or strongly positive. Nuclei of glomeruli, endothelial cells, and fibroblasts were negative in the normal kidney. Only some tubular cells had weak CDKN1A expression.

Like *CDKN1A* on chromosome 6—which is absent in 80% of chRCC—the tumor suppressor genes *PTEN* and *TP53* are located on chromosomes (chromosome 10 and 17) that are also frequently lost in chRCC. Whereas *PTEN* and *TP53* are mutated in up to 9% and 32% of chRCC [16,17], respectively, *CDKN1A* gene mutations are rare [16,33]. Although immunohistochemical analysis showed no correlation between CDKN1A, TP53 and PTEN expression in chRCC (TP53 and PTEN positivity was rare in our chRCC cohort; data not shown), the loss of function of the latter two tumor suppressors may have significant impact on *CDKN1A* regulation. One important downstream target of TP53 is *CDKN1A* [34]. The downregulation of CDKN1A may thus be caused through loss of functional TP53 in those chRCC in which *TP53* is inactivated by two hits, chromosomal loss and mutation. In addition, it was shown that interaction between PTEN and TP53 stimulates TP53-mediated transcription and stabilizes TP53 [35–37]. In a minor fraction of chRCC loss of PTEN function may therefore exert similar negative effects on CDKN1A expression. It is tempting to speculate that a combination of loss of chromosomes 6, 10, and 17 and molecular two-hit disruption of *PTEN* and *TP53* are the main drivers for the loss of CDKN1A expression and worse patient outcomes in chRCC.

Importantly, our survival analysis revealed a clear association between reduced *CDKN1A* mRNA expression levels and CDKN1A immuno-negativity with worse outcome. Data on the prognostic relevance of CDKN1A expression are controversial in the literature and seem to be dependent on cancer type. Increased CDKN1A levels are associated with poor outcome in esophageal, ovarian, prostate cancers as well as in gliomas [38–43], while loss of CDKN1A expression is associated with decreased survival in breast, cervical, gastric, and ovarian cancers [44–47]. In some cancers, the loss of CDKN1A expression upregulates genes that repress *CDKN1A* transcription, such as *MYC* [25,48]. Ubiquitin-dependent and -independent proteosomal degradation of CDKN1A may also contribute to tumorigenesis [25,49]. CDKN1A can also exhibit oncogenic activities in some cancers, which may explain the strong correlation of its overexpression with tumor grade, rapid progression, poor prognosis, and drug resistance [25,28,43,50]. This two-faced nature of CDKN1A seems to be dependent on its cellular location. Several IHC studies imply that nuclear expression of CDKN1A indicates its tumor-suppressive role, while its presence in the cytoplasm favors an oncogenic role [25,51–54]. We have observed a significant correlation between CN loss, decreased CDKN1A expression and poor prognosis, suggesting a tumor suppressive role of CDKN1A in chRCC. This is supported by the strong CDKN1A positivity seen in tumor cell nuclei of almost half of the analyzed chRCC.

Our proposed data mining strategy demonstrated its usefulness to identify expression patterns of 13 candidate genes with prognostic impact in chRCC. However, the validation of gene expression data using additional and independent patient cohorts and different technological platforms is of utmost importance to confirm the robustness of the data. Due to the lack of suitable antibodies and only low protein expression levels in RCC, we decided to forego an immunohistochemical in situ analysis of 12 of 13 candidates. In contrast to genes and proteins that are highly differentially expressed in cancer, the validation of low abundance genes as diagnostic and prognostic tools in tumor pathology is a big challenge. Branched probe-based or enzymatic amplification RNA-ISH methods for the detection and quantification of transcripts in FFPE tissues [55] may be ideally suited to evaluate cancer biomarker candidates on the mRNA level. Given the huge amount of survival-related gene expression data in the TCGA database, systematic and comprehensive gene expression profiling of such candidate genes are necessary to better understand the complex regulatory network along tumor progression, which may lead to new therapeutic strategies to treat aggressive chRCC.

From a clinical viewpoint time to progression or tumor-specific rather than overall survival after tumorectomy are the most important parameter for chRCC [30]. Biomarkers, which predict time to progression are therefore highly desirable to identify approximately 5%–10% of chRCC at risk for progression. Additional chRCC cohorts are needed to validate whether the loss of CDKN1A expression is a reliable molecular marker to detect chRCC patients with at greater risk of disease progression.

4. Materials and Methods

4.1. Data Acquisition and Processing Using the Cancer Genome Atlas Data Portal

Digital whole slide images of TCGA-KICH cases were reviewed using the Cancer Digital Slide Archive [56]. The corresponding clinical information of TCGA-KICH was obtained from the TCGA Data Portal [57]. Publically available Level 3 TCGA datasets comprising 66 primary chRCCs (TCGA-KICH) were downloaded from the Broad Institute TCGA Genome Data Analysis Center via FIREHOSE [24] including GISTIC copy number (CN) data, Next Generation Sequencing (NGS)-based whole genome sequencing data and RNA-sequencing data as previously described [14–16,58]. Two patients with missing or too short follow-up (less than 30 days) were excluded from the Cox regression analysis. TCGA CNV analysis was performed with Affimetrix SNP 6.0 with cutoff value −0.1 for copy number loss according to the Broad Institute FIREHOSE website description [24]. Gene expression values were log2-transformed to plot *CDKN1A* mRNA expression profiles of normal kidney and tumors with and without CN loss.

In the TCGA-KICH cohort, the median age at diagnosis was 49.5 years (range 17–86 years). The median follow-up of the entire cohort was 80.5 months. Nine patients (14.1%) died during follow-up. Forty-five chRCC were early stage (T1 and T2) and 19 late stage tumors (T3 and T4).

4.2. Strategy for Gene Candidate Selection

In a first step we used the Broad institute FIREHOSE website ("Correlate CopyNumber ys mRNAseq") [24] to download all 15,287 available human genes of the whole genome and extracted 4654 with significant positive correlation between gene copy number and mRNA expression (Pearson's correlation coefficient $R > 0$ and $p < 0.005$).

1631 of the 4654 genes were located on chromosomes 2, 6, 10, 13, 17 and 21. Since Figure 1 demonstrated chromosomal loss in 84% (79 of 94) chRCC, we hypothesized that by using a two-tiered separation based on presence or absence of chromosomal losses, the expression patterns of several genes on chromosomes 2, 6, 10, 13, 17 and 21 would fulfill the UALCAN [20,21] survival curve separation criteria: patients with high gene expression values > 3rd quartile versus patients with low gene expression (<3rd quartile). Obtaining survival curves separated by mRNA expression level in UALCAN [20,21] requires only minimal steps among three websites, UALCAN [20,21], the Human Protein Atlas [22,23] and FIREHOSE [24]. We entered all 1631 gene symbols in input fields of the UALCAN [20,21] and extracted the genes of > 3rd quartile high gene expression group with more than 80% overall survival rate. Next, we selected genes, of which the low gene expression was significantly correlated with poor prognosis ($p < 0.05$) and high mRNA expression group showed >80% overall survival rate using the Human Protein Atlas [22,23] (Table S1). Finally, 13 candidate genes were identified (Table 1).

4.3. Swiss Chromophobe Renal Cell Carcinomas

A total of 57 chRCCs were retrieved from the archives of the Department of Pathology and Molecular Pathology of the University Hospital Zurich (Zurich, Switzerland). Overall survival data were obtained from the Zurich Cancer Registry. The study was approved by the Cantonal Ethics Committee of Zurich (BASEC-No_2019-01959) in accordance with the Swiss Human Research Act and with the Declaration of Helsinki. All tumors were reviewed by two pathologists (Riuko Ohashi and Holger Moch) blinded to clinico-pathological information. The tumors were histologically classified according to the WHO classification [1]. In the Swiss cohort, the median age at diagnosis was 62 years (range 18–87 years). The median follow-up was 51.0 months and 14 patients (24.6%) died during follow-up. Tumors were staged according to the TNM staging system [59]. A total of 48 chRCC were early stage (T1 and T2) and 9 late stage tumors (T3 and T4).

4.4. OncoScan Assay

DNA from formalin-fixed, paraffin-embedded (FFPE) tumor tissue samples was obtained by punching 4 to 6 tissue cylinders (diameter 0.6 mm) from each sample. Punches were taken from tumor areas displaying >90% cancer cells which were marked previously on Hematoxylin and Eosin stained slides. DNA extraction from FFPE tissue was done as previously described [14,15,60]. The double-strand DNA (dsDNA) was quantified by the fluorescence-based Qubit dsDNA HS Assay Kit (Thermo Fisher Scientific, Inc., Waltham, MA, USA) according to manufacturer's instructions. Thirty chRCCs had sufficient DNA quality for copy number analysis. Genome-wide DNA copy-number alterations were analyzed by Affymetrix OncoScan® CNV FFPE Microarrays (Affymetrix, Santa Clara, CA, USA) as previously described [14,15,61]. The samples were processed by IMGM Laboratories GmbH (Martinsried, Germany). The data were analyzed by the OncoScan Console (Affymetrix) and Nexus Express for OncoScan 3 (BioDiscovery, Inc. El Segundo, CA, USA) software using the Affymetrix TuScan algorithm. The CNV cutoff value was -0.3 for copy number loss in Nexus Express for OncoScan 3 Software (BioDiscovery) default setting.

4.5. Immunohistochemistry

A tissue microarray (TMA) with 57 chRCC was constructed as described [29,62]. TMA sections (2.5µm) were transferred to glass slides and subjected to immunohistochemistry using Ventana Benchmark XT automated system (Roche Diagnostics, Rotkreuz, Switzerland). CDKN1A was immunostained using polyclonal anti-rabbit sc-397 (dilution 1:50; Santa Cruz Biotechnology, Inc.; Dallas, TX, USA). Immunostained slides were scanned using the NanoZoomer Digital Slide Scanner (Hamamatsu Photonics K.K., Shizuoka, Japan). Immunohistochemical evaluation was conducted by two pathologists (R.O. and H.M.) blinded to the clinical data. The criteria for protein expression analysis were as described in previous TMA studies [15,29]. A tumor was considered CDKN1A positive if ≥ 2% of the tumor cells showed unequivocal nuclear expression. A semi-quantitative approach (H-score) was also performed. The staining percentages (range 0–100%) and the intensity of nuclear expression of CDKN1A (range 0–3: 0, negative; 1, weak; 2, moderate; and 3, strong) in tumor cells were evaluated and the H-score was calculated using the formula 1 × (% of 1+ cells) + 2 × (% of 2+ cells) + 3 × (% of 3+ cells) (giving a score that ranged from 0 to 300) [63].

4.6. Statistical Analysis

All statistical analyses were conducted using R, 3.4.1 (R Foundation for Statistical Computing, Vienna, Austria) and EZR, Version 1.37 (Saitama Medical Center, Jichi Medical University, Saitama, Japan) [64]. The Fisher's exact test was used to assess association between two categorical variables. Overall survival rates were determined according to the Kaplan–Meier method and analyzed for statistical differences using a log rank test. Univariate and multivariate analyses were performed by using the Cox-proportional hazard model with Firth's penalized likelihood [65,66]. Cox regression analysis was performed using FIREHOSE mRNA expression data [24]. p-values < 0.05 were regarded as statistically significant.

5. Conclusions

In conclusion, chRCC without loss of chromosomes 2, 6, 10, 13, 17 and 21 have a favorable prognosis. CDKN1A mRNA and protein expression levels were of prognostic relevance independent from tumor stage. CDKN1A IHC is easily applicable in routine pathology and will help to stratify chRCC patients that have a significantly greater risk of disease progression.

Supplementary Materials: The following are available online at http://www.mdpi.com/2072-6694/12/2/465/s1, Figure S1: Loss of chromosome 6 harboring *CDKN1A* (A), chromosome 10 harboring *PTEN* (B), chromosome 17 harboring *TP53* (C), combined loss of chromosome 10 and 17 (D) and patient overall survival in chRCC. Figure S2: Correlation between CN loss and mRNA expression levels of 13 genes. Figure S3: Scatter plots showing the correlation between mRNA expression and copy number variation of the 13 genes using the TCGA-KICH dataset. Dotted line: log2 threshold at −0.1 between CN loss and no loss. Figure S4: Protein-protein interactions between the 13 gene products using STRING database. Figure S5: CDKN1A positive chRCC with weakly stained tumor cell nuclei (black arrows). Bar: 20 μm. Figure S6: Distribution of CDKN1A H-scores of chRCCs by immunohistochemistry. Table S1: Frequency of chromosomal loss in Swiss and TCGA chRCC cohorts. Table S2: Genes with correlation of expression levels, median and best separation cutoffs, and survival (Data from the Human Protein Atlas database).

Author Contributions: Conceptualization, R.O., P.S., and H.M.; methodology, R.O., S.A., A.A.B., and H.M.; software, R.O., S.A., A.A.B.; validation, R.O. and A.B.; formal analysis, R.O., S.A., A.A.B., and H.M.; investigation, R.O.; resources, R.O., N.J.R., P.S., and H.M.; data curation, R.O., P.S., N.J.R.; writing—original draft preparation, R.O. and P.S.; writing—review and editing, All authors; visualization, R.O. and A.A.B.; supervision, Y.A., P.S. and H.M.; project administration, P.S. and H.M.; funding acquisition, R.O. and H.M. All authors have read and agreed to the published version of the manuscript.

Funding: This work was supported in part by Niigata Foundation for the Promotion of Medicine (2015 to R.O.) and the Swiss National Science Foundation grant (No. S-87701-03-01 to H.M.).

Acknowledgments: The authors thank Susanne Dettwiler and Fabiola Prutek for their outstanding technical assistance. The results published here are in part based upon data generated by the TCGA Research Network: https://www.cancer.gov/tcga.

Conflicts of Interest: The authors have no conflict of interest and nothing to disclose.

References

1. Paner, G.; Amin, M.B.; Moch, H.; Störkel, S. Chromophobe renal cell carcinoma. In *WHO Classification of Tumours of the Urinary System and Male Genital Organs*, 4th ed.; Moch, H., Humphrey, P.A., Ulbright, T.M., Reuter, V.E., Eds.; International Agency for Research on Cancer: Lyon, France, 2016; pp. 27–28.
2. Thoenes, W.; Störkel, S.; Rumpelt, H.J.; Moll, R.; Baum, H.P.; Werner, S. Chromophobe cell renal carcinoma and its variants—A report on 32 cases. *J. Pathol.* **1988**, *155*, 277–287. [CrossRef]

3. Cheville, J.C.; Lohse, C.M.; Zincke, H.; Weaver, A.L.; Blute, M.L. Comparisons of outcome and prognostic features among histologic subtypes of renal cell carcinoma. *Am. J. Surg. Pathol.* **2003**, *27*, 612–624. [CrossRef] [PubMed]
4. Volpe, A.; Novara, G.; Antonelli, A.; Bertini, R.; Billia, M.; Carmignani, G.; Cunico, S.C.; Longo, N.; Martignoni, G.; Minervini, A.; et al. Chromophobe renal cell carcinoma (RCC): Oncological outcomes and prognostic factors in a large multicentre series. *BJU Int.* **2012**, *110*, 76–83. [CrossRef] [PubMed]
5. Yap, N.Y.; Rajandram, R.; Ng, K.L.; Pailoor, J.; Fadzli, A.; Gobe, G.C. Genetic and chromosomal aberrations and their clinical significance in renal neoplasms. *Biomed. Res. Int.* **2015**, *2015*, 476508. [CrossRef] [PubMed]
6. Przybycin, C.G.; Cronin, A.M.; Darvishian, F.; Gopalan, A.; Al-Ahmadie, H.A.; Fine, S.W.; Chen, Y.B.; Bernstein, M.; Russo, P.; Reuter, V.E.; et al. Chromophobe renal cell carcinoma: A clinicopathologic study of 203 tumors in 200 patients with primary resection at a single institution. *Am. J. Surg. Pathol.* **2011**, *35*, 962–970. [CrossRef] [PubMed]
7. Casuscelli, J.; Weinhold, N.; Gundem, G.; Wang, L.; Zabor, E.C.; Drill, E.; Wang, P.I.; Nanjangud, G.J.; Redzematovic, A.; Nargund, A.M.; et al. Genomic landscape and evolution of metastatic chromophobe renal cell carcinoma. *JCI Insight* **2017**, *2*. [CrossRef]
8. Delahunt, B.; Sika-Paotonu, D.; Bethwaite, P.B.; McCredie, M.R.; Martignoni, G.; Eble, J.N.; Jordan, T.W. Fuhrman grading is not appropriate for chromophobe renal cell carcinoma. *Am. J. Surg. Pathol.* **2007**, *31*, 957–960. [CrossRef]
9. Amin, M.B.; Paner, G.P.; Alvarado-Cabrero, I.; Young, A.N.; Stricker, H.J.; Lyles, R.H.; Moch, H. Chromophobe renal cell carcinoma: Histomorphologic characteristics and evaluation of conventional pathologic prognostic parameters in 145 cases. *Am. J. Surg. Pathol.* **2008**, *32*, 1822–1834. [CrossRef]
10. Paner, G.P.; Amin, M.B.; Alvarado-Cabrero, I.; Young, A.N.; Stricker, H.J.; Moch, H.; Lyles, R.H. A novel tumor grading scheme for chromophobe renal cell carcinoma: Prognostic utility and comparison with Fuhrman nuclear grade. *Am. J. Surg. Pathol.* **2010**, *34*, 1233–1240. [CrossRef]
11. Xie, Y.; Ma, X.; Li, H.; Gao, Y.; Gu, L.; Chen, L.; Zhang, X. Prognostic value of clinical and pathological features in chinese patients with chromophobe renal cell carcinoma: A 10-year single-center study. *J. Cancer* **2017**, *8*, 3474–3479. [CrossRef]
12. Finley, D.S.; Shuch, B.; Said, J.W.; Galliano, G.; Jeffries, R.A.; Afifi, A.A.; Castor, B.; Magyar, C.; Sadaat, A.; Kabbinavar, F.F.; et al. The chromophobe tumor grading system is the preferred grading scheme for chromophobe renal cell carcinoma. *J. Urol.* **2011**, *186*, 2168–2174. [CrossRef] [PubMed]
13. Leibovich, B.C.; Lohse, C.M.; Cheville, J.C.; Zaid, H.B.; Boorjian, S.A.; Frank, I.; Thompson, R.H.; Parker, W.P. Predicting oncologic outcomes in renal cell carcinoma after surgery. *Eur. Urol.* **2018**, *73*, 772–780. [CrossRef] [PubMed]
14. Ohashi, R.; Schraml, P.; Angori, S.; Batavia, A.A.; Rupp, N.J.; Ohe, C.; Otsuki, Y.; Kawasaki, T.; Kobayashi, H.; Kobayashi, K.; et al. Classic chromophobe renal cell carcinoma incur a larger number of chromosomal losses than seen in the eosinophilic subtype. *Cancers* **2019**, *11*, 1492. [CrossRef] [PubMed]
15. Ohashi, R.; Schraml, P.; Batavia, A.; Angori, S.; Simmler, P.; Rupp, N.; Ajioka, Y.; Oliva, E.; Moch, H. Allele Loss and reduced expression of CYCLOPS genes is a characteristic feature of chromophobe renal cell carcinoma. *Transl. Oncol.* **2019**, *12*, 1131–1137. [CrossRef] [PubMed]
16. Davis, C.F.; Ricketts, C.J.; Wang, M.; Yang, L.; Cherniack, A.D.; Shen, H.; Buhay, C.; Kang, H.; Kim, S.C.; Fahey, C.C.; et al. The somatic genomic landscape of chromophobe renal cell carcinoma. *Cancer Cell* **2014**, *26*, 319–330. [CrossRef] [PubMed]
17. Durinck, S.; Stawiski, E.W.; Pavía-Jiménez, A.; Modrusan, Z.; Kapur, P.; Jaiswal, B.S.; Zhang, N.; Toffessi-Tcheuyap, V.; Nguyen, T.T.; Pahuja, K.B.; et al. Spectrum of diverse genomic alterations define non-clear cell renal cancer subtypes. *Nat. Genet.* **2015**, *47*, 13–21. [CrossRef]
18. Brunelli, M.; Eble, J.N.; Zhang, S.; Martignoni, G.; Delahunt, B.; Cheng, L. Eosinophilic and classic chromophobe renal cell carcinomas have similar frequent losses of multiple chromosomes from among chromosomes 1, 2, 6, 10 and 17, and this pattern of genetic abnormality is not present in renal oncocytoma. *Mod. Pathol.* **2005**, *18*, 161–169. [CrossRef]
19. Quddus, M.B.; Pratt, N.; Nabi, G. Chromosomal aberrations in renal cell carcinoma: An overview with implications for clinical practice. *Urol. Ann.* **2019**, *11*, 6–14.

20. Chandrashekar, D.S.; Bashel, B.; Balasubramanya, S.A.H.; Creighton, C.J.; Ponce-Rodriguez, I.; Chakravarthi, B.V.S.K.; Varambally, S. UALCAN: A portal for facilitating tumor subgroup gene expression and survival analyses. *Neoplasia* **2017**, *19*, 649–658. [CrossRef]
21. UALCAN. TCGA Analysis. Available online: http://ualcan.path.uab.edu/analysis.html (accessed on 25 March 2018).
22. Thul, P.J.; Lindskog, C. The human protein atlas: A spatial map of the human proteome. *Protein Sci.* **2018**, *27*, 233–244. [CrossRef]
23. The Human Protein Atlas. Available online: https://www.proteinatlas.org/ (accessed on 25 March 2018).
24. Broad GDAC FIREHOSE-Broad Institute. Available online: http://gdac.broadinstitute.org/ (accessed on 23 March 2018).
25. Abbas, T.; Dutta, A. p21 in cancer: Intricate networks and multiple activities. *Nat. Rev. Cancer* **2009**, *9*, 400–414. [CrossRef] [PubMed]
26. NCBI > Genes & Expression > Gene. National Center for Biotechnology Information, U.S. National Library of Medicine. Available online: https://www.ncbi.nlm.nih.gov/gene/ (accessed on 16 April 2019).
27. GeneCards. The Human Gene Database. Available online: https://www.genecards.org/ (accessed on 21 November 2019).
28. Georgakilas, A.G.; Martin, O.A.; Bonner, W.M. p21: A two-faced genome guardian. *Trends Mol. Med.* **2017**, *23*, 310–319. [CrossRef] [PubMed]
29. Dahinden, C.; Ingold, B.; Wild, P.; Boysen, G.; Luu, V.D.; Montani, M.; Kristiansen, G.; Sulser, T.; Bühlmann, P.; Moch, H.; et al. Mining tissue microarray data to uncover combinations of biomarker expression patterns that improve intermediate staging and grading of clear cell renal cell cancer. *Clin. Cancer Res.* **2010**, *16*, 88–98. [CrossRef] [PubMed]
30. Ohashi, R.; Martignoni, G.; Hartmann, A.; Caliò, A.; Segala, D.; Stöhr, C.; Wach, S.; Erlmeier, F.; Weichert, W.; Autenrieth, M.; et al. Multi-institutional re-evaluation of prognostic factors in chromophobe renal cell carcinoma: Proposal of a novel two-tiered grading scheme. *Virchows Arch.* **2019**, 1–10. [CrossRef] [PubMed]
31. Kreis, N.N.; Friemel, A.; Zimmer, B.; Roth, S.; Rieger, M.A.; Rolle, U.; Louwen, F.; Yuan, J. Mitotic p21Cip1/CDKN1A is regulated by cyclin-dependent kinase 1 phosphorylation. *Oncotarget* **2016**, *7*, 50215–50228. [CrossRef]
32. Willenbring, H.; Sharma, A.D.; Vogel, A.; Lee, A.Y.; Rothfuss, A.; Wang, Z.; Finegold, M.; Grompe, M. Loss of p21 permits carcinogenesis from chronically damaged liver and kidney epithelial cells despite unchecked apoptosis. *Cancer Cell.* **2008**, *14*, 59–67. [CrossRef]
33. Roninson, I.B. Oncogenic functions of tumour suppressor p21$^{Waf1/Cip1/Sdi1}$: Association with cell senescence and tumour-promoting activities of stromal fibroblasts. *Cancer Lett.* **2002**, *179*, 1–14. [CrossRef]
34. Kreis, N.N.; Louwen, F.; Yuan, J. The multifaceted p21 (Cip1/Waf1/*CDKN1A*) in cell differentiation, migration and cancer therapy. *Cancers* **2019**, *11*, 1220. [CrossRef]
35. Freeman, D.J.; Li, A.G.; Wei, G.; Li, H.H.; Kertesz, N.; Lesche, R.; Whale, A.D.; Martinez-Diaz, H.; Rozengurt, N.; Cardiff, R.D.; et al. PTEN tumor suppressor regulates p53 protein levels and activity through phosphatase-dependent and -independent mechanisms. *Cancer Cell.* **2003**, *3*, 117–130. [CrossRef]
36. Tang, Y.; Eng, C. p53 down-regulates phosphatase and tensin homologue deleted on chromosome 10 protein stability partially through caspase-mediated degradation in cells with proteasome dysfunction. *Cancer Res.* **2006**, *66*, 6139–6148. [CrossRef]
37. Li, A.G.; Piluso, L.G.; Cai, X.; Wei, G.; Sellers, W.R.; Liu, X. Mechanistic insights into maintenance of high p53 acetylation by PTEN. *Mol. Cell* **2006**, *23*, 575–587. [CrossRef] [PubMed]
38. Sarbia, M.; Stahl, M.; zur Hausen, A.; Zimmermann, K.; Wang, L.; Fink, U.; Heep, H.; Dutkowski, P.; Willers, R.; Müller, W.; et al. Expression of p21WAF1 predicts outcome of esophageal cancer patients treated by surgery alone or by combined therapy modalities. *Clin. Cancer Res.* **1998**, *4*, 2615–2623. [PubMed]
39. Lin, Y.; Shen, L.Y.; Fu, H.; Dong, B.; Yang, H.L.; Yan, W.P.; Kang, X.Z.; Dai, L.; Zhou, H.T.; Yang, Y.B.; et al. P21, COX-2, and E-cadherin are potential prognostic factors for esophageal squamous cell carcinoma. *Dis. Esophagus* **2017**, *30*, 1–10. [CrossRef] [PubMed]
40. Ferrandina, G.; Stoler, A.; Fagotti, A.; Fanfani, F.; Sacco, R.; De Pasqua, A.; Mancuso, S.; Scambia, G. p21WAF1/CIP1 protein expression in primary ovarian cancer. *Int. J. Oncol.* **2000**, *17*, 1231–1235. [CrossRef] [PubMed]

41. Baretton, G.; Klenk, U.; Diebold, J.; Schmeller, N.; Löhrs, U. Proliferation-and apoptosis-associated factors in advanced prostatic carcinomas before and after androgen deprivation therapy: Prognostic significance of p21/WAF1/CIP1 expression. *Br. J. Cancer* **1999**, *80*, 546. [CrossRef]
42. Aaltomaa, S.; Lipponen, P.; Eskelinen, M.; Ala-Opas, M.; Kosma, V. Prognostic value and expression of p21 (waf1/cip1) protein in prostate cancer. *Prostate* **1999**, *39*, 8–15. [CrossRef]
43. Korkolopoulou, P.; Kouzelis, K.; Christodoulou, P.; Papanikolaou, A.; Thomas-Tsagli, E. Expression of retinoblastoma gene product and p21 (WAF1/Cip 1) protein in gliomas: Correlations with proliferation markers, p53 expression and survival. *Acta Neuropathol.* **1998**, *95*, 617–624. [CrossRef]
44. Caffo, O.; Doglioni, C.; Veronese, S.; Bonzanini, M.; Marchetti, A.; Buttitta, F.; Fina, P.; Leek, R.; Morelli, L.; Palma, P.D.; et al. Prognostic value of p21(WAF1) and p53 expression in breast carcinoma: An immunohistochemical study in 261 patients with long-term follow-up. *Clin. Cancer Res.* **1996**, *2*, 1591–1599. [CrossRef]
45. Lu, X.; Toki, T.; Konishi, I.; Nikaido, T.; Fujii, S. Expression of p21WAF1/CIP1 in adenocarcinoma of the uterine cervix: A possible immunohistochemical marker of a favorable prognosis. *Cancer* **1998**, *82*, 2409–2417. [CrossRef]
46. Ogawa, M.; Onoda, N.; Maeda, K.; Kato, Y.; Nakata, B.; Kang, S.M.; Sowa, M.; Hirakawa, K. A combination analysis of p53 and p21 in gastric carcinoma as a strong indicator for prognosis. *Int. J. Mol. Med.* **2001**, *7*, 479–483. [CrossRef]
47. Anttila, M.A.; Kosma, V.M.; Hongxiu, J.; Puolakka, J.; Juhola, M.; Saarikoski, S.; Syrjänen, K. p21/WAF1 expression as related to p53, cell proliferation and prognosis in epithelial ovarian cancer. *Br. J. Cancer.* **1999**, *79*, 1870. [CrossRef] [PubMed]
48. Mukherjee, S.; Conrad, S.E. c-Myc suppresses p21WAF1/CIP1 expression during estrogen signaling and antiestrogen resistance in human breast cancer cells. *J. Biol. Chem.* **2005**, *280*, 17617–17625. [CrossRef] [PubMed]
49. Alam, S.; Sen, E.; Brashear, H.; Meyers, C. Adeno-associated virus type 2 increases proteosome-dependent degradation of p21WAF1 in a human papillomavirus type 31b-positive cervical carcinoma line. *J. Virol.* **2006**, *80*, 4927–4939. [CrossRef] [PubMed]
50. El-Deiry, W.S. p21 (WAF1) mediates cell-cycle inhibition, relevant to cancer suppression and therapy. *Cancer Res.* **2016**, *76*, 5189–5191. [CrossRef] [PubMed]
51. Zhou, B.P.; Liao, Y.; Xia, W.; Spohn, B.; Lee, M.H.; Hung, M.C. Cytoplasmic localization of p21Cip1/WAF1 by Akt-induced phosphorylation in HER-2/neu-overexpressing cells. *Nat. Cell Biol.* **2001**, *3*, 245–252. [CrossRef] [PubMed]
52. Winters, Z.E.; Hunt, N.C.; Bradburn, M.J.; Royds, J.A.; Turley, H.; Harris, A.L.; Norbury, C.J. Subcellular localisation of cyclin B, Cdc2 and p21(WAF1/CIP1) in breast cancer. association with prognosis. *Eur. J. Cancer* **2001**, *37*, 2405–2412. [CrossRef]
53. Xia, W.; Chen, J.S.; Zhou, X.; Sun, P.R.; Lee, D.F.; Liao, Y.; Zhou, B.P.; Hung, M.C. Phosphorylation/cytoplasmic localization of p21Cip1/WAF1 is associated with HER2/neu overexpression and provides a novel combination predictor for poor prognosis in breast cancer patients. *Clin. Cancer Res.* **2004**, *10*, 3815–3824. [CrossRef]
54. Ohata, M.; Nakamura, S.; Fujita, H.; Isemura, M. Prognostic implications of p21 (Waf1/Cip1) immunolocalization in multiple myeloma. *Biomed. Res.* **2005**, *26*, 91–98. [CrossRef]
55. Voith von Voithenberg, L.; Fomitcheva Khartchenko, A.; Huber, D.; Schraml, P.; Kaigala, G.V. Spatially multiplexed RNA in situ hybridization to reveal tumor heterogeneity. *Nucleic Acids Res.* **2019**. [CrossRef]
56. Digital Slide Archive (DSA). Available online: https://cancer.digitalslidearchive.org/ (accessed on 9 May 2019).
57. GDC Data Portal-National Cancer Institute. Available online: https://portal.gdc.cancer.gov/ (accessed on 23 March 2019).
58. Sun, M.; Tong, P.; Kong, W.; Dong, B.; Huang, Y.; Park, I.Y.; Zhou, L.; Liu, X.D.; Ding, Z.; Zhang, X.; et al. HNF1B loss exacerbates the development of chromophobe renal cell carcinomas. *Cancer Res.* **2017**, *77*, 5313–5326. [CrossRef]
59. Brierley, J.D.; Gospodarowicz, M.K.; Wittekind, C. *TNM Classification of Malignant Tumours*; John Wiley & Sons: Hoboken, NJ, USA, 2016.

60. Deml, K.F.; Schildhaus, H.U.; Compérat, E.; von Teichman, A.; Storz, M.; Schraml, P.; Bonventre, J.V.; Fend, F.; Fleige, B.; Nerlich, A.; et al. Clear cell papillary renal cell carcinoma and renal angiomyoadenomatous tumor: Two variants of a morphologic, immunohistochemical, and genetic distinct entity of renal cell carcinoma. *Am. J. Surg. Pathol.* **2015**, *39*, 889–901. [CrossRef] [PubMed]
61. Noske, A.; Brandt, S.; Valtcheva, N.; Wagner, U.; Zhong, Q.; Bellini, E.; Fink, D.; Obermann, E.C.; Moch, H.; Wild, P.J. Detection of CCNE1/URI (19q12) amplification by in situ hybridisation is common in high grade and type II endometrial cancer. *Oncotarget* **2017**, *8*, 14794–14805. [CrossRef] [PubMed]
62. Bihr, S.; Ohashi, R.; Moore, A.L.; Rüschoff, J.H.; Beisel, C.; Hermanns, T.; Mischo, A.; Corrò, C.; Beyer, J.; Beerenwinkel, N.; et al. Expression and mutation patterns of PBRM1, BAP1 and SETD2 mirror specific evolutionary subtypes in clear cell renal cell carcinoma. *Neoplasia* **2019**, *21*, 247–256. [CrossRef] [PubMed]
63. McCarty, K.S., Jr.; Szabo, E.; Flowers, J.L.; Cox, E.B.; Leight, G.S.; Miller, L.; Konrath, J.; Soper, J.T.; Budwit, D.A.; Creasman, W.T.; et al. Use of a monoclonal anti-estrogen receptor antibody in the immunohistochemical evaluation of human tumors. *Cancer Res.* **1986**, *46*, 4244s–4248s. [PubMed]
64. Kanda, Y. Investigation of the freely-available easy-to-use software "EZR" (Easy R) for medical statistics. *Bone Marrow Transplant.* **2013**, *48*, 452–458. [CrossRef] [PubMed]
65. Firth, D. Bias reduction of maximum likelihood estimates. *Biometrika* **1993**, *80*, 27–38. [CrossRef]
66. coxphf: Cox Regression with Firth's Penalized Likelihood. Available online: https://CRAN.R-project.org/package=coxphf, https://cran.r-project.org/web/packages/coxphf/coxphf.pdf (accessed on 10 October 2018).

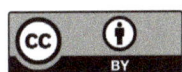

© 2020 by the authors. Licensee MDPI, Basel, Switzerland. This article is an open access article distributed under the terms and conditions of the Creative Commons Attribution (CC BY) license (http://creativecommons.org/licenses/by/4.0/).

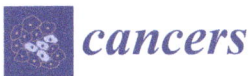

Article

Deletion of Von Hippel–Lindau Interferes with Hyper Osmolality Induced Gene Expression and Induces an Unfavorable Gene Expression Pattern

Alexander Groß, Dmitry Chernyakov, Lisa Gallwitz, Nicola Bornkessel and Bayram Edemir *

Department of Medicine, Hematology and Oncology, Martin Luther University Halle-Wittenberg, Ernst-Grube-Str. 40, 06120 Halle (Saale), Germany; alexander.gross.halle@gmx.net (A.G.); Dmitry.Chernyakov@uk-halle.de (D.C.); lgallwitz@biochem.uni-kiel.de (L.G.); nicola.bornkessel@student.uni-halle.de (N.B.)
* Correspondence: bayram.edemir@uk-halle.de; Tel.: +49-345-557-4890; Fax: +49-345-557-2950

Received: 6 December 2019; Accepted: 6 February 2020; Published: 12 February 2020

Abstract: Loss of von Hippel–Lindau (VHL) protein function can be found in more than 90% of patients with clear cell renal carcinoma (ccRCC). Mice lacking Vhl function in the kidneys have urine concentration defects due to postulated reduction of the hyperosmotic gradient. Hyperosmolality is a kidney-specific microenvironment and induces a unique gene expression pattern. This gene expression pattern is inversely regulated in patients with ccRCC with consequences for cancer-specific survival. Within this study, we tested the hypothesis if Vhl function influences the hyperosmolality induced changes in gene expression. We made use of the Clustered Regularly Interspaced Short Palindromic Repeats (CRISPR)/Cas9 technology to inhibit functional Vhl expression in murine collecting duct cell line. Loss of Vhl function induced morphological changes within the cells similar to epithelial to mesenchymal transition like phenotype. Vhl-deficient cells migrated faster and proliferated slower compared to control cells. Gene expression profiling showed significant changes in gene expression patterns in Vhl-deficient cells compared to control cells. Several genes with unfavorable outcomes showed induced and genes with favorable outcomes for patients with renal cancer reduced gene expression level. Under hyperosmotic condition, the expression of several hyperosmolality induced genes, with favorable prognostic value, was downregulated in cells that do not express functional Vhl. Taken together, this study shows that Vhl interferes with hyperosmotic signaling pathway and hyperosmolality affected pathways might represent new promising targets.

Keywords: von Hippel–Lindau; EMT like; hyperosmolality

1. Introduction

Renal cell carcinomas (RCC) are a heterogeneous group of cancers and are among the top 10 cancers worldwide. RCC arises from renal tubular epithelial cells and more than 80% of all renal neoplasms belong to RCC [1]. The major RCC subtypes are clear cell RCC (ccRCC) with a frequency of around 70–80%, papillary RCC with a frequency of around 10%–15%, and chromophobe RCC with a frequency of around 3–5% [2]. RCC incidence increases with age and is higher for men than women. Risk factors for RCC are, for example, obesity, hypertension, cigarette smoking, chronic kidney disease, hemodialysis, renal transplantation, or acquired kidney cystic disease [3]. Moreover, genetic risk factors are involved in the pathogenesis of RCC including the von Hippel–Lindau (VHL) gene, the protein polybromo-1 gene (PBRM-1), and the SET Domain Containing 2 (SETD2) gene [4,5].

VHL is a tumor suppressor that plays a pivotal role in the development of ccRCC and gene alterations can be found in up to 90% of ccRCC cases [6]. VHL can be altered and transmitted rarely in an autosomal dominant fashion, which is associated with the VHL disease, or in most cases to a sporadic manner [6].

Several studies have been performed to generate ccRCC in mouse kidneys by inactivating Vhl. The first study used the phosphoenolpyruvate carboxykinase (Pepck)-Cre to generate proximal tubule-specific knock out (KO) mice. These mice developed a modest phenotype and after 12 months 25% of the mice had renal microcysts [7]. Using Ksp1.3-Cre, as deleter Cre, led to generation of distal tubule and collecting duct (CD) specific deletion of Vhl. These mice developed hydronephrosis but no further abnormalities [8]. However, the combined KO of Vhl together with the phosphatase and tensin homolog (Pten) resulted in hyperproliferation and kidneys with multiple epithelial tubule cysts in the cortex and medulla. A further study on mouse showed that deletion of Vhl caused increased medullary vascularization and, as a physiological consequence, developed a diabetes insipidus like phenotype by excretion of highly diluted urine. The authors hypothesized that the increased medullary vasculature alters salt uptake from the renal interstitium, resulting in a disruption of the osmotic gradient and impaired urinary concentration [9]. The rate-limiting factor in the urine concentration is the expression of the aquaporin-2 (Aqp2) water channel. Aqp2 is expressed in the principal cells of the collecting duct, and the binding of the antidiuretic hormone vasopressin (AVP) to the vasopressin type 2 receptor induces the translocation of Aqp2 bearing vesicles to the apical plasma membrane [10]. The expression of Aqp2 in the mentioned mouse model was decreased [9]. The expression of Aqp2 on the mRNA level is regulated by the cAMP-responsive element-binding protein [11] and by the action of the nuclear factor of activated T cells 5 (Nfat5) [12]. Nfat5 is activated by hyperosmotic environment of the kidney [13]. It has been recently shown that in renal cancer Nfat5 expression is targeted by microRNAs that led to reduced expression of Nfat5 target genes [14].

The cells of the renal inner medulla are challenged with a hyperosmotic environment, the driving force for water retention. We have shown that this environment is also important to regulate a specific gene expression pattern of several kidney-specific genes [15]. Further, we have recently shown that the expression of osmolality affected genes is inversely regulated in the ccRCC samples compared to normal tissue, and we were able to generate an Osm-score that allows the prediction of patients' survival [16]. We were also able to induce the expression of the E74-like factor 5 (ELF5), a tumor suppressor in RCC [17], in the 786-0, VHL deficient, RCC cell line under hyperosmotic cell culture conditions. Interestingly, the expression level was higher in 786-0 that ectopically expressed wild type VHL [16], suggesting that VHL somehow interferes with hyperosmolality associated gene expression.

Based on these data we hypothesized that Vhl also plays an important role in the expression of hyperosmolality induced genes and that loss of Vhl function induces a ccRCC like phenotype in a normal murine collecting duct cell line. Indeed, the results of this study showed massive functional, morphological abnormalities and changes in gene expression that are Vhl and osmolality dependent.

2. Results

2.1. Generation of VHL-Deficient Cells

We have used the murine mpkCCD cells to analyze the role of Vhl in the collecting duct. This cell line has been intensively used to analyze the regulation of Aqp2 and the role of Nfat5 on hyperosmotic adaptation and they are capable of genetic manipulation [18,19]. We decided to use the CRISPR/Cas9 method to efficiently knock out functional Vhl protein expression. We used 3 different guide RNA sequences (Supplemental Table S1) and a non-targeting (Scr) sequence. Single cells were isolated and mutations within the Vhl locus were analyzed by Sanger sequencing using specific primer pairs (Supplemental Table S1 and Supplemental Figure S1). The type of mutation was analyzed by the online tool Tracking of InDels by Decomposition (TIDE) [20]. Based on this analysis, we selected single clones that showed InDels leading to a frameshift (Supplemental Figure S2).

Based on these results, the functional expression of Vhl should be lost in these clones. To validate this on protein level, Western blot experiments were performed. Since the loss of Vhl stabilizes the expression of Hif1a, we have also tested if this is the case in our model. As a control, we used Scr gRNA expressing cells and 5 Vhl-targeted single-cell clones. Vhl protein expression was lost in clones H6 and G10 (Figure 1). This was associated, as expected, with Hif1a expression.

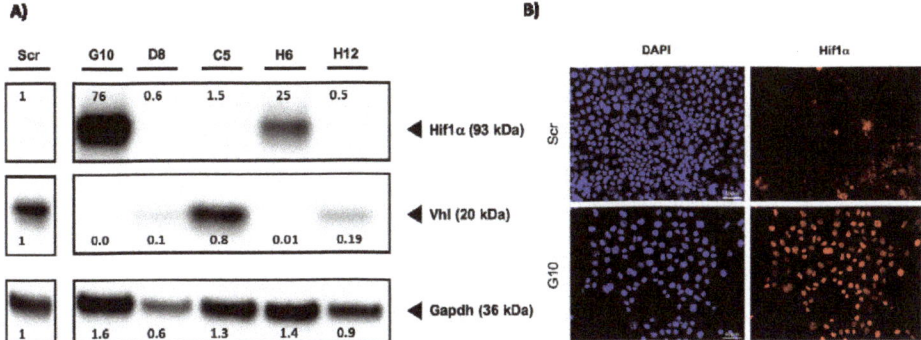

Figure 1. Loss of von Hippel–Lindau (VHL) protein induces nuclear Hif1A expression. (**A**) Cell lysates from control cells (Scr) and 5 VHL clones were prepared and the expression of VHL and Hif1a was analyzed by Western blot. An antibody directed against Gapdh served as control. The numbers indicate ratios in signal intensity compared to Scr. (**B**) Cells were cultivated on glass coverslips. After fixation, the cells were incubated with a specific Hif1a antibody. A secondary Alexa-568 labeled antibody was used to visualize the signals. The staining of the nuclei was done by incubation with 4′,6-diamidino-2-phenylindole (DAPI) (scale bar = 40 µm).

Hif1a was only detectable when Vhl protein expression was completely lost. For example, in clone D8 and C5, the expression of Vhl is weak compared to Scr. However, no stabilization of Hif1a was observed for these clones. This data shows that our cell model shows similar changes as described by other groups. In a second approach, we have analyzed the intracellular localization of Hif1a. Hif1a acts as a transcription factor and should be localized within the nucleus. We have, therefore, performed immunofluorescence analysis with Scr -cells and clone G10 using a specific Hif1a antibody. As expected, no Hif1a signal was detectable in the nucleus of Scr cells (Figure 1).

Since we were able to validate the loss of Vhl expression in these cells, we will name them as Vhl-KO hereafter.

2.2. Vhl Deletion Induces Loss of Epithelial Structures

Loss of Vhl is associated with an epithelial to mesenchymal transition (EMT) like phenotype [21]. We have, therefore, analyzed if this is also the case in the cell model that we used. We have performed immunofluorescence analysis using specific antibodies for markers of tight (Zona occludens 1, Zo1) and adherence junctions (β-catenin). While the control cells showed localization of ß-catenin at the cell–cell contacts, this was not the case in Vhl-KO cells (Figure 2).

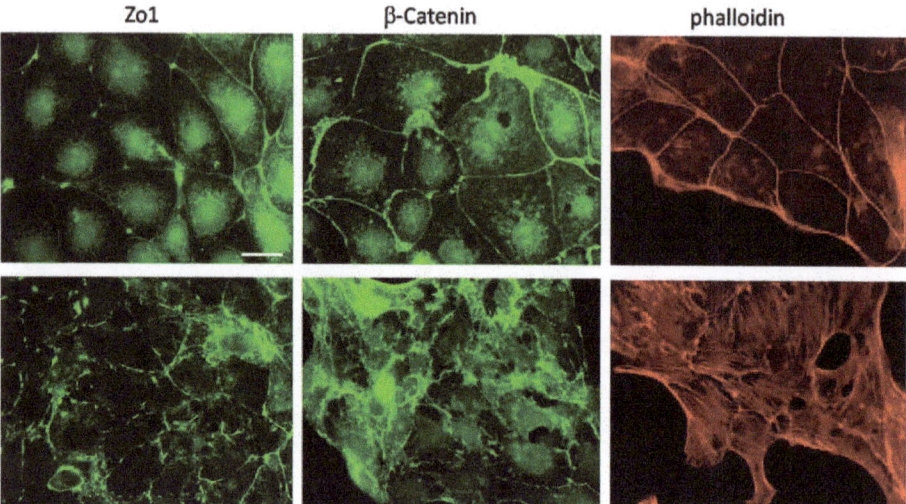

Figure 2. Loss of von Hippel–Lindau (Vhl) protein induces morphological changes. Cells were cultivated on glass coverslips. After fixation, the cells were incubated with specific antibodies directed against Zo1 and β-catenin. A secondary Alexa-488 labeled antibody was used to visualize the signals. For actin filament staining, after fixation, the cells were incubated with an Alexa-568 labeled phalloidin (scale bar = 20 μm).

Similar to β-catenin, loss of Vhl function disturbs proper tight junction assembly (Figure 2). The staining for Zo1 showed interruption of the tight junction band. This indicates that in Vhl-KO cells the epithelial cell to cell assembly is disturbed. This is also further supported by staining for the actin filaments (Figure 2). Scr cells showed actin enrichment predominantly at the cell–cell contacts, indicating an intact epithelial structure and polarity, which is not the case in the Vhl-KO cells. The cells develop a fibroblast-like phenotype with intracellular actin stress fibers and hardly any enrichment at the cell–cell contacts.

Since the changes in morphology are related to an EMT-like phenotype, we have also analyzed the mRNA expression of EMT marker genes like fibronectin, alpha smooth muscle actin, N-cadherin, and vimentin (Supplemental Figure S3). We observed significant differences in expression for fibronectin and alpha smooth muscle actin. However, the expression of N-cadherin and vimentin were not affected, which could implicate an incomplete EMT.

2.3. Vhl Deletion is Associated with Changes in Proliferation and Migration Behavior

In the next step, we analyzed if Vhl deletion is associated with functional changes. Given that the morphological and molecular changes might represent an incomplete EMT like phenotype, we set out to determine whether these changes are associated with other phenotypic changes. We have first tested if there are differences in the proliferation rate between Scr and Vhl-KO cells using the IncuCyte S3 live-cell analysis system. We have done this by calculation of the mean doubling time of the cells. The results showed that Vhl-KO cells had significant longer doubling time, resulting in a lower proliferation rate, compared to Scr cells (Figure 3).

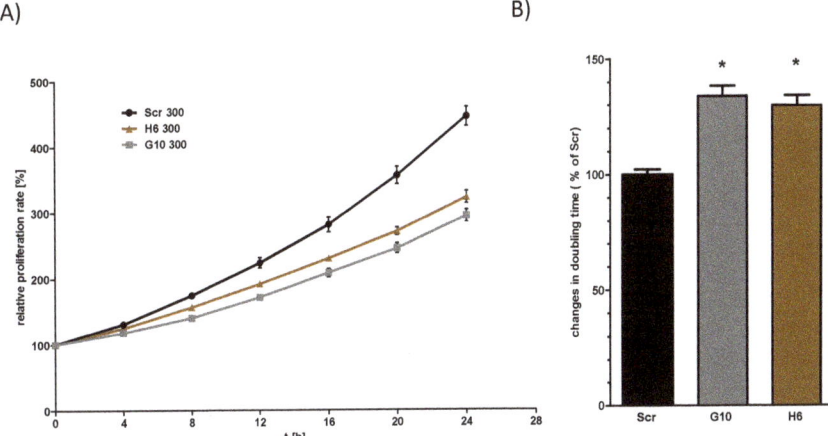

Figure 3. von Hippel–Lindau (Vhl) deletion is associated with longer doubling time. Cells were cultivated in 96-well plates and the proliferation was measured by live-cell imaging using IncuCyte S3 system taking an image every 4 h. The relative cell density was plotted and the doubling time was calculated by nonlinear exponential growth equation using GraphPad Prism (**A**). The doubling times were normalized to the Scr cells (**B**). One Way ANOVA was performed to identify statistically significant differences compared to Scr cell and are marked by * (p value < 0.05; n > 5).

Since we wanted to test if Vhl function is involved in hyperosmolality affected pathways, we tested the proliferation rate of Scr and Vhl-KO cells also under hyperosmotic conditions. Hyperosmolality alone reduced the proliferation of Scr cells (Supplemental Figure S4). This was also the case for the Vhl-KO cells. Under hyperosmotic conditions, however, the differences between Scr and Vhl-KO cells were still detectable. To test if the phenotype of Vhl deficient mpkCCD correlates with that of classical RCC cell lines, we tested the proliferation rate using the RCC cell line 786-0. We tested cells that do not express VHL and 786-0 cells that ectopically express human VHL (786-0-VHL). In contrast to the collecting duct cells, there were no differences between the 786-0 and 786-0-VHL expressing cells (Supplemental Figure S5).

Besides cell proliferation, we have analyzed the migration behavior of Scr and Vhl-KO as well as that of the 786-0 and 786-0-VHL RCC cells by scratch wound healing assay using the IncuCyte S3 live-cell imaging system. The results showed that Vhl-KO cells migrate at a significantly faster speed (~25% faster) compared to Scr cells (Figure 4A and Supplemental Figure S6). Similar to the results obtained for cell proliferation, VHL expression in 786-0 cells has a different effect on cell migration compared to the mpkCCD cells. The ectopic expression of VHL induced a significantly higher cell migration speed (Supplemental Figure S7).

So far the data showed that functional deletion of Vhl in mpkCCD cells is associated with massive changes in cell morphology, proliferation, and migration. These differences are cell context-specific since 786-0 RCC cell lines showed different effects. All these experiments were performed with cells cultivated under normal (isoosmotic) cell culture conditions. Since we postulate that Vhl has an osmolality dependent function, we have repeated the analysis under hyperosmotic conditions. In contrast to proliferation, the Vhl-KO cells behaved differently in the cell migration analysis under hyperosmotic conditions. While the Vhl-KO cells migrated faster under isotonic conditions, this was reversed under hyperosmotic conditions (Figure 4B).

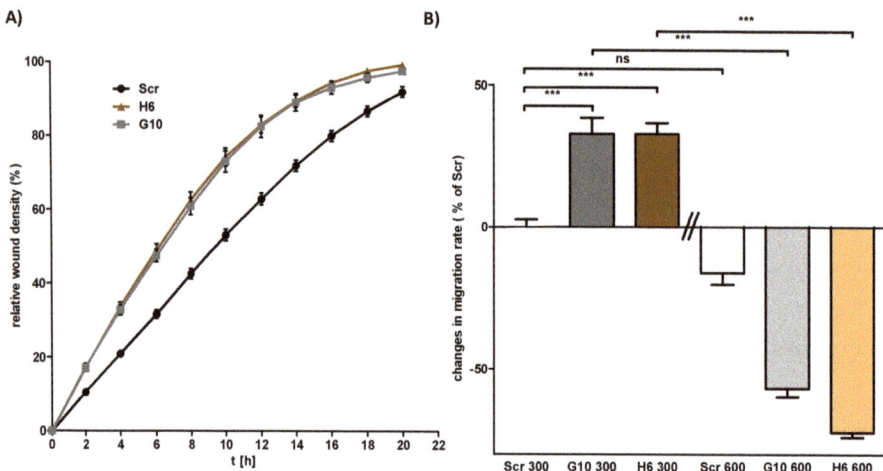

Figure 4. Loss of von Hippel–Lindau (Vhl) expression induces cell migration capacity. Cells were cultivated in 96-well plates until confluency and a wound to the cell monolayer was applied using the AutoScratch wound making tool. Cell migration was observed by live-cell imaging using the IncuCyte S3 system. (**A**) Representative plot of the wound density over time. (**B**) Cells were cultivated in 96-well plates until confluency either at 300 or 600 mosmol/kg. The relative wound density after 12 h was calculated by linear regression analysis using GraphPad Prism. The migration speed was normalized to Scr cells cultivated at 300 mosmol/kg. One Way ANOVA was performed to identify statistically significant differences and are marked by *** (p value < 0.001; $n > 3$).

2.4. Vhl Deletion Affects Expression of Hyperosmolality Regulated Genes

These results showed that Vhl deletion has a cell and osmolality specific effect on cellular behavior. We next asked if this is also associated with changes in the gene expression level. The expression level of Aqp2 served as a marker gene. The water channel Aqp2 expression in mpkCCD cells is either induced by vasopressin stimulation or by hyperosmotic cultivation conditions. Studies have shown that the expression of Aqp2 was decreased in Vhl deficient mice. Therefore, we cultivated the Scr and Vhl-KO cells under hyperosmotic conditions and analyzed Aqp2 gene expression by real-time PCR. The expression of Aqp2 is nearly lost in Vhl-deficient cells (Supplemental Figure S8). This indicates that Vhl deletion has a direct effect on AQP2 expression and probably interferes with hyperosmotic pathways. To identify additional genes that are differentially expressed in Vhl-KO cells, we cultivated Scr and Vhl-KO cells at 300 or 600 mosmol/kg, isolated total RNA, and performed gene expression profiling by RNA-Seq. In Scr cells, more than 2700 genes were differentially expressed between cells cultivated at 300 vs 600 mosmol/kg (Supplemental Figure S9). For example, Ranbp3l, Prss35, or Slc6a12 are within the top upregulated genes (Supplemental Excel File S1). These genes were also identified in primary cultured inner medullary collecting duct (IMCD) cells [15], which indicates that the mpkCCD cell line behaves similarly to primary cultured IMCD cells. We next compared Scr cells with Vhl-KO cells cultivated at 300 or 600 mosmol/kg. The deletion of Vhl was always associated with massive changes in gene expression. The total number of differentially expressed genes was over 4700 for the 300 and more than 4200 genes for the 600 mosmol/kg comparison (Figure 5).

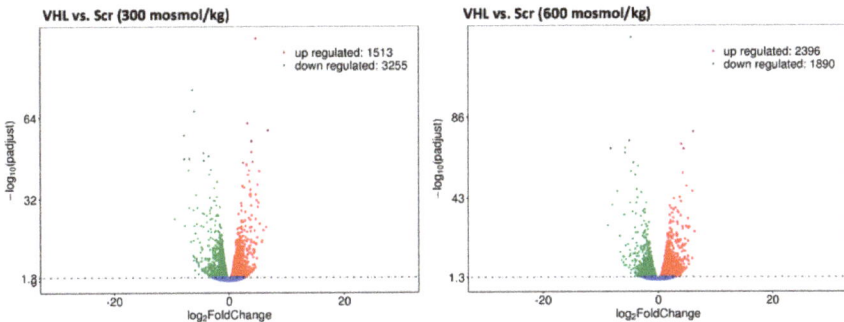

Figure 5. VHL (von Hippel–Lindau) deletion induces massive changes in gene expression. Scr- and Vhl-KO cells were cultivated at 300 or 600 mosmol/kg. Total RNA was isolated and gene expression was analyzed using Next-Generation Sequencing technology and differentially expressed genes were identified ($p < 0.05$, $n = 3$). The volcano plots show the number of genes, the p-values, and log$_2$ fold changes for cells cultivated at 300 (**left**) or 600 (**right**) mosmol/kg.

Functional analysis identified enrichment of genes in specific Kyoto Encyclopedia of Genes and Genomes (KEGG) pathways. Within the top 20 enriched KEGG pathways using the list of genes that were differentially expressed in the 300 mosmol/kg comparison only one cancer-associated pathway ("proteoglycans in cancer") was detected. The top enriched KEGG pathway was "metabolic pathways" (Supplemental Figure S10 and Supplemental Excel File S2). Similar analyses were performed with the differentially expressed genes in cells cultivated at 600 mosmol/kg. Again, the top enriched pathway was "metabolic pathways". In contrast to the 300 mosmol/kg comparison, more cancer-associated pathways were enriched namely "pathways in cancer", "viral carcinogenesis", "proteoglycans in cancer", and "central carbon metabolism in cancer". Two of the high-ranking pathways are "focal adhesion" and "regulation of actin cytoskeleton", revealing higher gene expression for f-actin proteins but also actin-binding factors like vinkulin or α-actinin. Furthermore, high ranking is the "PI3K-Akt pathway" that is strongly associated with ccRCC tumors [22]. Interestingly, these data support the observed morphological and functional changes in Vhl-KO cells since these pathways are associated with cell morphology and migration.

The screening of the gene expression data for classical EMT marker genes showed that the expression of desmin is significantly induced in Vhl-KO cells. The expressions of other markers like Snail1, Snail2, Zeb1, or Axl [23] were not affected (Supplemental Excel File S1). Again, this might be explained by an incomplete EMT like phenotype.

2.5. Loss of Vhl Function Leads to an Unfavorable Gene Expression Pattern

The data of TCGA and the Human Pathology Atlas [24] allowed the identification of prognostic genes that are associated with favorable or unfavorable clinical outcome. We have, therefore, analyzed if the loss of Vhl function has an impact on expression of genes that are prognostic for patients with renal cancer. However, the Human Pathology Atlas does not discriminate between the renal cancer entities.

We have used genes that showed at least 2/−2 log$_2$ fold changes in gene expression and that are prognostic on clinical outcome of the patients. About 151 genes fitted to the scheme. 91 genes were associated with unfavorable and 60 with a favorable clinical outcome (Figure 6).

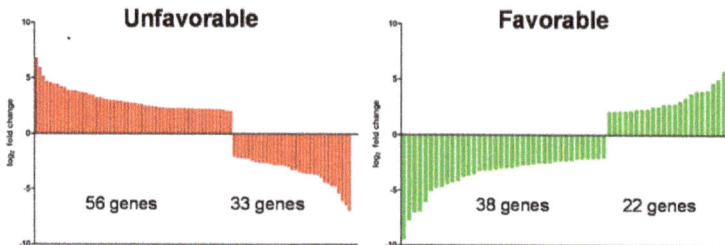

Figure 6. Deletion of VHL (von Hippel–Lindau) induces an unfavorable gene expression pattern. The list of genes with a $\log_2$ fold of 2 or higher and −2 or lower was compared with genes that have a prognostic impact on patient's outcome with renal cell carcinomas (RCC). The left panel shows genes with unfavorable and the right with favorable prognostic outcome. The expression level after Vhl deletion is plotted as $\log_2$ fold change.

When we compare the changes in expression, we observed that Vhl-KO cells showed reduced expression of 33 unfavorable and induced expression of 22 favorable genes. But the upregulated expression of more unfavorable genes (56) and predominantly reduced expression of favorable genes (38) indicates that, in summary, the loss of functional Vhl in the mpkCCD cells induces an unfavorable gene expression pattern.

We have shown that the expression of hyperosmolality induced genes is reduced in RCC samples and that a gene signature of osmolality affected genes can be used for the prediction of patient's clinical outcome [16]. We have, therefore, analyzed if this is also the case in the present study. We have generated a list of genes that are upregulated by hyperosmolality and have a favorable prognostic outcome for patients with RCC. This list was compared with the list of genes that were differentially expressed (and a $\log_2$ fold change of at least 1/−1) in Vhl-KO cells under hyperosmotic conditions. We identified 51 genes that met the criteria (Figure 7). Only 5 genes were higher expressed compared to Scr in Vhl-KO cells under hyperosmotic conditions. The majority, 46 genes, were downregulated in expression. This again demonstrates that loss of Vhl induces an unfavorable gene expression pattern. These data also show that Vhl has an influence on the expression of hyperosmolality affected genes.

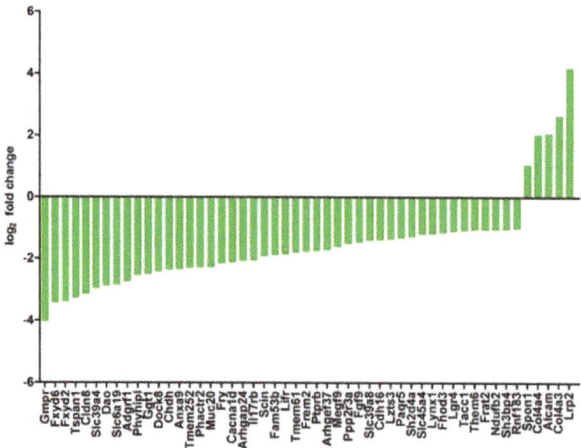

Figure 7. Deletion of von Hippel–Lindau (Vhl) reduces expression of hyperosmolality induced genes with favorable prognostic value. The list of genes that are (1) induced by hyperosmolality, (2) favorable for patients outcome, and (3) differentially expressed in Vhl-KO cell with a $\log_2$ fold change of 1 or higher and −1 or are plotted here.

Vhl-KO reduces, for example, the expression of Fxyd2, Fxyd4, Rnf183, and Ranbp3l, which are prognostically favorable in patients with ccRCC [16]. Since the Human Pathology Atlas does not discriminate between the RCC entities, we have used selected genes and queried the KIRC TCGA database if they could serve as prognostic markers for patients with ccRCC. In all cases, high expression of these genes was associated with a significant overall survival of the patients (Supplemental Figure S11).

Vice versa, we have also analyzed if the Vhl-KO leads to induced expression of unfavorable genes, which are downregulated by hyperosmolality. Moreover, 20 genes showed upregulation in expression and only 3 downregulated expression in Vhl-KO cells (Supplemental Figure S12).

3. Discussion

The CRISPR/Cas9 technology has been used in a study before to delete VHL in the RENCA renal cancer cell line [25] where the authors described an EMT like phenotype due to a Vhl knock out. To our knowledge, this study is the first one that used a healthy renal epithelial cell line to introduce CRISPR/Cas9-mediated Vhl deletion and characterizes the phenotype of the cells. The limitations of the study might be: 1. that we used renal collecting duct cells, although the ccRCC is originated from proximal tubulus and 2. The use of a murine cell line. However, we are convinced that this was the right strategy to test the hypothesis that Vhl function interferes with hyperosmolality affected gene expression.

We successfully introduced mutation into the Vhl locus, leading to a frameshift and expression of nonfunctional Vhl protein. Loss of Vhl function induced stabilization of Hif1a. The deletion of Vhl was associated with loss of epithelial structure that is similar to the phenotype observed in RENCA cells [25]. Similar to RENCA cells, loss of Vhl induces a more metastatic phenotype in mpkCCD cells as they migrate faster. However, the 786-0 RCC cell line showed different behavior. Ectopic expression of VHL was associated with an increased cell migration speed. In contrast to the cell migration analysis, Vhl-KO cells showed a slower doubling time. There were no differences observed between 786-0 and 786-0-VHL cells. This indicates that Vhl deletion has a cell type-specific effect on cellular function. However, the knockdown of Vhl in lung cancer cell lines showed similar effects to what we observed in the mpkCCD cells, higher migration and lower proliferation capacity [26]. These data show that the mpkCCD cell line is a suitable model to study the role of Vhl in renal cells. Traditionally it has been thought that ccRCC originates from cells of the proximal tubulus [1]. However, there is also evidence that subsets can also originate from distal tubulus or even collecting duct [27–30]. Therefore, these studies indicate that the use of the mpkCCD cells as a collecting duct cell line might not represent a major limitation. A mouse model using Hoxb7-Cre as driver to delete Vhl expression in the collecting duct developed epithelial disruption, fibrosis, and hyperplasia [31]. However, Vhl deletion alone is not sufficient and only in combination with deletion of other genetic factors it was possible to induce ccRCC. The combined loss of Vhl, Tp53, and Rb1 induced, for example, ccRCC [32]. The same group showed that renal Vhl deletion is associated with disturbed urine concentration capability [9]. More than 14 different cell types are involved in the urine concentration and water retention in the kidneys representing a specific transcriptome [33]. Most of the water retention is mediated by the action of aquaporin water channel family [10]. The driving force for water transport is a cortico-medullary osmotic gradient. The cells of the renal medulla are faced with a hyperosmotic environment. We have also shown that the hyperosmotic environment induces a kidney and even cell-specific gene expression pattern [15]. In a recent study, we have shown that the hyperosmotic gene expression pattern is lost in ccRCC samples and that this has also consequences for patients' outcome [16]. In the mentioned study, the initial gene list was generated in rat primary collecting duct cells [15,16] and we were able to develop a translational comparison from healthy rat cell to human renal cancer and survival prediction, showing the translational potential of the data [16].

In the collecting duct, the rate-limiting factor in water retention is the water channel Aqp2. The expression of Aqp2 is downregulated in Vhl-deficient mice [9,32]. Downregulation of Aqp2 has been also shown in patient-derived ccRCC samples [34,35]. The expression of Aqp2 is regulated by the action of Nfat5 transcription factor. Nfat5 is activated by the hyperosmotic environment [13]. The group of Schönenberger et al. postulated that Vhl deletion induces reduction of the osmotic gradient by the increased angiogenesis that could lead to decreased Aqp2 expression [9]. Loss of Aqp2 is also evident in a mice model that developed renal cancer [32]. We have shown that hyperosmolality regulates the expression of several hundred genes (including Aqp2), that this expression pattern inversely correlates with ccRCC tumor samples, and that this can be used for prediction of cancer-specific survival [15,16]. Within this study, we have shown that Vhl deletion has a direct negative effect on Aqp2 expression. Besides the massive morphological changes, loss of Vhl induced changes in gene expression. More than 4700 genes were differentially expressed compared to control cells under isosmotic conditions. Loss of Vhl function was associated with more than 8500 differentially expressed genes in the RENCA RCC cell line after CRIPSR/Cas9 deletion of Vhl [25]. Unfortunately, the total list of genes and the used significance level is not published to compare the list of genes. However, in both cases, loss of Vhl function alone induces massive changes in gene expression in either cancer or normal cell lines. KEGG Pathway analysis showed that loss of Vhl affects, for example, "PI3K-Akt signaling pathway" or "Regulation of actin cytoskeleton" pathway. Dysregulation of these pathways could explain the observed EMT like phenotype. Since we were able to detect increased expression of selected markers genes for EMT like fibronectin and smooth muscle actinin, no changes were observed for vimentin, E-cadherin, or Snail1. Therefore, the observed changes might represent an incomplete EMT. Since the expression of fibronectin is induced, the observed changes might be due to pro-fibrotic changes. Besides Col1a1 no other classical markers like Mmp9, Timp1, or Col3a1 were induced on gene expression level. As explained for EMT, this might indicate a partial or mild pro-fibrotic change. However, further studies are needed to specifically analyze if the observed changes might represent incomplete EMT, pro-fibrotic changes, or a mixture of both.

The KEGG pathway analysis might be used for the identification of novel therapeutic targets. For example, targeting PI3K-Akt pathways has been in focus in treatment of different cancer types including RCC [22,36]. These data show that Vhl deletion in mpkCCD cells induces a gene expression associated with a cancer-related phenotype and this is also supported by the enrichment of genes that are involved in "Pathways in cancer". This is also supported by the comparison of our data with the data from the Human Pathology Atlas [24]. Vhl deletion induced the expression of more genes that are unfavorable and predominantly reduced expression of genes that are associated with a favorable outcome of patients with RCC. Nonetheless, the data from the Human Pathology Atlas does not discriminate between the RCC entities. However, the query of the TCGA KIRC cohort for selected genes showed that they could serve as prognostic markers for patients with ccRCC.

Since the cells in the inner medulla of the kidneys are faced with a hyperosmotic environment, we also compared the gene expression pattern in Vhl-KO and Scr cells under hyperosmotic conditions. Several genes are regulated by changes in hyperosmolality and their expression is inversely regulated in ccRCC samples compared to normal tissue [15,16]. For example, the expression of the E74 like ETS transcription factor 5 is not detectable in ccRCC samples and ectopic ELF5 expression reduced tumor development in mice [17]. This indicates that ELF5 can act as a tumor suppressor in ccRCC. We have shown that Elf5 expression is highly induced by hyperosmotic environment [15]. The expression of ELF5 was also inducible in the 786-0 ccRCC cell line when the cells were cultivated under hyperosmotic conditions. However, the level of induction was even more striking in 786-0-VHL cells [16]. When we compare the influence of Vhl on hyperosmolality affected gene expression again several thousand genes are affected. KEGG pathway analysis showed that 4 cancer-associated pathways are within the top 20 enriched pathways compared to one in the isosmotic comparison. There are also several genes within the significantly downregulated genes that are known to be induced in expression by hyper osmolality. For example, the expression of gamma subunit of Na K-ATPase (Fxyd2) and the FXYD domain containing ion transport regulator 4 (Fxyd4) are upregulated by hyperosmolality [15,37]. The expressions of both genes are downregulated in human ccRCC and a mouse ccRCC model [32,35].

Other prominent genes are the ran-binding protein 3 like (RanBP3L) or the ring finger 183 (Rnf183). The expression of both genes is induced by hyperosmolality [15,38,39]. However, in Vhl-KO cells, the expression of both genes is significantly downregulated. FXYD2, RanBP3L, and Rnf183 expression level is associated with clinical outcome of patients with ccRCC [16]. This is also the case in the Vhl-KO cells. About 51 genes that are induced by hyperosmolality and have a favorable outcome for patients with RCC are differentially expressed in Vhl-KO vs. Scr cells under hyperosmotic conditions and 46 of them are downregulated in expression when Vhl function is missing. We have shown that the expression of hyperosmolality affected genes are inversely regulated in ccRCC samples and that high expression of genes in patients, which are downregulated by hyperosmolality, have an unfavorable outcome [16]. These data show that Vhl-KO cells under hyperosmotic conditions express a gene expression pattern that is described to be unfavorable for patients with ccRCC. These data also support our hypothesis that loss of Vhl function is associated with disturbed hyperosmotic adaptation capacity, as it is shown by differences in proliferation and migration capacity. Of course, we have to be aware of the fact that up to 30% of patients with ccRCC have functional VHL protein or at least no genetic alterations that would affect the functional expression of VHL.

The main transcription factor that is activated under hyperosmotic condition is Nfat5 [40], inducing the expression of osmoprotective genes [41]. As an example, NFAT5 induces the expression of the solute carrier SLC6a12 [41] and the expression of Slc6a12 is massively downregulated in Vhl-KO cells ($\log_2$ fold change of −3.3). This implicates that probably loss of Vhl function has an influence on Nfat5 activity. Nfat5 has also a function in the immune system for the macrophage and T lymphocyte function [42], and haploinsufficiency is associated with immunodeficiency [43]. However, the role of Nfat5 in cancer is controversial. Nfat5 deficiency promoted hepatocellular carcinogenesis and metastasis [44] in one study. Another study showed that Nfat5 promoted apoptosis and inhibited invasion in hepatocellular carcinoma cell lines [45]. A further study reports that S100a4 protein promoted proliferation and migration of ccRCC cell line through NFAT5 [46]. A recent study showed that NFAT5 is a target of metabolically active micro RNAs (miRNA) [14]. The gene expression of NFAT5 is downregulated in ccRCC samples compared to normal tumor samples [14] as well as expression of NFAT5 target genes. The authors postulate that the miR-106b-5p and miR-122-5p are involved in the downregulation of NFAT5 and also downstream of NFAT5 target genes [14]. However, VHL-dependent regulation of NFAT5 remained unclear. Our data indicates at least an interaction of VHL and NFAT5 functions and further analysis are needed to identify the molecular mechanisms in more detail. Since Vhl deletion alone did not induce renal cancer in mice model, it might be interesting to test if a Vhl/Nfat5 double KO develops renal cancer.

Taken together, we have shown that Vhl deletion in collecting duct cells induces an EMT like phenotype, an unfavorable gene expression pattern, and that loss of Vhl function significantly regulates the expression of hyperosmolality expressed genes that are favorable prognostic markers for patients with ccRCC.

4. Material and Methods

4.1. Cell Culture

HEK293T cells were obtained from the DSMZ-German Collection of Microorganisms and Cell Cultures and cultivated in Dulbecco's Modified Eagle's Medium (DMEM) supplemented with 10% serum (fetal calf serum (FCS)) and 1% penicillin/streptavidin. The 786-0 and ectopic VHL expressing 786-0-VHL cells were a kind gift of Prof. Barbara Seliger [47]. These cells were maintained in DMEM supplemented with 10% fetal calf serum (FCS), 2 mM glutamine, 1 mM pyruvate, and 1% penicillin/streptomycin. The mpkCCD cell line was a kind gift of Prof. Mark Knepper [48]. These cells were cultivated in DMEM Ham F-12 medium supplemented with 10% FCS and 1% penicillin/streptomycin. All cell lines were cultured at 37 °C and 5% CO_2. The medium osmolality was adjusted to 600 mosmol/kg by the addition of 100 mM NaCl and 100 mM urea to the corresponding medium.

4.2. Oligos and Primers

The selection of the sequences for the guide RNAs (gRNA) targeting Vhl was performed according to the DNA 2.0 online tool [49] Three different sequences were selected (Supplemental Table S1). Real-time PCR primers and the PCR primers for amplification of the targeted Vhl locus were designed by NCBI Primer BLAST [50]. All oligos were purchased from Biolegio B.V. (Nijmegen, The Netherlands).

4.3. Cloning of gRNAs and Vector Production in Escherichia coli

Three different gRNAs targeting murine Vhl locus and random scrambled (Scr) gRNA were cloned into lentiCRISPRv2. The lentiCRISPR v2 was a gift from Feng Zhang (Addgene plasmid # 52,961; Addgene, Watertown, MA, USA). The cloning was performed as described [49]. Plasmid isolation was performed using GeneJET Miniprep Kit (Thermo Scientific, Waltham, MA, USA). Isolated plasmids were analyzed by Sanger sequencing (Eurofins Genomics, Ebersberg, Germany) using human U6 primer. Positive plasmids were used for further experiments.

4.4. Vectors

The lentiviral particles were produced in HEK293T cells. For the production, the pLP1, pLP2, and pLP/VSVG vectors were used from ViraPower™ Lentiviral Packaging Mix (Thermo Fisher, Waltham, MA, USA). The HEK293T cells were cultivated to 70% confluency. Cell culture medium was reduced to starve cells and then lentiviral vectors pLP1 (7.2 µg), pLP2 (2.4 µg), pLP/VSVG (4.0 µg), and ligated lentiCRISPRv2 vector (10.4 µg) were added to the medium together with transfection reagent Turbofect™ (Thermo Fisher). Cells were incubated for 24 h. After exchange, medium cells were incubated for another 48 h. The conditioned virus-containing medium was removed, sterile filtrated, and kept at −20 °C.

4.5. Viral Transfection of mpkCCD Cells and Sequencing of Vhl Locus

The mpkCCD cell line was seeded into 6-well cell culture dishes and cultivated to 40–50% confluency. Medium was removed and conditioned medium containing the virus particles and fresh medium in a 1:1 ratio was added. After 48 h, medium containing 2 µg/mL puromycin for selection of transduced cells was added. Genomic DNA was isolated and targeted genomic regions were amplified by PCR using specific primers. The PCR products were purified using GenElute™ PCR Clean-up Kit (Sigma Aldrich, St. Louis, MO, USA) and analyzed by Sanger sequencing using the sequencing service of Eurofins Genomics GmbH (Eberberg, Germany).

4.6. Isolation of Single-Cell Clones and Tracking of Indels (TIDE)

Single-cell clones were isolated in 96-well cell culture plates by serial dilution. Total DNA was isolated and the targeting region was amplified by PCR and analyzed by Sanger sequencing. The sequences were analyzed by TIDE for the identification of specific mutations of Vhl gene [20]. Single clones harboring frameshift mutations on both alleles were finally selected and used for further analysis.

4.7. Western Blot

Total protein was isolated from cells using Pierce® RIPA lysis and extraction buffer with protease inhibitor mix (40 µL/mL, Thermo Fisher Scientific, Waltham, MA, USA). Protein lysates were separated by SDS-PAGE with 4–12% Novex™ Bis-Tris gradient gel (Thermo Fisher Scientific). Separated protein bands were then blotted onto 0.45 µm nitrocellulose membrane by Western blotting. Successful blotting was confirmed by Ponceau S staining. All washing steps of the membrane were performed with phosphate buffered saline + 0.1% Tween 20 (PBST). Unspecific binding sites were blocked with 5% BSA or milk solution. First and horse reddish peroxidase coupled secondary antibody were applied in milk or BSA solution and incubated for 1h at room temperature. Afterward, the membrane was incubated with ECL Western Blotting Substrate (Thermo Scientific) and signals were detected on the ChemiDoc Imager detecting system (BioRad, Hercules, CA, USA). The antibody directed against Vhl (sc-55506) was purchased from Santa Cruz Biotechnology, Inc. (Dallas, TX, USA). Against Hif1a (36169S) and Gapdh (2118S) from Cell Signaling Technology, Inc.(Danvers, MA, USA).

4.8. Immunofluorescence

Immunofluorescence was performed as described before [15]. Cells were seeded in 24-well cell culture plates on glass cover slips and cultured to desired confluency. Medium was then removed and cells were fixed in 4% formalin. Unspecific binding sites were blocked by incubation with fishskin-gelatine (0.3% in PBS). First antibody was applied in gelatine solution and incubated at 37 °C for 1 h. Three wash steps (15 min) were performed with PBS and the cells were incubated for 1 h with the secondary Alexa-labeled antibody solution in PBS. The cells were washed three times with PBS (15 min) and mounted on glass slides. Images were taken on a Keyence BZ-8100E microscope (Keyence Corporation, Osaka, Japan).

4.9. Proliferation and Migration

For proliferation and migration assays, cells were cultivated either at 300 or 600 mosmol/kg in 96-well cell culture dishes. For migration assays, the wells were grown to 100% confluency. Data were collected with IncuCyte® Live-Cell Analysis System (Essen BioScience, Inc., Ann Arbor, MI, USA) for 24 h. For migration analysis, a wound to the cell layer was created with WoundMaker™ (Essen BioScience) Migration capacity was evaluated by relative wound density (RWD) (Essen BioScience). Cell proliferation was also measured by live-cell imaging using the IncuCyte® Live-Cell Analysis System. In a 96-well plate 1000–2000 cells were cultivated either at 300 or 600 mosmol/kg and monitored for 48 h. The doubling time was calculated by using nonlinear regression analysis and exponential growth quotation with GraphPad Prism version 5.0 (GraphPad Software Company, San Diego, CA, USA).

4.10. Real-Time PCR (RT-PCR)

Real-time PCR was performed as described before [15]. The expression of *Aqp2* was acquired by real-time PCR using a specific primer pair (forward: 5′CAC CGG CTG CTC CAT GAA TCC3′, reverse: 5′TCC GCC TCC AGG CCC TTG AGC3′). As reference gene, *Gapdh* was used (forward: 5′TGG CCT TCC GTG TTC CTA CC3′, reverse: 5′GGT CCT CAG TGT AGC CCA AGA TG3′). Data acquisition was done with Bio-Rad CFX Manager 3.1 Software and quantified by $2^{-\Delta\Delta CT}$ method as described [51].

4.11. Preparation of Samples for Next-Generation Sequencing

For gene expression analysis using Next-Generation Sequencing RNA-Seq, the cells were cultivated for 5 days to 70–85% confluency at 300 and 600 mosmol/kg. Total RNA was isolated and reverse transcribed. Within these samples, the single clone specific *Vhl* mutations were confirmed via TIDE as described above. RNA samples from 3 independent separate isolations were used for analysis by RNA-Seq by Novogene Co, Ltd. (Cambridge, UK). The quality control, sequencing, and bioinformatics were performed by Novogene as service. The detailed description can be found in Supplemental Methods.

4.12. Favorable and Unfavorable Gene Expression in Kidney Cancer

A total of 2755 favorable and 3213 unfavorable genes for kidney cancer from the Human Protein Atlas Database were used. These two groups of genes were compared separately to differential expressed genes with a $\log_2$ fold change $\geq 2.0/<-2.0$ between Vhl-KO and Scr cells at 300 mosmol/kg.

Overlapping genes between the groups were selected and the changes in expression are displayed in waterfall plots.

4.13. Induced Gene Expression by Osmolality in Kidney Cancer

All induced genes with a $\log_2$ fold change ≥ 1.0 from the comparison of Scr 600 mosmol/kg (600) vs. 300 mosmol/kg (300) were compared to identify favorable genes from Human Protein Atlas database. The expression of these genes was compared with the list of differentially expressed genes (with a $\log_2$ fold change $\geq 1.0/<-1.0$) between Vhl-KO vs. Scr cultivated at 600 mosmol/kg. The overlapping genes with level of expression changes are displayed as a waterfall plot.

4.14. Statistics

Results are expressed as the mean ± standard error of mean (SEM). Statistical evaluation was performed using GraphPad Prism 5.0 software. Comparisons were analyzed using one-way analysis of variance (ANOVA) or by two-tailed Student's *t* test. The data were considered significant if *p*-values ≤ 0.05.

5. Conclusions

Our study demonstrates that loss of Vhl function alone induces massive morphological and functional changes in a healthy renal cell line. It induces an unfavorable gene expression pattern under isosmotic cell culture conditions. Vhl deletion massively interferes with the hyperosmotic gene expression program. It induces predominantly downregulation of hyperosmolality induced genes, which are predicted with favorable clinical outcome of patients with ccRCC.

Thus, targeting osmolality represents a novel promising therapeutic option for ccRCC therapy.

Supplementary Materials: The following are available online at http://www.mdpi.com/2072-6694/12/2/420/s1, Table S1: Sequences selected for cloning and amplification of targeted region, Figure S1: The selected gRNAs induced mutations in the Vhl locus, Figure S2: TIDE analysis leads to identification of clones with frame shift mutations, Figure S3: Effect of Vhl deletion on selected EMT marker genes, Figure S4: Hyper osmolality increases doubling time, Figure S5: VHL expression has no effect on proliferation rate of 786-0 RCC cell line, Figure S6: VHL deletion increases migration speed, Figure S7: Ectopic VHL expression induces cell migration capacity in 786-0 cells, Figure S8: The expression of Aqp2 mRNA is down regulated in Vhl-KO cells, Figure S9: Hyper osmolality causes massive changes in gene expression, Figure S10: KEGG pathway analysis, Figure S11: Kaplan-Meier analysis of survival probability for selected genes, Figure S12: Deletion of Vhl induces the expression of hyper osmolality suppressed genes with unfavorable prognostic value, Figure S13: Total Western blot membrane from Figure 1.

Author Contributions: A.G. performed research, analyzed data, and wrote the paper; L.G. performed research and wrote the paper; D.C. performed research and wrote the paper; N.B. performed research; B.E. designed research, performed research, analyzed data and wrote the paper. All authors have read and agreed to the published version of the manuscript.

Funding: This work was supported by the Deutsche Forschungsgemeinschaft (DFG, German Research Foundation) ED 181/9-1.

Acknowledgments: We would like to thank Barbara Seliger for providing the 786-0 cell line. The results shown here are in part based upon data generated by the TCGA Research Network. We would like to thank The Cancer Genome Atlas initiative, all tissue donors, and investigators who contributed to the acquisition and analyses of the samples used in this study. Information about TCGA and the investigators and institutions that constitute the TCGA research network can be found at http://cancergenome.nih.gov/.

Conflicts of Interest: The authors declare that they have no competing interests.

References

1. Hsieh, J.J.; Purdue, M.P.; Signoretti, S.; Swanton, C.; Albiges, L.; Schmidinger, M.; Heng, D.Y.; Larkin, J.; Ficarra, V. Renal cell carcinoma. *Nat. Rev. Dis. Primers* **2017**, *3*, 17009. [CrossRef] [PubMed]
2. Rini, B.I.; Campbell, S.C.; Escudier, B. Renal cell carcinoma. *Lancet* **2009**, *373*, 1119–1132. [CrossRef]
3. McLaughlin, J.; Lipworth, L.; Tarone, R.; Blot, W. *Cancer Epidemiology and Prevention*; Oxford University Press: Oxford, UK, 2006; pp. 1087–1100.

4. Hakimi, A.A.; Chen, Y.B.; Wren, J.; Gonen, M.; Abdel-Wahab, O.; Heguy, A.; Liu, H.; Takeda, S.; Tickoo, S.K.; Reuter, V.E.; et al. Clinical and pathologic impact of select chromatin-modulating tumor suppressors in clear cell renal cell carcinoma. *Eur. Urol.* **2013**, *63*, 848–854. [CrossRef] [PubMed]
5. Gnarra, J.R.; Tory, K.; Weng, Y.; Schmidt, L.; Wei, M.H.; Li, H.; Latif, F.; Liu, S.; Chen, F.; Duh, F.M.; et al. Mutations of the VHL tumour suppressor gene in renal carcinoma. *Nat. Genet.* **1994**, *7*, 85–90. [CrossRef]
6. Nickerson, M.L.; Jaeger, E.; Shi, Y.; Durocher, J.A.; Mahurkar, S.; Zaridze, D.; Matveev, V.; Janout, V.; Kollarova, H.; Bencko, V.; et al. Improved identification of von Hippel-Lindau gene alterations in clear cell renal tumors. *Clin. Cancer Res.* **2008**, *14*, 4726–4734. [CrossRef]
7. Rankin, E.B.; Tomaszewski, J.E.; Haase, V.H. Renal cyst development in mice with conditional inactivation of the von Hippel-Lindau tumor suppressor. *Cancer Res.* **2006**, *66*, 2576–2583. [CrossRef]
8. Frew, I.J.; Thoma, C.R.; Georgiev, S.; Minola, A.; Hitz, M.; Montani, M.; Moch, H.; Krek, W. pVHL and PTEN tumour suppressor proteins cooperatively suppress kidney cyst formation. *EMBO J.* **2008**, *27*, 1747–1757. [CrossRef]
9. Schönenberger, D.; Rajski, M.; Harlander, S.; Frew, I.J. Vhl deletion in renal epithelia causes HIF-1α-dependent, HIF-2α-independent angiogenesis and constitutive diuresis. *Oncotarget* **2016**, *7*, 60971–60985. [CrossRef]
10. Edemir, B.; Pavenstadt, H.; Schlatter, E.; Weide, T. Mechanisms of cell polarity and aquaporin sorting in the nephron. *Pflug. Arch.* **2011**, *461*, 607–621. [CrossRef]
11. Nielsen, S.; Frøkiær, J.; Marples, D.; Kwon, T.H.; Agre, P.; Knepper, M.A. Aquaporins in the kidney: From molecules to medicine. *Physiol. Rev.* **2002**, *82*, 205–244. [CrossRef]
12. Hasler, U.; Jeon, U.S.; Kim, J.A.; Mordasini, D.; Kwon, H.M.; Feraille, E.; Martin, P.Y. Tonicity-responsive enhancer binding protein is an essential regulator of aquaporin-2 expression in renal collecting duct principal cells. *J. Am. Soc. Nephrol.* **2006**, *17*, 1521–1531. [CrossRef] [PubMed]
13. Miyakawa, H.; Woo, S.K.; Dahl, S.C.; Handler, J.S.; Kwon, H.M. Tonicity-responsive enhancer binding protein, a rel-like protein that stimulates transcription in response to hypertonicity. *Proc. Natl. Acad. Sci. USA* **1999**, *96*, 2538–2542. [CrossRef] [PubMed]
14. Bogusławska, J.; Popławski, P.; Alseekh, S.; Koblowska, M.; Iwanicka-Nowicka, R.; Rybicka, B.; Kędzierska, H.; Głuchowska, K.; Hanusek, K.; Tański, Z.; et al. MicroRNA-Mediated Metabolic Reprograming in Renal Cancer. *Cancers* **2019**, *11*, 1825. [CrossRef] [PubMed]
15. Schulze Blasum, B.; Schroter, R.; Neugebauer, U.; Hofschroer, V.; Pavenstadt, H.; Ciarimboli, G.; Schlatter, E.; Edemir, B. The kidney-specific expression of genes can be modulated by the extracellular osmolality. *FASEB J.* **2016**, *30*, 3588–3597. [CrossRef]
16. Kandabarau, S.; Leiz, J.; Krohn, K.; Winter, S.; Bedke, J.; Schwab, M.; Schaeffeler, E.; Edemir, B. Hypertonicity-Affected Genes Are Differentially Expressed in Clear Cell Renal Cell Carcinoma and Correlate with Cancer-Specific Survival. *Cancers* **2019**, *12*, 6. [CrossRef]
17. Lapinskas, E.J.; Svobodova, S.; Davis, I.D.; Cebon, J.; Hertzog, P.J.; Pritchard, M.A. The Ets transcription factor ELF5 functions as a tumor suppressor in the kidney. *Twin Res. Hum. Genet.* **2011**, *14*, 316–322. [CrossRef]
18. Yu, M.J.; Miller, R.L.; Uawithya, P.; Rinschen, M.M.; Khositseth, S.; Braucht, D.W.; Chou, C.L.; Pisitkun, T.; Nelson, R.D.; Knepper, M.A. Systems-level analysis of cell-specific AQP2 gene expression in renal collecting duct. *Proc. Natl. Acad. Sci. USA* **2009**, *106*, 2441–2446. [CrossRef]
19. Hasler, U.; Vinciguerra, M.; Vandewalle, A.; Martin, P.Y.; Feraille, E. Dual effects of hypertonicity on aquaporin-2 expression in cultured renal collecting duct principal cells. *J. Am. Soc. Nephrol.* **2005**, *16*, 1571–1582. [CrossRef]
20. Brinkman, E.K.; Chen, T.; Amendola, M.; van Steensel, B. Easy quantitative assessment of genome editing by sequence trace decomposition. *Nucleic Acids Res.* **2014**, *42*, e168. [CrossRef]
21. Zhang, S.; Zhou, X.; Wang, B.; Zhang, K.; Liu, S.; Yue, K.; Zhang, L.; Wang, X. Loss of VHL expression contributes to epithelial-mesenchymal transition in oral squamous cell carcinoma. *Oral Oncol.* **2014**, *50*, 809–817. [CrossRef]
22. Guo, H.; German, P.; Bai, S.; Barnes, S.; Guo, W.; Qi, X.; Lou, H.; Liang, J.; Jonasch, E.; Mills, G.B.; et al. The PI3K/AKT Pathway and Renal Cell Carcinoma. *J. Genet. Genom.* **2015**, *42*, 343–353. [CrossRef] [PubMed]
23. Gurzu, S.; Turdean, S.; Kovecsi, A.; Contac, A.O.; Jung, I. Epithelial-mesenchymal, mesenchymal-epithelial, and endothelial-mesenchymal transitions in malignant tumors: An update. *World J. Clin. Cases* **2015**, *3*, 393–404. [CrossRef] [PubMed]

24. Uhlen, M.; Zhang, C.; Lee, S.; Sjostedt, E.; Fagerberg, L.; Bidkhori, G.; Benfeitas, R.; Arif, M.; Liu, Z.; Edfors, F.; et al. A pathology atlas of the human cancer transcriptome. *Science* **2017**, *357*, eaan2507. [CrossRef] [PubMed]
25. Schokrpur, S.; Hu, J.; Moughon, D.L.; Liu, P.; Lin, L.C.; Hermann, K.; Mangul, S.; Guan, W.; Pellegrini, M.; Xu, H.; et al. CRISPR-Mediated VHL Knockout Generates an Improved Model for Metastatic Renal Cell Carcinoma. *Sci. Rep.* **2016**, *6*, 29032. [CrossRef]
26. Zhou, Q.; Chen, T.; Ibe, J.C.F.; Usha Raj, J.; Zhou, G. Knockdown of von Hippel–Lindau protein decreases lung cancer cell proliferation and colonization. *FEBS Lett.* **2012**, *586*, 1510–1515. [CrossRef]
27. Ozcan, A.; Zhai, J.; Hamilton, C.; Shen, S.S.; Ro, J.Y.; Krishnan, B.; Truong, L.D. PAX-2 in the diagnosis of primary renal tumors: Immunohistochemical comparison with renal cell carcinoma marker antigen and kidney-specific cadherin. *Am. J. Clin. Pathol.* **2009**, *131*, 393–404. [CrossRef]
28. Kraus, S.; Abel, P.D.; Nachtmann, C.; Linsenmann, H.J.; Weidner, W.; Stamp, G.W.; Chaudhary, K.S.; Mitchell, S.E.; Franke, F.E.; El Lalani, N. MUC1 mucin and trefoil factor 1 protein expression in renal cell carcinoma: Correlation with prognosis. *Hum. Pathol.* **2002**, *33*, 60–67. [CrossRef]
29. Khurana, K.K.; Truong, L.D.; Verani, R.R. Image analysis of proliferating cell nuclear antigen expression and immunohistochemical profiles in renal cell carcinoma associated with acquired cystic kidney disease: Comparison with classic renal cell carcinoma. *Mod. Pathol.* **1998**, *11*, 339–346.
30. Shen, S.S.; Krishna, B.; Chirala, R.; Amato, R.J.; Truong, L.D. Kidney-specific cadherin, a specific marker for the distal portion of the nephron and related renal neoplasms. *Mod. Pathol.* **2005**, *18*, 933–940. [CrossRef]
31. Pritchett, T.L.; Bader, H.L.; Henderson, J.; Hsu, T. Conditional inactivation of the mouse von Hippel-Lindau tumor suppressor gene results in wide-spread hyperplastic, inflammatory and fibrotic lesions in the kidney. *Oncogene* **2015**, *34*, 2631–2639. [CrossRef]
32. Harlander, S.; Schönenberger, D.; Toussaint, N.C.; Prummer, M.; Catalano, A.; Brandt, L.; Moch, H.; Wild, P.J.; Frew, I.J. Combined mutation in Vhl, Trp53 and Rb1 causes clear cell renal cell carcinoma in mice. *Nat. Med.* **2017**, *23*, 869–877. [CrossRef] [PubMed]
33. Lee, J.W.; Chou, C.L.; Knepper, M.A. Deep Sequencing in Microdissected Renal Tubules Identifies Nephron Segment-Specific Transcriptomes. *J. Am. Soc. Nephrol.* **2015**, *26*, 2669–2677. [CrossRef] [PubMed]
34. Cancer Genome Atlas Research Network. Comprehensive molecular characterization of clear cell renal cell carcinoma. *Nature* **2013**, *499*, 43–49. [CrossRef] [PubMed]
35. Schrödter, S.; Braun, M.; Syring, I.; Klümper, N.; Deng, M.; Schmidt, D.; Perner, S.; Müller, S.C.; Ellinger, J. Identification of the dopamine transporter SLC6A3 as a biomarker for patients with renal cell carcinoma. *Mol. Cancer* **2016**, *15*, 10. [CrossRef] [PubMed]
36. Rafael, D.; Doktorovova, S.; Florindo, H.F.; Gener, P.; Abasolo, I.; Schwartz, S., Jr.; Videira, M.A. EMT blockage strategies: Targeting Akt dependent mechanisms for breast cancer metastatic behaviour modulation. *Curr. Gene Ther.* **2015**, *15*, 300–312. [CrossRef]
37. Wetzel, R.K.; Pascoa, J.L.; Arystarkhova, E. Stress-induced expression of the gamma subunit (FXYD2) modulates Na,K-ATPase activity and cell growth. *J. Biol. Chem.* **2004**, *279*, 41750–41757. [CrossRef]
38. Izumi, Y.; Yang, W.; Zhu, J.; Burg, M.B.; Ferraris, J.D. RNA-Seq analysis of high NaCl-induced gene expression. *Physiol. Genom.* **2015**, *47*, 500–513. [CrossRef]
39. Maeoka, Y.; Wu, Y.; Okamoto, T.; Kanemoto, S.; Guo, X.P.; Saito, A.; Asada, R.; Matsuhisa, K.; Masaki, T.; Imaizumi, K.; et al. NFAT5 up-regulates expression of the kidney-specific ubiquitin ligase gene Rnf183 under hypertonic conditions in inner-medullary collecting duct cells. *J. Biol. Chem.* **2019**, *294*, 101–115. [CrossRef]
40. Jeon, U.S.; Kim, J.A.; Sheen, M.R.; Kwon, H.M. How tonicity regulates genes: Story of TonEBP transcriptional activator. *Acta Physiol.* **2006**, *187*, 241–247. [CrossRef]
41. Burg, M.B.; Ferraris, J.D.; Dmitrieva, N.I. Cellular response to hyperosmotic stresses. *Physiol. Rev.* **2007**, *87*, 1441–1474. [CrossRef]
42. Tellechea, M.; Buxade, M.; Tejedor, S.; Aramburu, J.; Lopez-Rodriguez, C. NFAT5-Regulated Macrophage Polarization Supports the Proinflammatory Function of Macrophages and T Lymphocytes. *J. Immunol.* **2018**, *200*, 305–315. [CrossRef] [PubMed]
43. Boland, B.S.; Widjaja, C.E.; Banno, A.; Zhang, B.; Kim, S.H.; Stoven, S.; Peterson, M.R.; Jones, M.C.; Su, H.I.; Crowe, S.E.; et al. Immunodeficiency and autoimmune enterocolopathy linked to NFAT5 haploinsufficiency. *J. Immunol.* **2015**, *194*, 2551–2560. [CrossRef] [PubMed]

44. Lee, J.H.; Suh, J.H.; Choi, S.Y.; Kang, H.J.; Lee, H.H.; Ye, B.J.; Lee, G.R.; Jung, S.W.; Kim, C.J.; Lee-Kwon, W.; et al. Tonicity-responsive enhancer-binding protein promotes hepatocellular carcinogenesis, recurrence and metastasis. *Gut* **2019**, *68*, 347–358. [CrossRef] [PubMed]
45. Qin, X.; Wang, Y.; Li, J.; Xiao, Y.; Liu, Z. NFAT5 inhibits invasion and promotes apoptosis in hepatocellular carcinoma associated with osmolality. *Neoplasma* **2017**, *64*, 502–510. [CrossRef]
46. Kuper, C.; Beck, F.X.; Neuhofer, W. NFAT5-mediated expression of S100A4 contributes to proliferation and migration of renal carcinoma cells. *Front. Physiol.* **2014**, *5*, 293. [CrossRef]
47. Leisz, S.; Schulz, K.; Erb, S.; Oefner, P.; Dettmer, K.; Mougiakakos, D.; Wang, E.; Marincola, F.M.; Stehle, F.; Seliger, B. Distinct von Hippel-Lindau gene and hypoxia-regulated alterations in gene and protein expression patterns of renal cell carcinoma and their effects on metabolism. *Oncotarget* **2015**, *6*, 11395–11406. [CrossRef]
48. Rinschen, M.M.; Yu, M.J.; Wang, G.; Boja, E.S.; Hoffert, J.D.; Pisitkun, T.; Knepper, M.A. Quantitative phosphoproteomic analysis reveals vasopressin V2-receptor-dependent signaling pathways in renal collecting duct cells. *Proc. Natl. Acad. Sci. USA* **2010**, *107*, 3882–3887. [CrossRef]
49. Sanjana, N.E.; Shalem, O.; Zhang, F. Improved vectors and genome-wide libraries for CRISPR screening. *Nat. Methods* **2014**, *11*, 783–784. [CrossRef]
50. Ye, J.; Coulouris, G.; Zaretskaya, I.; Cutcutache, I.; Rozen, S.; Madden, T.L. Primer-BLAST: A tool to design target-specific primers for polymerase chain reaction. *BMC Bioinform.* **2012**, *13*, 134. [CrossRef]
51. Livak, K.J.; Schmittgen, T.D. Analysis of relative gene expression data using real-time quantitative PCR and the 2(-Delta Delta C(T)) Method. *Methods* **2001**, *25*, 402–408. [CrossRef]

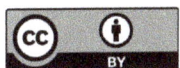

© 2020 by the authors. Licensee MDPI, Basel, Switzerland. This article is an open access article distributed under the terms and conditions of the Creative Commons Attribution (CC BY) license (http://creativecommons.org/licenses/by/4.0/).

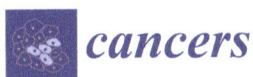

Article

Low Dosed Curcumin Combined with Visible Light Exposure Inhibits Renal Cell Carcinoma Metastatic Behavior in Vitros

Jochen Rutz [1,*], Sebastian Maxeiner [1], Saira Justin [1], Beatrice Bachmeier [2], August Bernd [3], Stefan Kippenberger [3], Nadja Zöller [3], Felix K.-H. Chun [1] and Roman A. Blaheta [1]

1. Department of Urology, Goethe-University, 60590 Frankfurt am Main, Germany; Sebastian.Maxeiner@kgu.de (S.M.); Justinsaira@hotmail.com (S.J.); Felix.Chun@kgu.de (F.K.-H.C.); Blaheta@em.uni-frankfurt.de (R.A.B.)
2. Institute of Laboratory Medicine, University Hospital, Ludwig-Maximilians-University, 80539 Munich, Germany; Beatrice.bachmeier@tum.de
3. Department of Dermatology, Venereology, and Allergology, Goethe-University, 60590 Frankfurt am Main, Germany; Bernd@em.uni-frankfurt.de (A.B.); Stefan.Kippenberger@kgu.de (S.K.); Nadja.Zoeller@kgu.de (N.Z.)
* Correspondence: jochen.rutz@kgu.de; Tel.: +49-69-6301-7109; Fax: +49-69-6301-7108

Received: 18 December 2019; Accepted: 25 January 2020; Published: 28 January 2020

Abstract: Recent documentation shows that a curcumin-induced growth arrest of renal cell carcinoma (RCC) cells can be amplified by visible light. This study was designed to investigate whether this strategy may also contribute to blocking metastatic progression of RCC. Low dosed curcumin (0.2 µg/mL; 0.54 µM) was applied to A498, Caki1, or KTCTL-26 cells for 1 h, followed by exposure to visible light for 5 min (400–550 nm, 5500 lx). Adhesion to human vascular endothelial cells or immobilized collagen was then evaluated. The influence of curcumin on chemotaxis and migration was also investigated, as well as curcumin induced alterations of α and β integrin expression. Curcumin without light exposure or light exposure without curcumin induced no alterations, whereas curcumin plus light significantly inhibited RCC adhesion, migration, and chemotaxis. This was associated with a distinct reduction of α3, α5, β1, and β3 integrins in all cell lines. Separate blocking of each of these integrin subtypes led to significant modification of tumor cell adhesion and chemotactic behavior. Combining low dosed curcumin with light considerably suppressed RCC binding activity and chemotactic movement and was associated with lowered integrin α and β subtypes. Therefore, curcumin combined with visible light holds promise for inhibiting metastatic processes in RCC.

Keywords: curcumin; renal cell cancer; tumor adhesion; tumor migration; integrins

1. Introduction

An estimated 18.1 million new patients worldwide were diagnosed with cancer in 2018, and of these, 9.6 million people died [1]. Characteristics of cancer are the loss of normal cell communication, unlimited cell growth, increased mobility, and the suppression of apoptosis [2]. Migration and motile spread are critical steps in tumor dissemination and progress. As with most tumors, metastasis plays an important role in renal cell carcinoma (RCC) and is the main cause of mortality [3]. Metastases infiltrate bones, lungs, lymph nodes, and less often brain and liver. At first diagnosis, one third of patients already suffer from lymph node and/or organ metastases [4] with another 20 to 30% developing metastases during therapy [5]. Without treatment, the probability of survival one year after diagnosis of metastasis is only about 50% [6], and the chances of recovery are poor. More than 5000 people died in Germany due to renal cell carcinoma in 2011 [7] and in a disseminated stage only palliative therapy can be provided. The incidence has been increasing in recent decades and has reached a constant level since the 1990s. The mortality is about 8/100,000 for men and 3/100,000 for women [8]. Targeted therapies have been introduced to improve the survival rate, but the prognosis for survival has hardly changed. Aspiring to active involvement, dissatisfaction with conventional medicine, and the hope to reduce unwanted side effects has made patients turn to complementary and alternative medicine (CAM). These approaches range from yoga to mind stimulating music to application of phytopharmacological agents. Up to 50% of cancer patients in Europe use CAM in addition to, or in place of, conventional medicine [9,10].

The natural compound curcumin (Figure 1) is a component of turmeric, a yellow-orange pigment harvested from the rhizomes of the plant Curcuma longa. Aside from its use as a spice in curry powder, anti-inflammatory, anti-oxidative, and anti-tumorigenic qualities have been demonstrated in vitro and in vivo [11–13], making it interesting for clinical application. Diverse biochemical processes and pathways associated with carcinogenesis are affected and modulated by curcumin [14]. In prostate, lung, breast, and colorectal cancers it has been shown [15] that curcumin affects growth and proliferation by inhibiting cell cycle progression, angiogenesis, and the expression of anti-apoptotic proteins [14,16,17].

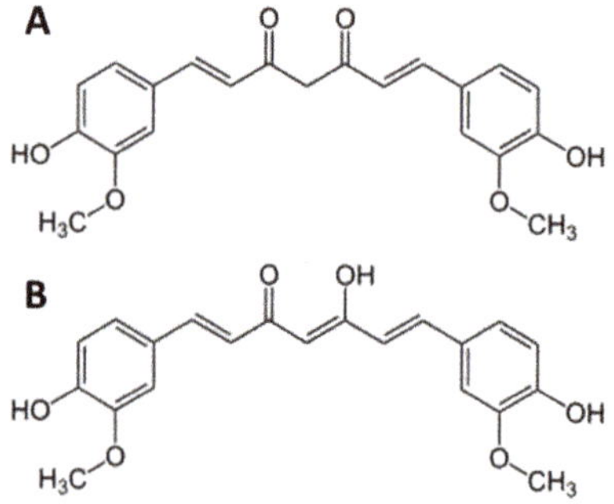

Figure 1. Chemical structure of curcumin ($C_{21}H_{20}O_6$), (**A**) shows keto and (**B**) enol form [18].

However, due to poor water solubility, low absorption, rapid metabolism and elimination, curcumin has low bioavailability, hampering its clinical use [19,20]. To improve bioavailability several approaches have been employed, such as wrapping lipophilic curcumin in liposomes, micelles, solid lipid nanoparticles, or polymer conjugates [21–23]. Likewise a range of analogues play a role in enhancing the bioavailability of curcumin [24]. Although some approaches have been successful, further improvement in bioavailability would be beneficial [22,25].

The present study continues a previous investigation on an RCC cell model demonstrating that exposing curcumin treated cells to visible light considerably enhances curcumin's potential to suppress tumor growth and proliferation [26]. Since metastasis, rather than that the growth of the primary tumor is the main cause of mortality, a therapeutic strategy blocking metastatic progression was investigated here. For this purpose, the influence of low dosed curcumin combined with visible light on adhesion and chemotaxis, as well as on intra- and extracellular integrin expression and signaling, was evaluated using a panel of three RCC cell lines.

2. Results

2.1. Curcumin Uptake

Curcumin uptake studies were carried out using 4 µg/mL curcumin instead of 0.2 µg/mL. This was necessary, since the fluorescence intensity of 0.2 µg/mL curcumin was too low to provide high quality images for confocal microscopy and optimum fluorescence detection by FACS analysis. Using 4 µg/mL, curcumin was rapidly incorporated into the cells following administration. In A498 cells, maximum fluorescence intensity was noted after 50 min, whereas a plateau phase was reached after 40 min in

Caki1 and already after 20 min in KTCTL-26 cells (Figure 2A). Confocal microscopy demonstrated homogenous cytoplasmic distribution of curcumin in all three cell lines with accumulation along the nuclear membrane (Figure 2B, solid arrows). Curcumin was also visualized within the nucleus (Figure 2B, dashed arrows).

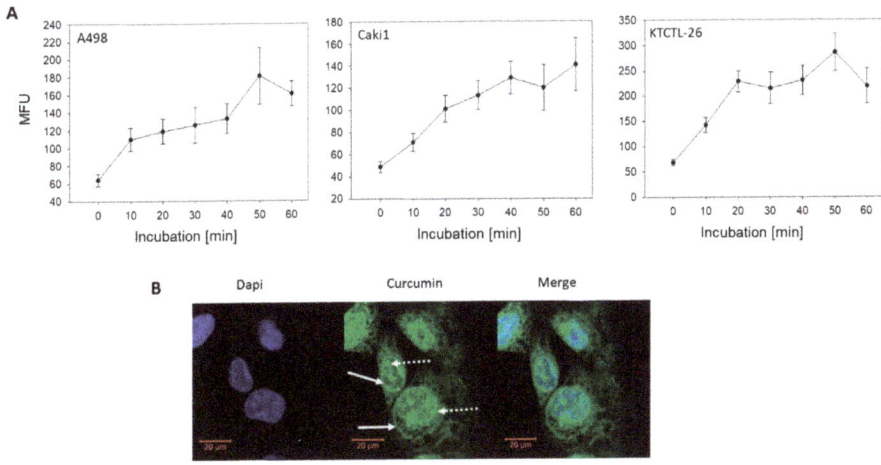

Figure 2. (**A**) Curcumin uptake in A498, Caki1, KTCTL-26 cells. Each value is the mean ± SD (standard deviation) of three independent experiments. (**B**) Intracellular distribution of curcumin (4 µg/mL) in A498 cells (representative for all three cell lines). Fluorescence shown by confocal laser-scanning microscopy after 60 min. Solid arrows: accumulation of curcumin along the nuclear membrane, dashed arrows: accumulation of curcumin within the nucleus. MFU = mean fluorescence units, DAPI = 4′,6-Diamidine-2′-phenylindole dihydrochloride.

2.2. Tumor Cell Adhesion and Binding Behavior

Adhesion of all three cell lines to HUVECs was blocked by combining 0.2 µg/mL curcumin with visible light (Figure 3A). The number of cells attached after 2 h (mean adhesion/mm^2, controls versus curcumin^{Light}) was: 62.8 ± 5.3 versus 20.6 ± 4.1 for A498; 40.6 ± 7.0 versus 9.2 ± 2.0 for Caki1; 40.6 ± 6.7 versus 14.4 ± 3.4 for KTCTL-26. Light exposure alone or curcumin alone had no more effect on adhesion than the addition of cell medium as a control. A similar response was seen in the binding behavior to immobilized collagen. Neither curcumin nor light exposure alone led to significant alterations of A498, Caki1, or KTCTL-26 cell binding, compared to the untreated controls. Combined use of curcumin and light was associated with a distinct attenuation in the tumor cell attachment rate, with maximum effects exerted on Caki1 cells (17.8 ± 6.0%, compared to the 100% control; Figure 3B).

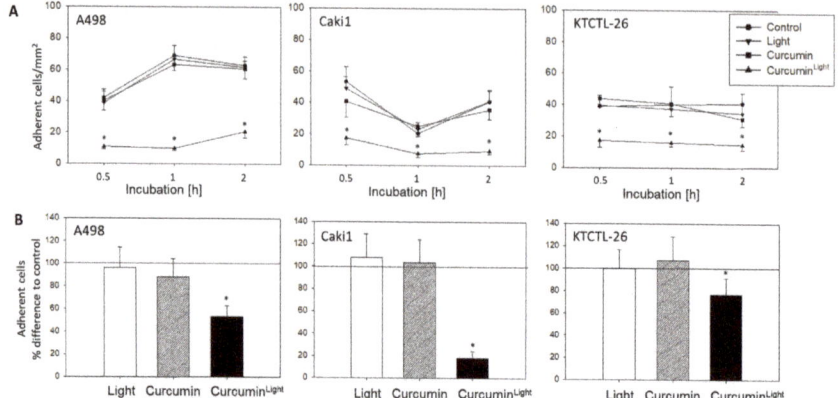

Figure 3. Influence of curcumin (0.2 µg/mL), light, or curcumin[Light] on adhesion of RCC cells to HUVECs (**A**) and (**B**) collagen. Five separate fields of 0.25 mm^2 were counted at 200× magnification (means ± SD, $n = 6$). Control was added cell medium and is indicated by the line at 100% in (**B**). * indicates significant difference to controls ($p = 0.00512$).

2.3. Chemotaxis and Migration

Figure 4A shows that neither treatment with light nor cultivation of the tumor cells with curcumin influenced chemotactic movement towards a serum gradient. A distinct down-regulation of chemotaxis was induced when the tumor cells were exposed to low-dosed curcumin with light. This response became evident in all three cell culture systems with the order KTCTL-26 (12.7 ± 3.6%) > Caki1 (20.9 ± 5.0%) > A498 (47.6 ± 9.6%), each compared to the 100% control; Figure 4A.

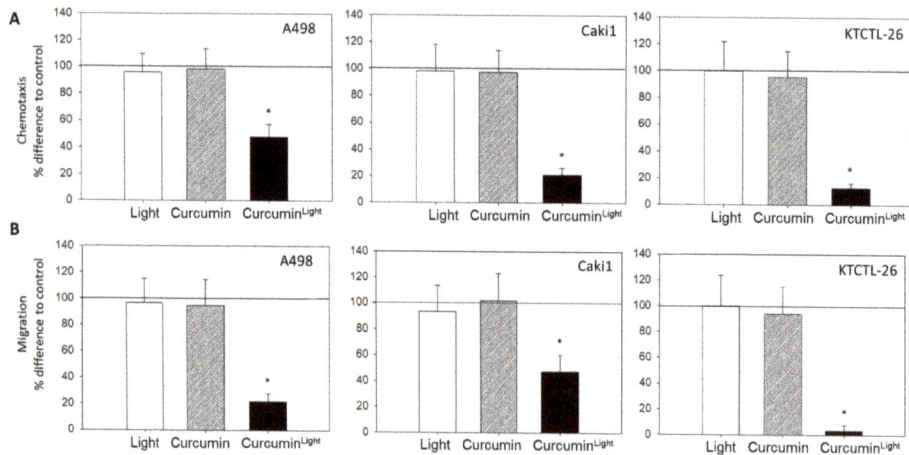

Figure 4. Influence of curcumin (0.2 µg/mL), light, or curcumin[Light] on chemotaxis towards a serum gradient (**A**) and migration through a collagen matrix (**B**). Endpoints after 24 h. Untreated control cells were set to 100%, indicated by a line drawn at 100%. 5 separate fields of 0.25 mm^2 were counted at 200× magnification (means ± SD, $n = 6$). * indicates significant difference to controls ($p = 0.00512$).

Tumor cell migration through a collagen matrix towards a serum gradient was also evaluated. Curcumin or light alone did not alter the trans-migration rate, whereas curcumin[Light] did (Figure 4B).

Migration was nearly completely abrogated in KTCTL-26 cells (3.4 ± 4.2%, compared to the 100% control).

2.4. FACS Analysis of Iintegrin Surface Expression

Different integrin expression patterns were apparent for the different tumor cell lines. In A498 cells, the integrin subtypes α3, β1, and β3 were expressed to the highest extent at the cell surface. Distinct fluorescence intensity was also recorded for α1 and α5. The subtypes α2, α4, and α6 were detected moderately, whereas β4 was not expressed at all (Figure 5).

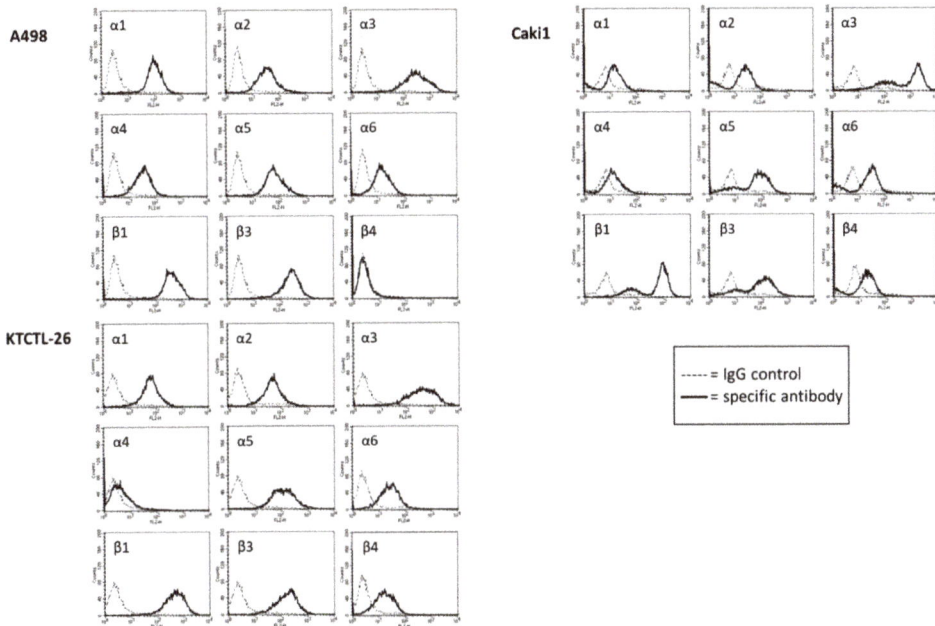

Figure 5. Surface expression of α and β integrins on A498, Caki1, and KTCTL-26 cells. Measured by Figure 1. PE, IgG2a-PE and IgG2b-PE (dashed line). The abscissa shows the relative logarithmic distribution of the relative fluorescence intensity of α1-α6 and β1, β3, and β4. The ordinate shows cell number. 10,000 cells were counted. Figure is representative for $n = 6$.

Caki1 cells were characterized by a very strong expression of α3 and β1, and a strong expression of α5 and β3. α2 and α6, as well as β4, were also present at the surface membrane. α1 and α4 were only marginally detectable (Figure 5).

Similar to Caki1, α3 and β1 were also expressed to the highest extent on KTCTL-26 cells. α5 and β3 were distinctly detectable. α1, α2, α6, and β4 were also detectable (Figure 5). α4 was barely detectable.

The integrin expression level was not modulated by curcumin or light, when applied separately, but significant alterations were evoked by curcumin^{Light}. The surface expression of α3, α5, β1, and β3 was diminished in all three tumor cell lines (A498: α3: −14.0 ± 1.3%, α5: −57.1 ± 3.7%, β1: −23.8 ± 1.5%, β3: −56.7 ± 4.4%; Caki1: α3: −15.9 ± 0.8%, α5: −18.0 ± 1.2%, β1: −37.3 ± 2.7%, β3: −20.4 ± 1.5%; KTCTL-26: α3: −41.1 ± 3.7%, α5: −40.2 ± 2.0%, β1: −45.8 ± 4.0%, β3: −25.6 ± 3.2%; each compared to the 100% control), while α1 was suppressed in A498 (−48.7 ± 2.4%) and KTCTL-26 cells (−37.0 ± 2.2%). α2 (−22.1 ± 1.8%) and α6 (−29.1 ± 1.8%) were exclusively down-regulated on KTCTL-26 (Figure 6). The influence of curcumin and/or light on α4 and β4 was not evaluated, since α4 was not expressed on all cell lines and β4 was not expressed on A498 and only slightly expressed on Caki1 and KTCTL-26 cells.

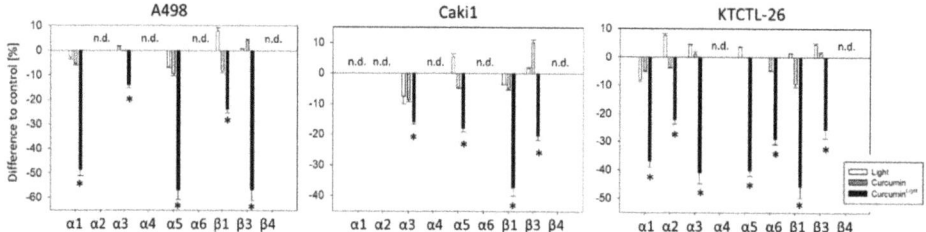

Figure 6. Influence of curcumin (0.2 µg/mL), light, or curcumin^{Light} on the integrin expression profile of A498, Caki1, and KTCTL-26 cells. The untreated control is set to 0% (line drawn at 0%). Values are means ± SD, $n = 6$. * indicates significant difference to controls ($p = 0.00512$). n.d. = not or hardly detectable.

2.5. Western Blot Analysis

Figure 7 illustrates changes in the integrin protein content including ILK, FAK, and pFAK after exposure to curcumin, light, or curcumin^{Light} (whole blots are shown in Figure S1). Figure 8 shows the respective pixel density data (pixel density and p-values are shown in Figure S2). Exposing the tumor cells to visible light did not lead to distinct protein modifications, excepting α2 and β1, both of which were up-regulated in KTCTL-26 cells, and pFAK which was diminished in KTCTL-26 and elevated in A498 cells, compared to the untreated controls. Curcumin alone also had no specific effect on protein expression, excepting β3, which was up-regulated in Caki1 cells, and α5, which was enhanced in KTCTL-26 cells. In contrast, a strong response became evident when the tumor cell lines were treated with curcumin^{Light}. Here, compared to the controls, exposure to light alone or treatment with curcumin alone, the following proteins were reduced: A498-α1, -β1, -β3; Caki1-α5, -β1; KTCTL-26-α1, -α2, -β1, -β3. ILK, FAK, and pFAK were suppressed in all cell lines when exposed to curcumin^{Light}.

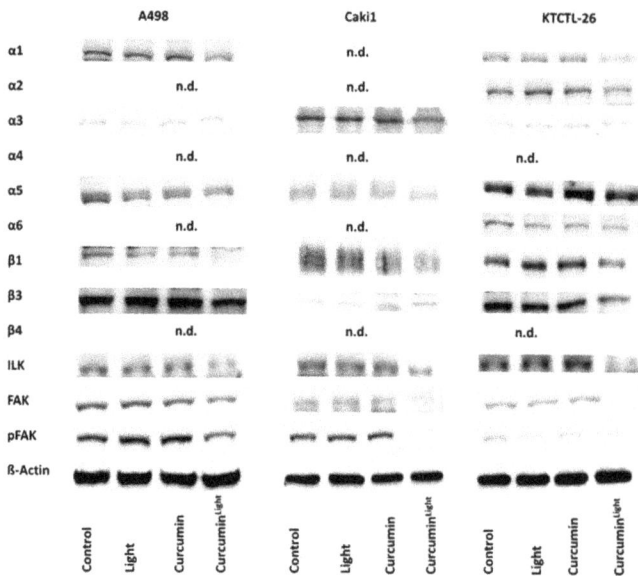

Figure 7. Western blot of α and β integrins, ILK and pFAK depending on the influence of curcumin (0.2 µg/mL), light, and curcumin^{Light} on A498, Caki1, and KTCTL-26 cells. Protein levels were measured 24 h after respective treatments. All bands are representative of $n = 3$. β-actin served as loading control and is representatively shown once. 50 µg were used per sample. n.d. = not detectable.

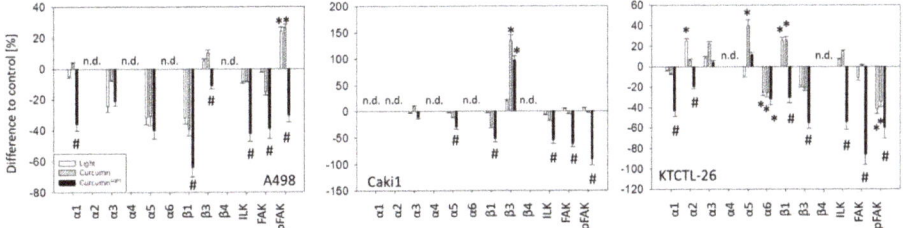

Figure 8. Pixel density of Western blot of α and β integrins, ILK and pFAK, depending on the influence of curcumin (0.2 µg/mL), light, or curcumin[Light] on A498, Caki1, and KTCTL-26 cells. Values are means ± SD, $n = 3$. * indicates significant difference to the untreated control (line drawn at 0%) and # indicates significant difference to light alone or curcumin alone. n.d. = not detectable.

2.6. Integrin Blockage

The FACS analysis demonstrated that curcumin[Light] induces the loss of α3, α5, β1, and β3 in all tumor cell lines. Therefore, the surface expression of α3, α5, β1, and β3 was blocked to evaluate the physiological and pathological relevance of these integrin subtypes on adhesion (Figure 9A) and chemotaxis (Figure 9B).

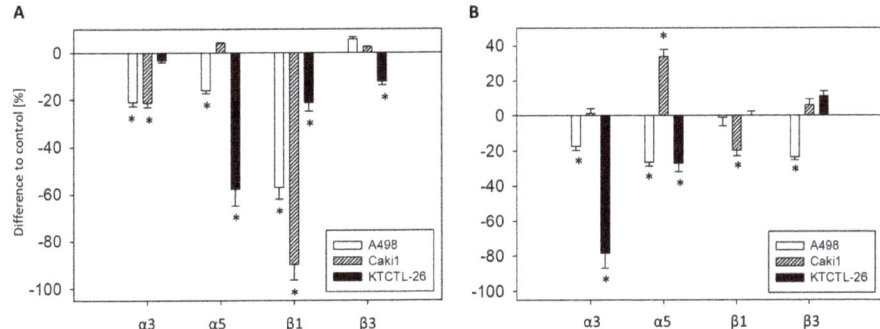

Figure 9. Adhesion to collagen (**A**) and chemotaxis (**B**) of A498, Caki1, and KTCTL-26 cells after blockade of integrins α3, α5, β1, or β3. The untreated control is set to 0% (line drawn at 0%). 5 separate fields of 0.25 mm² were counted at 200× magnification (means ± SD, $n = 6$). * indicates significant difference to controls ($p = 0.00512$).

Blocking integrin α3 was associated with reduced A498 and Caki1 adhesion (A498: −20.9 ± 1.9%; Caki1: −21.2 ± 2.0%) and diminished A498 and KTCTL-26 chemotaxis (A498: −17.5 ± 2.3%; KTCTL-26: −78.3 ± 8.6%). Blocking α5 down-regulated A498 and KTCTL-26 adhesion (A498: −16.0 ± 1.3%; KTCTL-26: −57.6 ± 7.3%) and chemotaxis (A498: −26.4 ± 2.4%; KTCTL-26: −27.0 ± 5.0%), whereas chemotaxis of Caki1 was enhanced (+33.7 ± 4.1%). Surface blocking of β1 suppressed adhesion of all cell lines in the order Caki1 (−89.7 ± 6.7%) > A498 (−57.1 ± 1.0%) > KTCTL-26 (−21.3 ± 3.6%), and diminished Caki1 chemotaxis (−19.7 ± 3.3%). β3 blockade down-regulated KTCTL-26 adhesion (−12.3 ± 1.0%) and A498 chemotaxis (−23.5 ± 1.9%).

3. Discussion

Exposing RCC cells to visible light significantly enhanced curcumin's potential to block adhesion and migration. While low dosed curcumin alone induced no alterations in tumor-endothelial or tumor-matrix interaction, the combination of curcumin plus light did. Photodynamic properties of curcumin are well documented, though the mechanistic background is not fully understood. In general, irradiation of a photodynamic molecule with a particular wavelength shifts electrons to higher energy orbitals. This singlet state is unstable, and the electrons return to their ground state by emitting light or heat. However, changes in electron spin can also shift a photodynamic molecule to the triplet state, which then triggers two reactions. The Type 1 reaction produces free radicals and, due to an interaction with oxygen, reactive oxygen species (ROS). The Type 2 reaction results in singlet oxygen that can interact with specific intracellular molecules [27]. Whether this mechanism also holds true for curcumin is not yet clear. Laubach et al. assumed a shift in the cellular redox balance by boosting H_2O_2 generation [28]. Bruzell et al. speculated that curcumin may photo-generate reduced forms of molecular oxygen [29]. In our own pilot experiments, treating curcumin with light prior to application did not enhance the anti-tumor effect of curcumin, compared to the application of curcumin without light. In line with this, intra-peritoneal injections of curcumin with or without light induced the same effect on nerve injury repair in a mouse model [30]. The phenomenon could be attributed to the unstable excitation state of irradiated curcumin with a very short half-life, although other mechanisms cannot be excluded. Bernd has suggested that a light-dependent energy transfer via curcumin may enhance the influence of this compound on tumor relevant protein functions [18]. Niu et al. assumed photo-activation to be an essential amplification factor when taking advantage of curcumin at low concentrations [31].

Low-dosed curcumin (0.2 µg/mL) combined with light profoundly blocked RCC cell adhesion to HUVEC, while even 5 µM of free curcumin without light could not alter the binding of prostate cancer cells to HUVEC [32]. In the present study, since the number of attached RCC cells was maximally reduced after 30 min, with no further diminishment at 1 or 2 h, curcumin^{Light} seems to exert its effect in the initial attachment phase. A strong benefit of adding light to a low curcumin concentration (0.2 µg/mL) was also evident in the tumor cell-matrix attachment, where curcumin^{Light} (but not curcumin alone) down-regulated the binding of all cell lines to immobilized collagen. Herman et al. have demonstrated adhesion blocking effects of curcumin on prostate cancer cells [33] and others have demonstrated that curcumin suppresses binding of esophageal [34], skin [35], or breast cancer [36] to extracellular matrix proteins. In all cases, high concentrations of 5–50 µM curcumin were necessary to exert therapeutic efficacy. Until now, the relevance of curcumin to RCC adhesive processes had not been documented.

The benefit of visual light on curcumin's bioavailability was also seen in regard to chemotaxis and migration. 0.2 µg/mL curcumin^{Light}, but not 0.2 µg/mL curcumin alone, profoundly reduced motile crawling of all three RCC cell lines. The invasion blocking effect of curcumin is important, since once metastasized, cancer is difficult to treat, and the extent of metastasis rather than the primary cancer determines survival. Therefore, application of curcumin^{Light} might be an innovative concept to accompany established RCC treatment protocols. The relevance of curcumin alone to act on tumor cell invasion has already been shown on other tumor entities, whereby curcumin concentrations of 10 µM, 15 µM, 50 µM, or higher have been applied to stop invasion of gastric [37], breast [38], prostate [39], or hepatic cancer cells [40]. Ongoing experiments should, therefore, deal with the question of whether the beneficial effects of light exposure on curcumin may also hold true for these tumor types.

When interpreting the influence of curcumin^{Light} on adhesion and chemotaxis, it is notable that curcumin^{Light} considerably blocked adhesion of Caki1, whereas KTCTL-26 adhesion was only slightly suppressed. In contrast, migration properties of KTCTL-26 were suppressed to a maximum, migration of Caki1 was suppressed moderately. Due to these differences, lowered migration does not seem to exclusively be just a consequence of a reduced attachment rate. Rather, curcumin^{Light} is involved in both the regulation of the mechanical tumor cell-matrix contact and modulation of cytoskeletal structures. Indeed, curcumin has been shown in tumor cell models to disorganize the architecture of actin microfilaments, leading to destabilization and a decrease in F-actin polymerization [41,42]. Dhar et al. assumed an allosteric effect in which curcumin binding at the "barbed end" of actin is transmitted to the "pointed end," where conformational changes disrupt interactions with the adjacent actin monomer to interrupt filament formation [43]. There is also evidence that curcumin stops the physical interaction of cortactin with p120 catenin, which then may inhibit migration [44].

Beyond intracellular components, membrane proteins expressed on the cell surface are also relevant for controlling cell movement. Alterations of the integrin α- and β-expression pattern have been closely associated with altered metastatic activity [45]. Therefore, integrins are considered to be highly relevant treatment targets [46]. The data presented here point to distinct changes of particular integrin subtypes in the presence of curcumin^{Light}, but not in the presence of curcumin alone. Of all integrin members evaluated, surface expression of four subtypes were modified in the same manner in all cell lines; α3, α5, β1, β3 were all down-regulated by curcumin^{Light}. Since the intracellular α3 protein content was neither reduced in Caki1, nor in KTCTL-26 and A498 cells, α3 might be shed from the surface without intracellular alteration. Shedding may also be relevant for α5 (KTCTL-26) and β1 (KTCTL-26). It is hypothesized that the β3 protein increase in Caki1 is caused by curcumin^{Light} inducing a translocation from the cell surface to the cytoplasm.

The relevance of integrins in tumor progression is not completely understood. Integrin α3 is thought to be closely associated with the capacity of RCC for local and distant spread [47]. The same attribute has been linked to integrin β3 [48], and based on clinical specimens from tumor patients, α3 as well as β3 have been proposed as potential prognostic markers [49,50]. Evidence indicates that the integrin subtype α5 correlates with poor survival [51]. In fact, α5 is the most highly expressed integrin in RCC tissue, compared with adjacent normal renal tissue, and knocking down α5 has been shown to significantly reduce cell migration [52].

Integrin β1 also plays an important role in the development of RCC tumors and advanced RCC with metastasis [53], the observation of which has led to the development of volociximab, an anti-α5β1 integrin monoclonal antibody [54]. The suppressive effect of low dosed curcumin plus light on the integrins α3, α5, β1, and β3 on RCC adhesion, chemotaxis, and migration could (at least in part) be attributed to inhibition of these integrins, which when blocked were shown to inhibit RCC binding and spreading. The inhibition of adhesion or chemotaxis depended on the cell line. β1, which was strongly reduced on Caki1 cells by curcumin^{Light}, was also prominently involved in regulating adhesion in this cell line. The integrin α5 subtype, the major regulator of KTCTL-26 adhesion, was also considerably suppressed by curcumin^{Light} in KTCTL-26 cells. α3 integrin served as a dominant element in reducing KTCTL-26 chemotaxis. The same integrin was also considerably suppressed by curcumin^{Light}. These data could indicate that metastatic tumor progression is controlled by different integrin members, depending on the tumor differentiation status, and that these specific integrins act as main targets for curcumin^{Light}. This is, however, speculative. A498 chemotaxis depended equally well on α3, α5, and β3. It must also be considered that quantitative alteration of the integrin surface expression, but not activity, was evaluated. Whether integrin loss is associated with a similar loss of activity cannot be judged.

Suppressed integrin α3 was associated with inhibited adhesion in A498 and Caki1 cells but not in KTCTL-26 cells. Chemotaxis was inhibited in A498 and KTCTL-26, but not in Caki1 cells. Suppression of β3 exclusively prevented A498 adhesion and KTCTL-26 chemotaxis. Blockade of α5 coupled to an increased chemotaxis rate of Caki1 is paradox and difficult to explain, since curcumin^{Light} evoked α5 inhibition would be expected to contribute to increased motile behavior, which was not the case. Rather, chemotaxis of Caki1 was considerably blocked by curcumin^{Light}. The extent to which α5 was diminished in Caki1 by curcumin^{Light} was only −20%, compared to an α5 reduction in A498 (−60%) and KTCTL-26 cells (−40%). Speculatively, the moderate alteration of Caki1's α5 surface level by curcumin^{Light} is of minor relevance for adhesion and migration. Counter regulation should be considered, and this α5 behavior in Caki1 may point to resistance induction.

Aside from the paradoxical role of α5 in Caki1 cells, curcumin^{Light} is shown here to act on a set of integrin receptors which, in combination, profoundly blocks metastatic progression in vitro. This indicates that the complex process of metastasis is not controlled by only one particular integrin subtype. Rather, several integrins seem to be regulatory elements driving the invasion cascade forward.

Consequently, blocking a set of relevant integrin members, as curcumin^{Light} did, might be more effective than blocking just a single integrin.

The therapeutic potential of curcumin is also reflected by its deactivation of FAK. FAK serves as a prominent linker molecule, connecting integrin related signaling with pro-mitogenic and pro-migratory pathways including the Ras-ERK and PI3K/AKT pathway [55]. Performing a mass spectrometry-based system-wide survey of tyrosine phosphorylation in clear cell and papillary RCC human tumors, distinct FAK phosphorylation has been found in all tumors [56]. FAK may also mediate resistance towards the tyrosine kinase inhibitor sorafenib in RCC patients [57]. This opens the possibility that light exposure to curcumin treated RCC cells might not only be an innovative strategy to fight metastatic progression but also to enhance or prolong the response towards a tyrosine kinase inhibitor-based regimen. Curcumin combined with sorafenib or sunitinib has already been demonstrated to synergistically inhibit cancer growth and metastasis in vitro and in vivo [58,59].

The technical aspect of curcumin–light application has been addressed. Introducing an optical fiber into RCC tumors in mice with subsequent laser illumination of the vascular-acting photosensitizer WST11 at 750 nm or multispectrally at 700–800 nm has been shown to induce significant necrosis in RCC tissue [60]. Kroeze et al. have suggested using the photosensitizer mTHPC (meso-tetra(hydroxyphenyl)chlorin), which targets both vasculature and tissue and, therefore, may produce a strong combined effect [61]. Exposing the tumor bed to light after tumor resection and curcumin administration has also been discussed in regard to eliminating invisible micro-metastases [62].

4. Materials and Methods

4.1. Cell Culture

Renal carcinoma Caki1 and KTCTL-26 cell lines, both derived from a clear cell renal cell carcinoma and von Hippel-Lindau (VHL) positive, were purchased from LGC Promochem (Wesel, Germany). A498 cells with disrupted VHL function were derived from Cell Lines Service (Heidelberg, Germany). The tumor cells were grown and subcultured in RPMI 1640 medium supplemented with 10% fetal calf serum (FCS), 1% Glutamax (all Gibco/Invitrogen, Karlsruhe, Germany), 2% HEPES (2-(4-(2-Hydroxyethyl)-1-piperazinyl)-ethansulfonsäure) buffer and 1% penicillin/streptomycin (both Sigma-Aldrich, München, Germany), at 37 °C in a humidified 5% CO_2 incubator. Subcultures from passages 5–30 were selected for experimental use.

Human umbilical vein endothelial cells (HUVEC), isolated from human umbilical veins, were grown in Medium 199 (M199; Biozol, Munich, Germany), 10% FCS, 10% pooled human serum, 20 µg/mL endothelial cell growth factor (Boehringer, Mannheim, Germany), 0.1% heparin, 100 ng/mL gentamycin and 20 mM HEPES-buffer. Subcultures from passages 2 to 6 were selected for experimental use.

4.2. Drug Dosage and Light Exposure

Curcumin (Biomol, Hamburg, Germany) was stored at −20 °C and diluted prior to use in cell culture medium to a final concentration of 0.2 µg/mL (0.54 µM). 4 µg/mL curcumin was used to provide high quality images for confocal microscopy and optimum fluorescence detection by FACS analysis. Cells were treated with curcumin for 1 h and then exposed to visible light for 5 min with 5500 lx (curcumin^{Light}; 10 × 40 W lamps, distance 45 cm, emission spectrum: 400–550 nm) using a Waldmann UV 801AL system (Waldmann, Villingen-Schwenningen, Germany) [18]. To prevent bias effects by the phenol red containing RPMI 1640 based cell culture medium, tumor cells were transferred to phenol red free PBS (phosphate-buffered saline) (Sigma-Aldrich) during light exposure. Thereafter, PBS was replaced by RPMI 1640 and supplements. Control cell cultures received PBS for 5 min without light exposure. To evaluate the effects of low dosed curcumin and light alone, two respective additional controls were employed; tumor cells exposed to light but not to curcumin, and tumor cells exposed to curcumin but no light. Following light exposure (including all controls), tumor cells were allowed to recover in complete cell culture medium for 24 h before starting adhesion and migration experiments.

4.3. Cellular Curcumin Uptake

5×10^4 RCC cells were plated on 6-well multiplates (Sarstedt, Nümbrecht, Germany) and, when grown to sub-confluency, incubated with 4 µg/mL curcumin for different time periods ranging from 10 to 60 min at 37 °C. Thereafter, the tumor cells were detached, washed three times with PBS (Ca^{2+} and Mg^{2+}) and subsequently added to FACS-buffer (PBS + 0.5% bovine serum albumin, BSA) at 0.5×10^5 cells/mL. Fluorescence intensity (mean fluorescence units, MFU) of curcumin exposed versus non-exposed cells was then measured by a FACS Canto (BD Biosciences, Heidelberg, Germany) at an absorption of 485 nm and emission of 514 nm.

4.4. Intracellular Distribution of Curcumin

To evaluate intracellular localization of curcumin, tumor cells were incubated with 4 µg/mL curcumin for 60 min, washed with PBS, fixed in cold (−20 °C) methanol/acetone (50/50 v/v) and then washed with blocking buffer (0.5% BSA in PBS). To prevent photobleaching of curcumin, tumor cells were embedded in Vectashield mounting medium including DAPI (Biozol, Munich, Germany), and viewed using a confocal laser scanning microscope (Zeiss, Oberkochen, Germany, equipped with Zen imaging software) with a plan-neofluar × 63/1.3 oil immersion objective.

4.5. Tumor Cell Endothelial Cell Interaction

To evaluate tumor cell adhesion, HUVEC were transferred to 6-well multiplates in complete HUVEC medium. Once the cells had reached confluence, A498, Caki-1, or KTCTL-26 cells were detached from the culture flasks by accutase treatment (PAA Laboratories, Cölbe, Germany), and 0.5×10^6 cells were added to the HUVEC monolayer. After 0.5, 1, or 2 h, non-adherent tumor cells were washed off using warmed (37 °C) PBS+ (Ca^{2+} and Mg^{2+}). The remaining cells were fixed with 1% glutaraldehyde. Adherent tumor cells were then counted in five different observation fields of a defined size (5×0.25 mm^2) using a phase contrast microscope and the mean cellular adhesion rate was calculated.

4.6. Attachment to Immobilized Collagen

Six-well plates were coated with collagen G (extracted from calfskin, consisting of 90% collagen type I and 10% collagen type III; Biochrom, Berlin, Germany; diluted to 400 µg/mL in PBS) overnight at 4 °C. Plastic dishes served as background control. Subsequently, plates were incubated for one h with 1% BSA in PBS to block nonspecific cell adhesion. 0.5×10^6 tumor cells were then added to each well and allowed to attach for 60 min at 37 °C. Subsequently, non-adherent tumor cells were washed off, the remaining adherent cells were fixed with 1% glutaraldehyde and counted microscopically. The mean cellular adhesion rate, defined by adherent cells$_{coated\ well}$ - adherent cells$_{background}$, was calculated from five different observation fields (5×0.25 mm^2).

4.7. Chemotaxis and Migration

Serum induced chemotactic movement was examined using 6-well Transwell chambers (Greiner, Frickenhausen, Germany) with 8 µm pores. 0.5×10^6 A498, Caki1, or KTCTL-26 cells/mL were placed in the upper chamber in serum-free medium. The lower chamber contained 10% serum. To evaluate cell migration, Transwell chambers were pre-coated with collagen (400 µg/mL) and tumor cells then added. After 24 h incubation, the upper surface of the Transwell membrane was gently wiped with a cotton swab to remove cells that had not migrated. Cells that had moved to the lower surface of the membrane were stained using hematoxylin and counted microscopically. The mean chemotaxis and migration rate were then calculated from five different observation fields (5×0.25 mm^2).

4.8. Integrin Surface Expression

Tumor cells were washed in blocking solution (PBS, 0.5% BSA) and then incubated for 60 min at 4 °C with phycoerythrin (PE)-conjugated monoclonal antibodies directed against the following integrin subtypes: anti-α1 (mouse IgG1; clone SR84; #559596), anti-α2 (mouse IgG2a; clone 12F1-H6; #555669), anti-α3 (mouse IgG1; clone C3II.1; #556025), anti-α4 (mouse IgG1; clone 9F10; #555503), anti-α5 (mouse IgG1; clone IIA1; #555617), anti-α6 (mouse IgG2a; clone GoH3; #555736), anti-β1 (mouse IgG1; clone MAR4; #555443), anti-β3 (mouse IgG1; clone VI-PL2; #555754) or anti-β4 (rat IgG2b; clone 439-9B; #555720) (all from BD Pharmingen, Heidelberg, Germany). Integrin expression of tumor cells was then measured using a FACScan (BD Biosciences; FL-2H (log) channel histogram analysis; 1×10^4 cells/scan) and expressed as mean fluorescence units (MFU). Mouse IgG1-PE (MOPC-21; #555749), IgG2a-PE (G155-178; #555574), and rat IgG2b-PE (R35-38; #555848; all from BD Biosciences) were used as isotype controls.

4.9. Western Blotting

To investigate integrin content, tumor cell lysates were applied to a 7–12% polyacrylamide gel (depending on the protein size) and electrophoresed for about 90 min at 100 V. The protein was then transferred to nitrocellulose membranes. After blocking with non-fat dry milk for 1 h, the membranes were incubated overnight with the following antibodies: integrin α1 (rabbit, polyclonal, 1:1,000; #AB1934; Chemicon/Millipore GmbH, Schwalbach, Germany), integrin α2 (mouse IgG1, 1:250, clone 2; #611017; BD Biosciences), integrin α3 (rabbit, polyclonal, 1:1000; #AB1920; Chemicon/Millipore GmbH), integrin α4 (mouse, 1:200, clone: C-20; #sc-6589; Santa Cruz Biotechnology, Inc., Santa Cruz, CA, USA), integrin α5 (mouse IgG2a, 1:5000, clone 1; #610634; BD Biosciences), integrin α6 (rabbit, 1:200, clone H-87; #sc-10730; Santa Cruz Biotechnology, Inc.,), and integrin β1 (mouse IgG1, 1:2500, clone 18; #610468), integrin β3 (mouse IgG1, 1:2500, clone 1; #611141) and integrin β4 (mouse IgG1, 1:250, clone 7; #611233) (all from BD Biosciences). HRP-conjugated goat anti-mouse IgG and HRP-conjugated goat anti-rabbit IgG (both 1:5000; Upstate Biotechnology, Lake Placid, NY, USA) served as secondary antibodies. Additionally, integrin-related signaling was explored by anti-integrin-linked kinase (ILK) (clone 3, dilution 1:1000; #611803), anti-focal adhesion kinase (FAK) (clone 77, dilution 1:1000; #610088), and anti-p-specific FAK (pY397; clone 18, dilution 1:1000; #611807) antibodies (all from BD Biosciences). HRP-conjugated goat-anti-mouse IgG (dilution 1:5000; Upstate Biotechnology) served as the secondary antibody. The membranes were briefly incubated with ECL detection reagent (ECL™; Amersham, GE Healthcare, München, Germany) to visualize the proteins and then analyzed with the Fusion FX7 system (Peqlab, Erlangen, Germany). β-actin (1:1000; Sigma-Aldrich) served as the internal control.

Gimp 2.8 software was used to perform pixel density analysis of the protein bands. The ratio of protein intensity/β-actin intensity was calculated and expressed as percentage difference, related to controls set to 100%.

4.10. Blocking Experiments

To determine whether the integrins α3, α5, β1, and β3 impact metastatic spread, A498, Caki-1, or KTCTL-26 cells were incubated for 60 min with 10 µg/mL function-blocking anti-integrin α3 (clone P1B5), anti-integrin α5 (clone P1D6), anti-integrin β1 (clone 6S6), or anti-integrin β3 (clone B3A) mouse mAb (all from Millipore). Controls were incubated with cell culture medium alone. Subsequently, tumor cell adhesion to immobilized collagen, as well as chemotaxis, was evaluated as described above.

4.11. Statistics

Curcumin uptake, adhesion, chemotaxis, and migration experiments were performed six times, and statistical significance was determined with the Wilcoxon–Mann-Whitney-U-test. Western bloting was done three times and statistics evaluated by t-test. Values are means ± SD. Differences were considered statistically significant at a p-value less than 0.05.

5. Conclusions

Since it is technically feasible to apply visible light during tumor resection, combining curcumin application with visible light could enhance the RCC treatment protocol, and compensate for the low bioavailability and rapid degradation of curcumin. The data presented here indicate a curcumin uptake within 1 h. This time window should be considered during surgery, e.g., by infusing curcumin 1 h prior to light application in future RCC in vivo models.

Supplementary Materials: The following are available online at http://www.mdpi.com/2072-6694/12/2/302/s1, Figure S1: Whole western blots for Figure 7, Figure S2: Pixel density values for Figure 8.

Author Contributions: Conceptualization, A.B. and R.A.B.; Investigation, J.R., S.J., S.M., S.K., and N.Z.; Methodology, S.K. and R.A.B.; Project administration, R.A.B.; Supervision, F.K.-H.C., A.B., and R.A.B.; Visualization, J.R., S.K., F.K.-H.C., and R.A.B.; Writing – original draft, J.R. and R.A.B.; Writing – review and editing, B.B., A.B., F.K.-H.C., and R.A.B. All authors have read and agreed to the published version of the manuscript.

Funding: This work was supported by the Brigitta & Norbert Muth Stiftung, Wiesbaden, Germany, the Friedrich-Spicker-Stiftung, Wuppertal, Germany, and a Wolfgang Lutzeyer grant of the Deutsche Gesellschaft für Urologie (German Society of Urology), grant ID RuJ1/WL-18.

Acknowledgments: The authors would like to thank Karen Nelson for language editing and proofreading.

Conflicts of Interest: The authors declare no conflict of interest.

References

1. Bray, F.; Ferlay, J.; Soerjomataram, I.; Siegel, R.L.; Torre, L.A.; Jemal, A. Global cancer statistics 2018: GLOBOCAN estimates of incidence and mortality worldwide for 36 cancers in 185 countries. *CA Cancer J. Clin.* **2018**, *68*, 394–424. [CrossRef]
2. Wang, D.-L.; Lan, J.-H.; Chen, L.; Huang, B.; Li, Z.; Zhao, X.-M.; Ma, Q.; Sheng, X.; Li, W.-B.; Tang, W.-X. Integrin-linked Kinase Functions as a Tumor Promoter in Bladder Transitional Cell Carcinoma. *Asian Pac. J. Cancer Prev.* **2012**, *13*, 2799–2806. [CrossRef]
3. Van Zijl, F.; Krupitza, G.; Mikulits, W. Initial steps of metastasis: Cell invasion and endothelial transmigration. *Mutat. Res.* **2011**, *728*, 23–34. [CrossRef]
4. Deutsche Krebshilfe, Deutschland. *Die blauen Ratgeber: Nierenkrebs. Antworten. Hilfen. Perspektiven*; Deutsche Krebshilfe, Deutschland: Bonn, Germany, 2014.
5. Kroeger, N.; Choueiri, T.K.; Lee, J.-L.; Bjarnason, G.A.; Knox, J.J.; MacKenzie, M.J.; Wood, L.; Srinivas, S.; Vaishamayan, U.N.; Rha, S.-Y.; et al. Survival outcome and treatment response of patients with late relapse from renal cell carcinoma in the era of targeted therapy. *Eur. Urol.* **2014**, *65*, 1086–1092. [CrossRef]
6. Umer, M.; Mohib, Y.; Atif, M.; Nazim, M. Skeletal metastasis in renal cell carcinoma: A review. *Ann. Med. Surg.* **2018**, *27*, 9–16. [CrossRef]
7. Zentrum fur Krebsregisterdaten. Available online: http://www.rki.de/Krebs/DE/Content/Krebsarten/Nierenkrebs/nierenkrebs_node.html (accessed on 12 December 2019).
8. Ljungberg, B.; Campbell, S.C.; Choi, H.Y.; Cho, H.Y.; Jacqmin, D.; Lee, J.E.; Weikert, S.; Kiemeney, L.A. The epidemiology of renal cell carcinoma. *Eur. Urol.* **2011**, *60*, 615–621. [CrossRef]
9. Mani, J.; Juengel, E.; Arslan, I.; Bartsch, G.; Filmann, N.; Ackermann, H.; Nelson, K.; Haferkamp, A.; Engl, T.; Blaheta, R.A. Use of complementary and alternative medicine before and after organ removal due to urologic cancer. *Patient Prefer. Adherence* **2015**, *9*, 1407–1412. [CrossRef]
10. Huebner, J.; Micke, O.; Muecke, R.; Buentzel, J.; Prott, F.J.; Kleeberg, U.; Senf, B.; Muenstedt, K. User rate of complementary and alternative medicine (CAM) of patients visiting a counseling facility for CAM of a German comprehensive cancer center. *Anticancer Res.* **2014**, *34*, 943–948.
11. Bose, S.; Panda, A.K.; Mukherjee, S.; Sa, G. Curcumin and tumor immune-editing: Resurrecting the immune system. *Cell Div.* **2015**, *10*, 6. [CrossRef]
12. Panda, A.K.; Chakraborty, D.; Sarkar, I.; Khan, T.; Sa, G. New insights into therapeutic activity and anticancer properties of curcumin. *J. Exp. Pharmacol.* **2017**, *9*, 31–45. [CrossRef]

13. Kronski, E.; Fiori, M.E.; Barbieri, O.; Astigiano, S.; Mirisola, V.; Killian, P.H.; Bruno, A.; Pagani, A.; Rovera, F.; Pfeffer, U.; et al. miR181b is induced by the chemopreventive polyphenol curcumin and inhibits breast cancer metastasis via down-regulation of the inflammatory cytokines CXCL1 and -2. *Mol. Oncol.* **2014**, *8*, 581–595. [CrossRef]
14. Bachmeier, B.E.; Killian, P.H.; Melchart, D. The Role of Curcumin in Prevention and Management of Metastatic Disease. *Int. J. Mol. Sci.* **2018**, *19*, 1716. [CrossRef]
15. Sa, G.; Das, T. Anti cancer effects of curcumin: Cycle of life and death. *Cell Div.* **2008**, *3*, 14. [CrossRef]
16. Aggarwal, B.B.; Sung, B. Pharmacological basis for the role of curcumin in chronic diseases: An age-old spice with modern targets. *Trends pharmacol. Sci.* **2009**, *30*, 85–94. [CrossRef]
17. Bhattacharyya, S.; Mandal, D.; Sen, G.S.; Pal, S.; Banerjee, S.; Lahiry, L.; Finke, J.H.; Tannenbaum, C.S.; Das, T.; Sa, G. Tumor-induced oxidative stress perturbs nuclear factor-kappaB activity-augmenting tumor necrosis factor-alpha-mediated T-cell death: Protection by curcumin. *Cancer Res.* **2007**, *67*, 362–370. [CrossRef]
18. Bernd, A. Visible light and/or UVA offer a strong amplification of the anti-tumor effect of curcumin. *Phytochem. Rev.* **2014**, *13*, 183–189. [CrossRef]
19. Anand, P.; Kunnumakkara, A.B.; Newman, R.A.; Aggarwal, B.B. Bioavailability of curcumin: Problems and promises. *Mol. Pharm.* **2007**, *4*, 807–818. [CrossRef]
20. Burgos-Morón, E.; Calderón-Montaño, J.M.; Salvador, J.; Robles, A.; López-Lázaro, M. The dark side of curcumin. *Int. J. Cancer* **2010**, *126*, 1771–1775. [CrossRef]
21. Muddineti, O.S.; Kumari, P.; Ray, E.; Ghosh, B.; Biswas, S. Curcumin-loaded chitosan-cholesterol micelles: Evaluation in monolayers and 3D cancer spheroid model. *Nanomedicine (Lond.)* **2017**, *12*, 12. [CrossRef]
22. Schiborr, C.; Kocher, A.; Behnam, D.; Jandasek, J.; Toelstede, S.; Frank, J. The oral bioavailability of curcumin from micronized powder and liquid micelles is significantly increased in healthy humans and differs between sexes. *Mol. Nutr. Food Res.* **2014**, *58*, 516–527. [CrossRef]
23. Bulboacă, A.E.; Boarescu, P.M.; Bolboacă, S.D.; Blidaru, M.; Feștilă, D.; Dogaru, G.; Nicula, C.A. Comparative Effect Of Curcumin Versus Liposomal Curcumin On Systemic Pro-Inflammatory Cytokines Profile, MCP-1 And RANTES In Experimental Diabetes Mellitus. *Int. J. Nanomed.* **2019**, *14*, 8961–8972. [CrossRef]
24. Wang, Z.S.; Chen, L.Z.; Zhou, H.P.; Liu, X.H.; Chen, F.H. Diarylpentadienone derivatives (curcumin analogues): Synthesis and anti-inflammatory activity. *Bioorganic Med. Chem. Lett.* **2017**, *27*, 1803–1807. [CrossRef]
25. Feng, T.; Wei, Y.; Lee, R.J.; Zhao, L. Liposomal curcumin and its application in cancer. *Int. J. Nanomed.* **2017**, *12*, 6027–6044. [CrossRef]
26. Rutz, J.; Maxeiner, S.; Juengel, E.; Bernd, A.; Kippenberger, S.; Zöller, N.; Chun, F.K.-H.; Blaheta, R.A. Growth and Proliferation of Renal Cell Carcinoma Cells Is Blocked by Low Curcumin Concentrations Combined with Visible Light Irradiation. *Int. J. Mol. Sci.* **2019**, *20*, 1464. [CrossRef]
27. Ghorbani, J.; Rahban, D.; Aghamiri, S.; Teymouri, A.; Bahador, A. Photosensitizers in antibacterial photodynamic therapy: An overview. *Laser Ther.* **2018**, *27*, 293–302. [CrossRef]
28. Laubach, V.; Kaufmann, R.; Bernd, A.; Kippenberger, S.; Zöller, N. Extrinsic or Intrinsic Apoptosis by Curcumin and Light: Still a Mystery. *Int. J. Mol. Sci.* **2019**, *20*, 905. [CrossRef]
29. Bruzell, E.M.; Morisbak, E.; Tønnesen, H.H. Studies on curcumin and curcuminoids. XXIX. Photoinduced cytotoxicity of curcumin in selected aqueous preparations. XXIX. Photoinduced cytotoxicity of curcumin in selected aqueous preparations. *Photochem. Photobiol. Sci.* **2005**, *4*, 523–530. [CrossRef]
30. Moharrami Kasmaie, F.; Jahromi, Z.; Gazor, R.; Zaminy, A. Comparison of melatonin and curcumin effect at the light and dark periods on regeneration of sciatic nerve crush injury in rats. *EXCLI J.* **2019**, *18*, 653–665.
31. Niu, T.; Tian, Y.; Cai, Q.; Ren, Q.; Wei, L. Red Light Combined with Blue Light Irradiation Regulates Proliferation and Apoptosis in Skin Keratinocytes in Combination with Low Concentrations of Curcumin. *PLoS ONE* **2015**, *10*, e0138754. [CrossRef]
32. Bessone, F.; Argenziano, M.; Grillo, G.; Ferrara, B.; Pizzimenti, S.; Barrera, G.; Cravotto, G.; Guiot, C.; Stura, I.; Cavalli, R.; et al. Low-dose curcuminoid-loaded in dextran nanobubbles can prevent metastatic spreading in prostate cancer cells. *Nanotechnology* **2019**, *30*, 214004. [CrossRef]
33. Herman, J.G.; Stadelman, H.L.; Roselli, C.E. Curcumin blocks CCL2 induced adhesion, motility and invasion, in part, through down-regulation of CCL2 expression and proteolytic activity. *Int. J. Oncol.* **2009**, *34*, 1319–1327. [PubMed]

34. Zheng, B.-Z.; Liu, T.-D.; Chen, G.; Zhang, J.-X.; Kang, X. The effect of curcumin on cell adhesion of human esophageal cancer cell. *Eur. Rev. Med. Pharmacol. Sci.* **2018**, *22*, 551–560. [PubMed]
35. Wu, J.; Lu, W.-Y.; Cui, L.-L. Inhibitory effect of curcumin on invasion of skin squamous cell carcinoma A431 cells. *Asian Pac. J. Cancer Prev.* **2015**, *16*, 2813–2818. [CrossRef] [PubMed]
36. Yodkeeree, S.; Ampasavate, C.; Sung, B.; Aggarwal, B.B.; Limtrakul, P. Demethoxycurcumin suppresses migration and invasion of MDA-MB-231 human breast cancer cell line. *Eur. J. Pharmacol.* **2010**, *627*, 8–15. [CrossRef]
37. Mu, J.; Wang, X.; Dong, L.; Sun, P. Curcumin derivative L6H4 inhibits proliferation and invasion of gastric cancer cell line BGC-823. *J. Cell. Biochem.* **2019**, *120*, 1011–1017. [CrossRef]
38. Hu, C.; Li, M.; Guo, T.; Wang, S.; Huang, W.; Yang, K.; Liao, Z.; Wang, J.; Zhang, F.; Wang, H. Anti-metastasis activity of curcumin against breast cancer via the inhibition of stem cell-like properties and EMT. *Phytomedicine* **2019**, *58*, 152740. [CrossRef]
39. Zhang, H.; Zheng, J.; Shen, H.; Huang, Y.; Liu, T.; Xi, H.; Chen, C. Curcumin Suppresses In Vitro Proliferation and Invasion of Human Prostate Cancer Stem Cells by Modulating DLK1-DIO3 Imprinted Gene Cluster MicroRNAs. *Genet. Test. Mol. Biomarkers* **2018**, *22*, 43–50. [CrossRef]
40. Wang, L.; Han, L.; Tao, Z.; Zhu, Z.; Han, L.; Yang, Z.; Wang, H.; Dai, D.; Wu, L.; Yuan, Z.; et al. The curcumin derivative WZ35 activates ROS-dependent JNK to suppress hepatocellular carcinoma metastasis. *Food Funct.* **2018**, *9*, 2970–2978. [CrossRef]
41. Li, Y.; Wang, P.; Chen, X.; Hu, J.; Liu, Y.; Wang, X.; Liu, Q. Activation of microbubbles by low-intensity pulsed ultrasound enhances the cytotoxicity of curcumin involving apoptosis induction and cell motility inhibition in human breast cancer MDA-MB-231 cells. *Ultrason. Sonochem.* **2016**, *33*, 26–36. [CrossRef]
42. Holy, J. Curcumin inhibits cell motility and alters microfilament organization and function in prostate cancer cells. *Cell Motil. Cytoskeleton.* **2004**, *58*, 253–268. [CrossRef]
43. Dhar, G.; Chakravarty, D.; Hazra, J.; Dhar, J.; Poddar, A.; Pal, M.; Chakrabarti, P.; Surolia, A.; Bhattacharyya, B. Actin-curcumin interaction: Insights into the mechanism of actin polymerization inhibition. *Biochemistry* **2015**, *54*, 1132–1143. [CrossRef] [PubMed]
44. Radhakrishnan, V.M.; Kojs, P.; Young, G.; Ramalingam, R.; Jagadish, B.; Mash, E.A.; Martinez, J.D.; Ghishan, F.K.; Kiela, P.R. pTyr421 cortactin is overexpressed in colon cancer and is dephosphorylated by curcumin: Involvement of non-receptor type 1 protein tyrosine phosphatase (PTPN1). *PLoS One* **2014**, *9*, e85796. [CrossRef] [PubMed]
45. Mierke, C.T.; Frey, B.; Fellner, M.; Herrmann, M.; Fabry, B. Integrin α5β1 facilitates cancer cell invasion through enhanced contractile forces. *J. Cell Sci.* **2011**, *124*, 369–383. [CrossRef] [PubMed]
46. Desgrosellier, J.S.; Cheresh, D.A. Integrins in cancer: Biological implications and therapeutic opportunities. *Nat. Rev. Cancer* **2010**, *10*, 9–22. [CrossRef] [PubMed]
47. Markovic-Lipkovski, J.; Brasanac, D.; Müller, G.A.; Müller, C.A. Cadherins and integrins in renal cell carcinoma: An immunohistochemical study. *Tumori* **2001**, *87*, 173–178. [CrossRef]
48. Feldkoren, B.; Hutchinson, R.; Rapoport, Y.; Mahajan, A.; Margulis, V. Integrin signaling potentiates transforming growth factor-beta 1 (TGF-β1) dependent down-regulation of E-Cadherin expression - Important implications for epithelial to mesenchymal transition (EMT) in renal cell carcinoma. *Exp. Cell res.* **2017**, *355*, 57–66. [CrossRef]
49. Wang, J.-R.; Liu, B.; Zhou, L.; Huang, Y.-X. MicroRNA-124-3p suppresses cell migration and invasion by targeting ITGA3 signaling in bladder cancer. *Cancer Biomark.* **2019**, *24*, 159–172. [CrossRef]
50. Sakaguchi, T.; Yoshino, H.; Yonemori, M.; Miyamoto, K.; Sugita, S.; Matsushita, R.; Itesako, T.; Tatarano, S.; Nakagawa, M.; Enokida, H. Regulation of ITGA3 by the dual-stranded microRNA-199 family as a potential prognostic marker in bladder cancer. *Br. J. Cancer* **2018**, *118*, e7. [CrossRef]
51. Bogusławska, J.; Rodzik, K.; Popławski, P.; Kędzierska, H.; Rybicka, B.; Sokół, E.; Tański, Z.; Piekiełko-Witkowska, A. TGF-β1 targets a microRNA network that regulates cellular adhesion and migration in renal cancer. *Cancer Lett.* **2018**, *412*, 155–169. [CrossRef]
52. Hase, H.; Jingushi, K.; Ueda, Y.; Kitae, K.; Egawa, H.; Ohshio, I.; Kawakami, R.; Kashiwagi, Y.; Tsukada, Y.; Kobayashi, T.; et al. LOXL2 status correlates with tumor stage and regulates integrin levels to promote tumor progression in ccRCC. *Mol. Cancer Res.* **2014**, *12*, 1807–1817.

53. Erdem, M.; Erdem, S.; Sanli, O.; Sak, H.; Kilicaslan, I.; Sahin, F.; Telci, D. Up-regulation of TGM2 with ITGB1 and SDC4 is important in the development and metastasis of renal cell carcinoma. *Urol. Oncol.* **2014**, *32*, 25.e13-20. [CrossRef] [PubMed]
54. Conti, A.; Santoni, M.; Amantini, C.; Burattini, L.; Berardi, R.; Santoni, G.; Cascinu, S.; Muzzonigro, G. Progress of molecular targeted therapies for advanced renal cell carcinoma. *BioMed Res. Int.* **2013**, *2013*, 419176. [CrossRef] [PubMed]
55. Cooper, J.; Giancotti, F.G. Integrin Signaling in Cancer: Mechanotransduction, Stemness, Epithelial Plasticity, and Therapeutic Resistance. *Cancer Cell* **2019**, *35*, 347–367. [CrossRef] [PubMed]
56. Haake, S.M.; Li, J.; Bai, Y.; Kinose, F.; Fang, B.; Welsh, E.A.; Zent, R.; Dhillon, J.; Pow-Sang, J.M.; Chen, Y.A.; et al. Tyrosine Kinase Signaling in Clear Cell and Papillary Renal Cell Carcinoma Revealed by Mass Spectrometry-Based Phosphotyrosine Proteomics. *Clin. Cancer Res.* **2016**, *22*, 5605–5616. [CrossRef]
57. Bao, Y.; Yang, F.; Liu, B.; Zhao, T.; Xu, Z.; Xiong, Y.; Sun, S.; Le, Q.; Wang, L. Angiopoietin-like protein 3 blocks nuclear import of FAK and contributes to sorafenib response. *Br. J. Cancer* **2018**, *119*, 450–461. [CrossRef]
58. Hu, B.; Sun, D.; Sun, C.; Sun, Y.-F.; Sun, H.-X.; Zhu, Q.-F.; Yang, X.-R.; Gao, Y.-B.; Tang, W.-G.; Fan, J.; et al. A polymeric nanoparticle formulation of curcumin in combination with sorafenib synergistically inhibits tumor growth and metastasis in an orthotopic model of human hepatocellular carcinoma. *Biochem. Biophys. Res. Commun.* **2015**, *468*, 525–532. [CrossRef]
59. Debata, P.R.; Begum, S.; Mata, A.; Genzer, O.; Kleiner, M.J.; Banerjee, P.; Castellanos, M.R. Curcumin potentiates the ability of sunitinib to eliminate the VHL-lacking renal cancer cells 786-O: Rapid inhibition of Rb phosphorylation as a preamble to cyclin D1 inhibition. *Anticancer Agents Med. Chem.* **2013**, *13*, 1508–1513. [CrossRef]
60. Neuschmelting, V.; Kim, K.; Malekzadeh-Najafabadi, J.; Jebiwott, S.; Prakash, J.; Scherz, A.; Coleman, J.A.; Kircher, M.F.; Ntziachristos, V. WST11 Vascular Targeted Photodynamic Therapy Effect Monitoring by Multispectral Optoacoustic Tomography (MSOT) in Mice. *Theranostics* **2018**, *8*, 723–734. [CrossRef]
61. Kroeze, S.G.C.; Grimbergen, M.C.M.; Rehmann, H.; Bosch, J.L.H.R.; Jans, J.J.M. Photodynamic therapy as novel nephron sparing treatment option for small renal masses. *J. Urol.* **2012**, *187*, 289–295. [CrossRef]
62. Ellerkamp, V.; Bortel, N.; Schmid, E.; Kirchner, B.; Armeanu-Ebinger, S.; Fuchs, J. Photodynamic Therapy Potentiates the Effects of Curcumin on Pediatric Epithelial Liver Tumor Cells. *Anticancer Res.* **2016**, *36*, 3363–3372.

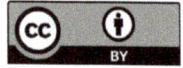

© 2020 by the authors. Licensee MDPI, Basel, Switzerland. This article is an open access article distributed under the terms and conditions of the Creative Commons Attribution (CC BY) license (http://creativecommons.org/licenses/by/4.0/).

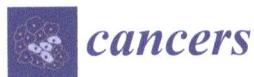

Article

EVI1 as a Prognostic and Predictive Biomarker of Clear Cell Renal Cell Carcinoma

Luis Palomero [1], Lubomir Bodnar [2,3,*], Francesca Mateo [1], Carmen Herranz-Ors [1], Roderic Espín [1], Mar García-Varelo [1], Marzena Jesiotr [4], Gorka Ruiz de Garibay [1], Oriol Casanovas [1], José I. López [5,*] and Miquel Angel Pujana [1,*]

1. ProCURE, Catalan Institute of Oncology (ICO), Bellvitge Institute for Biomedical Research (IDIBELL), L'Hospitalet del Llobregat, Barcelona 08908, Catalonia, Spain; lpalomero@iconcologia.net (L.P.); fmateo@iconcologia.net (F.M.); cherranz@iconcologia.net (C.H.-O.); rodericespin@gmail.com (R.E.); mgarciavaler@uoc.edu (M.G.-V.); grponce@iconcologia.net (G.R.d.G.); ocasanovas@iconcologia.net (O.C.)
2. Department of Oncology and Immunooncology, Hospital Ministry of the Interior and Administration with Warmia and Mazury Oncology Center, Olsztyn 10-719, Poland
3. Department of Oncology, University of Warmia and Masuria, Olsztyn 10-719, Poland
4. Department of Pathology, Military Institute of Medicine, Warsaw 04-141, Poland; marzena@obta.uw.edu.pl
5. Department of Pathology, Cruces University Hospital, Biocruces Institute, Barakaldo 48903, Spain
* Correspondence: lubomirbodnar.lb@gmail.com (L.B.); joseignacio.lopezfernandezdevillaverde@osakidetza.eus (J.I.L.); mapujana@iconcologia.net (M.A.P.); Tel.: +48-261817380 (L.B.); +34-946006336 (J.I.L.); +34-932607952 (M.A.P.)

Received: 20 November 2019; Accepted: 25 January 2020; Published: 28 January 2020

Abstract: The transcription factor EVI1 plays an oncogenic role in several types of neoplasms by promoting aggressive cancer features. EVI1 contributes to epigenetic regulation and transcriptional control, and its overexpression has been associated with enhanced PI3K-AKT-mTOR signaling in some settings. These observations raise the possibility that EVI1 influences the prognosis and everolimus-based therapy outcome of clear cell renal cell carcinoma (ccRCC). Here, gene expression and protein immunohistochemical studies of ccRCC show that EVI1 overexpression is associated with advanced disease features and with poorer outcome—particularly in the CC-e.3 subtype defined by The Cancer Genome Atlas. Overexpression of an oncogenic EVI1 isoform in RCC cell lines confers substantial resistance to everolimus. The *EVI1* rs1344555 genetic variant is associated with poorer survival and greater progression of metastatic ccRCC patients treated with everolimus. This study leads us to propose that evaluation of EVI1 protein or gene expression, and of *EVI1* genetic variants may help improve estimates of prognosis and the benefit of everolimus-based therapy in ccRCC.

Keywords: everolimus; EVI1; genetic association; mTOR; clear cell renal cell carcinoma

1. Introduction

The ecotropic viral integration site 1 gene (*Evi1*) locus was initially highlighted in mouse studies as a common retroviral integration genomic location causing myeloid tumors [1]. It encodes a dual-domain zinc-finger transcription factor with a fundamental role in regulating hematopoietic stem cell renewal and myeloid progenitor cell differentiation [2]. Abnormal overexpression of EVI1 and, therefore, activation of its underlying transcriptional program, are involved in up to a quarter of pediatric acute myeloid leukemia (AML), and influence prognosis and response to chemotherapy in this setting [3,4]. More recently, an oncogenic role for EVI1 has been broadened to include several epithelial cancers, similarly associated with aggressive features [5–13]. Analyses of genomic alterations across cancers have shown that chromosome 3q26.2, which harbors *EVI1*, is amplified in a variety of epithelial cancer types [14]. The specific locus is also known as the *MDS1* and *EVI1* complex locus (*MECOM*), and different isoforms may emerge with apparently opposite roles in tumorigenesis [5,15].

The oncogenic function of EVI1 is mediated by its established role on epigenetic regulation and transcriptional control [16–18]. EVI1 interacts with Polycomb-group (PcG) proteins to repress the expression of the tumor suppressor gene *PTEN* [19]. In parallel, it interacts with DNA methyltransferases causing a hypermethylation genomic signature [20]. In addition, EVI1 promotes specific gene silencing though interactions with histone methyltransferases [21–23]. As consequence of these functional associations, several key signaling pathways are altered promoting cancer. EVI1 negatively regulates TGF-β signaling through repression of *SMAD3* [24,25]. Furthermore, oncogenic EVI1 frequently enhances PI3K-AKT-mTOR signaling, as by repression of *PTEN* in leukemogenesis [19]. In intestinal epithelial cells, oncogenic EVI1 overactivates PI3K-AKT signaling in response to TGFβ-mediated and taxol-mediated apoptosis [6]. In breast cancer, overexpression of EVI1 is associated with poor prognosis [8], stem cell-like and lung-metastatic features, and resistance to allosteric mTOR inhibition [7]. Cancer stem cell-like and metastatic cells rely on enhanced mTOR activity, and EVI1 maintains this signaling by transcriptional upregulation of key pathway components and metastatic mediators [7].

The depicted associations between oncogenic EVI1 and abnormally enhanced mTOR activity raise the possibility that EVI1 influences cancer prognosis and therapeutic response in a clinical setting where this kinase plays a central role, that of ccRCC. This is the most frequent type of kidney cancer in adults, which is commonly caused by genetic alterations that hamper proper cellular response to hypoxia and, in turn, demand enhanced mTOR signaling [26,27]. Thus, everolimus, an allosteric mTOR inhibitor has been approved for the treatment of advanced ccRCC [28]. On the basis of these observations, we evaluated genetic variants and expression features of *EVI1*/EVI1 for their associations with ccRCC prognosis and therapeutic response. Our findings have the potential to improve estimates of ccRCC prognosis and the clinical benefit from everolimus.

2. Results

2.1. EVI1 Overexpression Is Associated with Progression Features and Poor Prognosis of ccRCC

In addition to myeloid leukemia, overexpression of EVI1 has been associated with aggressive phenotypes of breast cancer, colorectal, lung, ovarian, pancreatic, and prostate cancer [5–13]. To determine whether there is a similar link with ccRCC, EVI1-targeted immunohistochemistry assays were performed that included cases with tumor extension to the venous system (i.e., formation of venous tumor thrombus), since this is a feature of locally advanced disease [29]. Of 39 cases studied (Supplementary Table S1), 8 (20%) tumors and 18 (46%) venous tumor thrombi were found to be positive for EVI1 expression (Figure 1A). EVI1 was also found to be expressed in tumor-invasive areas of fat tissue (Figure 1A).

Analyses of histopathological data revealed a positive association between EVI1 expression and the presence of cancer-affected lymph nodes: odds ratio (OR) = 15.46, 95% confidence interval (CI) = 1.02-936.43, Fisher's exact test $p = 0.028$ (Figure 1B). Combined analysis of the immunohistochemistry results from the tumors and venous tumor thrombi showed a significant association between EVI1 positivity and poorer patient outcome: multivariate Cox regression (including age and gender) overall survival (OS) EVI1 positivity hazard ratio (HR) = 2.94, 95% CI = 1.13–7.63, $p = 0.027$ (Figure 1C). These data suggest that EVI1 overexpression also contributes to the aggressiveness of ccRCC.

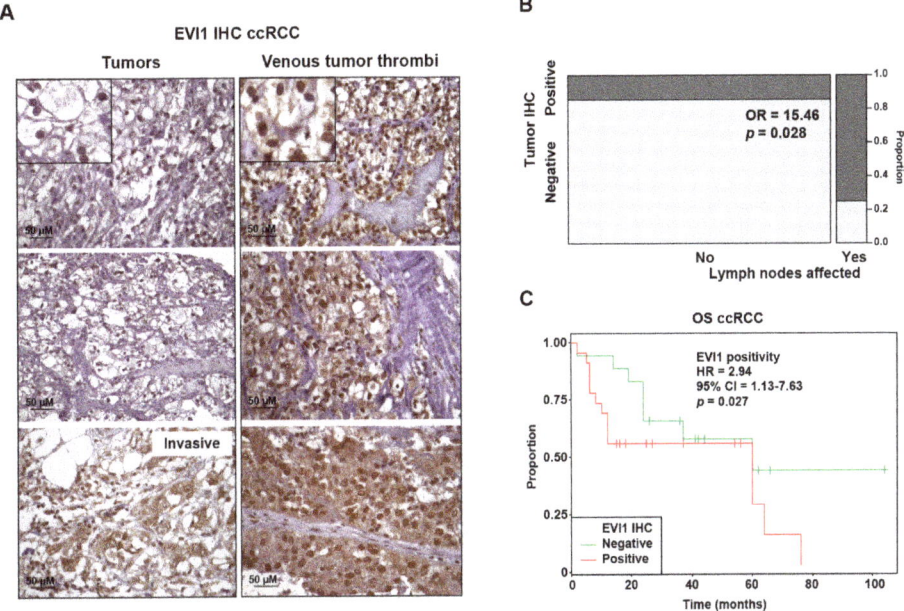

Figure 1. EVI1 expression in ccRCC tumors and venous tumor thrombi are associated with features of disease progression and poorer patient outcome. (**A**) Representative images of immunohistochemical detection of EVI1 in primary tumors (left panels) and venous tumor thrombi (right panels) from the cohort of 39 ccRCC cases (Supplementary Table S1). The top panel insets include magnified images showing nuclear positivity in cancer cells; weaker staining in the cytoplasm is also appreciated in some cases, which is consistent with observations in other cancer types [8,13]. (**B**) Grid showing the proportions of EVI1 IHC positivity in tumors relative to lymph node status in the same cohort. The odds ratio (OR) and corresponding p-value (Fisher's exact test) for the association between EVI1 positivity and cancer-affected lymph node are shown. (**C**) Kaplan–Meier curves showing the association between EVI1 positivity and poorer survival in the same cohort. The multivariate (including age and gender) Cox regression overall survival (OS) hazard ratio (HR) estimate, 95% CI, and p-value are shown. The estimations for age and gender (male as reference) in this model were, respectively: HR = 1.05, 95% CI = 0.99–1.10, p = 0.07; and HR = 0.20, 95% CI = 0.07–0.54, p = 0.002.

2.2. EVI1 Overexpression Confers ccRCC Cell Resistance to Everolimus

Somatic gain of the 3q26 genomic region including *EVI1* was noted in the original study of ccRCC of The Cancer Genome Atlas (TCGA KIRC) [30]. Analysis of TCGA data identified the CC-e.3 as the ccRCC subtype with the greater proportion of tumors showing *EVI1* locus gain (Figure 2A). A high level of expression of EVI1 in this subtype—but not in the other KIRC subtypes (CC-e.1-2) and complete cohort—was found to be significantly associated with poorer outcome, as measured by a multivariate (including age, gender, and tumor stage) Cox regression analysis of progression-free interval (PFI; Figure 2B). The CC-e.3 subtype was identified by TCGA as the subgroup with a higher relative level of expression of markers of the epithelial–mesenchymal transition [30], which is consistent with the functional associations of EVI1 described in some cancer settings [6,7,15]. Indeed, *EVI1* expression in CC-e.3 tumors was found to be positively co-expressed with several metastasis-, invasion- and integrin-related curated gene sets (Supplementary Table S2). We previously identified the mTOR pathway components RHEB and RPTOR as being positively regulated by EVI1 in metastatic breast cancer with stem cell-like features [7]. Next, PFI analyses that took into account the expression of *EVI1* and either of these mTOR pathway components showed that outcome was significantly poorer when both genes were overexpressed (Figure 2C). Therefore, over-expression of *EVI1* may contribute to progression of certain ccRCC tumors.

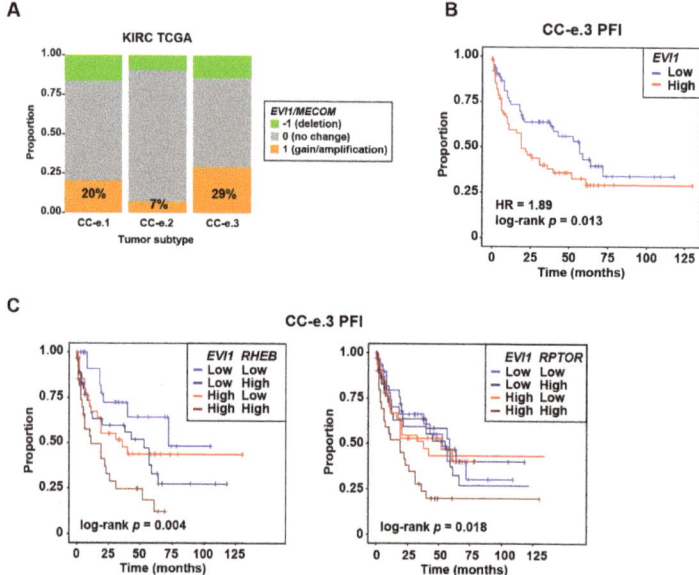

Figure 2. Frequent chromosome 3q26 *EVI1/MECOM* gain in the CC-e.3 KIRC/ccRCC subtype, gene expression association with poorer outcome in this subtype, and with *RHEB* and *RPTOR* influencing progression. (**A**) Graph showing the proportions of *EVI1/MECOM* genomic alterations (as depicted in the inset) in TCGA KIRC primary tumor subtypes (CC-e.1-3). The percentage of tumors with genomic gain in each subtype is shown. (**B**) Kaplan–Meier curves showing the association between *EVI1* overexpression and poorer PFI in the TCGA KIRC CC-e.3 cohort. This set was divided in two groups using the average expression value of *EVI1* as threshold (low or high *EVI1* tumor expression, being normally distributed). The multivariate (including age, gender, and tumor stage (I-II and III-IV) Cox regression HR estimate, 95% CI, and log-rank *p*-value are shown. (**C**) Kaplan–Meier curves showing the association between overexpression of *EVI1* and *RHEB* (left panel) or *RPTOR* (right panel) with poorer PFI in the TCGA KIRC CC-e.3 cohort. This set was divided in four groups using the average expression value of *EVI1* and *RHEB* or *RPTOR* as thresholds (low or high *EVI1* and low or high *RHEB/RPTOR* tumor expression). The log-rank *p*-values are shown.

Following on from the above observations, the responses of three RCC cell lines (ccRCC: 786-O and A498; and papillary RCC: ACHN) to everolimus upon ectopic overexpression of full-length EVI1 or EVI1$^{Del190-515}$—two isoforms identified as oncogenic in ovarian cancer [15]—were assessed. The ACHN cell line was included because advanced papillary RCC may also be treated with everolimus [31]. While the full-length isoform did not show any significant effects, all three cell lines were considerably less sensitive to everolimus when GFP-EVI1$^{Del190-515}$ was overexpressed relative to GFP alone, with >25-fold differences in the half-maximal inhibitory concentration (IC$_{50}$) observed (Figure 3A). Rapalogs are primarily cytostatic instead of cytotoxic [32] and, at the highest everolimus concentration (100 µM) tested for 72 hours, the percentages of cell viability were for the GFP alone and GFP-EVI1$^{Del190-515}$ conditions, respectively: 786-O, 26% and 21%; A498, 24% and 52%; and ACHN, 26% and 60%.

Molecular analyses showed that overexpression of GFP-EVI1$^{Del190-515}$ causes a robust increase of basal phospho-Ser235/236-ribosomal S6 protein (pS6) in two of the cell lines (786-O and ACHN; Figure 3B, left panels). In addition, an increase of total S6 was noted in ACHN cells (Figure 3B, left panels); however, no consistent changes were observed in the A498 assays (Figure 3B, right panels). Therefore, oncogenic EVI1 may be linked to enhanced mTOR signaling in some RCC cell models, which in turn might influence sensitivity to everolimus.

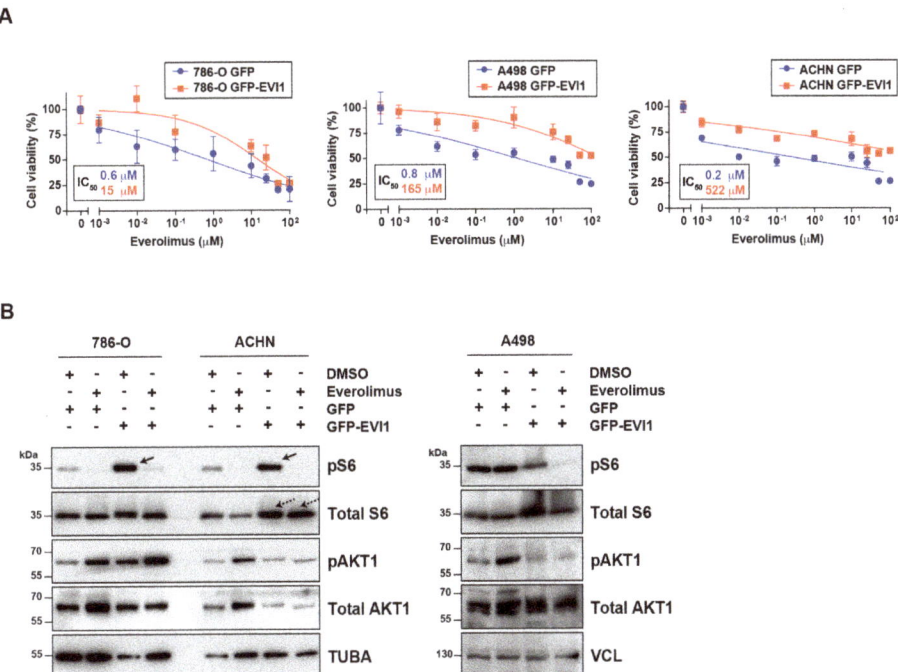

Figure 3. Ectopic oncogenic *EVI1* overexpression confers resistance to everolimus. (**A**) Graphs showing viability of RCC cells (Y-axis) transiently transfected and selected with GFP or GFP-EVI1$^{Del190-515}$ expression constructs, and exposed to different concentrations of everolimus for 72 hours (X-axis). The two cell line conditions (GFP and GFP-EVI1$^{Del190-515}$) are indicated in the insets and the estimated IC$_{50}$ values are shown in the graphs. Each measure shows the mean and standard deviation of quintuplicate values. The curve fitting regression was computed using the log value versus normalized response. (**B**) Western blot results from the three RCC cell lines and two conditions, treated with DMSO or everolimus (20 nM), and analyzed for the levels of total S6 and pS6, total AKT1 and pAKT1, and loading control (tubulin, TUBA; or vinculin, VCL). The solid arrows (top left panel) indicate increased levels of pS6 in GFP-EVI1$^{Del190-515}$ over-expressing 786-O and ACHN cells. The dashed arrows indicate increased levels of total S6 in GFP-EVI1$^{Del190-515}$ over-expressing ACHN cells. Molecular weight markers are shown on the left side and expressed in kiloDalton (kDa).

2.3. Common Genetic Variants in EVI1 Are Associated with Response to Everolimus of Metastatic ccRCC

The *EVI1* locus may be pleiotropic since at least 56 human traits have been linked to the corresponding genomic region (±50 kilobases of the *EVI1/MECOM* locus) in the results from diverse genome-wide association studies (Genome Browser GWAS catalog data, version GRCh37/hg19). Some of the identified traits might in turn be linked to known EVI1 functions. Variant forms at this locus have been associated with lung [33] and kidney function [34,35], and cancer risk, including breast and lung cancer susceptibility [36]. Therefore, we analyzed leading variants from these studies (rs1344555, rs16853722, and rs75316749, respectively) to establish their association with progression of metastatic ccRCC treated with everolimus (Supplementary Table S3).

The rs1344555 variant was significantly associated with progression-free survival (PFS) and OS of everolimus-treated metastatic ccRCC: CC versus CT/TT genotypes PFS, hazard ratio (HR) = 1.96, 95% CI = 1.01–3.81, p = 0.047; and OS HR = 2.09, 95% CI = 1.08–4.08, p = 0.029 (Figure 4A). In this setting, the T allele was associated with a higher probability of disease progression and patient death and, in the original lung study, was associated with inferior organ function [33]. A significant association between the genotypes of rs1344555 and the percentage of AKT1-positive metastatic ccRCC cells was revealed (Kruskal–Wallis test p = 0.018; Figure 4B). Notably, a TCGA-genotyped variant correlated with rs1344555, rs11718241 (r^2 = 0.94 in European populations), proved to be an expression quantitative locus (eQTL) for *EVI1* in the total KIRC cohort and in the CC-e.3 subtype (Figure 4C). Based on 1000 Genome Project data, the minor alleles of both variants (T) were correlated, and therefore one increased the risk of progression (rs1344555-T, Figure 4A) while the other was associated with a relatively higher level of expression of *EVI1* (rs11718241-T, Figure 4C).

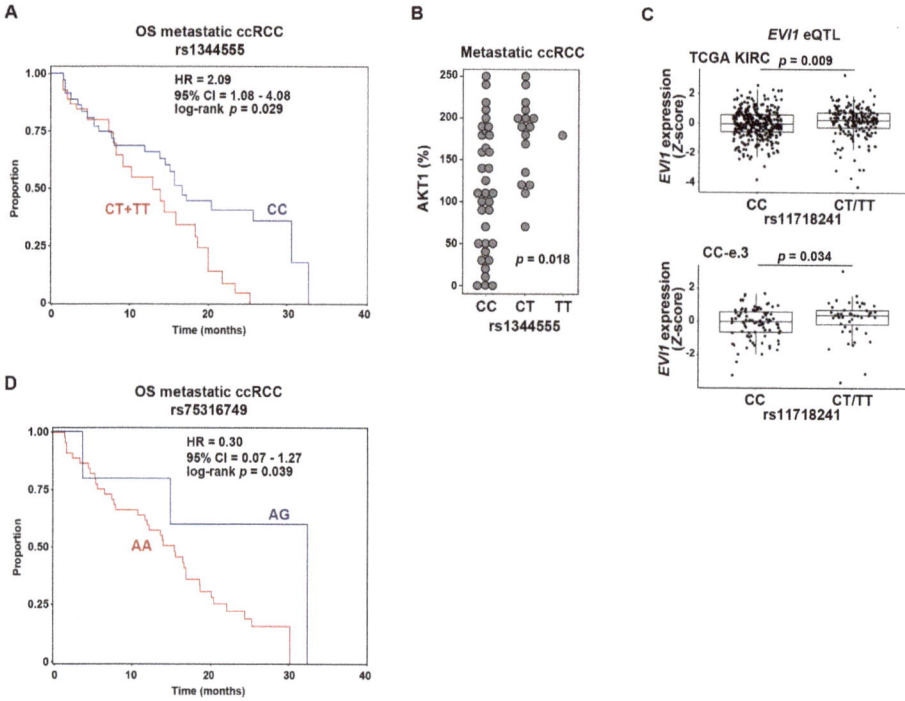

Figure 4. Common *EVI1* genetic variation is associated with response to everolimus of metastatic ccRCC. (**A**) Kaplan–Meier curves of OS based on rs1344555 C/C (n = 35) against C/T (n = 16) plus T/T (n = 1) genotypes. The univariate Cox regression HR estimate, 95% CI, and log-rank p are shown. (**B**) Graph showing the association between rs1344555 genotypes and AKT1 expression in metastatic RCC. The Kruskal–Wallis test p-value is shown. (**C**) Box plots showing the *EVI1* eQTL at rs11718241 in primary tumors from complete TCGA KIRC cohort (top panel) and from the CC-e.3 cohort (bottom panel). The Wilcoxon test p-values are shown. (**D**) Kaplan–Meier curves of OS of metastatic ccRCC based on rs75316749 A/G (n = 5) against A/A (n = 45) genotypes.

The rs16853722 variant did not show significant associations, while analyses of rs75316749 raised the possibility of associations with metastatic ccRCC OS, although the number of informative cases was too small for them to be statistically significant. Five rs75316749 heterozygous (AG) individuals were identified in the metastatic ccRCC cohort, with an estimated HR of 0.30 (log-rank p = 0.039; Figure 4C).

In this setting, the minor allele G, which has previously been linked to increased lung and breast cancer risk [36], may be associated with a lower probability of death.

3. Discussion

This study proposes that evaluation of EVI1 protein or gene expression, and of specific *EVI1* genetic variants, may help improve estimates of prognosis and of benefit from everolimus-based therapy in ccRCC. The connection with cancer progression is supported by immunohistochemical studies of tumors with advanced disease features, and by analyses of gene expression profiles in primary tumors from TCGA. The results are coherent with, and expand on, the proposed oncogenic role of EVI1 in other solid cancers [5–13]. However, its impact in ccRCC may be limited to tumors corresponding to the CC-e.3 subtype.

The influence of common genetic variation on everolimus-based therapy is based on the results of variants previously associated with lung function [34,35] and with pleiotropy, including cancer susceptibility [36]. Thus, the depicted genetic variants could also be relevant for predicting progression and/or therapeutic response in other cancer settings. Consistent with the observed genetic associations in metastatic ccRCC, ectopic overexpression of oncogenic EVI1$^{Del190-515}$ confers resistance to everolimus of RCC cell lines. In addition, the resistant phenotype is associated with enhanced pS6 in two models, which builds on previous AKT-mTOR signaling observations in breast and colorectal cancer cells [6,7], and with leukemia [19].

The oncogenic transcriptional program mediated by EVI1 in ccRCC and the potential differential role of *EVI1* isoforms remain to be determined. We may speculate that oncogenic EVI1 in ccRCC is linked to the acquisition of stem cell-like and/or EMT features, as described in other cancer types [5–10]. It is of particular note that EMT has also been associated with resistance to allosteric mTOR inhibition [37,38]. The precise causal variants linked to the observed genetic associations are also unknown. Based on data from other cancer models and from eQTL observations, associated risk alleles might increase *EVI1* expression and thereby enhance its function and activate the corresponding oncogenic transcriptional program [7,8,15]. Collectively, the prognostic and therapeutic predictive associations indicate that targeting EVI1 could improve the cure of advanced ccRCC. This may be accomplished by targeting known interactors of EVI1 involved in epigenetic and transcriptional regulation [17], or by targeting metabolic dependences centered on the creatine kinase pathway [39] and L-asparaginase function [40]. These strategies could be combined with allosteric mTOR inhibition; however, while rapalogs do not benefit all patients and do not always produce durable responses, immunotherapy with checkpoint inhibitors is becoming a major choice for the treatment of ccRCC [41]. Interestingly, simultaneously targeting TGF-β and checkpoint inhibitors confers marked inhibition of tumorigenesis in preclinical models [42–44]. Given that oncogenic EVI1 modulates TGF-β signaling [24,25], ccRCC cases with EVI1 over-expression might show differential benefit from immunotherapy, and further studies may warranted to assess the potential benefit of targeting EVI1.

4. Materials and Methods

4.1. Patients

A cohort of 39 ccRCC cases (Supplementary Table S1) collected at the Cruces University Hospital (Barakaldo, Spain) were analyzed for EVI1 expression by immunohistochemical assays. The cohort comprised 9 women and 30 men, who had a median age at diagnosis of 66 years. Their pathological data included tumor grade, diameter, stage, necrosis, sarcomatoid features, lymph nodes affected (yes/no), existence of metastases (yes/no), months of follow-up, and dead or alive status. The institutional ethics committee approved the study and all patients provided informed consent for the study (CEIC-PI2016096).

The cohort of patients genotyped for selected genetic variants corresponded to a prospective, single-arm phase II study of metastatic RCC (93.1% ccRCC) treated with everolimus [45] (Supplementary

Table S3). All enrolled patients received no more than two anti-angiogenic therapies before receiving everolimus. There were 19 women and 39 men, who had a median age at diagnosis of 60 years. Immunohistochemical results of AKT1 positivity were based on the H-score method. The ethics committee of the Military Institute of Medicine (Warsaw, Poland) approved the study and all patients provided informed consent for the study of genetic variants.

4.2. Immunohistochemistry Assays

The assays were performed on serial paraffin sections of a tissue microarray, applying a protocol including heat-induced epitope retrieval (35 min in a pressure cooker), citrate buffer, 1:50 dilution of anti-EVI1 delta 190–515 antibody (Novus Biologicals, Centennial, CO, USA), and Dako liquid DAB (diaminobenzidine) plus substrate chromogen system (Agilent, Santa Clara, CA, USA). In all experiments, analogous samples were processed without incubation with the primary antibody; no immunostaining was observed in any of these assays. Results were scored blind with respect to clinical information. Molecular analyses were carried out as part of the ProCURE research program, at the Catalan Institute of Oncology, IDIBELL (Barcelona, Spain), and followed the reporting recommendations for tumor marker prognostic studies [46].

4.3. Genetic Analyses

DNA was extracted from primary tumors. Samples were lysed using the PrepFiler™ buffer, and substrate was removed using LySep columns. The lysates were loaded onto an AutoMate Express instrument for DNA extraction. Quantitative and qualitative assays of the resulting DNA were carried out using Quantifiler Duo on the Applied Biosystems Real-Time PCR 7500 system. Genotyping was performed using TaqMan assays (Applied Biosystems, Foster City, CA, USA) in ABgene's Universal Master Mix (Thermo Scientific, Waltham, MA, USA). Replicate samples were assayed, with a template (buffer only) used as negative control. Duplicates consisting of DNA extracted from the same material, but at different times, were analyzed to assess the concordance and quality of the genotyping.

4.4. Statistical Analyses

Logistic regressions including age and gender as covariates, and 2 × 2 contingency Fisher's exact test were used to evaluate immunohistochemical results from tumor and thrombi. The association with survival was assessed by univariate and multivariate (including age, gender, and tumor stage) Cox regression analyses using the survival package in R software. For the genetic studies, the primary end point was PFS, defined as the time elapsed between the date of entry into the study and the date of disease progression or of the most recent follow-up. Secondary end points were OS, the probability of PFS for at least six months, objective response rate, and toxicity, determined by adverse events and laboratory measures. Statistical analyses were performed using STATA (10.0 STATA Corp.) and R software.

4.5. TCGA Data Analyses

Gene expression, genomic copy number, genotype, and clinical data were obtained from TCGA (data access #11689) and from the corresponding publications [30,47]. The genotype data corresponded to TCGA results using the Affymetrix Genome-Wide Human SNP Array 6.0 (SNP6). The GSEA tool was used with default parameters in the v4.0.3 Java desktop application [48], and the pre-ranked input corresponded to the Pearson's correlation coefficients computed between *EVI1* and any other gene analyzed by RNAseq (FPKM log2 scaled).

4.6. Cellular Assays

The 786-O, A498 and ACHN cell lines were cultured under standard conditions and confirmed to be free of *Mycoplasma* contamination. *EVI1* full-length and Del190–515 were ectopically overexpressed using a pEGFP-C1 construct [15]. Cells were transfected with GFP or GFP-EVI1-encoding vectors, sorted for GFP positivity at 24 hours and then plated for viability assays. The viability studies were based on colorimetric assays using a tetrazolium compound (MTT) and included exposure to different concentrations of everolimus (Selleck Chemicals, Houston, TX, USA).

4.7. Western Blot and Antibodies

To analyze extracts, cells were lysed in RIPA buffer, lysates were clarified twice by centrifugation, and protein concentrations were measured using the Bradford method (Bio-Rad, Hercules, CA, USA). Lysates were resolved in SDS-PAGE electrophoresis gels and transferred to Immobilon-P (Merck Millipore, Burlington, MA, USA) or PVDF membranes (Sigma-Aldrich, St. Luis, MO, USA). Target proteins were identified by detection of horseradish peroxidase-labeled antibody complexes with chemiluminescence using the ECL Western Blotting Detection Kit (GE Healthcare, Chicago, IL, USA). The antibodies were anti-total and anti-phospho-Ser473 AKT1 (#9272 and #9271, respectively, Cell Signaling Technology, Danvers, MA, USA), anti-total and anti-phospho-Ser235/236-ribosomal S6 protein (#SC-74459, Santa Cruz Biotechnology, Dallas, TX, USA; and #4858, Cell Signaling Technology, respectively), and anti-VCL (V9131, Sigma-Aldrich).

5. Conclusions

High levels of expression of *EVI1* in ccRCC are associated with features of cancer progression and invasion, and with poor patient outcome in the CC-e.3 subtype. Common genetic variants in *EVI1* are associated with the response to everolimus of metastatic ccRCC. Determination of EVI1 protein or gene expression, and of defined *EVI1* genetic variants could improve estimates of ccRCC patient outcome and benefit from everolimus in the clinical scenario.

Supplementary Materials: The following are available online: http://www.mdpi.com/2072-6694/12/2/300/s1. Table S1, Clinical and histopathological features of the retrospective ccRCC cohort used for immunohistochemical studies of EVI1; Table S2, Curated gene sets (GSEA MSigDB C2 set) positively co-expressed with *EVI1* in CC.e-3 tumors; and Table S3, Main clinical and histopathological characteristics of metastatic patients treated with everolimus, used for genetic analyses. Figure S1, The whole western blots.

Author Contributions: Conceptualization, M.A.P.; methodology, L.P., L.B., F.M., J.I.L., and M.A.P.; formal analysis, L.P., L.B., F.M., R.E., and M.A.P.; investigation, L.B., M.J., O.C., J.I.L., and M.A.P.; data curation, L.P., L.B., F.M., C.H.-O., M.G.-V., M.J, and G.R.d.G.; writing of original draft, M.A.P.; review and editing of manuscript, L.P., L.B., J.I.L., and M.A.P.; supervision, M.A.P.; funding acquisition, M.A.P. All authors have read and agreed to the published version of the manuscript.

Funding: This research was funded by: Generalitat de Catalunya grant SGR 2017-449; Spanish Ministry of Health ISCIII grants PI15/00854 and PI18/01029; and Telemaraton 2014 "Todos Somos Raros, Todos Somos Unicos" grant P35. This work was also supported by the CERCA Programme of the Generalitat de Catalunya and the European Regional Development Fund (ERDF/FEDER, "A way to make Europe").

Acknowledgments: We wish to thank Penny Soucy and Jacques Simard for their help with annotations of the genetic variants, and Roser Pons and Jordi Senserrich for advice about cancer cell lines. We would also like to thank all the participants for their contribution to the study, and the corresponding laboratory staff for their helpful comments. The results presented here are partly based on data generated by the TCGA Research Network (https://www.cancer.gov/tcga), and we would like to express our gratitude to the TCGA consortia and their coordinators for providing the data and clinical information used in this study.

Conflicts of Interest: O.C. and M.A.P. are recipients of an unrestricted grant from Roche Pharma to finance the ProCURE research program, which was paid to the Catalan Institute of Oncology (2017).

References

1. Mucenski, M.L.; Taylor, B.A.; Ihle, J.N.; Hartley, J.W.; Morse, H.C.; Jenkins, N.A.; Copeland, N.G. Identification of a common ecotropic viral integration site, Evi-1, in the DNA of AKXD murine myeloid tumors. *Mol. Cell. Biol.* **1988**, *8*, 301–308. [CrossRef] [PubMed]
2. Kataoka, K.; Kurokawa, M. Ecotropic viral integration site 1, stem cell self-renewal and leukemogenesis. *Cancer Sci.* **2012**, *103*, 1371–1377. [CrossRef] [PubMed]

3. Barjesteh van Waalwijk van Doorn-Khosrovani, S.; Erpelinck, C.; van Putten, W.L.J.; Valk, P.J.M.; van der Poel-van de Luytgaarde, S.; Hack, R.; Slater, R.; Smit, E.M.E.; Beverloo, H.B.; Verhoef, G.; et al. High *EVI1* expression predicts poor survival in acute myeloid leukemia: a study of 319 de novo AML patients. *Blood* **2003**, *101*, 837–845. [CrossRef] [PubMed]
4. Balgobind, B.V.; Lugthart, S.; Hollink, I.H.; Arentsen-Peters, S.T.J.C.M.; van Wering, E.R.; de Graaf, S.S.N.; Reinhardt, D.; Creutzig, U.; Kaspers, G.J.L.; de Bont, E.S.J.M.; et al. *EVI1* overexpression in distinct subtypes of pediatric acute myeloid leukemia. *Leukemia* **2010**, *24*, 942–949. [CrossRef] [PubMed]
5. Sayadi, A.; Jeyakani, J.; Seet, S.H.; Wei, C.-L.; Bourque, G.; Bard, F.A.; Jenkins, N.A.; Copeland, N.G.; Bard-Chapeau, E.A. Functional features of EVI1 and EVI1∆324 isoforms of *MECOM* gene in genome-wide transcription regulation and oncogenicity. *Oncogene* **2016**, *35*, 2311–2321. [CrossRef]
6. Liu, Y.; Chen, L.; Ko, T.C.; Fields, A.P.; Thompson, E.A. Evi1 is a survival factor which conveys resistance to both TGFb- and taxol-mediated cell death via PI3K/AKT. *Oncogene* **2006**, *25*, 3565–3575. [CrossRef]
7. Mateo, F.; Arenas, E.J.; Aguilar, H.; Serra-Musach, J.; de Garibay, G.R.; Boni, J.; Maicas, M.; Du, S.; Iorio, F.; Herranz-Ors, C.; et al. Stem cell-like transcriptional reprogramming mediates metastatic resistance to mTOR inhibition. *Oncogene* **2017**, *36*, 2737–2749. [CrossRef]
8. Wang, H.; Schaefer, T.; Konantz, M.; Braun, M.; Varga, Z.; Paczulla, A.M.; Reich, S.; Jacob, F.; Perner, S.; Moch, H.; et al. Prominent oncogenic roles of EVI1 in breast carcinoma. *Cancer Res.* **2017**, *77*, 2148–2160. [CrossRef]
9. Tanaka, M.; Suzuki, H.I.; Shibahara, J.; Kunita, A.; Isagawa, T.; Yoshimi, A.; Kurokawa, M.; Miyazono, K.; Aburatani, H.; Ishikawa, S.; et al. EVI1 oncogene promotes KRAS pathway through suppression of microRNA-96 in pancreatic carcinogenesis. *Oncogene* **2014**, *33*, 2454–2463. [CrossRef]
10. Queisser, A.; Hagedorn, S.; Wang, H.; Schaefer, T.; Konantz, M.; Alavi, S.; Deng, M.; Vogel, W.; von Mässenhausen, A.; Kristiansen, G.; et al. Ecotropic viral integration site 1, a novel oncogene in prostate cancer. *Oncogene* **2017**, *36*, 1573–1584. [CrossRef]
11. Choi, Y.-W.; Choi, J.S.; Zheng, L.T.; Lim, Y.J.; Yoon, H.K.; Kim, Y.H.; Wang, Y.-P.; Lim, Y. Comparative genomic hybridization array analysis and real time PCR reveals genomic alterations in squamous cell carcinomas of the lung. *Lung Cancer.* **2007**, *55*, 43–51. [CrossRef] [PubMed]
12. Starr, T.K.; Allaei, R.; Silverstein, K.A.T.; Staggs, R.A.; Sarver, A.L.; Bergemann, T.L.; Gupta, M.; O'Sullivan, M.G.; Matise, I.; Dupuy, A.J.; et al. A transposon-based genetic screen in mice identifies genes altered in colorectal cancer. *Science* **2009**, *323*, 1747–1750. [CrossRef] [PubMed]
13. He, D.; Wu, L.; Li, X.; Liu, X.; Ma, P.; Juang, Y. Ecotropic virus integration-1 and calreticulin as novel prognostic markers in triple-negative breast cancer: A retrospective cohort study. *Oncol. Lett.* **2019**, *18*, 1847–1855. [CrossRef] [PubMed]
14. Nanjundan, M.; Nakayama, Y.; Cheng, K.W.; Lahad, J.; Liu, J.; Lu, K.; Kuo, W.-L.; Smith-McCune, K.; Fishman, D.; Gray, J.W.; et al. Amplification of *MDS1/EVI1* and *EVI1*, located in the 3q26.2 amplicon, is associated with favorable patient prognosis in ovarian cancer. *Cancer Res.* **2007**, *67*, 3074–3084. [CrossRef] [PubMed]
15. Dutta, P.; Bui, T.; Bauckman, K.A.; Keyomarsi, K.; Mills, G.B.; Nanjundan, M. *EVI1* splice variants modulate functional responses in ovarian cancer cells. *Mol. Oncol.* **2013**, *7*, 647–668. [CrossRef]
16. Bard-Chapeau, E.A.; Gunaratne, J.; Kumar, P.; Chua, B.Q.; Muller, J.; Bard, F.A.; Blackstock, W.; Copeland, N.G.; Jenkins, N.A. EVI1 oncoprotein interacts with a large and complex network of proteins and integrates signals through protein phosphorylation. *Proc. Natl. Acad. Sci. USA* **2013**, *110*, E2885–E2894. [CrossRef]
17. Yoshimi, A.; Kurokawa, M. Evi1 forms a bridge between the epigenetic machinery and signaling pathways. *Oncotarget* **2011**, *2*, 575–586. [CrossRef]
18. Paredes, R.; Schneider, M.; Stevens, A.; White, D.J.; Williamson, A.J.K.; Muter, J.; Pearson, S.; Kelly, J.R.; Connors, K.; Wiseman, D.H.; et al. EVI1 carboxy-terminal phosphorylation is ATM-mediated and sustains transcriptional modulation and self-renewal via enhanced CtBP1 association. *Nucleic Acids Res.* **2018**, *46*, 7662–7674. [CrossRef]
19. Yoshimi, A.; Goyama, S.; Watanabe-Okochi, N.; Yoshiki, Y.; Nannya, Y.; Nitta, E.; Arai, S.; Sato, T.; Shimabe, M.; Nakagawa, M.; et al. Evi1 represses *PTEN* expression and activates PI3K/AKT/mTOR via interactions with polycomb proteins. *Blood* **2011**, *117*, 3617–3628. [CrossRef]

20. Lugthart, S.; Figueroa, M.E.; Bindels, E.; Skrabanek, L.; Valk, P.J.M.; Li, Y.; Meyer, S.; Erpelinck-Verschueren, C.; Greally, J.; Löwenberg, B.; et al. Aberrant DNA hypermethylation signature in acute myeloid leukemia directed by EVI1. *Blood* **2011**, *117*, 234–241. [CrossRef]
21. Cattaneo, F.; Nucifora, G. EVI1 recruits the histone methyltransferase SUV39H1 for transcription repression. *J. Cell. Biochem.* **2008**, *105*, 344–352. [CrossRef] [PubMed]
22. Goyama, S.; Nitta, E.; Yoshino, T.; Kako, S.; Watanabe-Okochi, N.; Shimabe, M.; Imai, Y.; Takahashi, K.; Kurokawa, M. EVI-1 interacts with histone methyltransferases SUV39H1 and G9a for transcriptional repression and bone marrow immortalization. *Leukemia* **2010**, *24*, 81–88. [CrossRef] [PubMed]
23. Spensberger, D.; Delwel, R. A novel interaction between the proto-oncogene Evi1 and histone methyltransferases, SUV39H1 and G9a. *FEBS Lett.* **2008**, *582*, 2761–2767. [CrossRef] [PubMed]
24. Kurokawa, M.; Mitani, K.; Irie, K.; Matsuyama, T.; Takahashi, T.; Chiba, S.; Yazaki, Y.; Matsumoto, K.; Hirai, H. The oncoprotein Evi-1 represses TGF-b signalling by inhibiting Smad3. *Nature* **1998**, *394*, 92–96. [CrossRef]
25. Izutsu, K.; Kurokawa, M.; Imai, Y.; Maki, K.; Mitani, K.; Hirai, H. The corepressor CtBP interacts with Evi-1 to repress transforming growth factor beta signaling. *Blood* **2001**, *97*, 2815–2822. [CrossRef]
26. Sabatini, D.M. mTOR and cancer: insights into a complex relationship. *Nat. Rev. Cancer* **2006**, *6*, 729–734. [CrossRef]
27. Keefe, S.M.; Nathanson, K.L.; Rathmell, W.K. The molecular biology of renal cell carcinoma. *Semin. Oncol.* **2013**, *40*, 421–428. [CrossRef]
28. Motzer, R.J.; Escudier, B.; Oudard, S.; Hutson, T.E.; Porta, C.; Bracarda, S.; Grünwald, V.; Thompson, J.A.; Figlin, R.A.; Hollaender, N.; et al. Efficacy of everolimus in advanced renal cell carcinoma: a double-blind, randomised, placebo-controlled phase III trial. *Lancet* **2008**, *372*, 449–456. [CrossRef]
29. Wagner, B.; Patard, J.-J.; Méjean, A.; Bensalah, K.; Verhoest, G.; Zigeuner, R.; Ficarra, V.; Tostain, J.; Mulders, P.; Chautard, D.; et al. Prognostic value of renal vein and inferior vena cava involvement in renal cell carcinoma. *Eur. Urol.* **2009**, *55*, 452–459. [CrossRef]
30. The Cancer Genome Atlas Research Network. Comprehensive molecular characterization of clear cell renal cell carcinoma. *Nature* **2013**, *499*, 43–49. [CrossRef]
31. Escudier, B.; Molinie, V.; Bracarda, S.; Maroto, P.; Szczylik, C.; Nathan, P.; Negrier, S.; Weiss, C.; Porta, C.; Grünwald, V.; et al. Open-label phase 2 trial of first-line everolimus monotherapy in patients with papillary metastatic renal cell carcinoma: RAPTOR final analysis. *Eur. J. Cancer. 1990* **2016**, *69*, 226–235. [CrossRef] [PubMed]
32. Zoncu, R.; Efeyan, A.; Sabatini, D.M. mTOR: from growth signal integration to cancer, diabetes and ageing. *Nat. Rev. Mol. Cell Biol.* **2011**, *12*, 21–35. [CrossRef] [PubMed]
33. Soler Artigas, M.; Loth, D.W.; Wain, L.V.; Gharib, S.A.; Obeidat, M.; Tang, W.; Zhai, G.; Zhao, J.H.; Smith, A.V.; Huffman, J.E.; et al. Genome-wide association and large-scale follow up identifies 16 new loci influencing lung function. *Nat. Genet.* **2011**, *43*, 1082–1090. [CrossRef] [PubMed]
34. Okada, Y.; Sim, X.; Go, M.J.; Wu, J.-Y.; Gu, D.; Takeuchi, F.; Takahashi, A.; Maeda, S.; Tsunoda, T.; Chen, P.; et al. Meta-analysis identifies multiple loci associated with kidney function-related traits in east Asian populations. *Nat. Genet.* **2012**, *44*, 904–909. [CrossRef]
35. Wain, L.V.; Vaez, A.; Jansen, R.; Joehanes, R.; van der Most, P.J.; Erzurumluoglu, A.M.; O'Reilly, P.F.; Cabrera, C.P.; Warren, H.R.; Rose, L.M.; et al. Novel blood pressure locus and gene discovery using genome-wide association study and expression data sets from blood and the kidney. *Hypertension* **2017**, *70*, e4–e19. [CrossRef]
36. Fehringer, G.; Kraft, P.; Pharoah, P.D.; Eeles, R.A.; Chatterjee, N.; Schumacher, F.R.; Schildkraut, J.M.; Lindström, S.; Brennan, P.; Bickeböller, H.; et al. Cross-cancer genome-wide analysis of lung, ovary, breast, prostate, and colorectal cancer reveals novel pleiotropic associations. *Cancer Res.* **2016**, *76*, 5103–5114. [CrossRef]
37. Holder, A.M.; Akcakanat, A.; Adkins, F.; Evans, K.; Chen, H.; Wei, C.; Milton, D.R.; Li, Y.; Do, K.-A.; Janku, F.; et al. Epithelial to mesenchymal transition is associated with rapamycin resistance. *Oncotarget* **2015**, *6*, 19500–19513. [CrossRef]
38. Valianou, M.; Filippidou, N.; Johnson, D.L.; Vogel, P.; Zhang, E.Y.; Liu, X.; Lu, Y.; Yu, J.J.; Bissler, J.J.; Astrinidis, A. Rapalog resistance is associated with mesenchymal-type changes in *Tsc2*-null cells. *Sci. Rep.* **2019**, *9*, 3015. [CrossRef]

39. Fenouille, N.; Bassil, C.F.; Ben-Sahra, I.; Benajiba, L.; Alexe, G.; Ramos, A.; Pikman, Y.; Conway, A.S.; Burgess, M.R.; Li, Q.; et al. The creatine kinase pathway is a metabolic vulnerability in EVI1-positive acute myeloid leukemia. *Nat. Med.* **2017**, *23*, 301–313. [CrossRef]
40. Saito, Y.; Sawa, D.; Kinoshita, M.; Yamada, A.; Kamimura, S.; Suekane, A.; Ogoh, H.; Matsuo, H.; Adachi, S.; Taga, T.; et al. EVI1 triggers metabolic reprogramming associated with leukemogenesis and increases sensitivity to L-asparaginase. *Haematologica* **2019**. [CrossRef]
41. Sánchez-Gastaldo, A.; Kempf, E.; González Del Alba, A.; Duran, I. Systemic treatment of renal cell cancer: A comprehensive review. *Cancer Treat. Rev.* **2017**, *60*, 77–89. [CrossRef] [PubMed]
42. Mariathasan, S.; Turley, S.J.; Nickles, D.; Castiglioni, A.; Yuen, K.; Wang, Y.; Kadel, E.E.; Koeppen, H.; Astarita, J.L.; Cubas, R.; et al. TGFβ attenuates tumour response to PD-L1 blockade by contributing to exclusion of T cells. *Nature* **2018**, *554*, 544–548. [CrossRef] [PubMed]
43. Ravi, R.; Noonan, K.A.; Pham, V.; Bedi, R.; Zhavoronkov, A.; Ozerov, I.V.; Makarev, E.; Artemov, A.V.; Wysocki, P.T.; Mehra, R.; et al. Bifunctional immune checkpoint-targeted antibody-ligand traps that simultaneously disable TGFβ enhance the efficacy of cancer immunotherapy. *Nat. Commun.* **2018**, *9*, 741. [CrossRef] [PubMed]
44. Lan, Y.; Zhang, D.; Xu, C.; Hance, K.W.; Marelli, B.; Qi, J.; Yu, H.; Qin, G.; Sircar, A.; Hernández, V.M.; et al. Enhanced preclinical antitumor activity of M7824, a bifunctional fusion protein simultaneously targeting PD-L1 and TGF-β. *Sci. Transl. Med.* **2018**, *10*, 424. [CrossRef] [PubMed]
45. Bodnar, L.; Stec, R.; Cierniak, S.; Synowiec, A.; Wcisło, G.; Jesiotr, M.; Koktysz, R.; Kozłowski, W.; Szczylik, C. Clinical usefulness of PI3K/Akt/mTOR genotyping in companion with other clinical variables in metastatic renal cell carcinoma patients treated with everolimus in the second and subsequent lines. *Ann. Oncol.* **2015**, *26*, 1385–1389. [CrossRef] [PubMed]
46. Sauerbrei, W.; Taube, S.E.; McShane, L.M.; Cavenagh, M.M.; Altman, D.G. Reporting recommendations for tumor marker prognostic studies (REMARK): an abridged explanation and elaboration. *J. Natl. Cancer Inst.* **2018**, *110*, 803–811. [CrossRef]
47. Ricketts, C.J.; De Cubas, A.A.; Fan, H.; Smith, C.C.; Lang, M.; Reznik, E.; Bowlby, R.; Gibb, E.A.; Akbani, R.; Beroukhim, R.; et al. The Cancer Genome Atlas comprehensive molecular characterization of renal cell carcinoma. *Cell Rep.* **2018**, *23*, e313–326.e5. [CrossRef]
48. Subramanian, A.; Tamayo, P.; Mootha, V.K.; Mukherjee, S.; Ebert, B.L.; Gillette, M.A.; Paulovich, A.; Pomeroy, S.L.; Golub, T.R.; Lander, E.S.; et al. Gene set enrichment analysis: a knowledge-based approach for interpreting genome-wide expression profiles. *Proc. Natl. Acad. Sci. USA* **2005**, *102*, 15545–15550. [CrossRef]

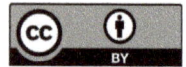

© 2020 by the authors. Licensee MDPI, Basel, Switzerland. This article is an open access article distributed under the terms and conditions of the Creative Commons Attribution (CC BY) license (http://creativecommons.org/licenses/by/4.0/).

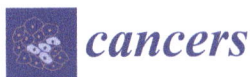

Article

In-Depth Mapping of the Urinary N-Glycoproteome: Distinct Signatures of ccRCC-related Progression

Lucia Santorelli [1,*,†], Giulia Capitoli [2,†], Clizia Chinello [1], Isabella Piga [1], Francesca Clerici [1], Vanna Denti [1], Andrew Smith [1], Angelica Grasso [3], Francesca Raimondo [1], Marco Grasso [4] and Fulvio Magni [1]

[1] Clinical Proteomics and Metabolomics Unit, School of Medicine and Surgery, University of Milano-Bicocca, 20854 Vedano al Lambro, Italy; clizia.chinello@gmail.com (C.C.); isabella.piga@unimib.it (I.P.); f.clerici10@campus.unimib.it (F.C.); v.denti@campus.unimib.it (V.D.); andrew.smith@unimib.it (A.S.); francesca.raimondo@unimib.it (F.R.); fulvio.magni@unimib.it (F.M.)
[2] Centre of Biostatistics for Clinical Epidemiology, School of Medicine and Surgery, University of Milano-Bicocca, 20854 Vedano al Lambro, Italy; g.capitoli@campus.unimib.it
[3] Urology Service, Department of Surgery, EOC Beata Vergine Regional Hospital, 23, 6850 Mendrisio, Switzerland; angelica_grasso@yahoo.it
[4] Urology Unit, S. Gerardo Hospital, 20900 Monza, Italy; m.grasso@hsgerardo.org
* Correspondence: luciasantorelli13@gmail.com; Tel.: +39-026-448-8246
† These authors contributed equally to this paper.

Received: 29 November 2019; Accepted: 14 January 2020; Published: 18 January 2020

Abstract: Protein N-glycosylation is one of the most important post-translational modifications and is involved in many biological processes, with aberrant changes in protein N-glycosylation patterns being closely associated with several diseases, including the progression and spreading of tumours. In light of this, identifying these aberrant protein glycoforms in tumours could be useful for understanding the molecular mechanism of this multifactorial disease, developing specific biomarkers and finding novel therapeutic targets. We investigated the urinary N-glycoproteome of clear cell renal cell carcinoma (ccRCC) patients at different stages ($n = 15$ at pT1 and $n = 15$ at pT3), and of non-ccRCC subjects ($n = 15$), using an N-glyco-FASP-based method. Using label-free nLC-ESI MS/MS, we identified and quantified several N-glycoproteins with altered expression and abnormal changes affecting the occupancy of the glycosylation site in the urine of RCC patients compared to control. In particular, nine of them had a specific trend that was directly related to the stage progression: CD97, COCH and P3IP1 were up-expressed whilst APOB, FINC, CERU, CFAH, HPT and PLTP were down-expressed in ccRCC patients. Overall, these results expand our knowledge related to the role of this post-translational modification in ccRCC and translation of this information into pre-clinical studies could have a significant impact on the discovery of novel biomarkers and therapeutic target in kidney cancer.

Keywords: clear cell Renal Cell Carcinoma; urine; glycoproteomics; N-glycomapping; label-free; glycomarkers

1. Introduction

Malignant transformation is a complex of heterogeneous cellular events that regulates the growth and survival cycle of affected cells. Among cancer-associated alterations, changes in protein N-glycosylation have recently received attention as one of the key events that are able to influence the onset of neoplasia and its consequent spreading [1].

N-glycosylation represents one of the most prominent protein post-translational modification (PTMs) and play a role in determining several protein properties, defining its correct tertiary structure, specific function as well as its cellular localisation [2]. Under physiological conditions, N-glycosylated proteins have various biological functions, including folding and quality control, cell adhesion and motility, molecular trafficking, cell signalling, immune recognition and clearance [3].

Moreover, the fundamental role of this PTM in oncogenesis has been widely documented over seven decades [4,5]. In fact, high levels of altered N-glycosylated proteins are demonstrated to promote tumour invasiveness as well as being correlated with a high frequency of tumour recurrence and metastasis. Furthermore, aberrant changes to N-glycosylated protein patterns frequently accompany the transformation of normal tissue towards neoplasia [6,7] and these abnormal changes essentially affect the occupancy of the glycosylation sites (glycan macro-heterogeneity) and/or the attached N-glycan structures (glycan micro-heterogeneity) [8,9].

Given their evident role in cancer development, a consistent group of glycoproteins have recently passed the discovery and validation phases and are regularly used in clinical practice as cancer biomarkers, successfully completing the research bench to the patient bedside program. Most of the approved cancer glycoprotein-based biomarkers (glycomarkers) are proteins derived from diverse bodily fluids. Prostate-specific antigen (PSA), for example, which is largely present in seminal fluids and plasma, has been used to screen and monitor prostate cancer patients for 20 years [10,11]. Cancer antigen 15-3 and cancer antigen 125, both detected in serum [12], are useful biomarkers for breast [12] and ovarian [13,14] tumours, respectively, and are particularly used for monitoring affected patients and evaluating the possibility of disease recurrence. Finally, N-glycosylated protein markers also include the carcinoembryonic antigen (CEA), detectable principally in blood [15,16], which has been correlated with colorectal, bladder, breast, pancreatic and lung cancers [17,18].

In this context, an easily accessible biological sample, such as urine, is a valuable source of glycomarkers for kidney cancer-related diseases. Urine can be collected non-invasively and in large quantities, with its molecular composition being less complex than other bodily fluids, and it is for these reasons that the use of the urinary proteomics has expanded exponentially in recent years [19,20]. Owing to the rapid development of MS-based technologies and their application in clinical research, the urinary proteome was extensively explored and numerous urinary glycoproteins were brought to light and characterised in healthy subjects [21]. Concerning, the typical proteome of healthy human urine counts almost 2500 proteins [22] and about 300 of these are reported to be N-glycosylated [23].

Whilst the urine proteome was widely investigated in clear cell renal cell carcinoma (ccRCC), the most aggressive RCC morphotype [24], limited information describing the urinary N-glycoproteome is available. Furthermore, despite ccRCC being commonly diagnosed at the early stages, its aggressiveness and clinical outcomes remain heterogeneous within each staging group, making the research for novel diagnostic and prognostic predictors an urgent priority.

Since cancer transformation causes alterations in the synthesis and expression of specific glycosylated proteins, evaluating the urinary glycoprotein content of ccRCC-affected patients represents a valid strategy to expand our knowledge regarding the role of this modification in the onset of cancer. In this context, we applied a glycoproteomic approach to study urine of ccRCC patients at early (pT1) and advanced (pT3) stages compared to urine of unaffected ccRCC subjects (controls, CTRL). Our final goal was to identify potential biologically relevant indicators of the development and progression of ccRCC in order to provide support for stage-related classification and defining the course of treatment.

2. Results

2.1. Clinical Data and Study Design

To identify potential protein N-glycoforms of interest, urine of 15 controls and 30 ccRCC patients were collected. Three urine pools were prepared, one representative of the CTRL and other two of ccRCC, one of pT1 and one of pT3 (15 subjects for each pool) (Table 1). Then, each pool was analysed by nUHPLC-MS/MS.

Table 1. Clinicopathological data regarding the patients enrolled in the study.

Group	# of Patients	Gender (Male-Female)	Age Mean (Range)	Tumour Dimension (cm)
CTRL	15	10–5	57.9 (39–77)	/
pT1	15	8–7	67.8 (42–82)	4
pT3	15	12–3	68.9 (45–81)	12

2.2. Mapping of the N-Glycosylation Sites

Urinary N-glycoproteins were extracted by an N-Glyco-FASP method [25]. Tryptic peptides (~100 µg) were incubated in the presence of a triad of lectins that are able to bind to different types of carbohydrates. By using filter units, the N-glycosylated peptides were then isolated and underwent enzymatic hydrolysis by PNGase F. This enzymatic reaction caused the release of the deglycosylated peptides from lectins and were then analysed by nanoLC-ESI-MS/MS. Those peptides that were present in the whole proteome and not deamidated as a result of the PNGase F treatment were removed from the list of the N-glycopeptides.

First, we investigated the whole N-glycopeptidome of the three groups of patients in order to uncover possible differences in terms of N-glycan macro-heterogeneity. More than 760 N-glycopeptides were comprehensively identified: 479 in CTRL, 484 in pT1 and 513 in pT3, respectively (Table S1). Among these, 35.1% were observed to be present in all the groups, 24% were exclusively present in two of the three groups (CTRL and pT1 3%; CTRL and pT3 10.7%, pT1 and pT3 10.3%), whilst the 14.2%, 15.3% and 11.4% were specifically related to CTRL, pT1 and pT3, respectively.

In order to determine the recurrence frequency of the consensus and non-consensus regions in the identified peptides, we subsequently evaluated the sites distribution of the N-glycosylation in the urinary proteome. Considering that the canonical N-glycosylation motif of proteins is N-x-S/T (where x are all the amino acids, with the exception of proline), we observed a variation of the glycosylated sites between the CTRL and ccRCC patients (Table 2a).

Initially, we compared the CTRL and the ccRCC subjects, without considering the pT feature as variable. We observed that the ratio between the number of asparagine modified (N̲) present in the glycopeptides-enriched fraction and the total number of asparagine, modified and unmodified (N) in the corresponding proteome was constant in the two groups. For both samples, threonine (T) and serine (S) were significantly overrepresented, meaning that most of the identified urinary N-glycosites were typical sites. Moreover, N-glycosites that matched with N-x-T (88% CTRL, 82% ccRCC) occurred more frequently than those that matched with N-x-S (71% CTRL, 69% ccRCC) (Table 2a). The differences between controls and affected subjects emerged by considering the sequence motif around the N-glycosites. For the ccRCC samples, we observed a general decrease in the frequency of the N̲ within the consensus regions and a corresponding increase of the frequency within the non-consensus regions (Table 2a).

Subsequently, we investigated the ccRCC samples cohort according to the pT feature, considering the two sub-groups pT1 and pT3, separately. The N-glycosites mapping analysis showed a global decrease in the N-glycosylation level for the pT1 compared to CTRL group (Table 2b, Figure S1a). In fact, we observed a reduction of 8% when considering the consensus sequence N-x-T, but an increment of the N̲ in the non-consensus sequences (14%) (Table 2b, Figure S1a).

The N̲ as a part of non-consensus motifs was observed to increase even further in the pT3 glycoproteome (29%), suggesting a correlation between an altered glycosylation of non-consensus sequences and ccRCC. We also detected a decrease of glycosylation frequency for the motif N-x-T (-7%) in pT3, despite an overall increment of the total modified asparagine on all the sequences (9%) (Table 2b, Figure S1a).

Considering the distribution of the N-glycosylation sites of the peptides present in of the three groups, it is worth noting that the percentages were very similar (Table 2c, Figure S1b); this indicates that the differences observed for all the identified glycosylated peptides are not due to differences in the quantities of the peptides tested. These data support the presence of alterations to the N-glycosylation pattern in ccRCC patients compared to healthy subjects.

Table 2. The N-glycomapping of the urinary peptidome of CTRL and clear cell renal cell carcinoma (ccRCC) patients.

(**a**) Comparison of the N-glycosylation distribution (%) between the CTRL and ccRCC patients cohorts.

N-glycosylated Asparagine Distribution	% CTRL	% ccRCC
N̲/N tot	21	21
N̲ in ncSeq/N ncSeq tot	5.6	6.8
N̲ in cSeq/N cSeq tot	81	77
N̲-x-T/N-x-T tot	88	82
N̲-x-S/N-x-S tot	71	69

(**b**) Comparison of the N-glycosylation distribution (%) between CTRL and pT1 and CTRL and pT3 patients cohorts, measured by considering all the identified peptides, shared and not shared in the three groups.

% CTRL	pT1	Variation		% CTRL	pT3	Variation
21	19	−10	N̲/N tot	21	23	9
5.6	6.4	14	N̲ in ncSeq/N ncSeq tot	5.6	7.2	29
81	75	−7	N̲ in cSeq/N cSeq tot	81	79	−2
88	81	−8	N̲-x-T/N-x-T tot	88	82	−7
71	66	7	N̲-x-S/N-x-S tot	71	73	3

(**c**) Comparison of the N-glycosylation distribution (%) between CTRL and pT1 and CTRL and pT3 patients cohorts, determined by taking into account the identified peptides common to all three groups.

% CTRL	pT1	Variation		% CTRL	pT3	Variation
66	66	0	N̲/N tot	66	66	0
31	37	19	N̲ in ncSeq/N ncSeq tot	31	37	19
91	88	−3	N̲ in cSeq/N cSeq tot	91	88	−3
92	88	−4	N̲-x-T/N-x-T tot	92	88	−4
89	88	−1	N̲-x-S/N-x-S tot	89	89	0

ncSeq: non-consensus sequence; cSeq: consensus sequence; N̲: asparagine glycomodified; N: asparagine glycomodified and non glycomodified.

In order to better characterise the N-glycosylated peptides, we determined the amino acid composition of the N-glycosylation motif. Then, we estimated the frequency of single amino acidic residues present at the +3 position in the modified triplet N̲-x-x (Figure 1).

Results clearly showed that the consensus sequences N-x-T/S were most frequently modified in both early and advanced cancer conditions (Figure 1).

However, some remarks can also be formulated regarding the frequency of any non-canonical motif. In the pT1 group, for example, a preference for the other amino acids at the +3 position was detectable. Specifically, we recorded an increased frequency of glutamic acid (E), glycine (G), histidine (H), leucine (L), isoleucine (I), methionine (M), asparagine (N) and valine (V). At the same time, we also highlighted a mild inflection for the non-consensus sequence containing cysteine (C), aspartic acid (D), lysine (K) and glutamine (Q) (Figure 1).

In the pT3 group, the non-canonical triplets contained an increased amount of the amino acids D, glutamine (Q) and arginine (R), in addition to those already detected in the pT1 group (Figure 1). Conversely, a consistent decrease in residue V was observed and comparable to both the CTRL and pT1 groups, whilst the amino acids G and L showed a similar level to that of control subjects (Figure 1).

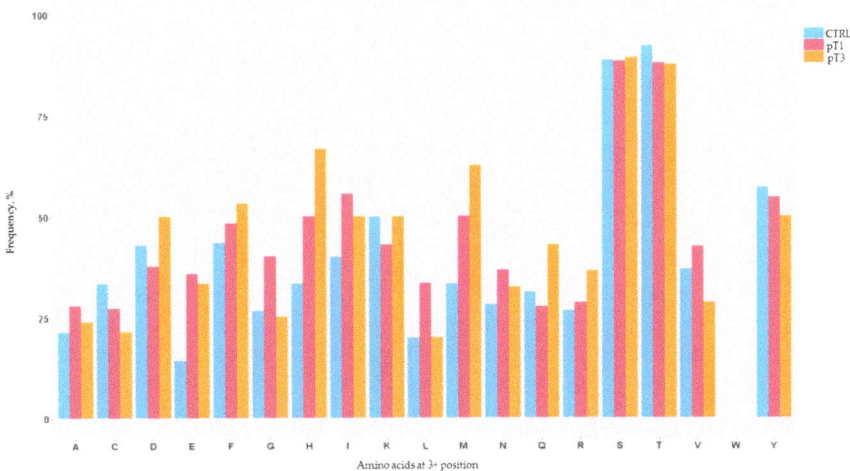

Figure 1. The frequencies of each amino acid in the +3 position in the triplet N-x-x presented in the urinary N-glycoproteome calculated for the CTRL, pT1 and pT3 groups. These frequencies were measured considering the identified peptides in all of the three cohorts.

2.3. Characterisation of the Urinary N-Glycoproteins: Identification

After characterising the number and distribution of the N-glycomodified sites, we evaluated the tryptic peptides identified by nUHPLC-MS/MS in term of proteins identification: 299 different N-glycoprotein species were identified with FDR peptide-spectrum matches of 1% and at least one unique peptide (Table S2).

Comparing lists of the identified proteins showed that half were shared among the three groups (50.2%). Moreover, we noticed three clusters of proteins that were specific for each group: 11% related to pT1, 8% to pT3 and 10.7% to CTRL (Figure 2).

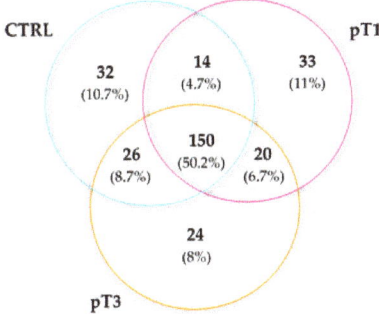

Figure 2. Distribution of the urine N-glycoproteins identified by shotgun LC-MS illustrated by a Venn diagram.

2.4. Characterisation of the Urinary N-Glycoproteins: Functional Analysis

To obtain an overview of the primary subcellular compartments, molecular functions and biological process in which the identified N-linked glycoproteins were implicated, we used Cytoscape tool (https://cytoscape.org/last access March 2019) to perform Gene Ontology (GO) function enrichment analysis.

Overall, the most represented subcellular compartments were the extracellular space, lysosomes, membranes, endocytic and extracellular vesicles, which are generally involved in the processes of

N-glycoprotein synthesis and transport blood components and plasma lipoprotein particles were also significantly enriched (Figure S2a).

Furthermore, many molecular functions that are known to be performed by N-glycoproteins were enriched. As shown in Figure S2, the principle clusters affected were binding activity (carbohydrate, chaperone, immune component), extracellular matrix remodelling and receptor activity (Figure S2b).

Finally, the major biological processes that were overrepresented included regulation of vesicle transport, tissue homeostasis, extracellular structure organisation and remodelling, aminoglycan and oligosaccharide metabolisms, endocytosis and blood vessel morphogenesis (Figure S2c).

The principal clusters that emerged for each GO class differed in terms of number of enriched proteins in the controls compared to ccRCC groups. In particular, a substantial increment of those N-glycoproteins that compromise a component of immunoglobulin complexes was observed for both early and advanced ccRCC stages whilst an overrepresentation of N-glycoproteins related to cellular membrane and immune secretory vesicles could be seen depending upon the pT1 status. For the process of vesiculation, the pT1 stage seemed decrease in terms of endocytic activity and increase in the corresponding secretory activity. This evidence was confirmed either by GO terms, cellular component or biological process (Figure S2a,c).

2.5. Characterisation of the Urinary N-Glycoproteins: Quantitative Analysis

A label-free quantitation approach was used to evaluate the relative glycoproteins content present in ccRCC and control urine. Differentially expressed proteins were selected based upon their fold change among the CTRL, pT1 and pT3 groups. We selected those marker-proteins that were detected in two analytical replicates with ≥ 2 or ≤ -2-fold changes (adjusted p-value ≤ 0.05).

The majority of potential candidate markers were upregulated in the disease N-glycoproteome (Figure 3). These included proteins implicated in lipid transport and metabolic processes (e.g., FOLR1, LRP2, PLTP, CATD), immune system processes (e.g., CD97, HPT, A1AT, CD63, PTGDS, CD276) as well as control and maintenance of the cellular shape (e.g., COCH, FINC).

Considering the abundance levels of the significantly dysregulated proteins, we observed a panel of glycoproteins whose specific trend in abundance was related to the stage progression. This panel includes nine proteins of interest, six of which were also identified and quantified in the whole urinary proteome. These nine proteins were differently expressed in the comparisons pT1 vs. CTRL and pT3 vs. CTRL; three of them showed an increasing pattern (CD97, COCH and P3IP1), whilst six presented a decreasing trend (APOB, FINC, CERU, HPT, CFAH and PLTP). It is noteworthy that all the down-regulated glycoproteins showed a considerable decrease in pT1 whilst their levels increased in the pT3 group (Figure 4).

(a)

pT1 vs CTRL		
Total Varied Proteins: 17		
Protein	p-Value adj	Fold Change
UP: 5		
• COCH	0.001	4.78
• CD97	0.005	3.03
• FOLR1	0.004	2.29
• LRP2	0.001	2.22
• P3IP1	0.01	2.18
DOWN: 12		
• APOB	0.004	−34.3
• FINC	0.001	−24.5
• HPT	0.000	−14.70
• CFAH	0.001	−11.61
• PLTP	0.001	−9.76
• A1AT	0.001	−6.13
• TRFE	0.000	−3.59
• CD63	0.004	−3.47
• CERU	0.001	−3.12
• IGHA2	0.000	−2.60
• HEMO	0.001	−2.55
• APOH	0.005	−2.52

(b)

pT3 vs CTRL		
Total Varied Proteins: 17		
Protein	p-Value adj	Fold Change
UP: 10		
• COCH	0.013	4.77
• CD97	0.000	3.82
• LAMP2	0.000	3.13
• AMBP	0.002	3.09
• P3IP1	0.001	2.60
• PTGDS	0.000	2.47
• WFDC2	0.000	2.44
• ZA2G	0.000	2.41
• CD276	0.000	2.3
• CATD	0.000	2.12
DOWN: 7		
• CERU	0.000	−2.06
• HPT	0.000	−2.41
• PERM	0.000	−2.52
• PLTP	0.000	−3.30
• FINC	0.000	−6.04
• CFAH	0.001	−6.16
• APOB	0.001	−9.59

(c)

pT3 vs pT1		
Total varied proteins: 14		
Protein	p-value adj	Fold change
UP: 13		
• KLK1	0.000	6.87
• HPT	0.003	6.10
• A1AT	0.002	4.18
• FINC	0.020	4.05
• TRFE	0.002	3.32
• PLTP	0.034	2.96
• AMBP	0.001	2.68
• ZA2G	0.000	2.54
• APOH	0.002	2.44
• PPAP	0.004	2.22
• CD63	0.002	2.11
• A1AG2	0.000	2.07
• CD276	0.002	2.06
DOWN: 1		
• PERM	0.006	−3.32

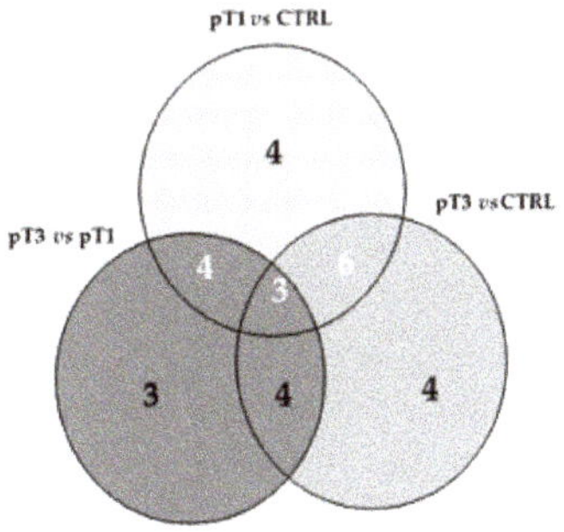

(d)

Figure 3. Lists of *N*-glycoproteins significantly varied in the comparisons: pT1 vs. CTRL (**a**), pT3 vs. CTRL (**b**), pT3 vs. Pt1 (**c**). The number of *N*-glycosylated proteins that significantly varied in each group represented by Venn diagram (**d**).

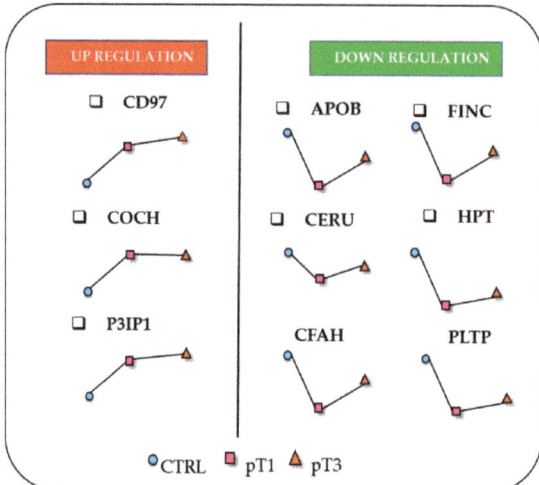

Figure 4. Panel of urinary N-glycosylated proteins with the relative abundance trend of each one in the three different sub-cohorts (CTRL, pT1, pT3).

3. Discussion

In this study, we detected alterations in the N-glycosylation pattern of proteins in ccRCC patient urine relative to healthy subjects. In fact, we observed an increased frequency of glycosylation in non-consensus regions in ccRCC, showing a specific distribution of glycosites related to patients at early (pT1) and advanced (pT3) stages.

Over the years, the N-glycan distribution on proteins has been extensively investigated. In fact, many efforts were spent in order to set up the most proficient MS-analytical strategy for mapping the N-glycoproteome, enabling the glycoprotein content of different kinds of samples, including cell lines, plants, tissue and bodily fluids to be analysed [25–30]. Currently, studies that aim to evaluate the occurrence of N-glycosylation within non-consensus sequences in disease conditions are rapidly increasing in number, but the process is still not completely understood. Notwithstanding, acquisition of unconventional N-glycosylation sites was described for diverse pathologies, such as follicular and Burkitt's lymphomas, pancreatic, ovarian, prostatic and gastric cancers [11,31–35].

Some amino acids, such as N, G, C and V were described as part of the N-glycosylation motif in several studies [36–38] and it was demonstrated that such atypical sites, when glycomodified, play a significant role in biological processes, as well as the canonical counterpart motif T/S [39,40]. As a whole, this suggests that the involvement of glycan macro-heterogeneity may also alter the pathogenesis and progression of ccRCC.

These findings were supported by the isolated N-glycoproteins that were identified and quantified in this study. We noted the presence of a group of glycoproteins common to healthy subjects and ccRCC patients at different stages, suggesting the existence of a glycoproteic core of the urinary proteome. In fact, considering the specific role and/or subcellular localisation that the N-glycosylation confers to the proteins, it is not surprising that the biological feature of the glycan macro-heterogeneity remains constant, even within a tumour environment [25]. At the same time, each group of samples contained specific proteins and these represented a disease-stage specific signature.

According to their localization, the identified glycoproteins belong to the subcellular compartments, sites of the N-glycoprotein formation process. In addition, blood components and plasma lipoprotein particles were significantly enriched since the proteins related to these classes are usually the most abundant ones isolated from the urine [41,42], especially in case of kidney impairment and pathological conditions. Regarding GO classification, as expected, the proteins involved in the immunological pattern were largely enriched, supporting the well-known role of immune response in the onset and progression of ccRCC [43].

In addition, we identified nine N-glycoproteins that could be characteristic of the early stage of tumourigenesis, and potentially a glycosignature of the tumour condition. Since ccRCC is a heterogeneous disease, it seems unlikely that only one biomarker will be uniformly elevated. Therefore, a panel of biomarkers may provide more accurate diagnosis than any given single marker.

It is remarkable that PLPT, CD97 and COCH were detected and quantified only after the glycopeptide enrichment, indicating further potential for this approach.

Haptoglobin (HPT), fibronectin (FINC), ceruplasmin (CERU), apolipoprotein-B (APOB), phospholipid transfer protein (PLTP) and complement factor H (CFAH) were down-expressed in urine of RCC patients (Figure 3a,b and Figure 4). Among them, HPT is one of the proteins that is most reported to be affected by oligosaccharide modifications in human malignancies, including ovarian, liver, colon and pancreatic cancers, and its N-glycosylation status is different from one type of cancer to another [44–48]. However, all those studies were particularly focused on the N-glycan portion of HPT present in serum or plasma samples. To the best of our knowledge, no data that focuses on the N-glycosylated isoform of HPT in the ccRCC tumour is currently available. Our result seems to be in contrast with another proteomic study that highlighted an over-secretion of HPT in the urine of ccRCC patients [49]. However, the data are not directly comparable with those of Sadim et al.'s work, where the patients were grouped according with the Fuhrman grade, mixing pT1, 2 and 3, and were of different age compared to our cohort.

Moreover, our data are supported by the findings reported by Bruneel et al. that showed decreased levels of glycosylated HPT in the serum of patients affected by congenital disorders of glycosylation, rare inherited diseases, suggesting that it can be valid as a biomarker with diagnostic relevance for this pathology [50].

A similar consideration can be done for FINC, an extracellular matrix glycoprotein that plays important roles in cellular adhesion and mediation of cell migration and metastasis formation [51,52]. These functions are exploited through N-glycosylation modifications, in synergy with integrin-mediated signals [53]. Several studies performed on tissue samples proposed that the overexpression of FINC is an unfavourable prognostic indicator for diverse cancer types, such as breast and pancreatic cancer, nasopharyngeal and neck squamous cell carcinomas [54–56]. Regarding RCC, this protein seems to promote cell growth and migration [57]. Moreover, Kondisette et al. investigated the relationship of FINC with the clinical stage of tumour, pinpointed the increase of FINC expression levels in RCC tissue compared to controls, as particularly significant for the early stage condition [58]. In our analysis, we observed a different correlation between the urinary abundance levels of FINC and the cancer stage. In fact, we noted a strong decrease of the N-glycosylated FINC levels in the pT1 group (Figures 3a and 4), both for the total protein and the glycosylated form. In light of this, it is arguable that FINC could be retained by cancer cells, and not secreted in urine. On the other hand, a sort of balance between the N-glycosylated and the non-glycosylated isoform of FINC could exist and may occur in order to decrease the expression of N-glycosylated FINC, in favour of the non-glycosylated form, and may represent a fundamental equilibrium in the early process of ccRCC tumorigenesis [59].

The glycoprotein CERU is normally synthesised in the liver and is involved in different cellular processes [60]. Several studies have demonstrated that CERU expression is required for the growth and survival of tumours. In fact, CERU protein levels were increased in various forms of human tumours, including breast (saliva and plasma), bile duct (tissue microarray), oral and gastrointestinal tract cancers (blood) [61–64]. On the contrary, CERU abundance was decreased in urine of the HER2-enriched subtype of breast cancer with respect to healthy controls [65]. Concerning ccRCC, it is reported that the expression of the *CERU* gene can distinguish a subset of RCC patients with poor outcome, independently from the known genetic aberrations [66]. In addition, a quantitative proteomic study associated the high serum levels of CERU with the histopathological classification of stage and/or grade of RCC [67]. Moreover, high levels of CERU were found in ccRCC patients at the level of urinary exosomes, a specific compartment of urine [68]. However, no previous studies that focused specifically on the role of the N-glycosylation of this protein in ccRCC are present in the literature.

Known as the primary apolipoprotein, APOB plays a key role in lipid transport, lipoprotein metabolism and the recognition of lipoprotein receptors. It is the major constituent of the atherogenic particles and its plasma concentration represents a useful marker for cardiovascular risk. Moreover, increasing evidence shows that high concentrations of plasma APOB are also associated with poor prognosis in patients with hepatocellular carcinoma [69] and breast cancer [70]. High levels of APOB in urine were proposed as a potential marker and a prognostic factor for bladder cancer [71]. The analysis of tissue microarrays highlighted the cytoplasmic expression of APOB in ccRCC, indicating the storage of lipoproteins rather than lipids [72]. Very recently, the APOB/A1 ratio in preoperative blood sample was proposed as an independent prognostic factor in metastatic renal cell carcinoma [73]. Here, we detected APOB in urine, focusing on its glycosylated isoform (Figure 3a,b and Figure 4). It is of particular relevance considering that there is a specific influence of N-linked glycosylation on LDL pathways and lipid metabolism [74].

Interestingly, among the candidate glycomarkers, there is another protein involved in lipoprotein metabolism. PLTP is a non-specific lipid transfer protein [75]. Remarkably, this is the first report of PLTP being present in urine and of its association with RCC. It seems to play a role in lipoprotein assembly, which also involves APOB, although there is no evidence of any direct interaction [76]. In this regard, since that both the proteins are part of the lipoprotein metabolism, the simultaneous reduction of PLTP and APOB in the urine of ccRCC patients could make sense (Figure 3a,b and Figure 4). Moreover, the differential expression of PLTP is documented in multiple types of tumours, including prostate, ovarian, breast, lung carcinoma and glioma. In particular, the study performed on brain tissue of glioma patients showed a correlation between PLTP expression and the tumour grade [77].

The plasma glycoprotein CFAH is the main regulator of the alternative complement pathway, inhibiting the activation of the complement system and thus protecting host cells [78]. Given its role, CFAH alterations can have serious implications and cause various diseases, including several cancers, such as non-small cell lung cancer, ovarian cancer, and colon cancer [79–81]. In particular, in human lung cancer tissues, CFAH over-expression was associated with a shorter survival time [82]. There are no relevant data regarding the expression of CFAH in relation with RCC, nor in tissue, nor in biological fluid studies. As hypothesised for FINC, cancer cells could modulate the secretion of CFAH in order to maintain high levels in the tumour microenvironment as a mechanism of protection.

Among the over-expressed proteins, PIK3IP1 is a cell-surface glycoprotein reported as a negative regulator of the PI3K pathway [83]. The transcriptional regulation and expression of PIK3IP1 directly affects the PI3K signalling in tumorigenesis. In fact, the downregulation of this inhibitor contributes to increased tumour growth [84], whilst its over-expression in mouse hepatocytes leads to the suppression of hepatocyte carcinoma development [85]. In this context, it is noteworthy that this protein was over-represented in the urine of ccRCC patients (Figure 3a,b and Figure 4). In this case, the assumption made for FINC, APOB and PLTP would be the opposite: cancer cells eliminate more PIK3IP1 protein in the urine, as a mechanism to down-regulate its expression, in order to survive.

Finally, we found CD97 and COCH over-expression in RCC patient urine (Figure 3a,b and Figure 4). There is currently no evidence of an association with RCC. CD97 is an adhesion G protein-coupled receptor (GPCR) that is expressed on multiple hematopoietic cell types. Favouring the migration and invasive properties of cancer cells, it is involved in various non-hematopoietic malignancies including breast, thyroid, gastric, and prostate carcinoma, as well as glioblastoma. Furthermore, the role of CD97 was explored in acute myeloid leukaemia and was also related to the PI3K/Akt pathway [86]. COCH is a protein of the extracellular matrix (ECM) that is expressed prevalently at the cochlea level and is associated mainly with hearing defects [87]. Its function is not completely understood, and it is presented in numerous heterogeneous isoforms because of N-glycosylation modification and proteolytic cleavage.

To conclude, we also investigated the gene expression of our putative glycomarkers in comparison with the Human Protein Atlas database (www.proteinatlas.org). We considered the mRNA expression in the cell-enriched group in order to verify the renal tissue specificity of the urinary dysregulated proteins identified in our study. Different mRNA expression levels of CD97, CERU, CFAH, COCH, FINC, HPT, PLTP and P3 IP1 were detected and confirmed in diverse cell lines related to the urinary tract, including normal human embryonic renal cell line (HEK 293), human embryonal carcinoma cell line (NTERA-2), normal human renal proximal tubule epithelial cell line (RPTEC/TERT1), human hypertriploid renal carcinoma cells (786-O cells), human renal cell line (Caki-1), human bladder cancer cell line (RT4) and human prostate cancer cell line (PC-3). To our knowledge, no data concerning the gene expression of APOB in other cell line models suitable for the in vitro study of ccRCC are available.

4. Materials and Methods

4.1. Urine Collection and Processing

Forty-five patients, 30 ccRCC and 15 non-RCC, were enrolled between 2011 and 2016 at San Gerardo hospital (Monza, Italy). All participants gave their informed consent prior to sample collection. Study protocols and procedures were approved by the local ethic committee (Comitato Etico Azienda Ospedaliera San Gerardo, Monza, Italy, BPCR 24-02-2011) and analysis were carried out in agreement with the Declaration of Helsinki. Second morning midstream urine before total or partial nephrectomy (for ccRCC patients) was collected in sterile urine tubes. The collected samples were cleared by centrifuging at 4 °C at $1000 \times g$ for 10 min to remove cells and debris and stored at −80 °C until the day of the analysis.

4.2. Sample Population

Three urine pools were prepared (15 subjects each), one for the CTRL, one for ccRCC at pT1 and one for ccRCC at pT3. The stage stratification was confirmed by radiological evaluation and pathological assessment of the surgical specimens. Each patient contributed to the pool sample with an equal amount of proteins (70 µg).

4.3. Urinary Proteins Digestion

Two milliliter of each of the urine samples was defrosted and urinary proteins were precipitated by nine volumes of cold 90% ethanol and pelleted at $3500 \times g$ for 30 min [88]. After drying, proteins were dissolved in bidistilled water, and protein concentration was assessed by BCA assay (Microplate BCA™ protein Assay Kit, Thermo Scientific, Waltham, MA, USA), using BSA as standard.

Approximately 400 µg of pooled proteins were digested following the FASP protocol, as already described [89]. Briefly, proteins were first reduced by incubation with 50 mM DL-dithiothreitol (Sigma Aldrich, Switzerland) and alkylated for 30 min with iodoacetamide 100 mM (Sigma Aldrich, Switzerland). Then, they were digested overnight on 30 kDa filters (Amicon Ultra-500 30 kDa, Millipore, New York, NY, USA) adding trypsin from porcine pancreas (Proteomics Grade, BioReagent, Dimethylated) in a ratio 1:100 to the initial protein concentration. After repeated washing of the filter, the eluted peptides were collected and lyophilised. The resulting peptides were resuspended in steril-filtered water (Sigma Aldrich, Buchs, Switzerland) and their concentration was determined by nanodrop spectrophotometer (Thermo Scientific™).

4.4. Urinary N-Glycopeptides Enrichment and Deglycosylation

After the whole urinary proteome digestion, the N-glycopeptides were enriched by the lectins-capture strategy, using a FASP-based method (so-called N-Glyco-FASP) that was first described by Zielinska et al. [25]. Briefly, a solution containing a pool of three different types of lectins, concavalin A (ConcA), wheat germ agglutinin (WGA) and agglutinin RCA_{120} (Sigma Aldrich) was mixed with approximately 100 µg of digested peptides with a mass proportion of 1:3. The mixture was loaded on a new 30 kDa filter unit (Amicon Ultra-500, 30 kDa, Millipore) and the lectins-glycopeptides incubation was performed at 4 °C for 2 h. Then, the unbound peptides were eluted by four steps of centrifugations at 14,000× g, each one for 10 min. The captured peptides underwent overnight deglycosylation with PNGase F (Roche, New York, NY, USA) at 37 °C. The deglycosylated peptides were eluted with another centrifugation series (14,000× g, 10 min), lyophilised and stored at -20 °C, until the following MS analysis.

4.5. Mass Spectrometric Analysis

Two microgram of N-glycopeptides was injected into nanoHPLC and separation was performed using 50 cm nanocolumn (Dionex, ID 75 µm, Acclaim PepMap100, C18, 2 µm, Sunnyvale, CA, USA). The separation was performed at 40 °C and at a flow rate of 300 nL/min, using a multistep 4-h gradients that increased the percentage of B from 4 to 66% in 204 min (mobile phase A, used for nano-pump H$_2$O w/0,1% formic acid and whilst mobile phase B was composed of 80:20 ACN: H$_2$O w/0.08% FA). An Impact HD™ Ultra High Resolution-QqTOF (Bruker Daltonics, Bremen, Germany), equipped with a nanoBoosterCaptiveSpray™ ESI source (Bruker Daltonics) was used in the Data-Dependent-Acquisition mode. The MS/MS data were acquired by targeting precursor ions (m/z 300–2000 range) with a charge state between +2 and +5. The fragmentation was performed by collision-induced dissociation (CID). Both the MS scans and MS/MS data were recorded as line spectra based on centroided data.

Internal calibration, using a lock mass of m/z 1221.9906, and a calibration segment based on a 10 mM sodium formiate cluster solution (15 min before each run) were used to correct the raw MS and MS/MS data Compass DataAnalysis v4.1 software (Bruker Daltonics) was used to calibrate, deconvolute and convert the acquired raw data prior to protein identification and quantification.

4.6. Data Processing

4.6.1. Protein Identification

Mascot (v 2.4.1, Matrix Science, London, UK) was used for protein identification. Trypsin was chosen as the enzyme and the number of missed cleavages was set to 1. The peptide charge was set to 2+ and 3+, and the peptide tolerance and MS/MS tolerance were 20 ppm and 0.05 Da, respectively. Cysteine carbamidomethylation was set as fixed modification, whilst methionine oxidation and asparagine deamidation were used as variable modifications. Swiss-prot was used as database (accessed May 2017, 555.594 total entries). The maximum false discovery rate (FDR) for peptide spectral match was set to 1%, using percolator algorithm and a minimum of one sequence-unique peptides was required for identification. Proteins of interest were analysed for cellular component, molecular functions and biological processes with ClueGO v2.5, Clupedia v1.5 and the Cytoscape tools [90].

4.6.2. Bioinformatics and Statistical Analysis

Progenesis QI for proteomics v.2.0.5387.52102 (Nonlinear Dynamics, Newcastle, UK) was used for the label-free protein quantification [91]. Data were imported as centroided data and automatic alignment with additional manual adjustment were performed to maximise the overlay between runs. Peak picking was achieved with a default sensitivity, a minimum peak width of 0.2 min and maximum charge of 8. Normalisation was applied using Progenesis software and calculated over all peptide ions by a global scaling factor between the samples based on selected reference.

Peptides were identified using an in-house Mascot search engine as described previously. Only non-conflicting peptides were used for the relative quantification. Protein abundance was calculated using the sum of all unique normalised peptide ion abundances for each specific protein in each single analysis. Statistical analyses for quantitative evaluation were performed using the open-source R software v.3.5.0. For the comparison between the different sample cohorts in terms of N-glycoprotein abundance the Anova test was used and a post-hoc Tukey test, with Benjamini and Hochberg adjustment, was applied for pairwise comparisons. For each test, the level of significance was set equal to 0.05.

Proteins with at least two-fold changes were considered differentially regulated. For N-glycomapping characterisation of the glycopeptides, all the potential N-glycosylation sites were investigated in order to recognise and count all the deamidated asparagine present in sequences obtained from Uniprot database (http://www.uniprot.org.), using R language. Peptides that were found to be already deamidated in the whole proteome were excluded from the further analysis.

5. Conclusions

Despite recent developments in our understanding of glycosylation processes, an in-depth comprehension of the N-glycoproteome in ccRCC is still lacking. N-glycoproteins are involved in numerous fundamental processes that occur during cancer, such as tumour cell invasion, cell-matrix interactions, tumour angiogenesis, immunomodulation and metastasis genesis and propagation. It is well-known that unusual glycosylation of the protein causes severe defects in protein localisation, trafficking, cellular adhesion and transduction pathways in disease conditions, which may lead to valuable diagnostic markers.

To the best of our knowledge, our study is the first that thoroughly investigates the urinary N-glycoproteome in patients with early and advanced ccRCC conditions and compares this with non-ccRCC subjects. We evaluated the urinary glycoprotein content both qualitatively (N-glycosites distribution) and quantitatively (N-glycoprotein expression) and highlight a specific distribution of glycosites that is related to patients at early (pT1) and advanced (pT3) stages. These alterations suggest that the N-glycosylation of motifs different from the most relevant N-x-T/S may have role in cancer status, as already shown in other studies. In fact, it is well known that some of the unconventional glycosylations are carried out by unique classes of glycosyltransferase enzymes. Therefore, it could be highly interesting to verify the existence of these *special enzymes* in a future study and explore the mechanisms that they adopt to recognise both consensus and non-consensus motifs, performing a targeted study in ccRCC cells lines or tissue biopsies.

Additionally, our investigation highlights the presence of a group of nine urinary N-glycoproteins with a specific abundance trend that could constitute a specific disease-related glycosignature and may be able to underlined the transition from early to the advanced stage. These dysregulated proteins may have important implications in the pathogenesis of this renal malignancy, potentially playing a role that is different from their corresponding non-glycosylated isoform in the process of tumourigenesis and may be useful for future diagnostic applications. Finally, our data encourage further investigations that target the in-depth characterisation of the N-glycans attached to the deregulated proteins identified in order to determine the precise role of this important PTM in the onset and development of ccRCC.

Supplementary Materials: The following are available online at http://www.mdpi.com/2072-6694/12/1/239/s1, Figure S1: Trend distribution of the N-glycosylation sites of the urinary glycoproteins, Figure S2: Gene ontology analysis of the N-glycoproteins identified from all sample groups by LC-MS , Table S1: List of N-glycoproteins identified in the CTRL, pT1, pT3 groups, Table S2: List of N-glycomodified peptides in the CTRL, pT1, pT3 groups.

Author Contributions: Methodology, A.G.; validation, C.C., I.P. and A.S.; formal analysis: G.C.; investigation, conceptualisation and writing—original draft: L.S.; writing—review and editing: F.R., V.D. and F.C.; supervision: F.M. and M.G. All authors have read and agreed to the published version of the manuscript.

Funding: This research was funded by University of Milano-Bicocca (Fondi di Ateneo per la Ricerca, FAR 2014-2017) and by a kind donation from the Gigi & Pupa Ferrari Foundation onlus (Fondazione Gigi & Pupa Ferrari onlus).

Acknowledgments: The authors thank Iris Marangia for management of clinical data of patients.

Conflicts of Interest: The authors declare no conflict of interest.

References

1. Chandler, K.B.; Costello, C.E.; Rahimi, N. Glycosylation in the Tumor Microenvironment: Implications for Tumor Angiogenesis and Metastasis. *Cells* **2019**, *8*, 544. [CrossRef] [PubMed]
2. Aebi, M. N-linked protein glycosylation in the ER. *Biochim. Biophys. Acta Mol. Cell Res.* **2013**, *1833*, 2430–2437. [CrossRef] [PubMed]
3. Ohtsubo, K.; Marth, J.D. Glycosylation in Cellular Mechanisms of Health and Disease. *Cell* **2006**, *126*, 855–867. [CrossRef] [PubMed]
4. Lander, E.S.; Linton, L.M.; Birren, B.; Nusbaum, C.; Zody, M.C.; Baldwin, J.; Devon, K.; Dewar, K.; Doyle, M.; FitzHugh, W.; et al. Initial sequencing and analysis of the human genome. *Nature* **2001**, *409*, 860–921. [CrossRef] [PubMed]
5. Taniguchi, N.; Kizuka, Y. Glycans and cancer: Role of N-Glycans in cancer biomarker, progression and metastasis, and therapeutics. *Adv. Cancer Res.* **2015**. [CrossRef]
6. Lau, K.S.; Dennis, J.W. N-Glycans in cancer progression. *Glycobiology* **2008**, *18*, 750–760. [CrossRef]
7. Häuselmann, I.; Borsig, L. Altered tumor-cell glycosylation promotes metastasis. *Front. Oncol.* **2014**, *4*, 28. [CrossRef]
8. Oliveira-Ferrer, L.; Legler, K.; Milde-Langosch, K. Role of protein glycosylation in cancer metastasis. *Semin. Cancer Biol.* **2017**, *44*, 141–152. [CrossRef]
9. Gilgunn, S.; Conroy, P.J.; Saldova, R.; Rudd, P.M.; O'Kennedy, R.J. Aberrant PSA glycosylation-A sweet predictor of prostate cancer. *Nat. Rev. Urol.* **2013**, *10*, 99. [CrossRef]
10. Ilic, D.; Neuberger, M.M.; Djulbegovic, M.; Dahm, P. Screening for prostate cancer. *Cochrane database Syst. Rev.* **2013**, CD004720. [CrossRef]
11. Drake, R.R.; Jones, E.E.; Powers, T.W.; Nyalwidhe, J.O. Altered Glycosylation in Prostate Cancer. *Adv. Cancer Res.* **2015**, 345–382. [CrossRef]
12. Duffy, M.J.; Shering, S.; Sherry, F.; McDermott, E.; O'Higgins, N. CA 15-3: A prognostic marker in breast cancer. *Int. J. Biol. Markers* **2000**, *15*, 330–333. [CrossRef]
13. Choi, J.W.; Moon, B.I.; Lee, J.W.; Kim, H.J.; Jin, Y.; Kim, H.J. Use of CA15-3 for screening breast cancer: An antibody-lectin sandwich assay for detecting glycosylation of CA15-3 in sera. *Oncol. Rep.* **2018**, *40*, 145–154. [CrossRef] [PubMed]
14. Yin, B.W.; Lloyd, K.O. Molecular cloning of the CA125 ovarian cancer antigen: Identification as a new mucin, MUC16. *J. Biol. Chem.* **2001**, *276*, 27371–27375. [CrossRef]
15. Duffy, M.J. Carcinoembryonic antigen as a marker for colorectal cancer: Is it clinically useful? *Clin. Chem.* **2001**, *47*, 624–630. [PubMed]
16. Saito, G.; Sadahiro, S.; Okada, K.; Tanaka, A.; Suzuki, T.; Kamijo, A. Relation between Carcinoembryonic Antigen Levels in Colon Cancer Tissue and Serum Carcinoembryonic Antigen Levels at Initial Surgery and Recurrence. *Oncology* **2016**, *91*, 85–89. [CrossRef] [PubMed]
17. Moertel, C.G.; Fleming, T.R.; Macdonald, J.S.; Haller, D.G.; Laurie, J.A.; Tangen, C. An Evaluation of the Carcinoembryonic Antigen (CEA) Test for Monitoring Patients with Resected Colon Cancer. *JAMA J. Am. Med. Assoc.* **1993**, *270*, 943–947. [CrossRef]
18. Hammarstrom, S. The carcinoembryonic antigen (CEA) family: Structures, suggested functions and expression in normal and malignant tissues. *Semin. Cancer Biol.* **1999**, *9*, 67–81. [CrossRef]
19. Davis, M.T.; Spahr, C.S.; McGinley, M.D.; Robinson, J.H.; Bures, E.J.; Beierle, J.; Mort, J.; Yu, W.; Luethy, R.; Patterson, S.D. Towards defining the urinary proteome using liquid chromatography-tandem mass spectrometry. II. Limitations of complex mixture analyses. *Proteomics* **2001**, *1*, 108–117. [CrossRef]
20. Sun, W.; Li, F.; Wu, S.; Wang, X.; Zheng, D.; Wang, J.; Gao, Y. Human urine proteome analysis by three separation approaches. *Proteomics* **2005**, *5*, 4994–5001. [CrossRef]
21. Arivusudar Marimuthu A Comprehensive Map of the Human Urinary Proteome. *J. Proteome Res.* **2011**, *23*, 1–7. [CrossRef]
22. Desiere, F.; Deutsch, E.W.; King, N.L.; Nesvizhskii, A.I.; Mallick, P.; Eng, J.; Chen, S.; Eddes, J.; Loevenich, S.N.; Aebersold, R. The PeptideAtlas project. *Nucleic Acids Res.* **2006**, *34*, D655–D658. [CrossRef] [PubMed]
23. Kawahara, R.; Saad, J.; Angeli, C.B.; Palmisano, G. Site-specific characterization of N-linked glycosylation in human urinary glycoproteins and endogenous glycopeptides. *Glycoconj. J.* **2016**, *33*, 937–951. [CrossRef] [PubMed]

24. Different collaborators Comprehensive Molecular Characterization of clear cell renal cell carcinoma. *Nature* **2014**, *499*, 43–49. [CrossRef]
25. Zielinska, D.F.; Gnad, F.; Wiśniewski, J.R.; Mann, M. Precision mapping of an in vivo N-glycoproteome reveals rigid topological and sequence constraints. *Cell* **2010**, *141*, 897–907. [CrossRef] [PubMed]
26. Fang, P.; Wang, X.-J.; Xue, Y.; Liu, M.-Q.; Zeng, W.-F.; Zhang, Y.; Zhang, L.; Gao, X.; Yan, G.-Q.; Yao, J.; et al. In-depth mapping of the mouse brain N-glycoproteome reveals widespread *N*-glycosylation of diverse brain proteins. *Oncotarget* **2016**, *7*, 38796–38809. [CrossRef]
27. Geng, F.; Wang, J.; Liu, D.; Jin, Y.; Ma, M. Identification of N-Glycosites in Chicken Egg White Proteins Using an Omics Strategy. *J. Agric. Food Chem.* **2017**, *65*, 5357–5364. [CrossRef]
28. Song, W.; Mentink, R.A.; Henquet, M.G.L.; Cordewener, J.H.G.; van Dijk, A.D.J.; Bosch, D.; America, A.H.P.; van der Krol, A.R. N-glycan occupancy of Arabidopsis N-glycoproteins. *J. Proteomics* **2013**, *93*, 343–355. [CrossRef]
29. Xu, Y.; Bailey, U.-M.; Punyadeera, C.; Schulz, B.L. Identification of salivary N-glycoproteins and measurement of glycosylation site occupancy by boronate glycoprotein enrichment and liquid chromatography/electrospray ionization tandem mass spectrometry. *Rapid Commun. Mass Spectrom.* **2014**, *28*, 471–482. [CrossRef]
30. Malerod, H.; Graham, R.L.J.; Sweredoski, M.J.; Hess, S. Comprehensive profiling of N-linked glycosylation sites in HeLa cells using hydrazide enrichment. *J. Proteome Res.* **2013**, *12*, 248–259. [CrossRef]
31. Hollander, N.; Haimovich, J. Altered N-Linked Glycosylation in Follicular Lymphoma and Chronic Lymphocytic Leukemia: Involvement in Pathogenesis and Potential Therapeutic Targeting. *Front. Immunol.* **2017**, *8*, 912. [CrossRef] [PubMed]
32. Mamessier, E.; Drevet, C.; Broussais-Guillaumot, F.; Mollichella, M.-L.; Garciaz, S.; Roulland, S.; Benchetrit, M.; Nadel, B.; Xerri, L. Contiguous follicular lymphoma and follicular lymphoma in situ harboring N-glycosylated sites. *Haematologica* **2015**, *100*, e155–e157. [CrossRef] [PubMed]
33. Pan, S.; Chen, R.; Tamura, Y.; Crispin, D.A.; Lai, L.A.; May, D.H.; McIntosh, M.W.; Goodlett, D.R.; Brentnall, T.A. Quantitative glycoproteomics analysis reveals changes in *N*-glycosylation level associated with pancreatic ductal adenocarcinoma. *J. Proteome Res.* **2014**, *13*, 1293–1306. [CrossRef] [PubMed]
34. Miyamoto, S.; Ruhaak, L.R.; Stroble, C.; Salemi, M.R.; Phinney, B.; Lebrilla, C.B.; Leiserowitz, G.S. Glycoproteomic Analysis of Malignant Ovarian Cancer Ascites Fluid Identifies Unusual Glycopeptides. *J. Proteome Res.* **2016**, *15*, 3358–3376. [CrossRef] [PubMed]
35. Wu, J.; Qin, H.; Li, T.; Cheng, K.; Dong, J.; Tian, M.; Chai, N.; Guo, H.; Li, J.; You, X.; et al. Characterization of site-specific glycosylation of secreted proteins associated with multi-drug resistance of gastric cancer. *Oncotarget* **2016**, *7*, 25315–25327. [CrossRef]
36. Valliere-Douglass, J.F.; Kodama, P.; Mujacic, M.; Brady, L.J.; Wang, W.; Wallace, A.; Yan, B.; Reddy, P.; Treuheit, M.J.; Balland, A. Asparagine-linked oligosaccharides present on a non-consensus amino acid sequence in the CH1 domain of human antibodies. *J. Biol. Chem.* **2009**, *284*, 32493–32506. [CrossRef]
37. Matsumoto, S.; Taguchi, Y.; Shimada, A.; Igura, M.; Kohda, D. Tethering an N-Glycosylation Sequon-Containing Peptide Creates a Catalytically Competent Oligosaccharyltransferase Complex. *Biochemistry* **2017**, *56*, 602–611. [CrossRef]
38. Trinidad, J.C.; Schoepfer, R.; Burlingame, A.L.; Medzihradszky, K.F. N-and O-glycosylation in the murine synaptosome. *Mol. Cell. Proteomics* **2013**, *12*, 3474–3488. [CrossRef]
39. Valliere-Douglass, J.F.; Eakin, C.M.; Wallace, A.; Ketchem, R.R.; Wang, W.; Treuheit, M.J.; Balland, A. Glutamine-linked and non-consensus asparagine-linked oligosaccharides present in human recombinant antibodies define novel protein glycosylation motifs. *J. Biol. Chem.* **2010**, *285*, 16012–16022. [CrossRef]
40. Vance, B.A.; Wu, W.; Ribaudo, R.K.; Segal, D.M.; Kearse, K.P. Multiple dimeric forms of human CD69 result from differential addition of N-glycans to typical (Asn-X-Ser/Thr) and atypical (Asn-X-cys) glycosylation motifs. *J. Biol. Chem.* **1997**, *272*, 23117–23122. [CrossRef]
41. Mooser, V.; Seabra, M.C.; Abedin, M.; Landschulz, K.T.; Marcovina, S.; Hobbs, H.H. Apolipoprotein (a) kringle 4-containing fragments in human urine. Relationship to plasma levels of lipoprotein (a). *J. Clin. Investig.* **1996**, *97*, 858–864. [CrossRef] [PubMed]
42. Bolenz, C.; Schröppel, B.; Eisenhardt, A.; Schmitz-Dräger, B.J.; Grimm, M.-O. Abklärung der Hämaturie. *Dtsch. Aerzteblatt Online* **2018**, *25*, 127–135. [CrossRef]
43. Tian, Z.-H.; Yuan, C.; Yang, K.; Gao, X.-L. Systematic identification of key genes and pathways in clear cell renal cell carcinoma on bioinformatics analysis. *Ann. Transl. Med.* **2019**, *7*, 89. [CrossRef] [PubMed]

44. Dobryszycka, W. Biological functions of haptoglobin–new pieces to an old puzzle. *Eur. J. Clin. Chem. Clin. Biochem.* **1997**, *35*, 647–654.
45. Liu, T.; Qian, W.J.; Gritsenko, M.A.; Camp, D.G.; Monroe, M.E.; Moore, R.J.; Smith, R.D. Human plasma N-glycoproteome analysis by immunoaffinity subtraction, hydrazide chemistry, and mass spectrometry. *J. Proteome Res.* **2005**, *4*, 2070–2080. [CrossRef]
46. Zhu, J.; Lin, Z.; Wu, J.; Yin, H.; Dai, J.; Feng, Z.; Marrero, J.; Lubman, D.M. Analysis of serum haptoglobin fucosylation in hepatocellular carcinoma and liver cirrhosis of different etiologies. *J. Proteome Res.* **2014**, *13*, 2986–2997. [CrossRef]
47. Park, S.Y.; Yoon, S.J.; Jeong, Y.T.; Kim, J.M.; Kim, J.Y.; Bernert, B.; Ullman, T.; Itzkowitz, S.H.; Kim, J.H.; Hakomori, S.I. N-glycosylation status of β-haptoglobin in sera of patients with colon cancer, chronic inflammatory diseases and normal subjects. *Int. J. Cancer* **2010**, *126*, 142–155. [CrossRef]
48. Lin, Z.; Simeone, D.M.; Anderson, M.A.; Brand, R.E.; Xie, X.; Shedden, K.A.; Ruffin, M.T.; Lubman, D.M. Mass spectrometric assay for analysis of haptoglobin fucosylation in pancreatic cancer. *J. Proteome Res.* **2011**, *10*, 2602–2611. [CrossRef]
49. Sandim, V.; de Abreu Pereira, D.; Kalume, D.E.; Oliveira-Carvalho, A.L.; Ornellas, A.A.; Soares, M.R.; Alves, G.; Zingali, R.B. Proteomic analysis reveals differentially secreted proteins in the urine from patients with clear cell renal cell carcinoma. *Urol. Oncol. Semin. Orig. Investig.* **2016**, *34*, e11–e15. [CrossRef]
50. Bruneel, A.; Habarou, F.; Stojkovic, T.; Plouviez, G.; Bougas, L.; Guillemet, F.; Brient, N.; Henry, D.; Dupre, T.; Vuillaumier-Barrot, S.; et al. Two-dimensional electrophoresis highlights haptoglobin beta chain as an additional biomarker of congenital disorders of glycosylation. *Clin. Chim. Acta.* **2017**, *470*, 70–74. [CrossRef]
51. To, W.S.; Midwood, K.S. Plasma and cellular fibronectin: Distinct and independent functions during tissue repair. *Fibrogenesis Tissue Repair* **2011**, *4*, 21. [CrossRef] [PubMed]
52. Kumra, H.; Reinhardt, D.P. Fibronectin-targeted drug delivery in cancer. *Adv. Drug Deliv. Rev.* **2016**, *97*, 101–110. [CrossRef] [PubMed]
53. Hsiao, C.T.; Cheng, H.W.; Huang, C.M.; Li, H.R.; Ou, M.H.; Huang, J.R.; Khoo, K.H.; Yu, H.W.; Chen, Y.Q.; Wang, Y.K.; et al. Fibronectin in cell adhesion and migration via N-glycosylation. *Oncotarget* **2017**, *8*, 70653–70668. [CrossRef] [PubMed]
54. Han, Z.; Cheng, H.; Parvani, J.G.; Zhou, Z.; Lu, Z.R. Magnetic resonance molecular imaging of metastatic breast cancer by targeting extradomain-B fibronectin in the tumor microenvironment. *Magn. Reson. Med.* **2018**, *79*, 3135–3143. [CrossRef] [PubMed]
55. Ludwig, K.F.; Du, W.; Sorrelle, N.B.; Wnuk-Lipinska, K.; Topalovski, M.; Toombs, J.E.; Cruz, V.H.; Yabuuchi, S.; Rajeshkumar, N.V.; Maitra, A.; et al. Small-Molecule Inhibition of Axl Targets Tumor Immune Suppression and Enhances Chemotherapy in Pancreatic Cancer. *Cancer Res.* **2018**, *78*, 246–255. [CrossRef] [PubMed]
56. Ma, L.J.; Lee, S.W.; Lin, L.C.; Chen, T.J.; Chang, I.W.; Hsu, H.P.; Chang, K.Y.; Huang, H.Y.; Li, C.F. Fibronectin overexpression is associated with latentmembrane protein 1 expression and has independent prognostic value for nasopharyngeal carcinoma. *Tumor Biol.* **2014**, *35*, 1703–1712. [CrossRef]
57. Gopal, S.; Veracini, L.; Grall, D.; Butori, C.; Schaub, S.; Audebert, S.; Camoin, L.; Baudelet, E.; Adwanska, A.; Beghelli-De La Forest Divonne, S.; et al. Fibronectin-guided migration of carcinoma collectives. *Nat. Commun.* **2017**, *8*. [CrossRef]
58. Ou, Y.C.; Li, J.R.; Wang, J.D.; Chang, C.Y.; Wu, C.C.; Chen, W.Y.; Kuan, Y.H.; Liao, S.L.; Lu, H.C.; Chen, C.J. Fibronectin Promotes Cell Growth and Migration in Human Renal Cell Carcinoma Cells. *Int. J. Mol. Sci.* **2019**, *20*, 2792. [CrossRef]
59. Kondisetty, S.; Menon, K.N.; Pooleri, G.K. Fibronectin protein expression in renal cell carcinoma in correlation with clinical stage of tumour. *Biomark. Res.* **2018**, *6*, 1–6. [CrossRef]
60. Hellman, N.E.; Gitlin, J.D. Ceruloplasmin metabolism and function. *Annu. Rev. Nutr.* **2002**, *22*, 439–458. [CrossRef]
61. Delmonico, L.; Bravo, M.; Silvestre, R.T.; Ornellas, M.H.F.; De Azevedo, C.M.; Alves, G. Proteomic profile of saliva and plasma from women with impalpable breast lesions. *Oncol. Lett.* **2016**, *12*, 2145–2152. [CrossRef] [PubMed]
62. Han, I.W.; Jang, J.-Y.; Kwon, W.; Park, T.; Kim, Y.; Lee, K.B.; Kim, S.-W. Ceruloplasmin as a prognostic marker in patients with bile duct cancer. *Oncotarget* **2017**, *8*, 29028–29037. [CrossRef] [PubMed]
63. Shah, P.H.; Venkatesh, R.; More, C.B. Determination of role of ceruloplasmin in oral potentially malignant disorders and oral malignancy-A cross-sectional study. *Oral Dis.* **2017**, *23*, 1066–1071. [CrossRef] [PubMed]

64. Boz, A.; Evliyaoglu, O.; Yildirim, M.; Erkan, N.; Karaca, B. The value of serum zinc, copper, ceruloplasmin levels in patients with gastrointestinal tract cancers. *Turk. J. Gastroenterol.* **2005**, *16*, 81–84.
65. Gajbhiye, A.; Dabhi, R.; Taunk, K.; Vannuruswamy, G.; RoyChoudhury, S.; Adhav, R.; Seal, S.; Mane, A.; Bayatigeri, S.; Santra, M.K.; et al. Urinary proteome alterations in HER2 enriched breast cancer revealed by multipronged quantitative proteomics. *Proteomics* **2016**, *16*, 2403–2418. [CrossRef]
66. Bleu, M.; Gaulis, S.; Lopes, R.; Sprouffske, K.; Apfel, V.; Holwerda, S.; Pregnolato, M.; Yildiz, U.; Cordo', V.; Dost, A.F.M.; et al. PAX8 activates metabolic genes via enhancer elements in Renal Cell Carcinoma. *Nat. Commun.* **2019**, *10*, 3739. [CrossRef]
67. Zhang, L.; Jiang, H.; Xu, G.; Chu, N.; Xu, N.; Wen, H.; Gu, B.; Liu, J.; Mao, S.; Na, R.; et al. iTRAQ-based quantitative proteomic analysis reveals potential early diagnostic markers of clear-cell Renal cell carcinoma. *Biosci. Trends* **2016**, *10*, 210–219. [CrossRef]
68. Raimondo, F.; Morosi, L.; Corbetta, S.; Chinello, C.; Brambilla, P.; Della Mina, P.; Villa, A.; Albo, G.; Battaglia, C.; Bosari, S.; et al. Differential protein profiling of renal cell carcinoma urinary exosomes. *Mol. Biosyst.* **2013**, *9*, 1220–1233. [CrossRef]
69. Yan, X.; Yao, M.; Wen, X.; Zhu, Y.; Zhao, E.; Qian, X.; Chen, X.; Lu, W.; Lv, Q.; Zhang, L.; et al. Elevated apolipoprotein B predicts poor postsurgery prognosis in patients with hepatocellular carcinoma. *Onco Targets Ther.* **2019**, *12*, 1957–1964. [CrossRef]
70. Liu, J.-X.; Yuan, Q.; Min, Y.-L.; He, Y.; Xu, Q.-H.; Li, B.; Shi, W.-Q.; Lin, Q.; Li, Q.-H.; Zhu, P.-W.; et al. Apolipoprotein A1 and B as risk factors for development of intraocular metastasis in patients with breast cancer. *Cancer Manag. Res.* **2019**, *11*, 2881–2888. [CrossRef]
71. Chen, C.-L.; Lin, T.-S.; Tsai, C.-H.; Wu, C.-C.; Chung, T.; Chien, K.-Y.; Wu, M.; Chang, Y.-S.; Yu, J.-S.; Chen, Y.-T. Identification of potential bladder cancer markers in urine by abundant-protein depletion coupled with quantitative proteomics. *J. Proteomics* **2013**, *85*, 28–43. [CrossRef] [PubMed]
72. Velagapudi, S.; Schraml, P.; Yalcinkaya, M.; Bolck, H.A.; Rohrer, L.; Moch, H.; von Eckardstein, A. Scavenger receptor BI promotes cytoplasmic accumulation of lipoproteins in clear-cell renal cell carcinoma. *J. Lipid Res.* **2018**, *59*, 2188–2201. [CrossRef] [PubMed]
73. Zhang, F.; Xie, Y.; Ma, X.; Gu, L.; Li, H.; Li, X.; Guo, G.; Zhang, X. Preoperative apolipoprotein B/A1 ratio is an independent prognostic factor in metastatic renal cell carcinoma. *Urol. Oncol.* **2019**, *37*, e9–e184. [CrossRef] [PubMed]
74. van den Boogert, M.A.W.; Larsen, L.E.; Ali, L.; Kuil, S.D.; Chong, P.L.W.; Loregger, A.; Kroon, J.; Schnitzler, J.G.; Schimmel, A.W.M.; Peter, J.; et al. N-Glycosylation Defects in Humans Lower Low-Density Lipoprotein Cholesterol Through Increased Low-Density Lipoprotein Receptor Expression. *Circulation* **2019**, *140*, 280–292. [CrossRef] [PubMed]
75. Jiang, X.-C. Phospholipid transfer protein: its impact on lipoprotein homeostasis and atherosclerosis. *J. Lipid Res.* **2018**, *59*, 764–771. [CrossRef] [PubMed]
76. Sirwi, A.; Hussain, M.M. Lipid transfer proteins in the assembly of apoB-containing lipoproteins. *J. Lipid Res.* **2018**, *59*, 1094–1102. [CrossRef]
77. Dong, W.; Gong, H.; Zhang, G.; Vuletic, S.; Albers, J.; Zhang, J.; Liang, H.; Sui, Y.; Zheng, J. Lipoprotein lipase and phospholipid transfer protein overexpression in human glioma cells and their effect on cell growth, apoptosis, and migration. *Acta Biochim. Et Biophys. Sin.* **2017**, *49*, 62–73. [CrossRef]
78. Cserhalmi, M.; Papp, A.; Brandus, B.; Uzonyi, B.; Jozsi, M. Regulation of regulators: Role of the complement factor H-related proteins. *Semin. Immunol.* **2019**, 101341. [CrossRef]
79. Ajona, D.; Castano, Z.; Garayoa, M.; Zudaire, E.; Pajares, M.J.; Martinez, A.; Cuttitta, F.; Montuenga, L.M.; Pio, R. Expression of complement factor H by lung cancer cells: effects on the activation of the alternative pathway of complement. *Cancer Res.* **2004**, *64*, 6310–6318. [CrossRef]
80. Bjorge, L.; Hakulinen, J.; Vintermyr, O.K.; Jarva, H.; Jensen, T.S.; Iversen, O.E.; Meri, S. Ascitic complement system in ovarian cancer. *Br. J. Cancer* **2005**, *92*, 895–905. [CrossRef]
81. Wilczek, E.; Rzepko, R.; Nowis, D.; Legat, M.; Golab, J.; Glab, M.; Gorlewicz, A.; Konopacki, F.; Mazurkiewicz, M.; Sladowski, D.; et al. The possible role of factor H in colon cancer resistance to complement attack. *Int. J. Cancer* **2008**, *122*, 2030–2037. [CrossRef] [PubMed]
82. Yoon, Y.-H.; Hwang, H.-J.; Sung, H.-J.; Heo, S.-H.; Kim, D.-S.; Hong, S.-H.; Lee, K.-H.; Cho, J.-Y. Upregulation of Complement Factor H by SOCS-1/3(-)STAT4 in Lung Cancer. *Cancers* **2019**, *11*. [CrossRef] [PubMed]

83. Zhu, Z.; He, X.; Johnson, C.; Stoops, J.; Eaker, A.E.; Stoffer, D.S.; Bell, A.; Zarnegar, R.; DeFrances, M.C. PI3K is negatively regulated by PIK3IP1, a novel p110 interacting protein. *Biochem. Biophys. Res. Commun.* **2007**, *358*, 66–72. [CrossRef] [PubMed]
84. Wong, C.C.; Martincorena, I.; Rust, A.G.; Rashid, M.; Alifrangis, C.; Alexandrov, L.B.; Tiffen, J.C.; Kober, C.; Green, A.R.; Massie, C.E.; et al. Inactivating CUX1 mutations promote tumorigenesis. *Nat. Genet.* **2014**, *46*, 33–38. [CrossRef] [PubMed]
85. He, X.; Zhu, Z.; Johnson, C.; Stoops, J.; Eaker, A.E.; Bowen, W.; DeFrances, M.C. PIK3IP1, a negative regulator of PI3K, suppresses the development of hepatocellular carcinoma. *Cancer Res.* **2008**, *68*, 5591–5598. [CrossRef] [PubMed]
86. Martin, G.H.; Roy, N.; Chakraborty, S.; Desrichard, A.; Chung, S.S.; Woolthuis, C.M.; Hu, W.; Berezniuk, I.; Garrett-Bakelman, F.E.; Hamann, J.; et al. CD97 is a critical regulator of acute myeloid leukemia stem cell function. *J. Exp. Med.* **2019**, *216*, 2362–2377. [CrossRef]
87. Chance, M.R.; Chang, J.; Liu, S.; Gokulrangan, G.; Chen, D.H.-C.; Lindsay, A.; Geng, R.; Zheng, Q.Y.; Alagramam, K. Proteomics, bioinformatics and targeted gene expression analysis reveals up-regulation of cochlin and identifies other potential biomarkers in the mouse model for deafness in Usher syndrome type 1F. *Hum. Mol. Genet.* **2010**, *19*, 1515–1527. [CrossRef]
88. Lee, R.S.; Monigatti, F.; Briscoe, A.C.; Waldon, Z.; Freeman, M.R.; Steen, H. Optimizing sample handling for urinary proteomics. *J. Proteome Res.* **2008**, *7*, 4022–4030. [CrossRef]
89. Chinello, C.; Stella, M.; Piga, I.; Smith, A.J.; Bovo, G.; Varallo, M.; Ivanova, M.; Denti, V.; Grasso, M.; Grasso, A.; et al. Proteomics of liquid biopsies: Depicting RCC infiltration into the renal vein by MS analysis of urine and plasma. *J. Proteomics* **2019**, *191*, 29–37. [CrossRef]
90. Doncheva, N.T.; Morris, J.H.; Gorodkin, J.; Jensen, L.J. Cytoscape StringApp: Network Analysis and Visualization of Proteomics Data. *J. Proteome Res.* **2019**, *18*, 623–632. [CrossRef]
91. Severi, L.; Losi, L.; Fonda, S.; Taddia, L.; Gozzi, G.; Marverti, G.; Magni, F.; Chinello, C.; Stella, M.; Sheouli, J.; et al. Proteomic and Bioinformatic Studies for the Characterization of Response to Pemetrexed in Platinum Drug Resistant Ovarian Cancer. *Front. Pharmacol.* **2018**, *9*, 454. [CrossRef] [PubMed]

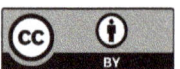

© 2020 by the authors. Licensee MDPI, Basel, Switzerland. This article is an open access article distributed under the terms and conditions of the Creative Commons Attribution (CC BY) license (http://creativecommons.org/licenses/by/4.0/).

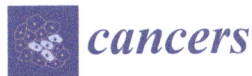

Article

Ex-Vivo Treatment of Tumor Tissue Slices as a Predictive Preclinical Method to Evaluate Targeted Therapies for Patients with Renal Carcinoma

Caroline Roelants [1,2], Catherine Pillet [3], Quentin Franquet [1,4], Clément Sarrazin [1,4], Nicolas Peilleron [1,4], Sofia Giacosa [1], Laurent Guyon [1], Amina Fontanell [4], Gaëlle Fiard [4], Jean-Alexandre Long [4], Jean-Luc Descotes [4], Claude Cochet [1] and Odile Filhol [1,*]

1. Université Grenoble Alpes, Inserm, CEA, IRIG-Biology of Cancer and Infection, UMR_S 1036, F-38000 Grenoble, France; caroline.roelants@inovarion.com (C.R.); qfranquet@chu-grenoble.fr (Q.F.); csarrazin1@chu-grenoble.fr (C.S.); nicolas.peilleron@gmail.com (N.P.); sofiagiacosa@gmail.com (S.G.); laurent.guyon@cea.fr (L.G.); claude.cochet@cea.fr (C.C.)
2. Inovarion, 75005 Paris, France
3. Université Grenoble Alpes, Inserm, CEA, IRIG-Biologie à Grande Echelle, UMR 1038, F-38000 Grenoble, France; catherine.pillet@cea.fr
4. Centre hospitalier universitaire Grenoble Alpes, CS 10217, 38043 Grenoble CEDEX 9, France; lafontanell@chu-grenoble.fr (A.F.); g.fiard@ucl.ac.uk (G.F.); JALong@chu-grenoble.fr (J.-A.L.); jldescotes@chu-grenoble.fr (J.-L.D.)
* Correspondence: odile.filhol-cochet@cea.fr; Tel.: +33-(0)4-38785645; Fax: +33-(0)4-38785058

Received: 30 November 2019; Accepted: 15 January 2020; Published: 17 January 2020

Abstract: Clear cell renal cell carcinoma (ccRCC) is the third type of urologic cancer. At time of diagnosis, 30% of cases are metastatic with no effect of chemotherapy or radiotherapy. Current targeted therapies lead to a high rate of relapse and resistance after a short-term response. Thus, a major hurdle in the development and use of new treatments for ccRCC is the lack of good pre-clinical models that can accurately predict the efficacy of new drugs and allow the stratification of patients into the correct treatment regime. Here, we describe different 3D cultures models of ccRCC, emphasizing the feasibility and the advantage of ex-vivo treatment of fresh, surgically resected human tumor slice cultures of ccRCC as a robust preclinical model for identifying patient response to specific therapeutics. Moreover, this model based on precision-cut tissue slices enables histopathology measurements as tumor architecture is retained, including the spatial relationship between the tumor and tumor-infiltrating lymphocytes and the stromal components. Our data suggest that acute treatment of tumor tissue slices could represent a benchmark of further exploration as a companion diagnostic tool in ccRCC treatment and a model to develop new therapeutic drugs.

Keywords: drug sensitivity; immune infiltration; renal cancer; targeted therapy; tumor slice culture

1. Introduction

Clear cell renal cell carcinoma (ccRCC) is the most frequent subtype of kidney cancer representing above 3% of all cancers. At the time of diagnosis, 30% of cases are metastatic and are associated with a poor prognosis and without long-lasting effects of traditional oncologic treatment such as chemotherapy or radiotherapy [1]. With the advance of targeted therapies for RCC, several agents targeting angiogenesis and signal transduction pathways such as sunitinib, temsirolimus, and pazopanib have appeared and showed improved clinical benefit and survival in randomized prospective clinical trials. Yet, improvements are still required, as many of these current therapies are limited by acquired resistance mostly through activation of alternative pathways [2]. The tumor immune microenvironment of ccRCC is known to be highly immunosuppressive and immune infiltration of tumors is closely associated with clinical outcome. Recently, immune checkpoint inhibitors have demonstrated significant anti-tumor activity in the first-line treatment of intermediate to poor risk RCC patients, but these therapies are only effective for a small fraction of patients, and are associated with problems, such as side effects and high costs [3–6]. Thus, new treatment strategies are needed to improve efficacy in a broader patient population. In the last decade, efforts have primarily focused on establishing a framework for predictions of anticancer drug responses using in vitro tumor cell line models [7–14]. These techniques are limited by the cell dissociation that selects the more robust cells and the ones that can attach to the cell culture substratum [15–17]. Moreover, in these conditions, inadequate representation of the tumor heterogeneity and microenvironment interactions during a preclinical screen can result in inaccurate predictions of drug candidate effects.

Organoids derived from patient tumors have recently gained much interest as promising tools for several translational applications, such as high-throughput drug screens and personalized medicine [18–20]. Tumor organoids grown with undefined natural (e.g., Matrigel®) or synthetic extracellular matrix gels show improved resemblance to the original tumor compared to 2D cultured cancer cell lines. However, they do not model tumor–stromal interactions (cancer cells, immune, and endothelial cells) and the growth selection pressures applied during their generation have the potential to introduce bias [13,21]. Consequently, the prediction of treatment outcome extrapolated from organoids may not recapitulate each cancer patient tumor. Moreover, it is not clear whether the timescales are quick enough to affect patient care [22].

Another approach often considered more representative is the use of patient-derived xenograft (PDX) systems. However, the generation of PDX models exhibits a low engraftment rate, and the timescales and costs involved in this process are very significant [23]. Furthermore, the PDX deviates from the original tumor over time [24], and difference in pathophysiology between animal models and humans contributes to high failure rates of current small-molecule inhibitors in preclinical trials [25–27]. Thus, predicting successful anticancer therapy remains extremely challenging, largely due to extensive inter- and intratumor heterogeneity [28] and there remains a need for alternative, innovative models that allow the precise balance between manipulability and biological complexity.

To address these challenges, ex-vivo culture of intact tumor slices is potentially an extremely attractive system that has been already validated in various types of cancers [29–38].

This method has several advantages: (1) it can be rapidly established using only small samples of fresh tissue with a limited cost, (2) it preserves the tumor architecture and the spatial interaction between tumor and stroma, (3) testing of drug susceptibility can be combined with gene sequencing and immunohistochemistry analysis. To the best of our knowledge, tumor slice culture has never been validated in renal carcinoma.

In this study, we developed different biological cell-based systems like 3D tumor spheroids, mice orthotopic tumor xenografts, and patient-derived tumor slice cultures (PDTSC) for ex-vivo assessment of drug effects in renal carcinoma. As we recently showed, a combination of two inhibitors targeting both the PI3K and Src kinases impedes cell viability of renal carcinoma cells [39], we compared the efficacy of this combination to standard-of-care-drugs for RCC like sunitinib, pazopanib, and temsirolimus using 3D tumor spheroids and PDTSC methods. We show that PDTSC has the potential to be exploited for cancer cell sensitivity assessment to novel molecularly targeted therapies among patients with ccRCC, and to identify suitable candidates for drug combinations in a cost-effective and patient-friendly manner. We also demonstrate that PDTSC faithfully preserves the molecular landscape of the original renal carcinoma, retaining histopathology, including the stromal components and the immune cells that innately infiltrate the patient's malignant epithelial cells, features that can be potentially useful to evaluate predictive biomarkers of treatment response and for patient stratification in prospective trials with immune checkpoint inhibitors.

2. Results

2.1. Evaluation of Drug Sensitivity on 786-0 Cell-Derived Spheroids

We first compared the induction of cell mortality in 786-O spheroids after their treatment with either a combination of GDC-0941 and saracatinib (GDC/SRC), two small-molecule inhibitors that target the PI3K and Src kinases respectively [39], or the currently clinically used inhibitors sunitinib, pazopanib, or temsirolimus at the indicated concentrations. Treated spheroids were recorded for 48 h using an Essen IncuCyte Zoom live-cell microscopy instrument (Figure 1A). Cell death induced by the different treatments at 6, 12, 24, and 48 h, was quantified through propidium iodide (PI) incorporation normalized by the surface of the spheroid. The results show that the drug effects on 786-O spheroids could be easily quantified using the Incucyte microscopy instrument (Figure 1B). Moreover, monitoring the size of the spheroids after 36 h of treatment showed that the GDC/SRC combination induces a significant reduction of the spheroid size (35%) while the effects of the other drugs were weaker compared to DMSO for which spheroid area declined by 15%, probably due to the maturation of the organoids that were under culture condition for five days (Figure 1C). During the last 12 h of treatment, cells in the spheroid center that was hypoxic, might have begun to die. Next, immunohistochemistry was performed on paraffin-embedded spheroids to visualize both the cellular architecture and the cell proliferation inside the 3D-spheroids. As shown in Figure 1D–F, both the integrity of the spheroids and the cell proliferation detected by PCNA labeling were affected by the GDC/SRC combination or Temsirolimus treatments confirming their effects on spheroids viability. Moreover, spheroid area measurements (Figure 1E) were consistent with the analysis of PI incorporation determined with the Incucyte microscope (Figure 1A). However, although promising, these data obtained with a 3D cancer cell line model suffered from inherent limitations due to inadequate representation of the heterogeneous architecture of human tumor and tumor–stromal interactions, which renders the interpretation on efficacy testing challenging. This is attested by the observation that among all the new molecules discovered for their action on cancer cell line models, only very few reached the FDA agreement. Therefore, implementation of physiologically relevant in- vitro models closer to patient-derived tumors is required.

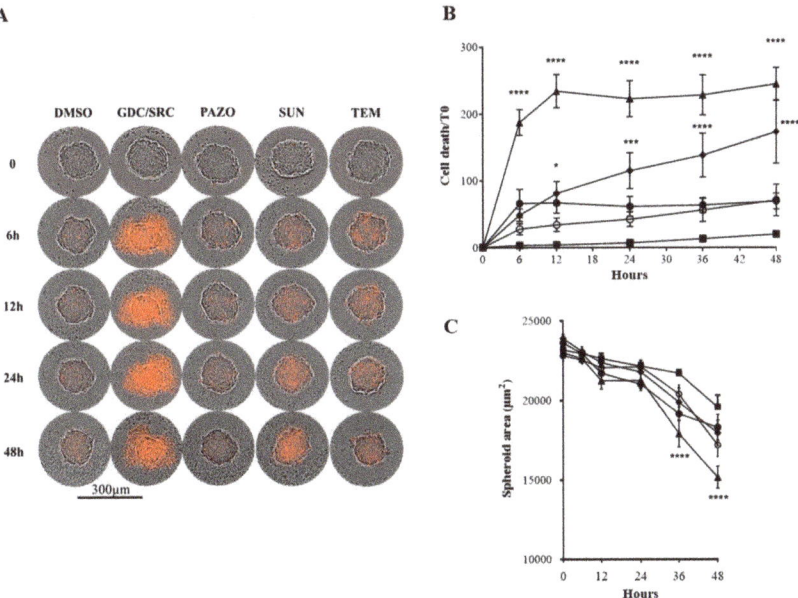

Figure 1. *Cont.*

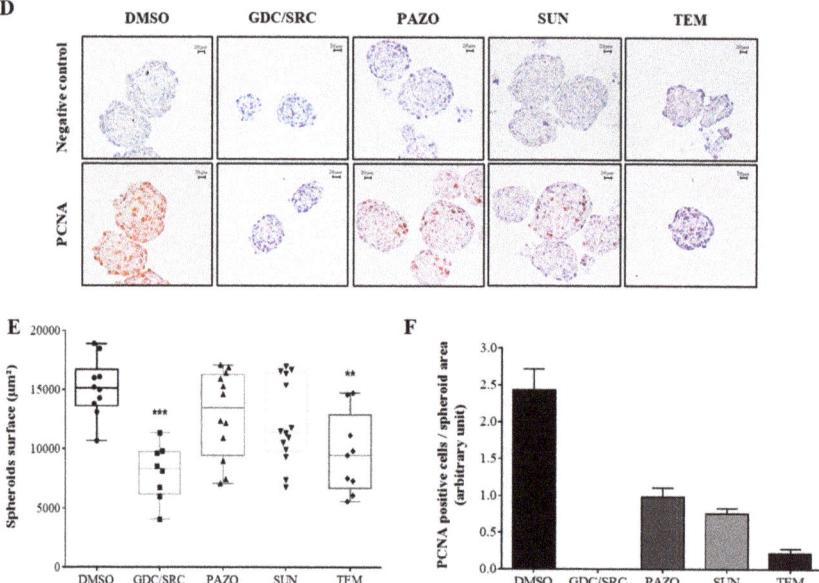

Figure 1. Treatment of 786-O spheroids. 786-O-WT (VHL⁻) cells were grown as spheroids and treated with 10 µM of either GDC-0941 + saracatinib (10 µM each, GDC/SRC, ▲), pazopanib (PAZO, ○), sunitinib (SUN, ♦), temsirolimus (TEM, ●), or vehicle (DMSO, ■) in the presence of propidium iodide. Cell death was monitored on spheroids using either an Essen IncuCyte Zoom live-cell microscopy incubator or by immunohistochemistry. (**A**) Bright field and fluorescent overlaid images show 786-O-treated spheroids at indicated times (0, 6, 12, 24, and 48 h). Bar scale 300 µm. (**B**) Images taken automatically every 6 h over 48 h of culture were analyzed for PI fluorescent area quantification. Cell death values (PI labeling area) was divided by the corresponding spheroid area and multiplied by 100. This percentage of cell death was divided by the one at T_0, for all the others time points and was expressed as mean ± SEM. The statistical analysis of dead cells was performed with 2 way ANOVA test for each time point compared to DMSO treatment. (**C**) The same images were analyzed for spheroid area quantification. Significant difference was observed between GDC/SRC (**** $p \leq 0.001$), SUN (**** $p \leq 0.01$), TEM (**** $p \leq 0.01$) versus DMSO after 36 h of treatment using a Kruskal-Wallis test. (**D**) PCNA staining to visualize proliferation of fixed paraffin-embedded (scale bar, 20 µm). (**E**) Spheroid area quantification by surface calculation of (**D**), ($n \geq 8$). Significant difference was observed between GDC/SRC (*** $p \leq 0.001$), TEM (** $p \leq 0.01$) versus DMSO in a Kruskal-Wallis test. (**F**) The number of PCNA positive cells was quantified in each spheroid and divided by the corresponding spheroid surface. Histogram plot represents mean of PCNA-stained cells pooled from 4 to 6 spheroids (biological replicated/condition) with error bar (±SEM).

2.2. Tissue Slice Cultures of Renal Tumors

We set out to determine whether an ex-vivo treatment protocol could be used as a means of determining ccRCC sensitivity to various cytotoxic agents. The PDTSC methodology has been previously used to evaluate the drug sensitivity of normal and tumor tissues [29–38]. Therefore, we set up an adaptation of this method outlined in Figure 2A, as an ex-vivo protocol to examine responses of ccRCC to different therapeutic agents. Cultures of slices, obtained either from 786-O-derived tumors generated in mouse xenografts or from human ccRCC surgical resection specimens, were prepared as detailed in the Methods section, and then subjected to a variety of tests. First, we noticed that over 96 h of culture, luminescence measurement of 786-O-luc cells in the tumor slice remained constant, attesting their viability during this time schedule (Figure 2B).

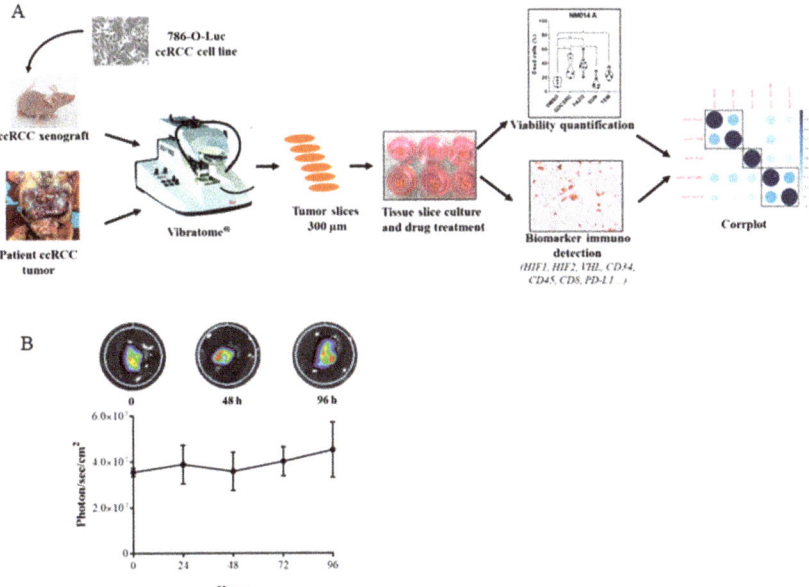

Figure 2. The procedure flowchart for renal tumor slice culture. (**A**) 786-O-derived tumors generated in mouse xenografts or human ccRCC surgical resection specimens are cut into 300 μm slices in buffer solution using a Vibratome®. The slices are transferred to culture medium and then carefully placed on membrane insert in 6-well plates to create an air-liquid interface. After 48 h of drug treatments, slices are analyzed for cell viability and biomarker immuno-detection. Correlation between drug sensitivity and biomarker expression is visualized with the graphical display of a correlation matrix (Corrplot, R package). (**B**) Tumor slices maintain cell survival over four days of culture. Slices from 786-O-luc-derived tumors were cultured for up to four days, with fresh media changes performed every two days. Each day, luminescence was recorded from slices after luciferin addition using IVIS imaging (upper panel). Plotted normalized photon quantification showed minimal changes over the culture periods.

2.3. The Cytotoxic Effects of Drug Treatments Can Be Evaluated in Tissue-Slice Cultures

In order to evaluate the PDTSC approach, we first used the renal carcinoma mouse xenograft model. The tumors were extracted from the mice, directly processed into 300 μm slices, and treated for 48 h as described in Materials and Methods and indicated in Figure 2A. Cell viability evaluated by ethidium homodimer staining of treated tumor-slice cultures are illustrated in Figure 3A. Mortality quantified on five to seven images using ImageJ, was reported as "Cell death/DMSO" that represents the percentage of dead cells in the different groups divided by the percentage of dead cells in the DMSO-treated slices. The mortality rate showed a significant difference between DMSO and drugs alone or the GDC/SRC combination ($p < 0.05$) (Figure 3A,B). Immuno-histochemistry (IHC) analysis was used to determine whether a differential proliferative (PCNA) response to drug treatment could be detected. For this, paraffin-embedded sections were stained with a PCNA antibody and counter-colored with hematoxylin. We found that the GDC/SRC combination caused a significant decrease in PCNA staining, while temsirolimus, sunitinib, and pazopanib were less efficient (Figure 3C). Taken together, these results demonstrate that PDTSC allows for the rapid investigation of ccCRCC sensitivity to targeted therapies.

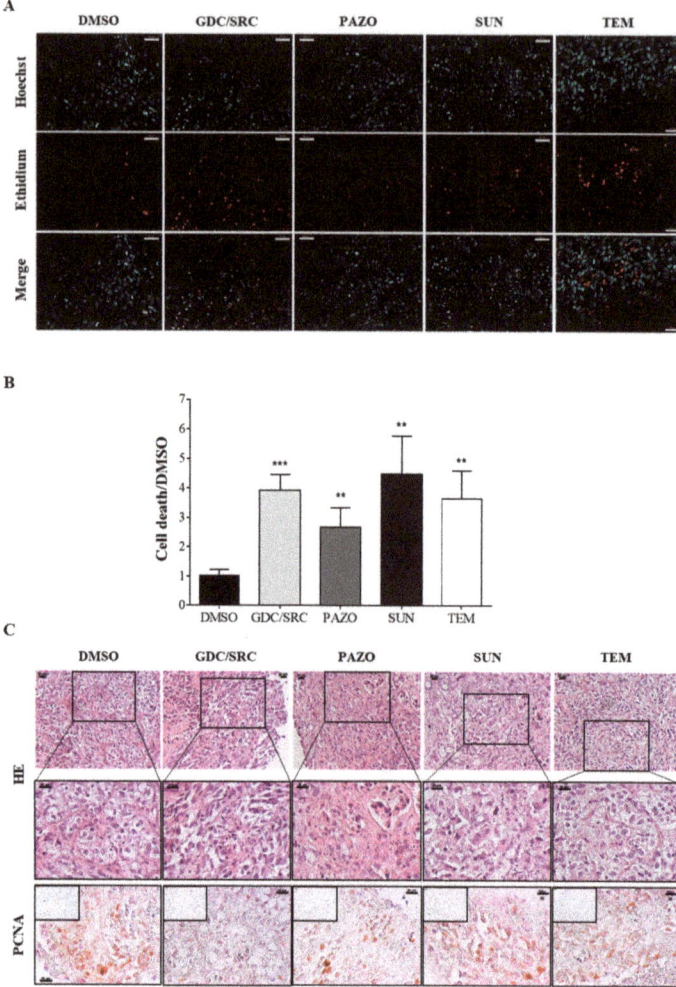

Figure 3. Treatment of slice cultures from 786-O tumor xenografts. 786-O cells were injected under the renal capsule of Balb/c nude mice. One month later, mice were euthanized, tumors were harvested and processed for tissue slice cultures. (**A**) Tissue slice cultures were treated with 10 µM of either GDC-0941 + saracatinib (10 µM each, GDC/SRC), pazopanib (PAZO), sunitinib (SUN), temsirolimus (TEM), or vehicle (DMSO 0.2%) for 48 h. Nuclei were stained with Hoechst 33342 and dead cells were visualized by Ethidium homodimer staining. Images were taken with an Apotome-equipped Zeiss microscope. Bar scale 50 µm. (**B**) The intensity of Ethidium homodimer positive cells was measured in each nucleus on five independent areas of the tumor slices as described in Material and Methods. The y-axis represents the ratio of the percentage of dead cells in the different groups divided by the corresponding value in the DMSO-treated-slices. Significant differences in cell death were observed between DMSO versus the GDC/SRC combination (*** $p \leq 0.001$) or each drug alone (** $p \leq 0.05$) using a Mann–Whitney test. (**C**) Tumor slices were treated as described in A, then fixed and embedded in paraffin. Fixed tissue slices were stained with Hematoxylin-Eosin (HE). Representative pictures of treated slices are shown at two magnifications (lower magnifications, upper images and higher magnifications, middle images). Tumor slices were also stained with the anti-PCNA antibody to visualize cell proliferation (lower panel). Negative controls (no primary antibody) are shown in the insets. Scale bars 20 µm.

To further evaluate the potential of this approach, slices from surgical resections of human ccRCC tumors were analyzed using the same optimized protocol. In this study, we focused on patient tumors that were later on characterized as renal clear cell carcinoma by a board certified histo-pathologist at the Urology Department—University Hospital Center of Grenoble-Alpes. We note that our protocol did not interfere with the pathologist's analysis. Warm ischemia was reduced to 15 min including tumor dissection and extraction during the surgery. Cold ischemia between extraction and the beginning of the culture was less than 2 h (including tumor sample dissection, transport and slicing). Two small pieces from two distinct regions (A and B) of each tumor were taken and processed in slices using a Vibratome®. Then, each tumor slice was cultured in the presence of the vehicle (0.2% DMSO) or the indicated therapeutic agents and assayed for cell viability after 48 h of drug treatment. Figure 4A shows that sample A disclosed high sensitivity to pazopanib or the GDC/SRC combination whereas sunitinib and temsirolimus were almost without effect. In contrast, sunitinib significantly compromised cell viability in sample B. Samples B-treated slices were further analyzed for their proliferation status after fixation and paraffin inclusion to assess functional response and cell viability. PCNA staining was detected in DMSO-treated slices (11.9%), whereas very few cells were stained in sunitinib-treated slices (0.2%). Moreover, a strong staining of cleaved-caspase-3 that reflects apoptotic cell death was observed in sunitinib-treated tumor slices (42.1%) but almost undetectable in DMSO-treated samples (4.2%) (Figure 4B).

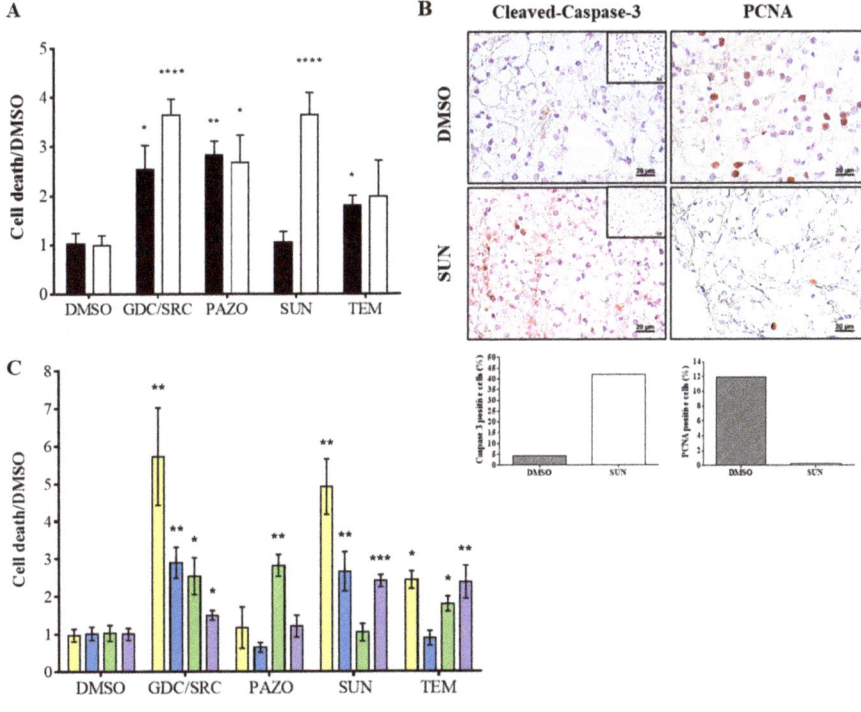

Figure 4. *Cont.*

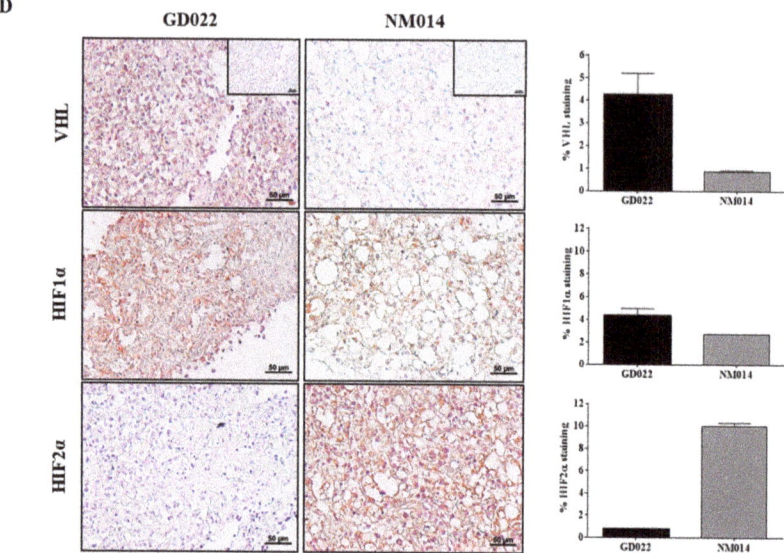

Figure 4. Treatment of slice cultures from human renal tumors. Tissue slice cultures from human renal tumors were treated for 48 h with a panel of drugs (10 µM each) and cell viability assayed as in Figure 3A. (**A**) Intra-tumor heterogeneity. Two fragments A and B of the same tumor (NM014) were analyzed for their sensitivity to indicated drug treatments. Mean DMSO was normalized to 1 to compare the two fragments of NM014. The *y*-axis represents the ratio of the percentage of dead cells in the different groups divided by the corresponding value in the DMSO-treated-PDTSC. Cell death measurement in fragment A (black bars) from NM014 shows significant differences between DMSO versus the combination (GDC/SRC, * $p < 0.5$), pazopanib (PAZO, ** $p < 0.01$) and temsirolimus (TEM, * $p < 0.5$) but not versus sunitinib (SUN). The same analysis of fragment B (white bars) from the same NM014 tumor, shows similar profile except for sunitinib that in this case induced significant cell death (SUN, **** $p < 0.0005$). (**B**) Apoptosis and proliferation assays. Representative pictures of tumor slices from fragment B of NM014 treated for 48 h with DMSO (**upper panels**) or 10 µM sunitinib (SUN, **lower panels**) and stained with Cleaved-Caspase-3 (**left panel**) or with anti-PCNA antibody (**right panel**). The PCNA stain identifies cells that are proliferating while the Cleaved-Caspase-3 stain shows cells undergoing apoptosis. The percentages of PCNA and Cleaved-Caspase 3 positive cells were plotted below each set of pictures. Scale bars, 20 µm. Negative controls (no primary antibody) are shown in insets. (**C**) Inter-tumor heterogeneity. Four different tumors were treated and analyzed as in Figure 3A showing distinct drug sensitivity profiles. Each color represents one patient tumor (Yellow, NB029; Blue, YL024; Green, NM014; Purple, MD034). (**D**) VHL and HIF expressions. Representative pictures of two untreated tumor slices GD022 and NM014 stained with anti-VHL, anti-HIF1α or anti-HIF2α antibodies. Scale bars, 50 µm. For each staining, images taken from five independent areas of a tumor slice were quantified with ImageJ and plotted as percentage of specific staining relative to tumor area (respective right panels).

These results highlight the intra-tumor heterogeneity of ccRCC, a property that has been well documented by extensive multi-regional whole-genome and -exome sequencing [40]. Collectively, these data demonstrated that PDTSC can be used to assess functional response and cell survival of human renal carcinoma specimens to drug treatments, reinforcing its value as a companion diagnostic tool in ccRCC treatment.

2.4. Acute Ex-Vivo Drug Treatments Identify Renal Tumor Subsets with Distinct Therapeutic Profiles

We compared the cell death rate of four different patient tumors upon the same panel of drug treatments (Figure 4C). Interestingly, this approach allowed for the identification of differential patient responses revealing sensitive and resistant tumors. For example, pazopanib was completely inactive on NB029, YL024 and MD034, whereas it was the most efficient on NM014. Temsirolimus was without effect on YL024.

Inactivation of the Von Hippel–Lindau (VHL) tumor suppressor gene has been shown to play an important role in the process of angiogenesis in RCC. As a component of an E3 ubiquitin ligase complex, the VHL protein targets the hypoxia-inducible transcription factors (HIF1α and HIF2α) for degradation. Loss of VHL function in ccRCC leads to the constitutive stabilization of these transcription factors, leading to a highly angiogenic environment [41] and HIF2α has recently emerged as a therapeutic target in ccRCC [42]. In line with this, we determined the protein expression level of VHL, HIF1α and HIF2α in human renal tumor slices (Figure 4D, left panels). Immuno-staining quantification shows that in slice NM014 where VHL expression was undetectable, HIF1α and mainly HIF2α were more abundant than in slice GD022 where VHL was present (Figure 4D, right panels).

2.5. Predictive Biomarkers in Renal Tumor Slice Cultures

The trafficking of immune cells in human cancers affects their immunobiology but also could have a major prognostic and predictive impact on the efficacy of the patient treatment. Indeed, renal cell carcinoma is an immunogenic tumor that characteristically harbors abundant infiltrating lymphocytes [43] and it has been shown that across renal tumors, there is a wide range of immune infiltrates [44]. Therefore, we tracked immune cells and their interaction with cancer cells within fixed slice cultures of different patient tumor samples (Figure 5). As an example, Figure 5A shows representative images of two non-treated tumor slices ML025 and DP027 in which the microvessel density labeled by CD34 staining was similar (Figure 5, right panel). Tumor slice DP027 was infiltrated with fewer cytotoxic CD8$^+$ T cells than the tumor slice ML025. Interestingly, it has been suggested that in highly infiltrated ccRCC tumors, T-cell activation state is a key determinant of ccRCC prognosis and likely of immunotherapy response. Given the variety of mechanisms triggered by molecularly targeted agents in cancers and their late-stage clinical trials, the validation of drug sensitivity predictive models may be critical to identify the right drug for the right patients and help to understand determinants of responsiveness, wherein alternative treatments could potentially overcome resistance [45]. There is a recently growing body of literature describing PDTSC from different normal and tumor tissues [34–38]. However, to our knowledge, the present study is the first to demonstrate the potential use of this approach to evaluate renal cancer response to novel therapies while modeling the tumor immune microenvironment. An important benefit of the PDTSC strategy is that it provides a rapid and easy readout of the functional effects and drug responses that result from a complex array of molecular alterations among patients with ccRCC. PDTSC delivers a much faster timeline than PDX animal models, which require at least 6 to 7 weeks to become established versus 48 h for the PDTSC method. There is an important limitation inherent to PDTSC: the frequent intra-tumor heterogeneity may not be represented in individual slices from specific regions of a surgical resection specimen. However, this can be taken into account by a careful geographical collection of replicated tumor slices. In agreement with the key role played by the immune infiltrate in ccRCC, a phase 3 clinical trial (CheckMate214) showed benefits in terms of overall survival and objective response rate using an immunotherapy combination (ipilinumab plus nivolumab) versus sunitinib for intermediate and poor-risk patients with previously untreated advanced renal cell carcinoma [46].

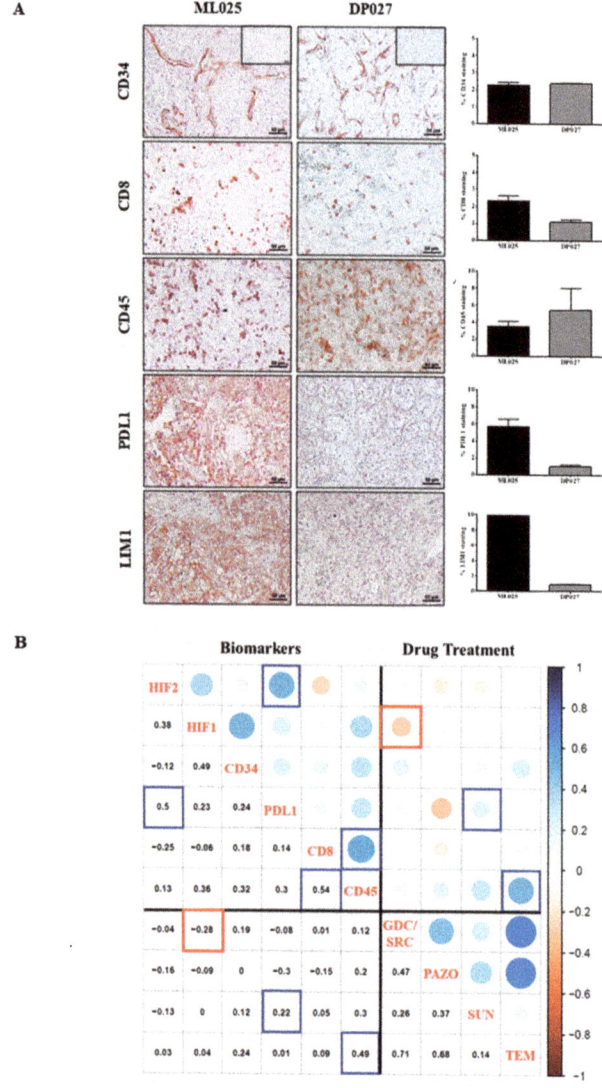

Figure 5. Predictive biomarkers in renal tumor slice cultures. (**A**) Vascular, immune and stem cell type characterization. Representative pictures of untreated tumor slices ML025 and DP027 stained with the following antibodies: anti-CD34, anti-CD8, anti-CD45, anti-PDL1, anti-LIM1. Scale bars, 50 μm. For each staining, images taken from five independent areas of a tumor slice were quantified with ImageJ and plotted (**right panels**). (**B**) Correlation plot between the percentage of positive cells following various IHC staining and the normalized proportion of dying cells following application of drug treatments. The Spearman rank correlation was used. The diagonal indicates the biomarker used for the IHC staining (**left part**) or the drug treatment (**right part**). Below the diagonal is the pairwise correlation value, and above the diagonal is the corresponding representation, with the color legend that is the bar on the right side of the plot. Blue (resp. red) colors correspond to positive (resp. negative) correlations. Boxes correspond to cases described in the text. For example, the two blue boxes on the top-left side highlight a correlation of 0.5 of the percentage of positive cells between HIF2 and PDL1 staining.

In both tumor slices, we also detected a differential intra-tumor positive staining for the protein tyrosine phosphatase receptor CD45, one of the key players in the initiation of T cell receptor signaling [47]. CD45$^+$ cells were abundant in DP027 tumor and localized in close proximity with microvessels and red blood cells. These cells were more intricately distributed in the ML025 slice than in DP027 reflecting a potential immune infiltration.

The tumor microenvironment deploys various immune escape mechanisms that neutralize CD8 T cell-mediated tumor rejection. One mechanism implies the aberrant expression of programmed death-ligand 1 (PD-L1) that targets the neutralization of activated CD8 T cells. PD-L1 has been reported in several human cancers including RCC [48]. This ligand is aberrantly expressed on the surface of both primary and metastatic RCC tumor cells [49] and several studies have described a positive correlation between PD-L1 expression, metastasis, and poor outcomes in ccRCC [50]. Consistent with this, we found that PD-L1 was strongly expressed in the ML025 tumor slice while undetectable in the DP027 tumor slice. Of note, ML025 slices were both positive for PD-L1 and cytotoxic CD8$^+$ T cells. Interestingly, it has been suggested that metastatic melanoma that are both expressing PD-L1 and CD8$^+$ T cells will likely respond to immunotherapy [51].

The LIM1 transcription factor which is essential for the development of human kidney is reactivated in nephroblastomas [52] and implicated in the metastatic spread of ccRCC [53]. While being undetectable in the DP027 slice, a strong intratumor LIM1 expression was observed in the ML025 slice. Altogether, these data support the contention that the PDTSC method allows for precise, short-term modeling of the stromal/immune microenvironment of renal tumors.

2.6. Prediction of Potential Correlations between Drug Sensitivity Responses and Tumor Immune Infiltration

To investigate whether there are links between drug-sensitivity and specific biomarkers previously analyzed in Figure 5A, we performed correlation analysis (Figure 5B). Eighteen human renal tumors (26 tumor specimens) that have been challenged for both drug-sensitivity and IHC- specific labeling were compared. Pairwise correlated variables were plotted in a graph of correlation matrix according to correlation coefficients indicated either by colored circles or numbers. This analysis highlights three subgroups/clusters of correlations between biomarkers only, drugs only and both drugs and biomarkers. In the first cluster, we visualized a strong positive correlation between CD8 and CD45 expressions (correlation coefficient, 0.54) and between HIF2α and PD-L1 (correlation coefficient, 0.5). These results are consistent with the literature as CD8 cytotoxic T cells are a subpopulation of CD45 positive leucocytes [54] and HIF2α as a transcription factor, binds to the PD-L1 promotor to induce its expression [55]. Inside the "drug" cluster, correlation are high (correlation coefficients > 0.35 except for the temsirolimus compared to the sunitinib situations). This result can be explained because the four treatments tested have similar action mechanisms (all are kinase inhibitors), however, they are not equal and more samples could help to find differences. Finally, the most informative cluster that compares biomarkers and drug treatments highlights two positive correlations between CD45 and temsirolimus (TEM) (correlation coefficient, 0.49) and PD-L1 and SUN (correlation coefficient, 0.22) and a negative correlation between GDC/SRC and HIF1α (correlation coefficient, −0.28). TEM has been demonstrated to have immune-modulating activity [56]. Obviously, the degree of correlation should be established by increasing the amount of tumor tissue samples for IHC analysis but even with this small cohort of tumor samples, potential valuable correlations dawned in this analysis and warrants further investigations.

3. Discussion

Given the variety of mechanisms triggered by molecularly targeted agents in cancers and their late-stage clinical trials, the validation of drug sensitivity predictive models may be critical to identify the right drug for the right patients and help to understand determinants of responsiveness, wherein alternative treatments could potentially overcome resistance [45]. There is a recently growing body of literature describing PDTSC from different normal and tumor tissues [29–38]. However, to our knowledge, the present study is the first to demonstrate the potential use of this approach to evaluate renal cancer response to novel therapies while modeling the tumor immune microenvironment. An important benefit of the PDTSC strategy is that it provides a rapid and facile readout of the functional effects and drug responses that result from a complex array of molecular alterations among patients with ccRCC. PDTSC delivers a much faster timeline than PDX animal models, which require at least 6 to 7 weeks to become established versus 48 h for the PDTSC method. There are several limitations inherent to PDTSC: (1) the frequent intra-tumor heterogeneity may not be represented in individual slices from specific regions of a surgical resection specimen. However, this can be taken into account by a careful geographical collection of replicated tumor slices; (2) fresh primary tissue may not be available when needed (in case of recurrent disease) and radical nephrectomy is not always performed on metastasized patients, whereas screening of these patients would be highly beneficial in the context of a predictive assay. The proof that the PDTSC can identify the best treatment need further investigations. In particular, as 30% of ccRCC becomes metastatic, one third of the patients will probably need specific treatments. In this context, the therapeutic profiling generated from the PDTSC may be informative after a retrospective clinical follow-up from patients who will develop metastasis; (3) PDTSC may be not relevant for some active drugs that are metabolites (e.g., for sunitinib).

4. Materials and Methods

4.1. Reagents, Drugs and Antibodies

Saracatinib (SRC) and GDC-0941(GDC) were obtained from LC Laboratories (Woburn, MA, USA). temsirolimus (TEM), pazopanib (PAZO), and sunitinib (SUN) were purchased from Selleck Chemicals (Houston, TX, USA), propidium iodide and Hoechst 33342 from Sigma-Aldrich (St Louis, MO, USA), and Live & Dead kit from Life Technologies (Carlsbad, CA, USA). The antibodies against the following targets were used: PCNA, CD8, CD34, PD-L1 (Ab29, Ab101500, Ab81289, Ab205921, Abcam, Cambridge, UK), Cleaved-Caspase-3, CD45 (#9664, #13971, Cell Signaling, Danvers, MA, USA); HIF1α, HIF2α (NB100-479, NB100-122, Novus Biologicals, Centennial, CO, USA), VHL (MA-1-12638, Thermo Scientific, Waltham, MA, USA).

4.2. 3D-Spheroid Culture and Live Cell Tracking

786-O cells (ATCC-CRL-1932) are derived from a human primary clear cell adenocarcinoma. This highly metastatic cell line is negative for VHL and is cultured in RPMI-1640 Medium supplemented with 10% SVF and penicillin [100 U/mL], streptomycin [100 µg/mL].

Spheroids were prepared in 96-wells U-bottom with low evaporation lid (MicrotestTM, Becton Dickinson Labware, San Jose, CA, USA) coated with 20 mg/mL poly-HEMA (Sigma-Aldrich). A 786-O cell suspension (1×10^3 cells) was seeded in each well and cells were allowed to form spheroids within three days. Then, they were treated with indicated inhibitors for 48 h in the presence of Propidium iodide (0.5 µg/mL) to visualize dead cells and video recorded every hour using an Incucyte microscope, an automated live cell imager with high-throughput capabilities and built-in data analysis (Essen Biosciences, Welwyn Garden City, UK). Experiments were conducted at 37 °C and 5% CO_2. Quantification of cell death was measured after 48 h as a percentage of confluence in the red channel (PI%) using the software incorporated into the IncuCyte Zoom. To normalize the data, all values for each time point was divided by the value at T_0. Experimental data are shown as mean ± standard error mean (SEM) except for Figure 1E for which whole the points are shown overlaid on boxplots and whiskers. Classically, the box corresponds to the first and third quartiles, and the horizontal bar is the median, whereas the whiskers demarcate here the extreme values.

4.3. Mice Orthotopic Tumor Xenograft Models

All animal studies were approved by the institutional guidelines and those formulated by the European Community for the Use of Experimental Animals. Six week-old BALB/c female nude mice (Charles River Laboratories, Wilmington, MA, USA) with a mean body weight of 18–20 g were used to establish orthotopic xenograft tumor models. The mice were housed and fed under specific pathogen-free conditions. To produce tumors, renal cancer cells 786-O-luc (Roelants et al.) were harvested from sub-confluent cultures by a brief exposure to 0.25% trypsin-EDTA. Trypsinization was stopped with medium containing 10% FBS, and the cells were washed once in serum-free medium and resuspended in 500 µL PBS. Renal orthotopic implantation was carried out by injection of 3×10^6 786-O luc cells into the left kidney of athymic nude mice. Mice were weighed once a week to monitor their health and tumor growth was measured by imaging luminescence of 786-O-luc cells (IVIS).

4.4. Patients and Clinical Samples

All human renal carcinoma samples were obtained from patients, with their informed consent and all procedures were approved by the ethic committee (Patient protection committee No 2017 A0070251). All patients had serology to detect blood transmissible diseases before surgery and all samples were anonymized. Fresh renal tumor tissues were obtained from patient undergoing a partial or a total nephrectomy for cancer at the Urology Department—University Hospital Center of Grenoble-Alpes (CHUGA). The minimal size of tumor samples for inclusion was 2 cm. After resection, tissue samples were directly transported to the pathology department of the CHUGA in a cold saline solution (Sterile 0.9% NaCl). A macroscopic dissection was performed by a pathologist and as far as possible two distinct tumor samples (A and B) were placed in a sterile conical tube containing a conservation medium (ice-cold sterile balanced salt HBSS solution containing [100 U/mL] penicillin and [100 µg/mL] streptomycin) on wet ice during transport from the pathology department to the INSERM research laboratory (CEA).

4.5. Preparation of Tissue Slices and Organotypic Culture

Upon arrival, resections were manually minced using a sterile scalpel and samples were soaked in ice-cold sterile HBSS, orientated, mounted in low-melting agarose (5%), and immobilized using cyanoacrylate glue. Thick tissue slices (300 µm) were prepared from fresh tissue under sterile conditions using a Vibratome VT1200 (Leica Microsystems, Wetzlar, Germany). Slicing speed was optimized according to tissue density and type; in general, slower slicing speed was used on the softer tissues and vice versa (0.2–0.7 mm/s). Vibration amplitude was set between 1.85 to 2.45 mm.

Tissue slices were then carefully placed on 0.4 µm pore size Teflon membrane culture inserts (Millipore Corporation, Burlington, MA, USA) containing one slice per insert and cultured for up to 96 h. at 37 °C in a 5% CO_2 humidified incubator using 2 mL of DMEM media supplemented with 20% inactivated FBS (GIBCO), 100 U/mL penicillin (Invitrogen, Carlsbad, CA, USA). Inserts were placed in a rotor agitator to allow gas and fluid exchanges with the medium. For each tumor, two slice samples (A and B) were treated with the inhibitors at the indicated concentrations for 48 h.

4.6. Slice Viability Assay

At the end of treatment, lived slices were stained with the Live & Dead kit (Life Technologies) as recommended and nuclei were labeled with Hoechst 33342. Images were taken with an Apotome-equipped Zeiss Axio-Imager microscope with a 20× PlanApochromat objective (Numerical Aperture 0.8). A minimum of three regions of interest (ROI) were taken, at three positions in z with 7 µm intervals to avoid counting the same nuclei twice. Dead cells in the tissue slices were quantified with scripts of ImageJ and further processed with R version 3.4.3 [57]. The histogram of red fluorescence intensity shows a peak of low intensity corresponding to live cells, and high and widely spread intensity values, corresponding to dying cells., called M_{raw}. A minimum of 1200 total cells was analyzed for each group. Experimental data are shown as mean ± standard error mean (SEM). As the percentage of dead cells varies significantly between different untreated tumor specimen due to variation inherent to surgery, the percentage of dead cells in the different groups was divided by the corresponding value in the DMSO-treated-PDTSC. Thus, the y-axis untitled "Cell death/DMSO" represents arbitrary units corresponding to this ratio.

For Figure 5B, mortality in a given condition is obtained by taking the median value among the different z acquisition and ROI. Only conditions associated with a mortality below 55% were kept for further analysis (four slices removed). As there is a correlation between cell mortality on a given slide treated with the DMSO and the other drugs, we normalized cell mortality values using the following formulae:

$$M_{norm} = (M_{raw} - M_{DMSO})/f(M_{DMSO})$$

where M_{norm} is the normalized mortality for a given drug, typically between 0 and 1, M_{raw} is the raw mortality of the given drug, between 0 and 100, M_{DMSO} is the raw mortality of the $DMSO$ for the nearby slice, between 0 and 100, $f(M_{DMSO})$ is the normalization function, depending on the $DMSO$, which evaluates the maximum amplitude of the drug effect on a given slice. It is given by:

$$f(M_{DMSO}) = a - M_{DMSO} + (100 - a) * (1 - \exp(-M_{DMSO}/b)),$$

where $a = 15$ and $b = 10$, chosen to fit with the maximal mortality.

The correlation analysis was performed using R version 3.4.3 [57], pairwise. The Spearman's rank correlation coefficient was used to perform a robust analysis. The figure was generated using the corrplot package version 0.84.

4.7. Immunohistochemistry Analysis

Sections (5 µm thick) of formalin-fixed, paraffin embedded tumor tissue samples were dewaxed, rehydrated through graded ethanol and subjected to heat-mediated antigen retrieval in citrate buffer (Antigen Unmasking Solution, Vector Laboratories, Burlingame, CA, USA). Slides were incubated for 10 min in hydrogen peroxide H_2O_2 to block endogenous peroxidases and then 30 min in saturation solution (Histostain, Invitrogen) to block nonspecific antibody binding. This was followed by overnight incubation with indicated primary antibodies at 4 °C. After washing, sections were incubated with a suitable biotinylated secondary antibody (Histostain, Invitrogen) for 10 min. Antigen-antibody complexes were visualized by applying a streptavidin-biotin complex (Histostain, Invitrogen) for 10 min followed by NovaRED substrate (Vector Laboratories). Sections were counterstained with hematoxylin to visualize nucleus. Control sections were incubated with pool secondary antibodies without primary antibody.

4.8. Statistical and Correlation Analyses

Experimental data are shown as mean ± standard error mean (SEM). Statistical analyses were performed using one-way analysis of variance (ANOVA) with multiple comparisons test (GraphPad Prism 6). A *p*-value of less than 0.05 was considered statistically significant.

5. Conclusions

Because the PDTSC strategy maintains the landscape of the original tumor sample, including the stromal and the immune tumor compartment, this approach is a relevant model for individualized testing of drug susceptibility to improve clinical success rates [22,58]. In agreement with the key role played by the immune infiltrate in ccRCC, a phase 3 clinical trial (CheckMate214) showed benefits in term of overall survival and objective response rate using an immunotherapy combination (ipilinumab plus nivolumab) versus sunitinib for intermediate and poor-risk patients with previously untreated advanced renal cell carcinoma [46]. Therefore, PDTSC also warrants further investigations to confirm potential correlations between drug sensitivity responses and the level of tumor vascularization and tumor-infiltrating immune cell populations. Finally, a recent study [59] suggests that further work will eventually make this technique useful for personalized clinical immunotherapy.

Author Contributions: Conceptualization, C.C. and O.F.; investigation and methodology, C.R., C.P., S.G., Q.F., N.P., C.S., and O.F.; validation, C.P., Q.F., C.S., L.G., C.C., and O.F.; formal analysis, C.R., Q.F., L.G., C.S., and O.F.; software, L.G. and C.S.; resources, C.R., C.P., S.G., Q.F., N.P., A.F., C.S., O.F., G.F., J.-A.L., and J.-L.D.; data curation, C.R., L.G., Q.F., C.S., and O.F.; visualization, C.R., C.S., L.G., and O.F.; writing—review and editing, Q.F., C.R., C.S., L.G., O.F., and C.C.; supervision, O.F., C.C., and J.-L.D.; project administration and funding acquisition, C.C.; O.F., and J.-L.D. All authors have read and agreed to the published version of the manuscript.

Funding: This work was supported by recurrent institutional funding from INSERM, CEA, Ligue Nationale contre le Cancer (accredited team 2010–2012) and Ligue Comité de l'Isère, University Grenoble Alpes, Centre Hospitalier Universitaire de Grenoble-Alpes (CHUGA), Groupement des Entreprises Françaises dans la LUtte contre le Cancer (GEFLUC), Grenoble Alliance for Integrated Structural & Cell Biology (GRAL) and Association Française d'Urologie (AFU).

Acknowledgments: We thank the animal unit staff (Jeannin I., Bama S., Magallon C., Chaumontel N. and Pointu H.) at Interdiciplinary Research Institute of Grenoble (IRIG) for animal husbandry.

Conflicts of Interest: The authors declare no financial or commercial conflict of interest.

References

1. Negrier, S.; Escudier, B.; Lasset, C.; Douillard, J.Y.; Savary, J.; Chevreau, C.; Ravaud, A.; Mercatello, A.; Peny, J.; Mousseau, M.; et al. Recombinant human interleukin-2, recombinant human interferon alfa-2a, or both in metastatic renal-cell carcinoma. Groupe Francais d'Immunotherapie. *N. Engl. J. Med.* **1998**, *338*, 1272–1278. [CrossRef]
2. Figlin, R.; Sternberg, C.; Wood, C.G. Novel agents and approaches for advanced renal cell carcinoma. *J. Urol.* **2012**, *188*, 707–715. [CrossRef]
3. Atkins, M.B.; Clark, J.I.; Quinn, D.I. Immune checkpoint inhibitors in advanced renal cell carcinoma: Experience to date and future directions. *Ann. Oncol. Off. J. Eur. Soc. Med Oncol.* **2017**, *28*, 1484–1494. [CrossRef]
4. Motzer, R.J.; Penkov, K.; Haanen, J.; Rini, B.; Albiges, L.; Campbell, M.T.; Venugopal, B.; Kollmannsberger, C.; Negrier, S.; Uemura, M.; et al. Avelumab plus Axitinib versus Sunitinib for Advanced Renal-Cell Carcinoma. *N. Engl. J. Med.* **2019**, *380*, 1103–1115. [CrossRef] [PubMed]
5. Rini, B.I.; Plimack, E.R.; Stus, V.; Gafanov, R.; Hawkins, R.; Nosov, D.; Pouliot, F.; Alekseev, B.; Soulieres, D.; Melichar, B.; et al. Pembrolizumab plus Axitinib versus Sunitinib for Advanced Renal-Cell Carcinoma. *N. Engl. J. Med.* **2019**, *380*, 1116–1127. [CrossRef] [PubMed]
6. Cella, D.; Grunwald, V.; Escudier, B.; Hammers, H.J.; George, S.; Nathan, P.; Grimm, M.O.; Rini, B.I.; Doan, J.; Ivanescu, C.; et al. Patient-reported outcomes of patients with advanced renal cell carcinoma treated with nivolumab plus ipilimumab versus sunitinib (CheckMate 214): A randomised, phase 3 trial. *Lancet Oncol.* **2019**, *20*, 297–310. [CrossRef]
7. Garnett, M.J.; Edelman, E.J.; Heidorn, S.J.; Greenman, C.D.; Dastur, A.; Lau, K.W.; Greninger, P.; Thompson, I.R.; Luo, X.; Soares, J.; et al. Systematic identification of genomic markers of drug sensitivity in cancer cells. *Nature* **2012**, *483*, 570–575. [CrossRef] [PubMed]
8. Barretina, J.; Caponigro, G.; Stransky, N.; Venkatesan, K.; Margolin, A.A.; Kim, S.; Wilson, C.J.; Lehar, J.; Kryukov, G.V.; Sonkin, D.; et al. The Cancer Cell Line Encyclopedia enables predictive modelling of anticancer drug sensitivity. *Nature* **2012**, *483*, 603–607. [CrossRef] [PubMed]
9. Shoemaker, R.H. The NCI60 human tumour cell line anticancer drug screen. *Nat. Rev. Cancer* **2006**, *6*, 813–823. [CrossRef]
10. Basu, A.; Bodycombe, N.E.; Cheah, J.H.; Price, E.V.; Liu, K.; Schaefer, G.I.; Ebright, R.Y.; Stewart, M.L.; Ito, D.; Wang, S.; et al. An interactive resource to identify cancer genetic and lineage dependencies targeted by small molecules. *Cell* **2013**, *154*, 1151–1161. [CrossRef]
11. Holbeck, S.L.; Collins, J.M.; Doroshow, J.H. Analysis of Food and Drug Administration-approved anticancer agents in the NCI60 panel of human tumor cell lines. *Mol. Cancer Ther.* **2010**, *9*, 1451–1460. [CrossRef] [PubMed]
12. Garnett, M.J.; McDermott, U. The evolving role of cancer cell line-based screens to define the impact of cancer genomes on drug response. *Curr. Opin. Genet. Dev.* **2014**, *24*, 114–119. [CrossRef] [PubMed]

13. Van de Wetering, M.; Francies, H.E.; Francis, J.M.; Bounova, G.; Iorio, F.; Pronk, A.; van Houdt, W.; van Gorp, J.; Taylor-Weiner, A.; Kester, L.; et al. Prospective derivation of a living organoid biobank of colorectal cancer patients. *Cell* **2015**, *161*, 933–945. [CrossRef] [PubMed]
14. Iorio, F.; Knijnenburg, T.A.; Vis, D.J.; Bignell, G.R.; Menden, M.P.; Schubert, M.; Aben, N.; Goncalves, E.; Barthorpe, S.; Lightfoot, H.; et al. A Landscape of Pharmacogenomic Interactions in Cancer. *Cell* **2016**, *166*, 740–754. [CrossRef] [PubMed]
15. Koerfer, J.; Kallendrusch, S.; Merz, F.; Wittekind, C.; Kubick, C.; Kassahun, W.T.; Schumacher, G.; Moebius, C.; Gassler, N.; Schopow, N.; et al. Organotypic slice cultures of human gastric and esophagogastric junction cancer. *Cancer Med.* **2016**, *5*, 1444–1453. [CrossRef]
16. Merz, F.; Gaunitz, F.; Dehghani, F.; Renner, C.; Meixensberger, J.; Gutenberg, A.; Giese, A.; Schopow, K.; Hellwig, C.; Schafer, M.; et al. Organotypic slice cultures of human glioblastoma reveal different susceptibilities to treatments. *Neuro Oncol.* **2013**, *15*, 670–681. [CrossRef]
17. Senkowski, W.; Zhang, X.; Olofsson, M.H.; Isacson, R.; Hoglund, U.; Gustafsson, M.; Nygren, P.; Linder, S.; Larsson, R.; Fryknas, M. Three-Dimensional Cell Culture-Based Screening Identifies the Anthelmintic Drug Nitazoxanide as a Candidate for Treatment of Colorectal Cancer. *Mol. Cancer Ther.* **2015**, *14*, 1504–1516. [CrossRef]
18. Sachs, N.; Clevers, H. Organoid cultures for the analysis of cancer phenotypes. *Curr. Opin. Genet. Dev.* **2014**, *24*, 68–73. [CrossRef]
19. Weeber, F.; Ooft, S.N.; Dijkstra, K.K.; Voest, E.E. Tumor Organoids as a Pre-clinical Cancer Model for Drug Discovery. *Cell Chem. Biol.* **2017**, *24*, 1092–1100. [CrossRef]
20. Bleijs, M.; van de Wetering, M.; Clevers, H.; Drost, J. Xenograft and organoid model systems in cancer research. *EMBO J.* **2019**, *38*, e101654. [CrossRef]
21. Lancaster, M.A.; Renner, M.; Martin, C.A.; Wenzel, D.; Bicknell, L.S.; Hurles, M.E.; Homfray, T.; Penninger, J.M.; Jackson, A.P.; Knoblich, J.A. Cerebral organoids model human brain development and microcephaly. *Nature* **2013**, *501*, 373–379. [CrossRef] [PubMed]
22. Pauli, C.; Hopkins, B.D.; Prandi, D.; Shaw, R.; Fedrizzi, T.; Sboner, A.; Sailer, V.; Augello, M.; Puca, L.; Rosati, R.; et al. Personalized In Vitro and In Vivo Cancer Models to Guide Precision Medicine. *Cancer Discov.* **2017**, *7*, 462–477. [CrossRef] [PubMed]
23. Lang, H.; Beraud, C.; Bethry, A.; Danilin, S.; Lindner, V.; Coquard, C.; Rothhut, S.; Massfelder, T. Establishment of a large panel of patient-derived preclinical models of human renal cell carcinoma. *Oncotarget* **2016**, *7*, 59336–59359. [CrossRef] [PubMed]
24. Morgan, K.M.; Riedlinger, G.M.; Rosenfeld, J.; Ganesan, S.; Pine, S.R. Patient-Derived Xenograft Models of Non-Small Cell Lung Cancer and Their Potential Utility in Personalized Medicine. *Front. Oncol.* **2017**, *7*, 2. [CrossRef]
25. Maeda, H.; Khatami, M. Analyses of repeated failures in cancer therapy for solid tumors: Poor tumor-selective drug delivery, low therapeutic efficacy and unsustainable costs. *Clin. Transl. Med.* **2018**, *7*, 11. [CrossRef]
26. Wong, C.C.; Cheng, K.W.; Rigas, B. Preclinical predictors of anticancer drug efficacy: Critical assessment with emphasis on whether nanomolar potency should be required of candidate agents. *J. Pharmacol. Exp. Ther.* **2012**, *341*, 572–578. [CrossRef]
27. Ward, C.; Meehan, J.; Gray, M.; Kunkler, I.H.; Langdon, S.P.; Murray, A.; Argyle, D. Preclinical Organotypic Models for the Assessment of Novel Cancer Therapeutics and Treatment. *Curr. Top. Microbiol. Immunol.* **2019**. [CrossRef]
28. Altman, R.B. Predicting cancer drug response: Advancing the DREAM. *Cancer Discov.* **2015**, *5*, 237–238. [CrossRef]
29. Guyot, C.; Combe, C.; Clouzeau-Girard, H.; Moronvalle-Halley, V.; Desmouliere, A. Specific activation of the different fibrogenic cells in rat cultured liver slices mimicking in vivo situations. *Virchows Arch.* **2007**, *450*, 503–512. [CrossRef]
30. Schmeichel, K.L.; Bissell, M.J. Modeling tissue-specific signaling and organ function in three dimensions. *J. Cell. Sci.* **2003**, *116*, 2377–2388. [CrossRef]
31. Vaira, V.; Fedele, G.; Pyne, S.; Fasoli, E.; Zadra, G.; Bailey, D.; Snyder, E.; Faversani, A.; Coggi, G.; Flavin, R.; et al. Preclinical model of organotypic culture for pharmacodynamic profiling of human tumors. *Proc. Natl. Acad. Sci. USA* **2010**, *107*, 8352–8356. [CrossRef] [PubMed]

32. De Hoogt, R.; Estrada, M.F.; Vidic, S.; Davies, E.J.; Osswald, A.; Barbier, M.; Santo, V.E.; Gjerde, K.; van Zoggel, H.; Blom, S.; et al. Protocols and characterization data for 2D, 3D, and slice-based tumor models from the PREDECT project. *Sci. Data* **2017**, *4*, 170170. [CrossRef] [PubMed]
33. Misra, S.; Moro, C.F.; Del Chiaro, M.; Pouso, S.; Sebestyen, A.; Lohr, M.; Bjornstedt, M.; Verbeke, C.S. Ex vivo organotypic culture system of precision-cut slices of human pancreatic ductal adenocarcinoma. *Sci. Rep.* **2019**, *9*, 2133. [CrossRef] [PubMed]
34. Gerlach, M.M.; Merz, F.; Wichmann, G.; Kubick, C.; Wittekind, C.; Lordick, F.; Dietz, A.; Bechmann, I. Slice cultures from head and neck squamous cell carcinoma: A novel test system for drug susceptibility and mechanisms of resistance. *Br. J. Cancer* **2014**, *110*, 479–488. [CrossRef] [PubMed]
35. Marciniak, A.; Cohrs, C.M.; Tsata, V.; Chouinard, J.A.; Selck, C.; Stertmann, J.; Reichelt, S.; Rose, T.; Ehehalt, F.; Weitz, J.; et al. Using pancreas tissue slices for in situ studies of islet of Langerhans and acinar cell biology. *Nat. Protoc.* **2014**, *9*, 2809–2822. [CrossRef]
36. Rebours, V.; Albuquerque, M.; Sauvanet, A.; Ruszniewski, P.; Levy, P.; Paradis, V.; Bedossa, P.; Couvelard, A. Hypoxia pathways and cellular stress activate pancreatic stellate cells: Development of an organotypic culture model of thick slices of normal human pancreas. *PLoS ONE* **2013**, *8*, e76229. [CrossRef]
37. Kang, C.; Qiao, Y.; Li, G.; Baechle, K.; Camelliti, P.; Rentschler, S.; Efimov, I.R. Human Organotypic Cultured Cardiac Slices: New Platform For High Throughput Preclinical Human Trials. *Sci. Rep.* **2016**, *6*, 28798. [CrossRef]
38. Jiang, T.; Zhou, C.; Ren, S. Role of IL-2 in cancer immunotherapy. *Oncoimmunology* **2016**, *5*, e1163462. [CrossRef]
39. Roelants, C.; Giacosa, S.; Pillet, C.; Bussat, R.; Champelovier, P.; Bastien, O.; Guyon, L.; Arnoux, V.; Cochet, C.; Filhol, O. Combined inhibition of PI3K and Src kinases demonstrates synergistic therapeutic efficacy in clear-cell renal carcinoma. *Oncotarget* **2018**, *9*, 30066–30078. [CrossRef]
40. Ricketts, C.J.; Linehan, W.M. Multi-regional Sequencing Elucidates the Evolution of Clear Cell Renal Cell Carcinoma. *Cell* **2018**, *173*, 540–542. [CrossRef]
41. Kaelin, W.G., Jr. The von Hippel-Lindau tumour suppressor protein: O_2 sensing and cancer. *Nat. Rev. Cancer* **2008**, *8*, 865–873. [CrossRef] [PubMed]
42. Ricketts, C.J.; Crooks, D.R.; Linehan, W.M. Targeting HIF2alpha in Clear-Cell Renal Cell Carcinoma. *Cancer Cell* **2016**, *30*, 515–517. [CrossRef] [PubMed]
43. Webster, W.S.; Lohse, C.M.; Thompson, R.H.; Dong, H.; Frigola, X.; Dicks, D.L.; Sengupta, S.; Frank, I.; Leibovich, B.C.; Blute, M.L.; et al. Mononuclear cell infiltration in clear-cell renal cell carcinoma independently predicts patient survival. *Cancer* **2006**, *107*, 46–53. [CrossRef] [PubMed]
44. Vuong, L.; Kotecha, R.R.; Voss, M.H.; Hakimi, A.A. Tumor Microenvironment Dynamics in Clear-Cell Renal Cell Carcinoma. *Cancer Discov.* **2019**, *9*, 1349–1357. [CrossRef]
45. Kraus, V.B. Biomarkers as drug development tools: Discovery, validation, qualification and use. *Nat. Rev. Rheumatol.* **2018**, *14*, 354–362. [CrossRef]
46. Motzer, R.J.; Tannir, N.M.; McDermott, D.F.; Aren Frontera, O.; Melichar, B.; Choueiri, T.K.; Plimack, E.R.; Barthelemy, P.; Porta, C.; George, S.; et al. Nivolumab plus Ipilimumab versus Sunitinib in Advanced Renal-Cell Carcinoma. *N. Engl. J. Med.* **2018**, *378*, 1277–1290. [CrossRef]
47. Rheinlander, A.; Schraven, B.; Bommhardt, U. CD45 in human physiology and clinical medicine. *Immunol. Lett.* **2018**, *196*, 22–32. [CrossRef]
48. Wu, P.; Wu, D.; Li, L.; Chai, Y.; Huang, J. PD-L1 and Survival in Solid Tumors: A Meta-Analysis. *PLoS ONE* **2015**, *10*, e0131403. [CrossRef]
49. Thompson, R.H.; Gillett, M.D.; Cheville, J.C.; Lohse, C.M.; Dong, H.; Webster, W.S.; Chen, L.; Zincke, H.; Blute, M.L.; Leibovich, B.C.; et al. Costimulatory molecule B7-H1 in primary and metastatic clear cell renal cell carcinoma. *Cancer* **2005**, *104*, 2084–2091. [CrossRef]
50. Thompson, R.H.; Dong, H.; Lohse, C.M.; Leibovich, B.C.; Blute, M.L.; Cheville, J.C.; Kwon, E.D. PD-1 is expressed by tumor-infiltrating immune cells and is associated with poor outcome for patients with renal cell carcinoma. *Clin. Cancer Res. Off. J. Am. Assoc. Cancer Res.* **2007**, *13*, 1757–1761. [CrossRef]
51. Tumeh, P.C.; Harview, C.L.; Yearley, J.H.; Shintaku, I.P.; Taylor, E.J.; Robert, L.; Chmielowski, B.; Spasic, M.; Henry, G.; Ciobanu, V.; et al. PD-1 blockade induces responses by inhibiting adaptive immune resistance. *Nature* **2014**, *515*, 568–571. [CrossRef] [PubMed]

52. Guertl, B.; Senanayake, U.; Nusshold, E.; Leuschner, I.; Mannweiler, S.; Ebner, B.; Hoefler, G. Lim1, an embryonal transcription factor, is absent in multicystic renal dysplasia, but reactivated in nephroblastomas. *Pathobiology* **2011**, *78*, 210–219. [CrossRef] [PubMed]
53. Hamaidi, I.; Coquard, C.; Danilin, S.; Dormoy, V.; Beraud, C.; Rothhut, S.; Barthelmebs, M.; Benkirane-Jessel, N.; Lindner, V.; Lang, H.; et al. The Lim1 oncogene as a new therapeutic target for metastatic human renal cell carcinoma. *Oncogene* **2019**, *38*, 60–72. [CrossRef] [PubMed]
54. Schnizlein-Bick, C.T.; Mandy, F.F.; O'Gorman, M.R.; Paxton, H.; Nicholson, J.K.; Hultin, L.E.; Gelman, R.S.; Wilkening, C.L.; Livnat, D. Use of CD45 gating in three and four-color flow cytometric immunophenotyping: Guideline from the National Institute of Allergy and Infectious Diseases, Division of AIDS. *Cytometry* **2002**, *50*, 46–52. [CrossRef]
55. Zerdes, I.; Matikas, A.; Bergh, J.; Rassidakis, G.Z.; Foukakis, T. Genetic, transcriptional and post-translational regulation of the programmed death protein ligand 1 in cancer: Biology and clinical correlations. *Oncogene* **2018**, *37*, 4639–4661. [CrossRef]
56. Wang, Y.; Wang, X.Y.; Subjeck, J.R.; Shrikant, P.A.; Kim, H.L. Temsirolimus, an mTOR inhibitor, enhances anti-tumour effects of heat shock protein cancer vaccines. *Br. J. Cancer* **2011**, *104*, 643–652. [CrossRef]
57. R Core Team. *R: A Language and Environment for Statistical Computing*; R Foundation for Statistical Computing: Vienna, Austria; Available online: https://www.R-project.org/ (accessed on 17 February 2018).
58. Dienstmann, R.; Tabernero, J. Cancer: A precision approach to tumour treatment. *Nature* **2017**, *548*, 40–41. [CrossRef]
59. Jiang, X.; Seo, Y.D.; Chang, J.H.; Coveler, A.; Nigjeh, E.N.; Pan, S.; Jalikis, F.; Yeung, R.S.; Crispe, I.N.; Pillarisetty, V.G. Long-lived pancreatic ductal adenocarcinoma slice cultures enable precise study of the immune microenvironment. *Oncoimmunology* **2017**, *6*, e1333210. [CrossRef]

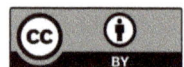

© 2020 by the authors. Licensee MDPI, Basel, Switzerland. This article is an open access article distributed under the terms and conditions of the Creative Commons Attribution (CC BY) license (http://creativecommons.org/licenses/by/4.0/).

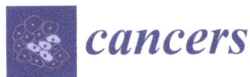

Article

RNA Sequencing of Collecting Duct Renal Cell Carcinoma Suggests an Interaction between miRNA and Target Genes and a Predominance of Deregulated Solute Carrier Genes

Sven Wach [1,†], Helge Taubert [1,*,†], Katrin Weigelt [1], Nora Hase [2], Marcel Köhn [2], Danny Misiak [2], Stefan Hüttelmaier [2], Christine G. Stöhr [3], Andreas Kahlmeyer [1], Florian Haller [3], Julio Vera [4], Arndt Hartmann [3], Bernd Wullich [1] and Xin Lai [4,*]

[1] Department of Urology and Pediatric Urology, University Hospital Erlangen, Friedrich-Alexander University Erlangen-Nürnberg, 91054 Erlangen, Germany; sven.wach@uk-erlangen.de (S.W.); Katrin.Weigelt@uk-erlangen.de (K.W.); Andreas.Kahlmeyer@uk-erlangen.de (A.K.); Bernd.Wullich@uk-erlangen.de (B.W.)
[2] Institute of Molecular Medicine, Section for Molecular Cell Biology, Faculty of Medicine, Martin Luther University Halle-Wittenberg, 06120 Halle, Germany; nora.hase@medizin.uni-halle.de (N.H.); marcel.koehn@medizin.uni-halle.de (M.K.); danny.misiak@medizin.uni-halle.de (D.M.); stefan.huettelmaier@medizin.uni-halle.de (S.H.)
[3] Department of Pathology, University Hospital Erlangen, Friedrich-Alexander University Erlangen-Nürnberg, 91054 Erlangen, Germany; Christine.Stoehr@uk-erlangen.de (C.G.S.); Florian.Haller@uk-erlangen.de (F.H.); arndt.hartmann@uk-erlangen.de (A.H.)
[4] Laboratory of Systems Tumor Immunology, Department of Dermatology, University Hospital Erlangen, FAU Erlangen-Nürnberg, 91054 Erlangen, Germany; julio.Vera-Gonzalez@uk-erlangen.de
* Correspondence: helge.taubert@uk-erlangen.de (H.T.); xin.lai@uk-erlangen.de (X.L.); Tel.: +49-9131-85-42658 (H.T.); +49-9131-85-45888 (X.L.); Fax: +49-9131-85-23374 (H.T.)
† These authors contributed equally to this work.

Received: 28 November 2019; Accepted: 22 December 2019; Published: 24 December 2019

Abstract: Collecting duct carcinoma (CDC) is a rare renal cell carcinoma subtype with a very poor prognosis. There have been only a few studies on gene expression analysis in CDCs. We compared the gene expression profiles of two CDC cases with those of eight normal tissues of renal cell carcinoma patients. At a threshold of |log2fold-change| ≥1, 3349 genes were upregulated and 1947 genes were downregulated in CDCs compared to the normal samples. Pathway analysis of the deregulated genes revealed that cancer pathways and cell cycle pathways were most prominent in CDCs. The most upregulated gene was *keratin 17*, and the most downregulated gene was *cubilin*. Among the most downregulated genes were four solute carrier genes (*SLC3A1, SLC9A3, SLC26A7,* and *SLC47A1*). The strongest negative correlations between miRNAs and mRNAs were found between the downregulated miR-374b-5p and its upregulated target genes *HIST1H3B, HK2,* and *SLC7A11* and between upregulated miR-26b-5p and its downregulated target genes *PPARGC1A, ALDH6A1,* and *MARC2*. An upregulation of HK2 and a downregulation of PPARGC1A, ALDH6A1, and MARC2 were observed at the protein level. Survival analysis of the cancer genome atlas (TCGA) dataset showed for the first time that low gene expression of *MARC2, cubilin,* and *SLC47A1* and high gene expression of *KRT17* are associated with poor overall survival in clear cell renal cell carcinoma patients. Altogether, we identified dysregulated protein-coding genes, potential miRNA-target interactions, and prognostic markers that could be associated with CDC.

Keywords: collecting duct carcinoma; RNA sequencing; solute carrier proteins

1. Introduction

Collecting duct renal cell carcinoma (CDC; also known as Bellini duct carcinoma, collecting duct carcinoma of the kidney) is a very rare (approximately 1–2%) but also very aggressive renal cell carcinoma with a median survival time of 11 months [1–3]. Tumors concerning the collecting duct were first described independently by Mancilla-Jimenez et al. and by Cromie et al. [4,5]. The putative cell of origin is in the distal convoluted tubules, a segment between the proximal tubules and the distal part of the nephron [6]. There are several cytogenetic abnormalities known, i.e., mostly loss of 11, 6p, 8p, 9p, and 21q and the Y chromosome as reviewed in [3]). However, there have been only a few reports about chromosomal aberrations, mutations in CDCs, and RNA expression changes [6–8]. Pal et al. identified clinically relevant genomic alterations mostly in genes *NF2*, *SETD2*, *SMARCH1*, and *CDKN2A* (29% to 12%) but also in 6% of genes *PIK3CA*, *PIK3R2*, *FBXW7*, *BAP1*, *DNMT3A*, *VHL*, and *HRAS* [7]. Furthermore, amplifications of *ERBB2* and genomic alterations of *SMARCB1* have been described [7]. Malouf et al. performed the first transcriptomic analysis of CDC and compared it with upper tract urothelial carcinomas (UTUCs) [6]. In addition to the finding that the CDC transcriptome is unique and clustered with that of clear cell renal cell carcinoma (ccRCC) patients rather than UTUC patients, the authors compared CDCs with UTUCs and identified *CDH6* and *POU3F3* as the top upregulated genes and *GATA3*, *TP63*, *KRT17*, *KRT7*, *KRT20*, *UPK2*, *UPK1A*, and *UPK3A* as the top downregulated genes in CDCs [6]. Based on the transcriptomic signature, they concluded that CDC is a disease characterized by metabolic and immunogenic aberrations. Wang et al. reported in a combined whole-exome sequencing and transcriptome sequencing study of CDC that many single nucleotide variations in cancer census genes, but also deletions of *CDKN2A*. In addition, RNA expression changes in members of the solute carrier (SLC) family, such as overexpression of *SLC7A11* (cystine transporter, *xCT*), have been reported [8].

Promising treatment schemes for metastasized renal cell carcinoma have been reported [9,10], but they mostly concern ccRCC, and there is still no specific therapy for CDC. However, there are treatment suggestions for metastatic CDC, i.e., first-line therapy with a combination of chemotherapy (gemcitabine) plus cisplatin/carboplatin, and second-line therapy as a targeted therapy [2,3]. Suggestions to treat CDC patients with drugs that target solute carriers, such as SLC7A11 or SLC6A7, have been made previously [11]. However, further molecular characterization of CDC is needed to better understand its tumor biology and to identify potential therapeutic targets.

In our study, we performed RNA transcriptome sequencing of two CDC cases and eight normal tissues in an effort to better characterize this rare tumor entity. We investigated differences in gene expression and sought to describe single nucleotide variation patterns and utilized pre-miRNA expression data in an effort to identify potentially regulated target proteins. Based on the finding of a predominance of gene expression changes in solute carriers in CDC, and our previous results concerning miRNAs and their target gene expression as biomarkers in urologic cancers, we focused our analysis on these two research fields. We found that several solute carrier genes are significantly dysregulated in CDC. In addition, we showed that the low expression of *SLC47A1* leads to poor survival of clear cell renal cell carcinoma patients, suggesting it as a prognostic marker for CDC.

2. Results

2.1. RNA Sequencing Revealed Up- and Downregulated Genes

RNA transcriptome sequencing was performed for two CDC cases and eight histologically normal tissue samples (Figure 1). Upon analyzing the read counts, a total of 7093 coding genes were detected as being significantly deregulated between the CDC and normal tissue samples ($p < 0.05$). After hierarchical clustering, it became evident that the two CDC samples formed a cluster that was very distinct from the normal tissue samples (Figure 2). Interestingly, the normal tissue samples, which were also derived from tumor-bearing kidneys of different entities, did not show any tendency to cluster according to their corresponding tumor entity, which strongly suggests the absence of any field effect. For filtering purposes, the differential expression measure was log2 transformed. Application of a |log2fold change| ≥1 cutoff revealed that 1,947 genes were downregulated and 3,349 genes were upregulated in CDCs vs. normal samples (Table S1). The clustering results were comparable to the result without filtering.

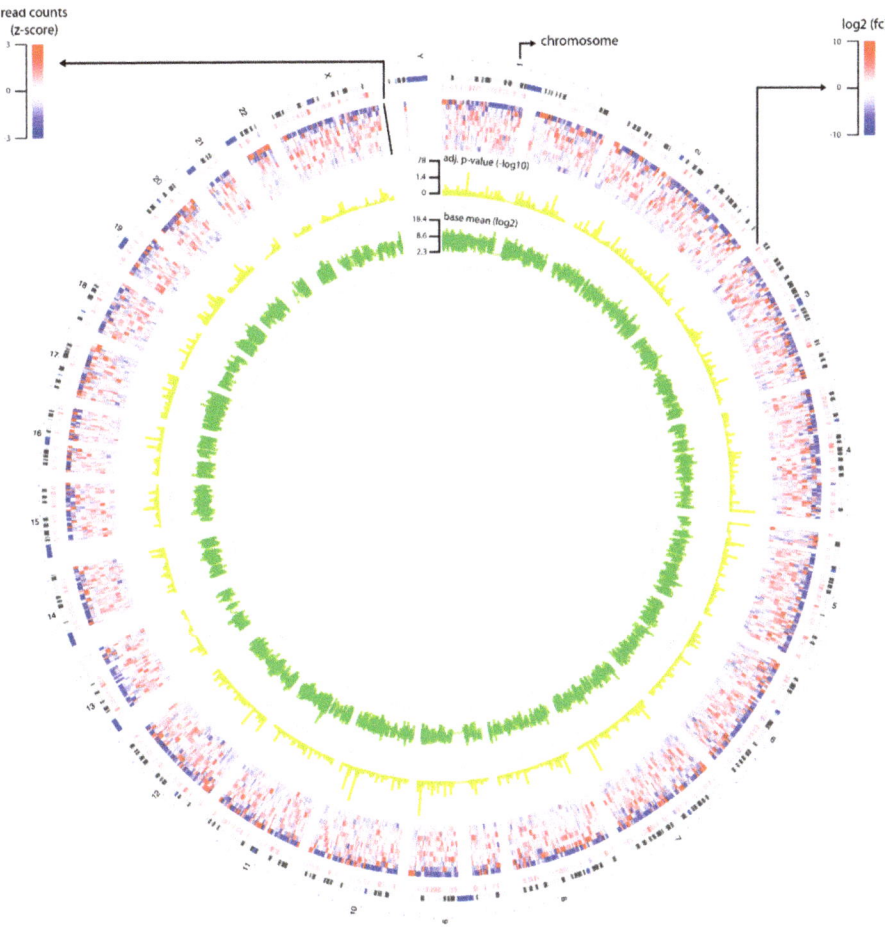

Figure 1. Overview of RNA sequencing data. The circus plot shows statistics of the genes ($n = 16,672$) that were selected for differential gene expression analysis. The plot contains four circles: Layer 1 is log2fold-change of the genes; Layer 2 is read counts of the genes that were transformed to z-score; Layer 3 is adjusted p-value of the genes that were transformed by $-\log10$; and Layer 4 is the base mean of the genes that were transformed by log2.

After applying a |log2fold change|≥3 cutoff, only 316 genes were detected as downregulated and 599 genes as upregulated in the CDC compared to the normal tissue samples (Table S1). The clustering analysis still demonstrated a clear distinction between the two CDC samples on one side and the normal samples on the other side. Among the 915 significantly deregulated genes with a |log2fold change| ≥3 were 15 downregulated and 11 upregulated SLC genes, which comprised 2.8% of all genes.

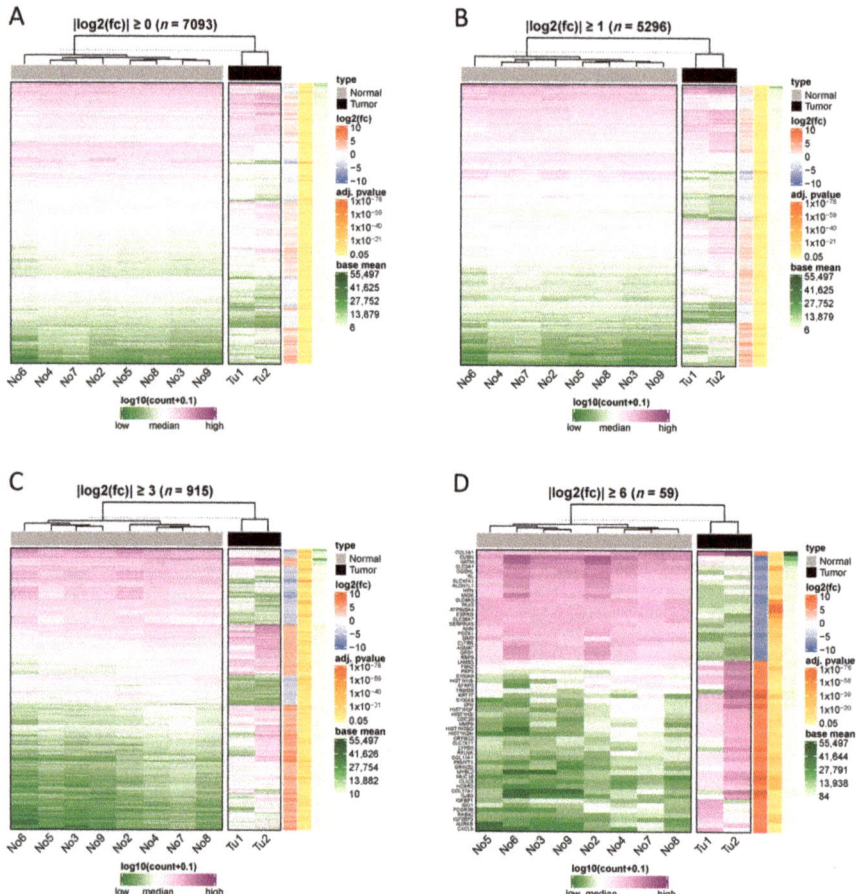

Figure 2. Hierarchical clustering of samples using differentially expressed protein-coding genes. We used different-fold changes as a threshold to filter significantly differentially expressed protein-coding genes (adjusted p-value ≤ 0.05). Read counts of the genes were used to cluster normal and tumor samples based on their Euclidian distance. In addition, we annotated the selected genes with their log2fold-change, adjusted p-value and base mean of their read counts. The thresholds used were (**A**) |log2fold-change| ≥0, (**B**) |log2fold-change| ≥1, (**C**) |log2fold-change| ≥3, and (**D**) |log2fold change| ≥6.

With even more strict filtering criteria for differential expression, |log2fold change| ≥6 (which corresponds to a 64-fold difference), we could still identify 57 deregulated genes, of which 22 genes were downregulated and 37 genes were upregulated in CDC compared to normal samples (Table S1). Again, the CDC samples formed a cluster distinct from the normal tissue samples, but subtle differences in their gene expression patterns were more obvious. Again, the normal tissue clustered closer together. Of note, among the upregulated genes were five histone 1 genes (*HIST1H2BO*, *HIST1H3I*, *HIST1H3F*, *HIST1H1B*, and *HIST1H2AI*) and three collagen genes (*COL1A1*, *COL11A1*, and *COL17A1*). Remarkably, among the |log2fold change| ≥6 deregulated genes, four solute carrier genes were found to be downregulated (*SLC3A1*, *SLC9A3*, *SLC26A7*, and *SLC47A1*), and one solute carrier gene was found to be upregulated (*SLC7A11*). The fact that a total of 8.8% of the genes with a |log2fold change| ≥6 belong either to histone 1 genes or to SLC genes is very remarkable. We will return to *SLC7A11* and *SLC47A1* later in our study.

On a global scale, the top downregulated gene in the CDC samples compared to the normal tissue samples was *cubilin* (*CUBN*) (Table S1), which is highly expressed in normal renal proximal tubules [12]. The top upregulated gene in the CDC samples was *keratin 17* (*KRT17*; Table S1). KRT17 is an intermediate filament protein rapidly induced in wounded stratified epithelia. It regulates cell growth and stimulates the Akt/mTOR pathway and glucose uptake [13–15].

2.2. Pathway Analyses

To gain a more comprehensive insight into the signaling pathways that are potentially affected in CDC, we first applied a |log2fold change| ≥1 cutoff and then performed a gene set enrichment analysis with pathways derived from three independent databases, KEGG, WikiPathway, and Reactome (Table S2). After mapping against the KEGG database, the terms "pathways in cancer", "cell cycle", and "small cell lung cancer" were found among the top 10 affected pathways. When mapping against the WikiPathway database, the terms "retinoblastoma in cancer", "integrated pancreatic cancer pathway", and "cell cycle" were found among the top 20 enriched pathways. Finally, the Reactome database revealed that "collagen" and "mitotic cell cycle" were among the top 10 enriched pathways. In summary, using different pathway databases, we were able to demonstrate that the genes deregulated in CDC are enriched in distinct cancer-related signaling pathways and pathways affecting cell cycle regulation.

2.3. Investigation of SNPs and Mutations

In an effort to identify a possible association between single nucleotide variants and the occurrence of CDC, we screened the RNA transcriptome sequencing data for single nucleotide variations between the CDC and the normal samples (Table S3). The identified variations were first mapped against the NCBI SNP database to identify known variants with accession numbers. To define the potential clinical relevance, every identified variant was queried against the NCBI ClinVar database to check whether the variations were pathogenic, likely pathogenic, or confer sensitivity or drug response [16]. However, none of the identified variations were indicated to have these features.

2.4. Correlations of miRNAs and Target mRNA Expression

Correlations between miRNAs and their corresponding target genes can reveal regulatory mechanisms in tumor biology. From the RNA transcriptome sequencing data, we were able to extract information about the expression of pre-miRNAs. Correlations between the mature miRNAs that could be processed from the assessed pre-miRNAs and target mRNAs are shown in Table 1 and Table S4. The strongest correlations between miRNAs and mRNA expression levels were found for miR-374b-5p and miR-26b-5p and their respective target genes (Table 1 and Table S4). Whereas miR-374b-5p was downregulated (1.65-fold; adjusted *p*-value = 0.155) in CDC samples, miR-26b-5p (1.55-fold; adjusted *p*-value = 0.021) was upregulated in CDC samples compared to normal samples. Accordingly, the target genes of miR-374b-5p were upregulated, and those of miR-26b-5p were downregulated in CDC samples. The associations derived from transcriptome sequencing data were further validated in the original RNA preparations by qRT-PCR. We could verify the upregulation of the target genes of miR-374b-5p, i.e., *HK2* and, in one CDC sample, *SLC7A11*, but not *HIST1H3B* (Figure 3A–C). Furthermore, the downregulation of the target genes of miR-26b-5p, i.e., *PPARGC1A*, *ALDH6A1*, and *MARC2*, could be validated (Figure 3D–F). Interestingly, *SLC7A11* is a predicted target of both miRNAs, raising the possibility of competitive binding of both miRNAs to their respective binding sites in the 3'UTR of the *SLC7A11* gene. There are four potential binding sites for miR-26b-5p and four potential binding sites for miR-374b-5p in the 3'UTR of the *SLC7A11* gene. However, the closest distance between any binding sites of these two miRNAs is 55 nt (Table S5), which argues against a competition between these two miRNAs for binding sites in the 3'UTR of the *SLC7A11* gene.

Table 1. Computational correlation analysis of miRNAs and their target genes.

miRNA	Target Gene	Correlation Coefficient	p-Value	log2fold Change of Target Genes	qRT-PCR of Target Genes
miR-374b-5p	SLC7A11	−0.67	0.034	6.41	up
miR-374b-5p	HIST1H3B	−0.71	0.021	5.87	up
miR-374b-5p	HK2	−0.74	0.013	5.72	up
miR-26b-5p	PPARGC1A	−0.70	0.020	−4.87	down
miR-26b-5p	ALDH6A1	−0.66	0.039	−4.71	down
miR-26b-5p	MARC2	−0.68	0.030	−4.08	down
miR-26b-5p	SLC7A11	+0.82	0.004	6.41	up

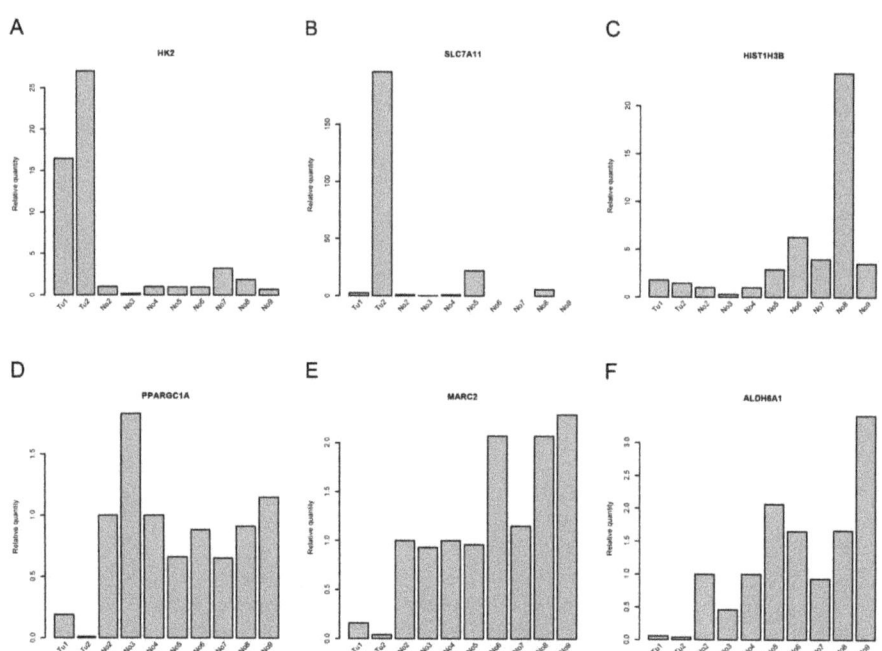

Figure 3. Quantitative RT-PCR for deregulated genes in collecting duct renal cell carcinoma (CDC). Gene expression of (**A**) *HK2*, (**B**) *SLC7A11*, (**C**) *HIST1H3B*, (**D**) *PPARGC1A*, (**E**) *MARC2*, and (**F**) *ALDH6A1* in the samples that were used for RNA sequencing.

2.5. Protein Expression of miRNA Target Genes

To further validate the expression of the potential miRNA target genes, we also assessed the protein expression of the target genes by western blotting (Figure 4 and Figure S2). HK2 protein expression was increased in at least one CDC sample compared to the normal samples. HIST1H3B was not detectable in our samples and, unexpectedly, SLC7A11 protein expression was decreased in the CDC samples compared to the normal samples. As expected, PPARGC1A, ALDH6A1, and MARC2 protein expression was downregulated in the CDC samples compared to most of the normal samples.

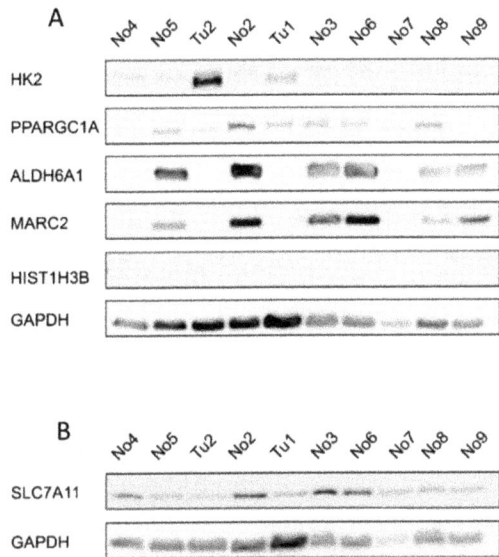

Figure 4. Protein expression of selected genes with deregulated expression in CDCs. (**A**) Western blot for HK2, PPARGC1A, ALDH6A1, MARC2, and HIST1H3B with GAPDH as the reference protein and (**B**) for SLC7A11 with GAPDH as the reference protein. Tu-tumor tissue sample; No-normal tissue sample.

2.6. Solute Carrier Genes

As previously described, many SLC genes in CDC are dysregulated in comparison to normal tissue samples [8,11]. Therefore, we decided to investigate the expression of SLC genes in more detail. After applying a |log2fold change| ≥3 cutoff, a total of 15 SLC genes (*SLC3A1*, *SLC4A4*, *SLC6A12*, *SLC9A3*, *SLC14A1*, *SLC22A13*, *SLC23A1*, *SLC23A3*, *SLC25A27*, *SLC26A1*, *SLC26A7*, *SLC27A2*, *SLC38A11*, *SLC47A1*, and *SLCO4C1*) were found to be significantly downregulated, and 11 SLC genes (*SLC1A4*, *SLC1A5*, *SLC2A1*, *SLC2A14*, *SLC5A6*, *SLC6A9*, *SLC7A5*, *SLC7A11*, *SLC11A1*, *SLC16A3*, and *SLC38A5*) were significantly upregulated in CDC samples compared to normal samples (Figure 5). With even more stringent criteria of a |log2fold change| ≥6, four SLC genes (*SLC3A1*, *SLC9A3*, *SLC26A7*, and *SLC47A1*) were still significantly downregulated.

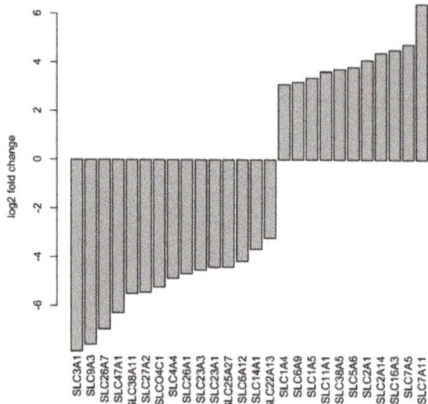

Figure 5. Deregulated solute carrier genes at |log2fold change| ≥3 in CDC samples compared to normal tissues.

2.7. Survival Analysis of Deregulated Genes

As we have described several distinct differences between CDC and normal tissue samples both in gene expression and in miRNA target gene expression, we sought to investigate whether these markers might provide any prognostic information. We used the TCGA dataset of renal cell carcinoma patients [17] and generated Kaplan-Meier analyses for the two most deregulated transcripts (*CUBN* and *KRT17*) as well as for the identified miRNA target genes. As the TCGA cohort did not contain any specified CDC patients, we performed this analysis independently for the two main histological subtypes of clear cell renal cell carcinoma patients (ccRCC; KIRC dataset) and for papillary renal cell carcinoma patients (pRCC; KIRP dataset) (Figure 6). The gene expression values, if available in the TCGA dataset, were separated at the median to generate a low-expression and a high-expression subgroup, which were analyzed for differences in patient survival.

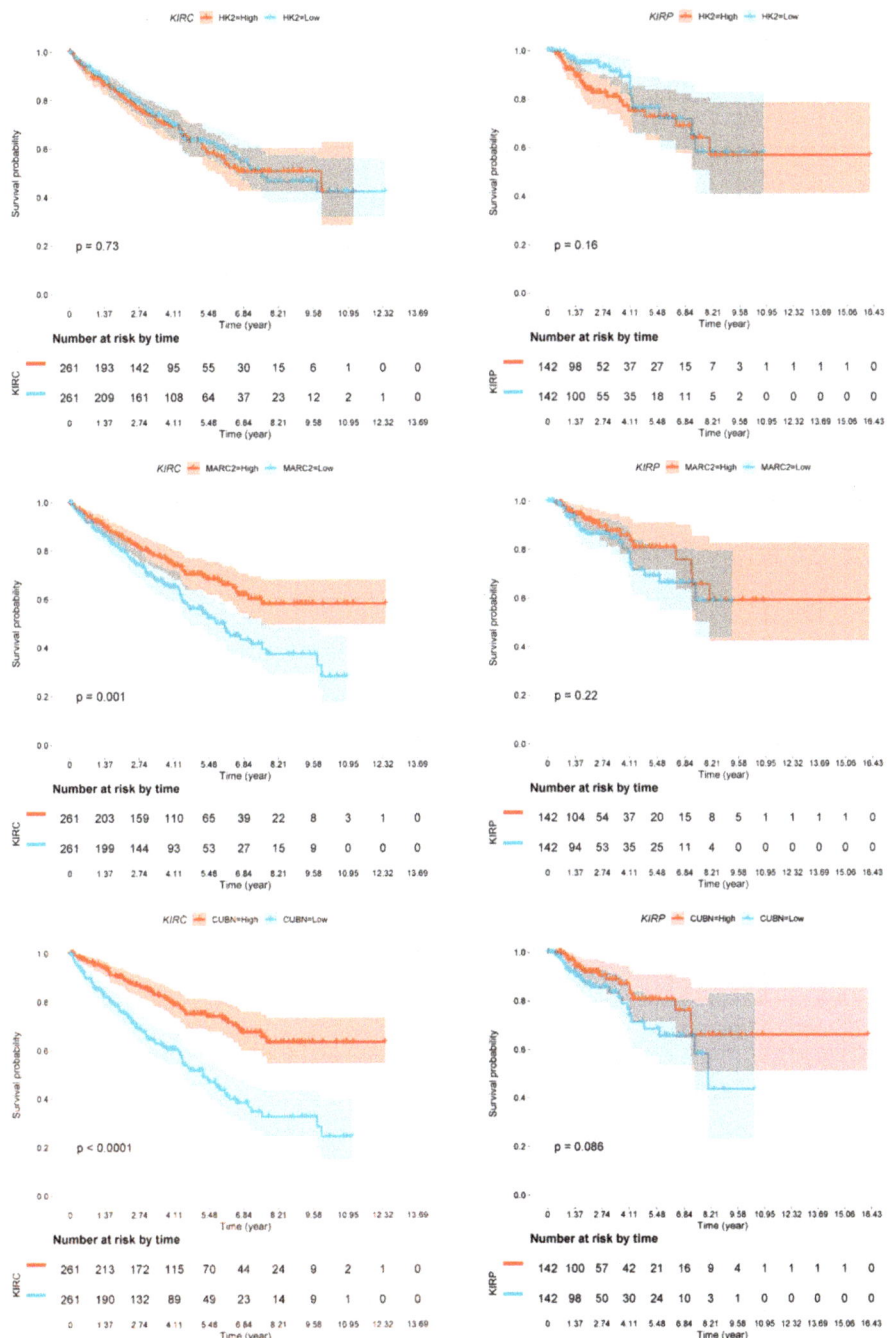

Figure 6. *Cont.*

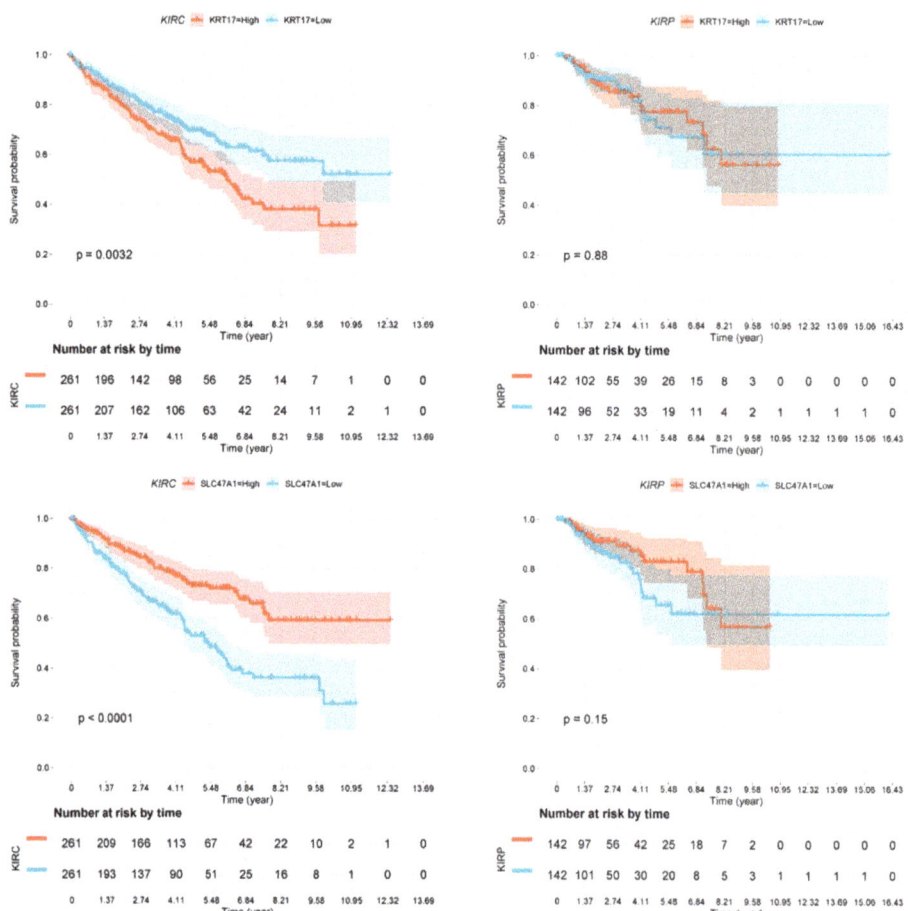

Figure 6. Kaplan-Meier analyses. Association of deregulated gene expression in CDCs with overall survival in clear cell renal cell carcinoma (ccRCC patients; KIRC dataset) and in papillary renal cell carcinoma (pRCC patients; KIRP dataset). Expression of none of the genes was significantly associated with overall survival in pRCC patients. However, the expression of all genes but *HK2* was significantly associated with overall survival, as shown for *HK2* (nonsignificant), *MARC2* ($p = 0.001$), *CUBN* ($p \leq 0.0001$), *KRT17* ($p = 0.0032$), and *SLC47A1* ($p \leq 0.0001$).

Several of the genes identified by our approach were confirmed to be of prognostic relevance in the ccRCC patient cohort (KIRC). Low *MARC2* gene expression was significantly associated with poor overall survival ($p = 0.001$). Moreover, low expression of *CUBN* ($p < 0.0001$) and *SLC47A1* ($p < 0.0001$) and high expression of the gene *KRT17* ($p = 0.0032$) were significantly associated with poor overall survival (Figure 6). However, none of the genes analyzed were associated with overall survival in the pRCC (KIRP) patient cohort.

Survival analysis data of genes *PPARGC1A*, *ALDH6A1*, and *SLC7A11* in the same TCGA KIRC dataset have already been published by other authors and are therefore not repeated by us. Significant associations of low *PPARGC1A*, low *ALDH6A1*, and high *SLC7A11* gene expression with poor outcomes in ccRCC patients have been reported [8,16,17].

3. Discussion

CDC is a rare and highly aggressive variant of renal cell carcinoma, and is associated with a mean survival of approximately 11 months. The molecular pathways responsible for the tumor biology of CDCs are still mainly unresolved. As expected, after RNA transcriptome sequencing, we observed several cancer pathways and cell cycle regulation pathways that might predominantly be affected in CDCs compared to normal samples. Altogether, more genes were upregulated than downregulated in CDCs, which is in line with previous findings [6,8].

In our study, the most pronounced downregulated gene in CDC was *CUBN*. This gene is normally highly expressed in renal proximal tubules [12]. *CUBN* has not been previously described as deregulated in CDCs. However, we found a significant association of low *CUBN* gene expression with poor overall survival of ccRCC patients in the TCGA ccRCC dataset. In addition, this gene has already been identified as an independent prognostic marker for renal cell carcinoma at the protein level [18]. Interestingly, *CUBN* has been suggested as a predictive marker for the treatment of renal cancer patients with sunitinib and sorafenib [19]. So far, there are only case reports for CDCs treated with sunitinib or sorafenib, but there have been some promising results concerning partial responses [3].

In our study, the most pronounced upregulated gene in CDC was *KRT17*. *KRT17* is normally expressed in the basal cells of complex epithelia, but not in stratified or simple epithelia. Furthermore, it is an intermediate filament protein that is rapidly induced in wounded stratified epithelia and regulates cell growth by binding to the adaptor protein 14-3-3-sigma [13]. This finding is relevant to the consideration that "tumors are wounds that do not heal" [20]. *KRT17* expression is known to be associated with disease severity in oral submucosa fibrosis [14]. In line with this finding, *keratin 17* is induced in oral cancer and facilitates tumor growth [15]. Remarkably, Malouf and colleagues found in their functional enrichment analysis of CDC that response to wounding was the predominant pathway; however, when comparing CDCs with UTUCs, *KRT17* was among the top downregulated genes in CDC [6]. In our study, we observed a significant association between high *KRT17* gene expression and shorter overall survival in ccRCC patients in the KIRC dataset.

Solute carriers (SLCs) have been described as biomarkers for RCC patients [21,22]. Strikingly, SLC gene expression is changed in CDCs [8]. Wang and colleagues found several members of the SLC family among the top deregulated genes, either upregulated, i.e., *SLC6A11*, *SLC6A15*, *SLC7A3*, *SLCO1B1*, and *SLCO1B3* or downregulated, i.e., *SLC5A12*, *SLC12A1*, *SLC22A12*, *SLC47A2*, and *SLC22A6* [8]. In our study, four SLC transporter genes were strongly (|log2fold change| ≥6) downregulated (*SLC3A1*, *SLC9A3*, *SLC26A7*, and *SLC47A1*). *SLC7A11* was detected to be among the most upregulated at the RNA level in the study by Wang and colleagues [8]. We confirmed this gene as upregulated in one of two CDC samples. However, at the protein level, SLC7A11 was detected as downregulated in both CDCs compared to the normal samples. The observed discrepancy between the RNA and protein levels could be explained by post-transcriptional regulation of *SLC7A11*, since alternative 3'UTRs for *SLC7A11* have been described, but this has not been further studied [23]. In contrast to our findings, Wang et al. detected a protein upregulation of *SLC7A11* in 12 out of 15 CDC cases, and they stated that *SLC7A11* upregulation at the RNA level was associated with poor survival in ccRCC [8]. Their suggestion to target *SLC7A11* as a therapy option has to be, in our opinion, based on testing SLC7A11 protein expression on a case-by-case basis and needs further investigation. Wang et al. reported that two SLC members, *SLC47A2* and *SLC47A1*, were downregulated (|log2fold change| >6 and >5, respectively) in CDCs [8]. In line with this observation, we found that *SLC47A1* was also strongly downregulated at the RNA level (|log2fold change| ≥6). *SLC47A1* and *SLC47A2* are transporters that excrete endogenous and exogenous toxic electrolytes through urine and bile [24]. In addition, the *SLC47A* gene may affect renal excretion of substrate drugs, such as metformin [25]. It is tempting to speculate that treatment of tumors with a downregulated *SLC47A* gene, e.g., CDCs, with metformin could have toxic effects; however, polymorphisms in the *SLC47A* gene may affect renal excretion of substrate drugs such as metformin, resulting in inadequate pharmacotherapy or toxic effects [25]. Therefore, before considering the application of metformin in tumor patients, these somatic polymorphisms should be tested. Notably, our two CDC patients did not possess single nucleotide variants in the *SLC47A* gene.

We utilized RNA sequencing information about pre-miRNAs or miRNA host genes as an alternative approach to identify target genes or proteins deregulated in CDC. In this way, we identified strong correlations between downregulated miR-374b-5p and its upregulated target genes *HIST1H3B*, *HK2*, and *SLC7A11*, and also between upregulated miR-26b-5p and its downregulated target genes *PPARGC1A*, *ALDH6A1*, and *MARC2*. Among the upregulated target genes, *HIST1H3B* has not yet been described to play any role in renal cell carcinomas. HK2 is well known as an enzyme in glycolysis that catalyzes the phosphorylation of glucose into glucose-6-phosphate [26]. HK2 has been described as a target of the HIF1a protein in several cancers, including RCC [27,28]. Recently, Nam et al. showed that HK2 plays a pivotal role in renal tumor progression to metastasis [29]. SLC7A11 (xCT) is an anionic amino acid transporter that is highly specific for the amino acids cysteine and glutamate [30]. Increased expression of *SLC7A11* at the RNA and protein levels in CDCs has been shown previously [8,11].

In our set of downregulated genes, *PPARGC1A* (*PGC-1α*) is a central regulator of mitochondrial energy metabolism and functions in renoprotection against ischemia [31]. LaGory and coworkers found that ccRCC cells expressing *PGC-1α* showed impaired tumor growth and enhanced sensitivity to cytotoxic therapies [32]. In line with this, RCC patients with low levels of *PGC-1α* expression displayed a poor outcome in the TCGA ccRCC dataset [32]. *ALDH6A1* catalyzes the oxidative decarboxylation of malonate and methylmalonate semialdehydes to acetyl- and propionyl-CoA in the valine and pyrimidine catabolic pathways [33]. Recently, Zhang et al. identified six genes, including *ALDH6A1*, as biomarkers for ccRCC, and demonstrated that downregulation of the *ALDH6A1* gene was associated with shorter overall survival of ccRCC patients in the TCGA dataset [34]. *MARC2* (*MOSC2*) has been suggested to play a role in the mitochondrial nitric oxidase pathway and in the detoxification of xenobiotics [35]. MARC2 associates with MARC1 in the mitochondrial amidoxime-reducing component (mARC), i.e., mammalian molybdenum-containing enzymes [35]. Rixen and coworkers recently showed that *MARC2* KO mice had decreased levels of total cholesterol and increased glucose levels, suggesting that *MARC2* affects energy pathways [36]. However, Li et al. showed that reduced *MARC2* expression was associated with an increased sensitivity to paclitaxel-based neoadjuvant therapy in human *EGFR-2*-negative breast cancer patients [37] but, to the best of our knowledge, there have been no previous reports on a role of *MARC2* in RCC.

In our survival analysis, we showed for the first time that low gene expression for *MARC2*, *CUBN*, and *SLC47A1* and high gene expression of *KRT17* were associated with poor overall survival of ccRCC patients. The limitations of our study were the small number of CDCs studied and the lack of an available validation set. The strength of our study is that we considered miRNA-mRNA correlations and could further confirm the role of SLC in CDCs. Based on the finding that among the deregulated genes in CDCs were genes that regulate (i) the transport of amino acids or electrolytes (*SLC7A11*, *SLC47A1*), (ii) mitochondrial pathways (*MARC2*, *PPARGC1A*), and (iii) catabolic pathways (*HK2*, *ALDH6A1*), we can support the statement that CDC is a metabolic disease [6].

4. Material and Methods

4.1. Patients and Tumor Material

The snap-frozen tissue samples were obtained from the Comprehensive Cancer Center tissue biobank of the University Hospital Erlangen. The tumor histology was reviewed by experienced uropathologists (AH and FH). All procedures were performed in accordance with the ethical standards established in the 1964 Declaration of Helsinki and its later amendments. All patients gave informed consent. The study was based on the approval of the Ethics Commissions of the University Hospital Erlangen (No. 4607). The CDC case Tu1 (pT3a, pN2, G3–G4) and CDC case Tu2 (pT3a, cN2, cM1, G3) presented with liver metastases at diagnosis and had a survival time of 2 months. The normal tissue samples originated in one case (No2) from CDC Tu2 adjacent tissue, in five cases from tumor-adjacent tissues from ccRCC patients (No3, No4, No7, No8, No9), in one case from tumor adjacent tissue from a chromophobe renal cell carcinoma patient (No5), and in one case from tumor adjacent tissue from an oncocytoma patient (No6) (Table S1).

4.2. RNA and Protein Isolation

Total RNA and protein were isolated using TRIzol (Invitrogen, Darmstadt, Germany) according to the manufacturer's instructions. Tissue samples were mechanically disrupted in TRIzol reagent prior to RNA and protein isolation. RNA preparations were treated with recombinant DNase I (Sigma Aldrich, Taufkirchen, Germany) before use. The RNA yield and purity were determined using a microliter spectrophotometer (NanoDrop 1000, Thermo Fisher Scientific, Wilmington, DE, USA).

4.3. Quantitative Real-Time PCR

The mRNA transcripts were detected using TaqMan gene expression assays (Thermo Fisher Scientific) according to the manufacturer's protocol. Briefly, 1 µg of RNA was reverse transcribed using the Maxima cDNA synthesis kit (Thermo Fisher Scientific). The reactions were carried out using the StepOne Plus Real-Time PCR System (Thermo Fisher Scientific) in triplicate in a final volume of 10 µL with cDNA equivalent to 25 ng RNA, using TaqMan gene expression assays (SLC7A11, Hs00921938_m1; HIST1H3B, Hs00605810_s1; HK2, Hs00606086_m1; PPARGC1A, Hs00173304_m1; ALDH6A1, Hs00194421_m1; MARC2, Hs01550747_m1; SLC47A1, Hs00217320_m1) and PCR reagents according to the manufacturer's instructions. No template controls were included in the reaction plates. Thermal cycling conditions were 95 °C for 20 s, followed by 40 cycles of 95 °C for 1 s and 60 °C for 20 s. GAPDH (Hs99999905_m1, Thermo Fisher Scientific) served as the endogenous reference. Relative mRNA expression levels were calculated according to the $\Delta\Delta Ct$ method [38].

4.4. Western Blotting

Twenty-five µg of protein extract was separated by SDS-PAGE (8% gels) and transferred to nitrocellulose membranes (GE Healthcare, Freiburg, Germany) by semidry electroblotting. The primary antibodies used were against *SLC7A11* (rabbit mAb, clone *D2M7A*, 1:1000, Cell Signaling, Frankfurt, Germany), *HIST1H3B* (rabbit pAb, PA5-111876, 1:1000, Thermo Fisher Scientific), *HK2* (rabbit mAb, clone C64G5, 1:1000, Cell Signaling), *PPARGC1A* (mouse mAb, clone 1C1B2, 1:3000, Proteintech, Manchester, UK), *ALDH6A1* (rabbit pAb, 20452-1-AP, 1:6000, Proteintech), *MARC2* (rabbit pAb, 24782-1-AP, 1:1000, Proteintech), *SLC47A1* (rabbit mAb, clone D4C62, 1:500, Cell Signaling), and GAPDH (rabbit mAb, clone 14C10, 1:10,000, Cell Signaling). Secondary horseradish peroxidase-conjugated antibodies against rabbit or mouse were purchased from Jackson ImmunoResearch (Suffolk, UK) and used at a concentration of 1:5000. Protein bands were detected by enhanced chemiluminescence in an LAS-4000 chemiluminescence detection system (GE Healthcare, Munich, Germany).

4.5. RNA Sequencing Data Processing

Total RNA sequencing library preparation and sequencing was performed at Core Facility Genomik (University of Münster, Münster, Germany). After rRNA depletion (NEBNext; New England Biolabs, Ipswich, MA, USA), library preparation was performed according to the manufacturer's protocols (NEBNext Ultra II, New England Biolabs). RNA sequencing was performed using the Illumina NextSeq 500 platform. Processing of 75 bp single-end reads of mRNA sequence data was quality checked using FastQC (v 0.11.8) [39]. Low-quality read ends and remaining sequencing adapters were clipped off using Cutadapt (v1.14) (https://cutadapt.readthedocs.io/en/stable/). Trimmed reads were aligned to the human genome (UCSC GRCh38) using HiSat2 (v2.1.0) (https://ccb.jhu.edu/software/hisat2/index.shtml). Annotation and counting of the processed reads was performed using featureCounts (v 1.5.3) (http://subread.sourceforge.net/) and Ensembl annotations (90, GRCh38.p10). Mapping results can be assessed in Table S6. Read counts of all genes can be found in Table S7.

4.6. Differential Gene Expression Analysis

Differential gene expression analysis was performed in R using DESeq2 v1.16.1 [40]. We first filtered genes by keeping those with at least five read counts in at least three normal tissues, and at least five read counts in both tumor samples. As a result, 16,672 out of 58,395 genes were used for follow-up analysis (Figure S1). Finally, we used an algorithm to estimate variance-mean dependence in read counts and test for differential expression based on a model using a negative binomial distribution. The Benjamini-Hochberg correction was used to correct for multiple comparisons. Genes with an adjusted p-value ≤ 0.05 were regarded as significantly differentially expressed. Statistics of the differential gene expression results including base mean, fold-change, and adjusted p-values of genes were visualized in a circos plot using OmicCircos. Hierarchical clustering of samples was performed and visualized using ComplexHeatmap [41].

4.7. Gene Enrichment Analyses

Significantly differentially expressed protein-coding genes with at least a 2-fold increase or a half-fold change were used to perform gene enrichment analysis using Enrichr [42]. This tool applies Fisher's exact test to determine whether a given set of genes is significantly associated with curated biological pathways from databases such as KEGG [43], WikiPathways [44], or Reactome [45]. The Benjamini-Hochberg correction was used to correct for multiple comparisons. The pathways with adjusted p-values ≤ 0.05 were regarded as significant. The results can be found in Table S2.

4.8. Survival Analysis

We extracted RNA sequencing data from 522 clear cell renal cell carcinoma (KIRC) patients and 284 papillary cell renal cell carcinoma (KIPR) patients from the TCGA database [17]. Patients were divided into two groups (high or low) based on their expression levels of the genes of interest (i.e., *HK2, MARC2, CUBN, KRT17, SLC47A1*). Patients at the top 50% expression level of a gene were assigned to the high group, and the other patients were assigned to the low group. Patient survival times were calculated as the number of days from initial pathological diagnosis to death, or the number of days from initial pathological diagnosis to the last time the patient was known to be alive. These times were used to generate the Kaplan-Meier survival plots using RTCGA (https://rtcga.github.io/RTCGA).

4.9. miRNA Target Genes

To derive miRNA-gene interactions, we combined results from three databases. We first obtained predictive miRNA-gene interactions from TargetScan v7.2 [46]. The data were further annotated with StarBase v2.0 [47] and miRTarbase 2018 [48], which provide experimental evidence for the putative miRNA-gene interactions. As a result, we obtained a list of miRNA-gene interactions that not only contained putative miRNA binding sites in 3′ UTR of target genes, but also experimental evidence validating such interactions. The list can be found in Table S4.

5. Conclusions

The RNA sequencing analysis of CDCs in comparison to normal tissues revealed a large number of dysregulated protein-coding genes with a predominance of solute carrier transporters, potential miRNA-target interactions and prognostic markers that could be associated with CDC.

Supplementary Materials: The following are available online at http://www.mdpi.com/2072-6694/12/1/64/s1, Figure S1: Analysis of the expression of the selected 16,672 genes, Figure S2: Western blots and densitometry, Table S1: Results of differential gene expression analysis. The table contains four sub-tables that are statistics of all selected genes (n = 16,672), significantly (adjusted p-value ≤ 0.05) differentially expressed protein-coding genes with |log2fold-change $\geq$1|, |log2fold-change $\geq$3| and |log2fold-change $\geq$6|, Table S2: Results of gene set enrichment analysis, Table S3: RNA transcriptome sequencing data for single nucleotide variations, Table S4: miRNA-gene interactions and correlation analysis, Table S5: Putative miRNA binding sites on 3′ UTR of *SLC7A11*, Table S6:

Statistics of the read counts that were mapped and identified in the RNA sequencing data, Table S7: Read counts of all identified genes ($n = 58,396$).

Author Contributions: H.T., S.W., M.K. and X.L. designed the study. C.G.S., A.K., F.H., A.H. and B.W. acquired the clinical samples and patient information. F.H. and A.H. performed the pathological review of all cases. K.W., N.H., and S.W. carried out the RNA isolation, protein isolation, qRT-PCR and Western blots. X.L., J.V., H.T., M.K., D.M., S.H. and S.W. performed RNA sequence analyses and the statistical analyses. X.L., H.T., and S.W. prepared the tables and figures. H.T., X.L., B.W., S.W., A.K., and A.H. wrote the main manuscript. All authors have read and agreed to the published version of the manuscript.

Funding: This research was funded by the Rudolf und Irmgard Kleinknecht-Stiftung, the Johannes und Frieda Marohn-Stiftung and the Wilhelm Sander-Stiftung [2015.171.1]. Xin Lai acknowledges ELAN-fund of Universitätsklinikum Erlangen [16-08-16-1-Lai]. The authors also acknowledge support by Deutsche Forschungsgemeinschaft and Friedrich-Alexander-Universität Erlangen-Nürnberg within the funding program Open Access Publishing.

Acknowledgments: Many thanks to N. Savaskan and E. Yakubov for helpful discussions. The authors would like to thank American Journal Experts for providing English language editing for our manuscript.

Conflicts of Interest: The authors declare no conflicts of interest.

Abbreviations

CDC	collecting duct renal cell carcinoma
SLC	solute carrier
SLC7A11	solute carrier family 7, member 11
SLC47A1	solute carrier family 47, member 1

References

1. Ciszewski, S.; Jakimow, A.; Smolska-Ciszewska, B. Collecting (Bellini) duct carcinoma: A clinical study of a rare tumour and review of the literature. *Can. Urol. Assoc. J.* **2015**, *9*, E589–E593. [CrossRef]
2. Ito, K. Recent advances in the systemic treatment of metastatic non-clear cell renal cell carcinomas. *Int. J. Urol.* **2019**, *26*, 868–877. [CrossRef]
3. Pagani, F.; Colecchia, M.; Sepe, P.; Apollonio, G.; Claps, M.; Verzoni, E.; de Braud, F.; Procopio, G. Collecting ducts carcinoma: An orphan disease. Literature overview and future perspectives. *Cancer Treat. Rev.* **2019**, *79*, e101891. [CrossRef]
4. Mancilla-Jimenez, R.; Stanley, R.J.; Blath, R.A. Papillary renal cell carcinoma: A clinical, radiologic, and pathologic study of 34 cases. *Cancer* **1976**, *38*, 2469–2480. [CrossRef]
5. Cromie, W.J.; Davis, C.J.; DeTure, F.A. Atypical carcinoma of kidney: Possibly originating from collecting duct epithelium. *Urology* **1979**, *1*, 315–317. [CrossRef]
6. Malouf, G.G.; Compérat, E.; Yao, H.; Mouawad, R.; Lindner, V.; Rioux-Leclercq, N.; Verkarre, V.; Leroy, X.; Dainese, L.; Classe, M.; et al. Unique transcriptomic profile of collecting duct carcinomas relative to upper tract urothelial carcinomas and other kidney carcinomas. *Sci. Rep.* **2016**, *6*, e30988. [CrossRef]
7. Pal, S.K.; Choueiri, T.K.; Wang, K.; Khaira, D.; Karam, J.A.; Van Allen, E.; Palma, N.A.; Stein, M.N.; Johnson, A.; Squillace, R.; et al. Characterization of clinical cases of collecting duct carcinoma of the kidney assessed by comprehensive genomic profiling. *Eur. Urol.* **2015**. [CrossRef]
8. Wang, J.; Papanicolau-Sengos, A.; Chintala, S.; Wei, L.; Liu, B.; Hu, Q.; Miles, K.M.; Conroy, J.M.; Glenn, S.T.; Costantini, M.; et al. Collecting duct carcinoma of the kidney is associated with CDKN2A deletion and SLC family gene up-regulation. *Oncotarget* **2016**, *7*, 29901–29915. [CrossRef]
9. Kröger, N.; Merseburger, A.S.; Bedke, J. Current recommendations for the systemic treatment of metastatic renal cell carcinoma. *Aktuelle Urol.* **2019**. [CrossRef]
10. Stukalin, I.; Wells, J.C.; Graham, J.; Yuasa, T.; Beuselinck, B.; Kollmansberger, C.; Ernst, D.S.; Agarwal, N.; Le, T.; Donskov, F.; et al. Real-world outcomes of nivolumab and cabozantinib in metastatic renal cell carcinoma: Results from the international metastatic renal cell carcinoma database consortium. *Curr. Oncol.* **2019**, *26*, e175–e179. [CrossRef]
11. Chintala, S.; Pili, R. Genomic profiling of collecting duct renal carcinoma. *Aging* **2016**, *8*, 2260–2261. [CrossRef]

12. Nykjaer, A.; Fyfe, J.C.; Kozyraki, R.; Leheste, J.-R.; Jacobsen, C.; Nielsen, M.S.; Verroust, P.J.; Aminoff, M.; de la Chapelle, A.; Moestrup, S.K.; et al. Cubilin dysfunction causes abnormal metabolism of the steroid hormone 25(OH) vitamin D3. *Proc. Natl. Acad. Sci. USA* **2001**, *98*, 13895–13900. [CrossRef]
13. Kim, S.; Wong, P.; Coulombe, P.A. A keratin cytoskeletal protein regulates protein synthesis and epithelial cell growth. *Nature* **2006**, *441*, 362–365. [CrossRef]
14. Lalli, A.; Tilakaratne, W.M.; Ariyawardana, A.; Fitchett, C.; Leigh, I.M.; Hagi-Pavli, E.; Cruchley, A.T.; Parkinson, E.K.; Teh, M.T.; Fortune, F.; et al. An altered keratinocyte phenotype in oral submucous fibrosis: Correlation of keratin K17 expression with disease severity. *J. Oral. Pathol. Med.* **2008**, *37*, 211–220. [CrossRef]
15. Khanom, R.; Nguyen, C.T.; Kayamori, K.; Zhao, X.; Morita, K.; Miki, Y.; Katsube, K.; Yamaguchi, A.; Sakamoto, K. Keratin 17 is induced in oral cancer and facilitates tumor growth. *PLoS ONE* **2016**, *11*, e0161163. [CrossRef]
16. Landrum, M.J.; Lee, J.M.; Benson, M.; Brown, G.R.; Chao, C.; Chitipiralla, S.; Gu, B.; Hart, J.; Hoffman, D.; Jang, W.; et al. ClinVar: Improving access to variant interpretations and supporting evidence. *Nucleic Acids Res.* **2018**, *46*, D1062–D1067. [CrossRef]
17. Ricketts, C.J.; De Cubas, A.A.; Fan, H.; Smith, C.C.; Lang, M.; Reznik, E.; Bowlby, R.; Gibb, E.A.; Akbani, R.; Beroukhim, R.; et al. The Cancer genome atlas comprehensive molecular characterization of renal cell carcinoma. *Cell Rep.* **2018**, *23*, e3698. [CrossRef]
18. Gremel, G.; Djureinovic, D.; Niinivirta, M.; Laird, A.; Ljungqvist, O.; Johannesson, H.; Bergman, J.; Edqvist, P.H.; Navani, S.; Khan, N.; et al. A systematic search strategy identifies cubilin as independent prognostic marker for renal cell carcinoma. *BMC Cancer* **2017**, *17*, e9. [CrossRef]
19. Niinivirta, M.; Enblad, G.; Edqvist, P.H.; Pontén, F.; Dragomir, A.; Ullenhag, G.J. Tumoral cubilin is a predictive marker for treatment of renal cancer patients with sunitinib and sorafenib. *J. Cancer Res. Clin. Oncol.* **2017**, *143*, 961–970. [CrossRef]
20. Dvorak, H.F. Tumors: Wounds that do not heal. Similarities between tumor stroma generation and wound healing. *New Engl. J. Med.* **1986**, *315*, 1650–1659.
21. Schrödter, S.; Braun, M.; Syring, I.; Klümper, N.; Deng, M.; Schmidt, D.; Perner, S.; Müller, S.C.; Ellinger, J. Identification of the dopamine transporter SLC6A3 as a biomarker for patients with renal cell carcinoma. *Mol. Cancer* **2016**, *15*, e10. [CrossRef]
22. Hansson, J.; Lindgren, D.; Nilsson, H.; Johansson, E.; Johansson, M.; Gustavsson, L.; Axelson, H. Overexpression of functional SLC6A3 in clear cell renal cell carcinoma. *Clin. Cancer Res.* **2017**, *23*, 2105–2115. [CrossRef]
23. Lewerenz, J.; Maher, P.; Methner, A. Regulation of xCT expression and system x (c) (-) function in neuronal cells. *Amino Acids* **2012**, *42*, 171–179. [CrossRef]
24. Otsuka, M.; Matsumoto, T.; Morimoto, R.; Arioka, S.; Omote, H.; Moriyama, Y. A human transporter protein that mediates the final excretion step for toxic organic cations. *Proc. Natl. Acad. Sci. USA* **2005**, *102*, 17923–17928. [CrossRef]
25. Staud, F.; Cerveny, L.; Ahmadimoghaddam, D.; Ceckova, M. Multidrug and toxin extrusion proteins (MATE/SLC47); role in pharmacokinetics. *Int. J. Biochem. Cell Biol.* **2013**, *45*, 2007–2011. [CrossRef]
26. Shuch, B.; Linehan, W.M.; Srinivasan, R. Aerobic glycolysis: A novel target in kidney cancer. *Expert Rev. Anticancer Ther.* **2013**, *13*, 711–719. [CrossRef]
27. Smith, T.A. Mammalian hexokinases and their abnormal expression in cancer. *Br. J. Biomed. Sci.* **2000**, *57*, 170–178.
28. Masoud, G.N.; Li, W. HIF-1α pathway: Role, regulation and intervention for cancer therapy. *Acta Pharm. Sin. B* **2015**, *5*, 378–389. [CrossRef]
29. Nam, H.Y.; Chandrashekar, D.S.; Kundu, A.; Shelar, S.; Kho, E.Y.; Sonpavde, G.; Naik, G.; Ghatalia, P.; Livi, C.B.; Varambally, S.; et al. Integrative epigenetic and gene expression analysis of renal tumor progression to metastasis. *Mol. Cancer Res.* **2019**, *17*, 84–96. [CrossRef]
30. Sato, H.; Tamba, M.; Ishii, T.; Bannai, S. Cloning and expression of a plasma membrane cystine/glutamate exchange transporter composed of two distinct proteins. *J. Biol. Chem.* **1999**, *274*, 11455–11458. [CrossRef]
31. Tran, M.T.; Zsengeller, Z.K.; Berg, A.H.; Khankin, E.V.; Bhasin, M.K.; Kim, W.; Clish, C.B.; Stillman, I.E.; Karumanchi, S.A.; Rhee, E.P.; et al. PGC1-alpha drives NAD biosynthesis linking oxidative metabolism to renal protection. *Nature* **2016**, *531*, 528–532. [CrossRef]

32. LaGory, E.L.; Wu, C.; Taniguchi, C.M.; Ding, C.C.; Chi, J.T.; von Eyben, R.; Scott, D.A.; Richardson, A.D.; Giaccia, A.J. Suppression of PGC-1α is critical for reprogramming oxidative metabolism in renal cell carcinoma. *Cell Rep.* **2015**, *12*, 116–127. [CrossRef]
33. Kedishvili, N.Y.; Popov, K.M.; Rougraff, P.M.; Zhao, Y.; Crabb, D.W.; Harris, R.A. CoA-dependent methylmalonate-semialdehyde dehydrogenase, a unique member of the aldehyde dehydrogenase superfamily: CDNA cloning, evolutionary relationships, and tissue distribution. *J Biol. Chem.* **1992**, *267*, 19724–19729.
34. Zhang, B.; Wu, Q.; Wang, Z.; Xu, R.; Hu, X.; Sun, Y.; Wang, Q.; Ju, F.; Ren, S.; Zhang, C.; et al. The promising novel biomarkers and candidate small molecule drugs in kidney renal clear cell carcinoma: Evidence from bioinformatics analysis of high-throughput data. *Mol. Genet. Genom. Med.* **2019**, *7*, e607. [CrossRef]
35. Kotthaus, J.; Wahl, B.; Havemeyer, A.; Kotthaus, J.; Schade, D.; Garbe-Schonberg, D.; Mendel, R.; Bittner, F.; Clement, B. Reduction of N(omega)-hydroxy-L-arginine by the mitochondrial amidoxime reducing component (mARC). *Biochem. J.* **2011**, *433*, 383–391. [CrossRef]
36. Rixen, S.; Havemeyer, A.; Tyl-Bielicka, A.; Pysniak, K.; Gajewska, M.; Kulecka, M.; Ostrowski, J.; Mikula, M.; Clement, B. Mitochondrial amidoxime-reducing component 2 (mARC2) has a significant role in N-reductive activity and energy metabolism. *J. Biol. Chem.* **2019**, *294*, 17593–17602. [CrossRef]
37. Li, Z.; Zhang, Y.; Zhang, Z.; Zhao, Z.; Lv, Q. A four-gene signature predicts the efficacy of paclitaxel-based neoadjuvant therapy in human epidermal growth factor receptor 2-negative breast cancer. *J. Cell. Biochem.* **2019**, *120*, 6046–6056. [CrossRef]
38. Schmittgen, T.D.; Livak, K.J. Analyzing real-time PCR data by the comparative C(T) method. *Nat. Protoc.* **2008**, *3*, 1101–1108. [CrossRef]
39. Andrews, S. FastQC: A Quality Control Tool for High Throughput Sequence Data. 2010. Available online: http://www.bioinformatics.babraham.ac.uk/projects/fastqc (accessed on 10 January 2019).
40. Love, M.I.; Huber, W.; Anders, S. Moderated estimation of fold change and dispersion for RNA-seq data with DESeq2. *Genome Biol.* **2014**, *15*, e550. [CrossRef]
41. Gu, Z.; Eils, R.; Schlesner, M. Complex heatmaps reveal patterns and correlations in multidimensional genomic data. *Bioinformatics* **2016**, *32*, 2847–2849. [CrossRef]
42. Chen, E.Y.; Tan, C.M.; Kou, Y.; Duan, Q.; Wang, Z.; Meirelles, G.V.; Clark, N.R.; Ma'ayan, A. Enrichr: Interactive and collaborative HTML5 gene list enrichment analysis tool. *BMC Bioinform.* **2013**, *14*, e128. [CrossRef] [PubMed]
43. Kanehisa, M.; Sato, Y.; Kawashima, M.; Furumichi, M.; Tanabe, M. KEGG as a reference resource for gene and protein annotation. *Nucleic Acids Res.* **2016**, *44*, D457–D462. [CrossRef] [PubMed]
44. Kutmon, M.; Riutta, A.; Nunes, N.; Hanspers, K.; Willighagen, E.L.; Bohler, A.; Mélius, J.; Waagmeester, A.; Sinha, S.R.; Miller, R.; et al. WikiPathways: Capturing the full diversity of pathway knowledge. *Nucleic Acids Res.* **2016**, *44*, D488–D494. [CrossRef] [PubMed]
45. Fabregat, A.; Sidiropoulos, K.; Garapati, P.; Gillespie, M.; Hausmann, K.; Haw, R.; Jassal, B.; Jupe, S.; Korninger, F.; McKay, S.; et al. The reactome pathway knowledgebase. *Nucleic Acids Res.* **2016**, *44*, D481–D487. [CrossRef]
46. Agarwal, V.; Bell, G.W.; Nam, J.W.; Bartel, D.P. Predicting effective microRNA target sites in mammalian mRNAs. *eLife* **2015**. [CrossRef]
47. Li, J.H.; Liu, S.; Zhou, H.; Qu, L.H.; Yang, J.H. starBase v2.0: Decoding miRNA-ceRNA, miRNA-ncRNA and protein-RNA interaction networks from large-scale CLIP-Seq data. *Nucleic Acids Res.* **2014**, *42*, D92–D97. [CrossRef]
48. Chou, C.H.; Shrestha, S.; Yang, C.D.; Chang, N.W.; Lin, Y.L.; Liao, K.W.; Huang, W.C.; Sun, T.H.; Tu, S.J.; Lee, W.H.; et al. miRTarBase update 2018: A resource for experimentally validated microRNA-target interactions. *Nucleic Acids Res.* **2018**, *46*, D296–D302. [CrossRef]

© 2019 by the authors. Licensee MDPI, Basel, Switzerland. This article is an open access article distributed under the terms and conditions of the Creative Commons Attribution (CC BY) license (http://creativecommons.org/licenses/by/4.0/).

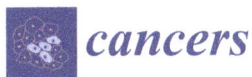

Article

*GSTO1**CC Genotype (rs4925) Predicts Shorter Survival in Clear Cell Renal Cell Carcinoma Male Patients

Tanja Radic [1,2], Vesna Coric [1,2], Zoran Bukumiric [2,3], Marija Pljesa-Ercegovac [1,2], Tatjana Djukic [1,2], Natasa Avramovic [2,4], Marija Matic [1,2], Smiljana Mihailovic [5], Dejan Dragicevic [2,6], Zoran Dzamic [2,6], Tatjana Simic [1,2,7] and Ana Savic-Radojevic [1,2,*]

[1] Institute of Medical and Clinical Biochemistry, 11000 Belgrade, Serbia; tanjajevtic@gmail.com (T.R.); drcoricvesna@gmail.com (V.C.); m.pljesa.ercegovac@gmail.com (M.P.-E.); tatjana.djukic@med.bg.ac.rs (T.D.); marija_opacic@yahoo.com (M.M.); tatjana.simic@med.bg.ac.rs (T.S.)
[2] Faculty of Medicine, University of Belgrade, 11000 Belgrade, Serbia; zoran.bukumiric@med.bg.ac.rs (Z.B.); natasa.avramovic@med.bg.ac.rs (N.A.); dpdragicevic@gmail.com (D.D.); slavica.lisicic@kcs.ac.rs (Z.D.)
[3] Institute of Medical Statistics and Informatics, 11000 Belgrade, Serbia
[4] Institute of Medical Chemistry, 11000 Belgrade, Serbia
[5] Clinic for Gynecology and Obstetrics "Narodni front", 11000 Belgrade, Serbia; smiljanamihailovic@gmail.com
[6] Clinic of Urology, Clinical Center of Serbia, 11000 Belgrade, Serbia
[7] Serbian Academy of Sciences and Arts, 11000 Belgrade, Serbia
[*] Correspondence: ana.savic-radojevic@med.bg.ac.rs; Tel.: +381-11-3643-271

Received: 19 November 2019; Accepted: 13 December 2019; Published: 17 December 2019

Abstract: Omega class glutathione transferases, GSTO1-1 and GSTO2-2, exhibit different activities involved in regulation of inflammation, apoptosis and redox homeostasis. We investigated the the prognostic significance of *GSTO1* (rs4925) and *GSTO2* (rs156697 and rs2297235) polymorphisms in clear cell renal cell carcinoma (ccRCC) patients. GSTO1-1 and GSTO2-2 expression and phosphorylation status of phosphoinositide 3-kinase (PI3K)/protein kinase B (Akt)/ /mammalian target of rapamycin (mTOR) and Raf/MEK/extracellular signal-regulated kinase (ERK) signaling pathways in non-tumor and tumor ccRCC tissue, as well as possible association of GSTO1-1 with signaling molecules were also assessed. GSTO genotyping was performed by quantitative PCR in 228 ccRCC patients, while expression and immunoprecipitation were analyzed by Western blot in 30 tissue specimens. Shorter survival in male carriers of *GSTO1**C/C wild-type genotype compared to the carriers of at least one variant allele was demonstrated ($p = 0.049$). *GSTO1**C/C genotype independently predicted higher risk of overall mortality among male ccRCC patients ($p = 0.037$). Increased expression of GSTO1-1 and GSTO2-2 was demonstrated in tumor compared to corresponding non-tumor tissue ($p = 0.002, p = 0.007$, respectively), while GSTO1 expression was correlated with interleukin-1β (IL-1β)/pro-interleukin-1β (pro-IL-1β) ratio ($r = 0.260, p = 0.350$). Interaction of GSTO1 with downstream effectors of investigated pathways was shown in ccRCC tumor tissue. This study demonstrated significant prognostic role of *GSTO1* polymorphism in ccRCC. Up-regulated GSTO1-1 and GSTO2-2 in tumor tissue might contribute to aberrant ccRCC redox homeostasis.

Keywords: glutathione transferase omega 1; glutathione transferase omega 2; polymorphism; PI3K/Akt/mTOR; Raf/MEK/ERK; IL-1β; pro-IL-1β

1. Introduction

Being the most common and the most aggressive subtype among renal cancers, clear cell renal cell carcinoma (ccRCC) accounts for most RCC fatal outcomes [1]. Such outcomes probably arise from significant intra-tumor and inter-tumor genetic diversity of ccRCC, revealed in recent genomic studies [1–3]. Indeed, among genetic factors that contribute to RCC risk, the most investigated is mutation of *VHL* gene [1], underlying the abnormal accumulation of hypoxia-inducible factor α (HIFα) proteins in normoxia [4]. Namely, downstream over-expression of HIF-targeted genes is involved in the regulation of angiogenesis, proliferation, invasion and survival [4], as well as in the metabolism of glucose, influencing the characteristic metabolic phenotype of the disease [5]. Among the most investigated HIF-targeted genes is vascular endothelial growth factor (VEGF). It binds to specific tyrosine kinase receptor, VEGF-R2, expressed on both endothelial and ccRCC cells [6], further resulting in downstream signaling which mediates the activation of Ras/MEK/ extracellular signal-regulated kinase (ERK) and phosphoinositide 3-kinase (PI3K)/protein kinase B (Akt)/ mammalian target of rapamycin (mTOR) pathway. In this way, tumor progression is promoted by additional HIFα production [5] as a part of positive feedback loop which contributes to constitutive activation of the signaling network [7]. In addition, multiple other mechanisms could contribute to constitutive activation of the PI3K/Akt pathway in ccRCC [7], including epigenetic regulatory mechanisms, specifically microRNAs (miRNAs) [7], as well as protein complex formation with phosphoinositide-dependent kinase-1 (PDK1) and 78-kDa glucose-regulated protein [7]. Interestingly, it has been shown that deglutathionylation type of modification mediated by glutaredoxin 1 was implicated in the activation of Akt, thus, protecting the cells from oxidative stress–induced apoptosis [8].

The role of glutathione transferases (GST) in redox regulation has already been taken into consideration as a contributing mechanism both in cancer development and progression [9,10]. Representing a set of cytosolic, mitochondrial and microsomal proteins with versatile catalytic and noncatalytic functions [11], GSTs have been readily studied in the light of their bio-transformational capacities towards potent xenobiotics, as well as endogenous reactive oxygen species [12]. This may not come as a surprise, since most of the genes encoding for members of GST enzyme superfamily are highly polymorphic, therefore, altering the individual susceptibility to environmental and oxidative stress [9,13]. Additionally, their functional repertoire comprises the ability to form protein-protein interactions, independently of their catalytic functions, thus negatively regulating certain protein kinases involved in cell proliferation and apoptosis [9,13]. In the case of RCC, a growing body of evidence suggests that cytosolic GSTs might be involved not exclusively in the development, but also in the progression of RCC [12,14,15]. However, a couple of studies have tackled the problem of GST polymorphisms with regard to RCC patients' survival [15,16], proposing the aforementioned protein-protein interactions as the underlying molecular mechanism in RCC progression.

Omega class members, GSTO1-1 and GSTO2-2 isoenzymes, are unique in terms of presence of cysteine in the active site [17], thus, manifesting the whole range of specific activities not associated with other human GSTs [18]. Cysteine residue in the active site allows these isoenzymes to catalyze specific spectrum of glutathione-dependent thiol exchange and reduction reactions [17]. Namely, among other, GST omega class members possess thioltransferase and dehydroascorbate reductase activities, similarly to glutaredoxins [18]. Indeed, GSTO1-1 exhibits deglutathionylase activity [18], and seems to be involved in the modulation of ryanodine receptors, as well as the activation of IL1-β [19,20]. On the other hand, GSTO2-2 is the enzyme with the highest dehydroascorbate-reductase (DHAR) activity, in that way preserving reduced form of ascorbic acid [21]. It has also been shown that in contrast to GSTO2-2, GSTO1-1 plays important role in the glutathionylation cycle by its deglutathionylase and glutathionylase activity, depending on different conditions [22]. Additionally, it has been suggested that GSTO1-1 alters cell survival signaling pathways by inhibiting apoptotic MAPK signaling pathways [23,24].

Recently, novel aspect of GSTO1-1 role in cancer progression is shown to be mediated by interaction with type 1 ryanodine receptor, RyR1 [25]. Namely, Lu et al. showed HIF-dependent expression of GSTO1-1 in breast cancer cells exposed to carboplatin with consequent breast cancer stem cell enrichment, mediated by interaction between GSTO1-1 and RyR1 and downstream activation of PYK2/SRC/STAT3 signaling [25]. Additionally, they demonstrated that GSTO1-1 knockdown blocks cancer stem cell enrichment, tumor initiation and metastasis [25]. The overexpression of GSTO1-1 has been also reported in esophageal squamous cell carcinoma, pancreatic cancer, and ovarian cancer [18]. The study by Piaggi et al. showed that overexpression of GSTO1-1 following cisplatin treatment of HeLa cells seems to be associated with the activation of survival signaling pathways and inhibition of apoptotic MAPK pathway [23].

Based on the association between structure and function, three GSTO polymorphisms seem to be of greatest importance: one transition polymorphism in the position 183 at 5' untranslated region (5' UTR) of *GSTO2* gene (*GSTO2**A183G, rs2297235), as well as two single nucleotide polymorphisms *GSTO1**C419A (rs4925) and GSTO2*A424G (rs156697). *GSTO1* rs4925 polymorphism, causing alanine to aspartate substitution in amino acid 140 (*Ala140Asp), results in a change in its deglutathionylase activity. Namely, *GSTO1**C wild-type allele exhibits higher deglutathionylase activity and lower activity in the forward glutathionylation reaction in contrast to GSTO1*A variant allele [22]. Regarding *GSTO2* rs156697 polymorphism, which causes an asparagine to aspartate substitution in amino acid 142 (* Asn142Asp), a strong association between variant *GSTO2**G allele and lower *GSTO2* gene expression has been shown [26,27]. These GSTO polymorphisms were independent predictors of a higher risk of death among patients with muscle invasive bladder cancer [28].

Regarding GST omega class polymorphisms in ccRCC, haplotype comprised of all three variant alleles (*GSTO1**A (rs4925), *GSTO2**G (rs156697) and *GSTO2**G (rs2297235)) showed significantly higher risk of disease development compared to haplotype consisting of all three referent alleles [29]. However, their potential functional significance in terms of ccRCC prognosis have not been studied, as yet. Therefore, we aimed to evaluate the effect of specific GSTO gene variants on the postoperative prognosis in patients with ccRCC. Furthermore, we evaluated GSTO1-1 and GSTO2-2 expression in ccRCC and adjacent non-tumor tissue, as well as phosphorylation status of two important survival pathways, PI3K/Akt/mTOR and Raf/MEK/ERK. Potential association of GSTO1-1 with downstream effectors of these signaling pathways was also investigated.

2. Results

2.1. The Relevance of GSTO1 and GSTO2 Polymorphisms in Overall Survival of ccRCC Patients

The effect of *GSTO1* and *GSTO2* polymorphisms on overall survival was investigated in 228 ccRCC patients during median follow-up period of 67 months ranging from 1 to 153 months. Considering the higher prevalence of disease in men, the overall survival was also studied in male and female subpopulations separately. As presented in Table 1, tumor grade II was shown to be the most frequent among ccRCC patients (G2, 55%). Regarding pT stage, the majority of patients had pT1 and pT3 tumors (45% and 42%, respectively). Similar distribution is observed among male patients (Table 1).

Table 1. Clinicopathological characteristics of the 228 patients with ccRCC.

Characteristics	Patients, n (%)	Male Patients, n (%)
Age, years (mean ± SD)	59.19 ± 11.58	57.79 ± 11.22
Gender, n (%)		
Female	74 (32)	
Male	154 (68)	
Fuhrman nuclear grade, n (%)		
G1	28 (14)	17 (12)
G2	111 (56)	76 (57)
G3	50 (26)	36 (27)
G4	8 (4)	5 (4)
pT stage, n (%)		
pT1	97 (45)	61 (40)
pT2	24 (11)	14 (10)
pT3	90 (42)	69 (47)
pT4	5 (2)	4 (3)

Among 228 ccRCC patients with successfully acquired follow-up data there were 79 (35%) deaths throughout the follow-up period. Kaplan-Meier survival analysis did not show statistically significant effect of either *GSTO1* (rs4925) or *GSTO2* (rs156697 and rs2297235) polymorphisms on overall survival among ccRCC patients (Figure 1a). Considering the higher propensity to RCC among men, we further focused on estimation of the potential effect of different GSTO genotypes on overall survival in male and female ccRCC patients separately. There were 61 (40%) deaths among 154 men and 18 (24%) deaths among 74 women during the follow-up period. Kaplan-Meier survival analysis demonstrated statistically significant shorter overall survival (log-rank: $p = 0.049$) in male carriers of *GSTO1**C/C wild-type genotype in comparison with the male carriers of at least one variant allele (Figure 1b). However, *GSTO2* rs156697 and rs2297235 polymorphisms did not show effect on overall survival among male ccRCC patients (Figure 1b). Furthermore, our results did not exhibit effect of either *GSTO1* (rs4925) or *GSTO2* (rs156697 and rs2297235) polymorphisms on overall survival among female ccRCC patients (Figure 1c).

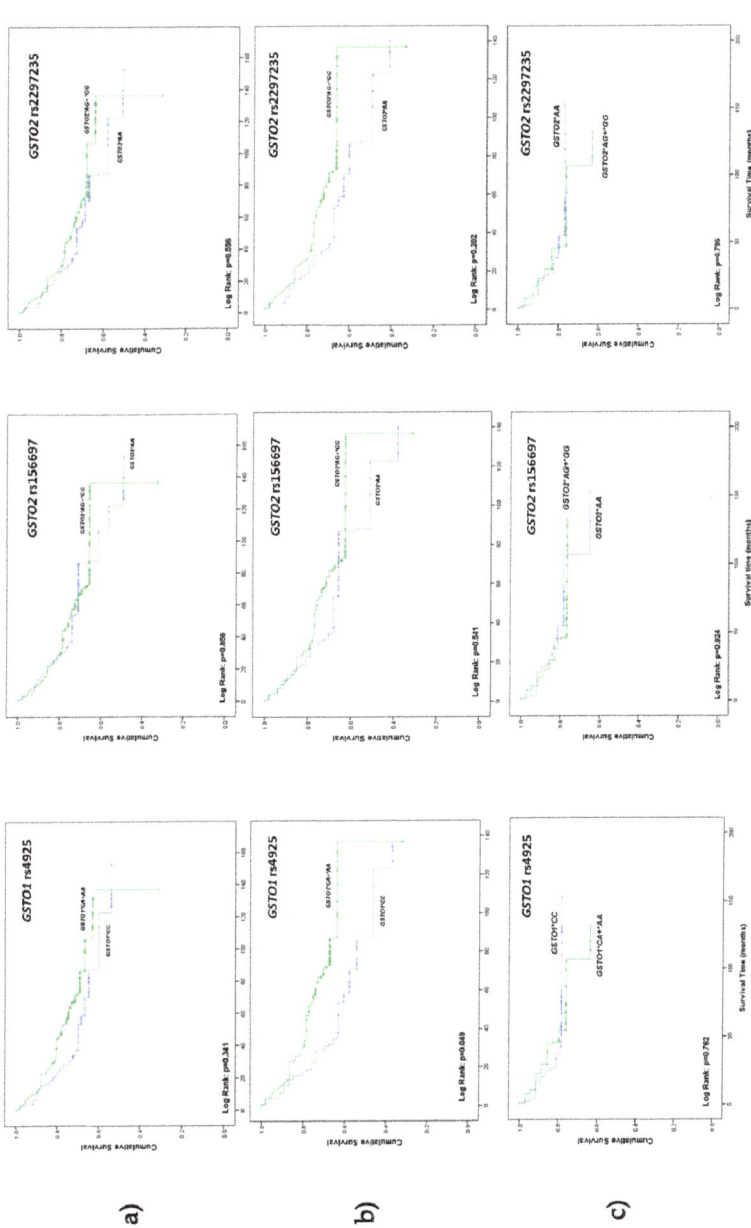

Figure 1. (a) Overall survival of clear cell renal cell carcinoma (ccRCC) patients stratified by *GSTO1* (rs4925) and *GSTO2* (rs156697 and rs2297235) polymorphisms; (b) overall survival of male ccRCC patients stratified by *GSTO1* (rs4925) and *GSTO2* (rs156697 and rs2297235) polymorphisms; (c) overall survival of female ccRCC patients stratified by *GSTO1* (rs4925) and *GSTO2* (rs156697 and rs2297235) polymorphisms.

2.2. Predicting Effect of GSTO1 and GSTO2 Polymorphisms on Overall Mortality in ccRCC Patients

The multivariate Cox regression analysis did not show statistically significant association between either *GSTO1* (rs1495) or *GSTO2* (rs156697 and rs2297235) genotypes and overall mortality, adjusted by recognized prognostic factors, Fuhrman nuclear grade and pT stage, among ccRCC patients (Table 2).

Table 2. Predicting effect of glutathione transferase omega (GSTO) polymorphisms on overall mortality in ccRCC patients.

Variable	Category	Events, n (%)	HR (95% CI) [b]	p
GSTO1 rs4925				
FNR [a]	G1/G2/G3/G4	2 (7)/32 (29)/29 (58)/5 (63)	1.57 (1.08–2.27)	0.017
pT stage	pT1/pT2/pT3/pT4	14 (14)/8 (33)/ 51 (57)/3 (60)	2.01 (1.46–2.76)	<0.001
GSTO1 rs4925				
*CC		32 (38)	1.53 (0.91–2.58)	0.107
*CA + *AA		47 (34)	1.00	
GSTO2 rs156697				
FNR	G1/G2/G3/G4	2 (7)/32 (29)/29 (58)/5 (63)	1.58 (1.09–2.27)	0.015
pT stage	pT1/pT2/pT3/pT4	14 (14)/8 (33)/51 (57)/3 (60)	1.97 (1.43–2.70)	<0.001
GSTO2 rs156697				
*AA		31 (35)	1.11 (0.66–1.88)	0.689
*AG + *GG		48 (34)	1.00	
GSTO2 rs2297235				
FNR	G1/G2/G3/G4	2 (7)/32 (29)/29 (58)/5 (63)	1.57 (1.08–2.27)	0.016
pT stage	pT1/pT2/pT3/pT4	14 (14)/8 (33)/51 (57)/3 (60)	1.96 (1.43–2.69)	<0.001
GSTO2 rs2297235				
*AA		34 (36)	1.24 (0.74–2.07)	0.425
*AG + *GG		44 (34)	1.00	

[a] Fuhrman nuclear grade; [b] HR, odds ratio adjusted to Fuhrman nuclear grade and pT stage; CI, confidence interval; $p < 0.05$ was considered to be statistically significant.

However, when we analyzed this association among male patients, the multivariate Cox regression analysis confirmed GSTO1*CC genotype as an independent predictor of higher risk for overall mortality in those patients. Namely, male carriers of GSTO1*CC genotype had an almost two-fold higher mortality risk compared to the carriers of GSTO1*A variant allele (HR = 1.89, 95%CI: 1.04–3.42, $p = 0.037$). Regarding both investigated GSTO2 polymorphisms (rs156697 and rs2297235), the results did not reach statistical significance ($p > 0.05$, Table 3).

Table 3. Predicting effect of GSTO polymorphisms on overall mortality in male ccRCC patients.

Variable	Category	Events, n (%)	HR (95% CI) [b]	p
GSTO1 rs4925				
FNR [a]	G1/G2/G3/G4	2 (12)/23 (30)/26 (72)/2 (40)	1.58 (1.03–2.43)	0.037
pT stage	pT1/pT2/pT3/pT4	10(16)/5 (36)/42 (61)/2 (50)	1.83 (1.28–2.62)	0.001
GSTO1 rs4925				
*CC		23 (49)	1.89 (1.04–3.42)	0.037
*CA + *AA		38 (36)	1.00	
GSTO2 rs156697				
FNR	G1/G2/G3/G4	2 (12)/23 (30)/26 (72)/2 (40)	1.56 (1.02–2.38)	0.040
pT stage	pT1/pT2/pT3/pT4	10(16)/5 (36)/42 (61)/2 (50)	1.83 (1.29–2.60)	0.001
GSTO2 rs156697				
*AA		21 (43)	1.32 (0.71–2.43)	0.380
*AG + *GG		40 (38)	1.00	
GSTO2 rs2297235				
FNR	G1/G2/G3/G4	2 (12)/23 (30)/26 (72)/2 (40)	1.59 (1.04–2.46)	0.034
pT stage	pT1/pT2/pT3/pT4	10(16)/5 (36)/42 (61)/2 (50)	1.81 (1.27–2.59)	0.001
GSTO2 rs2297235				
*AA		24 (45)	1.60 (0.88–2.92)	0.127
*AG + *GG		36 (37)	1.00	

[a] Fuhrman nuclear grade; [b] HR, odds ratio adjusted to Fuhrman nuclear grade and pT stage; CI, confidence interval; $p < 0.05$ was considered to be statistically significant.

The analysis of overall mortality did not show statistically significant association between either investigated GSTO genotypes among female ccRCC patients ($p > 0.05$, Table 4).

Table 4. Predicting effect of GSTO polymorphisms on overall mortality in female ccRCC patients.

Variable	Category	Events, n (%)	HR (95% CI) [b]	p
GSTO1 rs4925				
FNR [a]	G1/G2/G3/G4	0 (0)/9 (26)/3 (21)/3 (100)	1.92 (0.87–4.26)	0.107
pT stage	pT1/pT2/pT3/pT4	4 (11)/3 (30)/9 (43)/1 (100)	2.20 (1.08–4.46)	0.029
GSTO1 rs4925				
*CC		9 (24)	1.01 (0.34–3.00)	0.992
*CA + *AA		9 (26)	1.00	
GSTO2 rs156697				
FNR	G1/G2/G3/G4	0 (0)/9 (26)/3 (21)/3 (100)	1.95 (0.89–4.27)	0.098
pT stage	pT1/pT2/pT3/pT4	4 (11)/3 (30)/9 (43)/1 (100)	2.23 (1.11–4.47)	0.024
GSTO2 rs156697				
*AA		10 (26)	0.78 (0.27–2.28)	0.654
*AG+*GG		8 (23)	1.00	
GSTO2 rs2297235				
FNR	G1/G2/G3/G4	0 (0)/9 (26)/3 (21)/3 (100)	1.99 (0.90–4.38)	0.089
pT stage	pT1/pT2/pT3/pT4	4 (11)/3 (30)/9 (43)/1 (100)	2.11 (1.05–4.24)	0.035
GSTO2 rs2297235				
*AA		10 (24)	0.77 (0.26–2.31)	0.645
*AG+*GG		8 (27)	1.00	

[a] Fuhrman nuclear grade; [b] HR, odds ratio adjusted to Fuhrman nuclear grade and pT stage; CI, confidence interval; $p < 0.05$ was considered to be statistically significant.

2.3. Expression of Glutathione Transferase Omega Class Enzymes and Downstream Effectors of PI3K/Akt and Raf/MEK/ERK Signaling Pathway in ccRCC

Tumor and adjacent non-tumor tissue samples were acquired during total nephrectomy from 30 patients with ccRCC. All tumor samples were stratified by their pT stage to early-stage (pT1 and pT2) and late-stage (pT3 and pT4) ccRCC. Cytocolic fractions were used for determination of protein expression and immunoprecipitation analysis.

Densitometry analysis following Western blot showed 1.5-fold higher expression of GSTO1 in tumor ccRCC compared to non-tumor tissue ($p = 0.002$, Figure 2a, Figure S1, Table S1). Likewise, 2.2-fold higher expression of GSTO2 protein in tumor ccRCC in comparison with non-tumor tissue was found ($p = 0.007$, Figure 2b, Figure S1, Table S1). Since β-actin has been identified as a target for deglutathionylation by GSTO1-1, we used tubulin as a loading control. Representative blots demonstrating higher expression of GSTO1 and GSTO2 in tumor samples compared to respective non-tumor samples are presented in the Figure 2a,b.

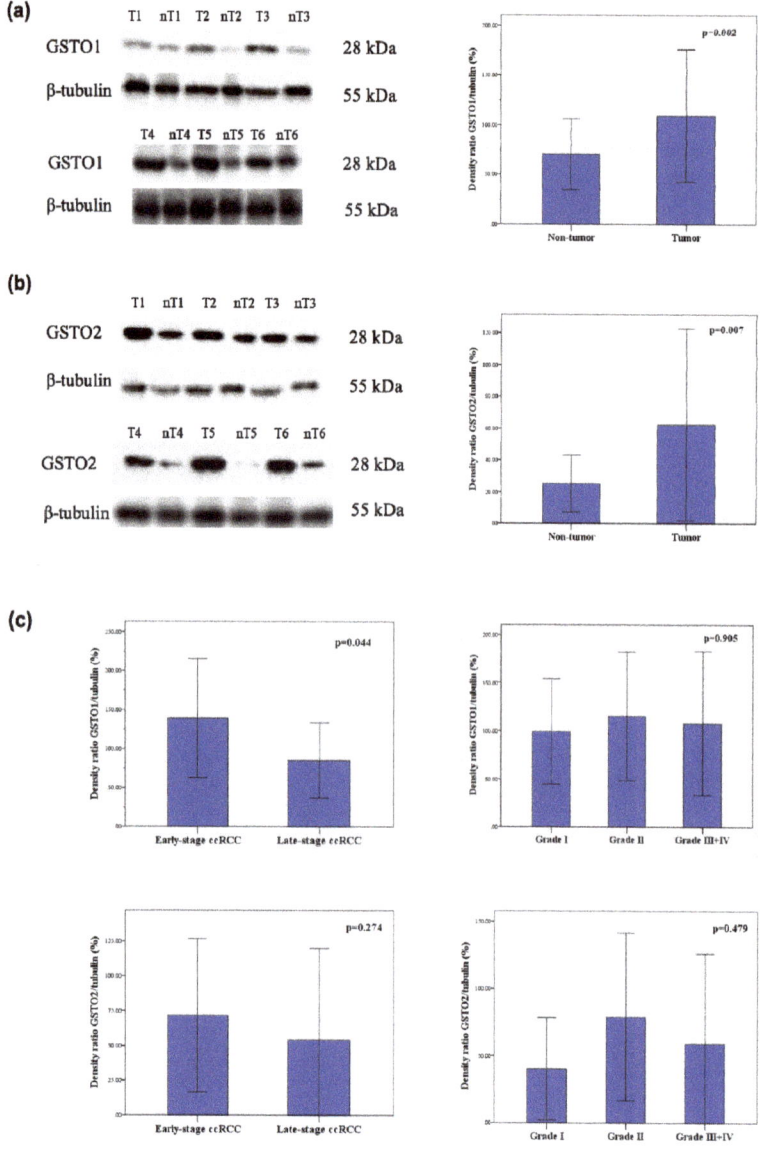

Figure 2. *Cont.*

(d)

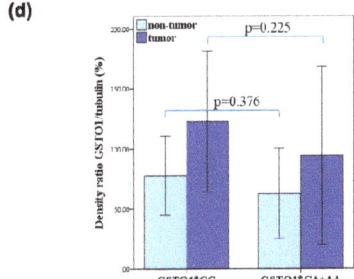 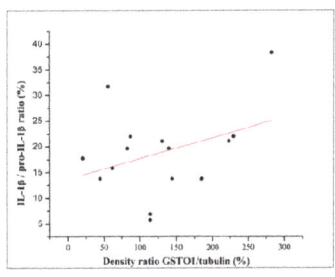

Figure 2. (**a**) Expression of GSTO1 (28 kDa) in ccRCC tumor (T) and corresponding non-tumor (nT) tissue samples; (**b**) expression of GSTO2 (28 kDa) in ccRCC tumor (T) and corresponding non-tumor (nT) tissue samples; (**c**) expression of GSTO1 and GSTO2 (28 kDa) in tumor ccRCC tissue samples according to pT stage and Fuhrman nuclear grade of ccRCC; early-stage ccRCC- pT1 and pT2; late-stage ccRCC- pT3 and pT4; (**d**) expression of GSTO1 stratified according to *GSTO1* polymorphism; correlation between GSTO1 and IL-1β/ pro-IL-1β ratio in tumor ccRCC tissue samples.

Moreover, in ccRCC samples categorized by their pT stage, statistically significant decrease of GSTO1 expression in the late-stage compared to early-stage of disease was found (p = 0.044, Figure 2c, Figure S1, Table S1). Similarly, GSTO2 expression was decreased in the late-stage compared to early-stage ccRCC, although without statistical significance (p = 0.274, Figure 2c, Figure S1, Table S1). On the contrary, no statistical significance regarding GSTO1 and GSTO2 expression was observed when stratified according to Fuhrman nuclear grade (Figure 2c). Interestingly, in tumor specimens of *GSTO1**CC wild-type genotype carriers, higher GSTO1 expression was found in comparison with those carrying at least one variant allele. However, this difference did not reach statistical significance (p = 0.225, Figure 2d, Figure S1, Table S1). Considering the role of GSTO1 in modulation of posttranslational processing of IL1-β, we determined the levels of pro-IL-1β and IL-1β in ccRCC tissue. We evaluated correlation between GSTO1 expression and IL-1β/pro-IL-1β ratio in tumor ccRCC tissue samples and observed weak positive correlation (r = 0.260, p = 0.350) (Figure 2d).

Considering the important role of PI3K/Akt/mTOR and Raf/MEK/ERK signaling pathways in ccRCC, we assessed the phosphorylation status of their downstream effectors. Downstream effectors of PI3K/Akt/mTOR pathway, targeted by the antibody cocktail used in Western blot analysis, comprise Akt1 phospho-S473 and ribosomal protein S6 (RPS6) phospho-S235/236, as well as ERK1/2 phospho-Y204/197 and ribosomal protein S6 kinase p90RSK phospho-S380 of Raf/MEK/ERK pathway. Increased expression of RSK1p90 phospho-S380 (p = 0.010), Akt1 phospho-S473 (p = 0.026) and ERK1/2 phospho-Y204/197 (p = 0.015) in tumor ccRCC compared to respective non-tumor tissue has been shown (Figure 3, Figure S1, Table S1).

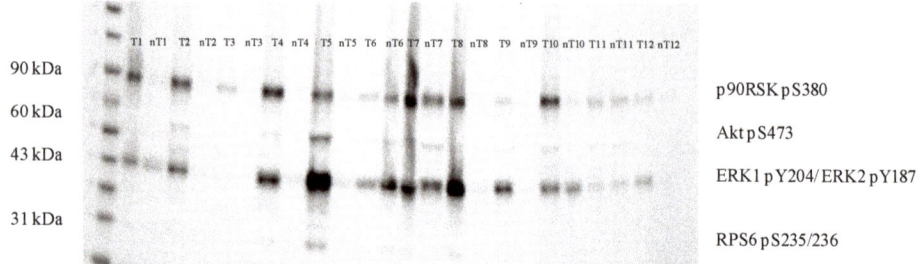

Figure 3. Phosphorylation status of downstream effectors of PI3K/Akt/mTOR and Raf/MEK/ERK signaling pathways in ccRCC tumor (T) and corresponding non-tumor (nT) tissue samples; RSK1p90-90 kDa ribosomal protein S6 kinase 1; Akt—protein kinase B; ERK—extracellular signal-regulated kinase; RPS6—ribosomal protein S6.

2.4. Immunoprecipitation of GSTO1 and Associated Proteins in Tumor ccRCC Tissue

Furthermore, we investigated potential association of GSTO1 with signaling molecules of PI3K/Akt/mTOR and Raf/MEK/ERK pathways, shown to be upregulated in ccRCC tissue (Figure 3). Western blot analysis, following protein immunoprecipitation of ccRCC tissue samples by anti-GSTO1 antibody, showed association of GSTO1 with RPS6 phospho-S235/236 and Akt phospho-S473, downstream effectors of PI3K/Akt/mTOR pathway (Figure 4, Figure S1). Interestingly, regarding downstream effectors of Raf/MEK/ERK pathway, ERK1/2 phospho-Y204/197 was not co-immunoprecipitated with GSTO1, in contrast to RSK1p90 phospho-S380. Although increased expression of ERK1/2 phospho-Y204/197 was found in tumor ccRCC tissue (Figure 3), the association of this protein with GSTO1 was not observed. Moreover, we demonstrated association of GSTO1 with Akt phospho-T308 and total Akt (panAkt) (Figure 4, Figure S1). Additionally, β-actin co-immunoprecipitated with GSTO1 (Figure 4, Figure S1) as expected considering that β-actin is the target for GSTO1-mediated deglutathionylation.

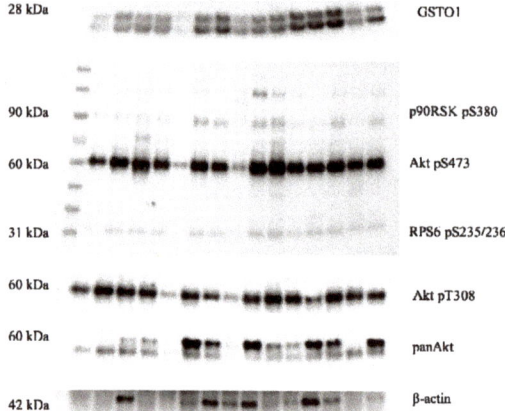

Figure 4. Immunoprecipitation of GSTO1 and associated proteins in tumor ccRCC tissue samples; RSK1p90- 90 kDa ribosomal protein S6 kinase 1; Akt—protein kinase B; RPS6—ribosomal protein S6. Their cytosolic expression was shown in Figure 3.

3. Discussion

The results of this study, for the first time, demonstrated statistically significant shorter survival in male carriers of *GSTO1**C/C wild-type genotype compared to the carriers of at least one variant allele. In addition, *GSTO1**C/C genotype independently predicted higher risk of overall mortality among male ccRCC patients when the association between different gene variants and overall mortality, adjusted by established prognostic factors, was analyzed. In ccRCC tumor tissue, in comparison with the corresponding non-tumor tissue, increased expression of both GSTO1 and GSTO2 was determined. Moreover, interaction of GSTO1 with activated downstream effectors of PI3K/Akt/mTOR and Raf/MEK/ERK pathway was shown in ccRCC tumor tissue.

Analysis of the role of investigated polymorphisms as determinants of postoperative prognosis and the risk of overall mortality in the whole group of ccRCC patients, regardless of gender, did not show a statistically significant effect. Considering that men are predominantly affected by the disease and slightly different modulating effect of risk factors in terms of gender [1], it is plausible that some mechanisms underlying ccRCC progression might also be different. Namely, in many cancers sex-biased disparities have been determined [30]. Until now, increased BMI and hypertension have been shown to increase the long-term RCC risk in men, whereas central adiposity and the waist to hip ratio were positively associated with disease risk in women [1]. Accumulating evidence also indicates that certain genes and proteins that are differentially expressed in male and female ccRCC might further influence sex-biased differences regarding tumor progression. Thus, upregulation of phosphoribosylanthranilate isomerase 1 (PAI-1), protein kinase C alpha (PKC-alpha), vascular endothelial growth factor receptor 2 (VEGFR2), androgen receptor (AR), Ras homologue gene family member J (ARHJ), insulin receptor substrate 1 (IRS1) and C-Jun activation domain-binding protein-1 (JAB1) genes was found in males with ccRCC, while increased expression of N-myc downstream regulated 1 (NDRG1), Akt, phosphatase and tensin homolog (PTEN), DJ-1, 4E binding protein 1 (4E-BP1), Src and p38 was shown in females [30]. Our results on different prognostic significance of GSTO1 polymorphism in male and female patients with ccRCC is a further proof of gender-specific molecular patterns in ccRCC. Exploring molecular mechanisms of the gender effect on cancer progression is important, especially regarding the monitoring of high risk patients. Possible underlying mechanism of prognostic significance of *GSTO1* polymorphism in male ccRCC might be the role of GSTO1 in IL-1β posttranslational processing [20]. Indeed, literature data indicate that GSTO1 might be a component of the inflammasomes, multi-protein complexes regulating the production of this pro-inflammatory cytokine [31]. Petrella and Vincenti elucidated that previously established association between high levels of IL-1β and RCC progression [32] might be explained by the stimulation of tumor cell invasion. Namely, IL-1β induces the expression of matrix metaloproteinases (MMP) through the activation of the transcription factor CCAAT enhancer binding protein β (CEBP β) [33]. Considering that GSTO1-1 activity is affected by GSTO1 allelic variant, it seems plausible that GSTO1 polymorphism might also influence activation of IL-1β. Considering recognized variance in immune response capacity of males and females, it might be hypothesized that one of molecular mechanisms involved in gender-specific survival difference observed in our study is contributing role of GSTO1-1 in inflammation [20,34].

We conducted additional investigations to elucidate the potential molecular mechanisms underlying the GSTO contribution to ccRCC progression. Additionally, to clarify the clinical meaning of *GSTO1* polymorphism, we assessed the expression of GSTO1 in relation to SNP status. Moreover, phosphorylation status of two constitutively active survival pathways in ccRCC, PI3K/Akt and MAPK/ERK, which potentiate cell growth, proliferation and invasion in cancer, were also studied [6].

Our results showed significantly higher protein expression of GSTO1 and GSTO2 in tumor ccRCC tissue compared to non-tumor tissue. We found slightly different GSTO1 expression in relation to its most investigated polymorphism, which is in concordance with the study of Mukherjee et al. investigating functional implications of GSTO1 variants [27]. Moreover, decrease of GSTO1 and GSTO2 expression in the late-stage compared to early-stage ccRCC was observed. However, the change between different stages of disease did not reach statistical significance regarding GSTO2 expression.

The GSTO1 upregulation has been reported in different cancers, including bladder [35], pancreatic, ovarian cancer [24,36] and esophageal adenocarcinoma [37]. Moreover, nuclear localization of GSTO1 in Barrett's esophagus [38] and colorectal carcinoma [39] suggests its probable involvement in the protection of specific nuclear components in conditions of oxidative stress, thus promoting malignant transformation. Unfortunately, there are no literature data on GSTO2 expression in cancer, as yet.

Significant change between early-stage and late-stage ccRCC regarding GSTO1 expression levels might be explained by complex changes of redox homeostasis throughout ccRCC progression [40]. Modification of cancer cells' metabolic phenotype enables maintenance of high ROS levels within a narrow range, allowing them to enhance growth and invasion, together with limitation of their apoptotic potential [41]. Distinctive for RCC is the shift in ratio of reduced and oxidized form of glutathione (GSH/GSSG) between early- and late-stage of disease, which is accompanied by the decrease of enzymes involved in GSH metabolism only in the early-stage RCC [40,42]. It could be speculated that GSTO1-1 affects progression of ccRCC by at least two mechanisms. Namely, higher deglutathionylase activity might increase exposure of proteins to oxidative modifications in early-stage ccRCC. Additionally, deglutathionylation seem to regulate and modulate function of the affected proteins. Considering the role of GSTO1-1 in glutathionylation cycle [22], it can be assumed that increased GSTO1-1 expression in ccRCC might be involved in regulation of redox-sensitive signaling pathways by its deglutathionylase activity. The relevance of glutathionylation status in redox signaling regulation was confirmed in investigations concerning glutaredoxins, as the major intracellular enzymes with deglutathionylase activity [22]. Numerous proteins involved in signaling (kinases and phosphatases), protein folding and stability, redox homeostasis, calcium homeostasis, energy metabolism and glycolysis, as well as cytoskeletal proteins, transcription factors and heat shock proteins are regulated via S-glutathionylation [43,44]. β-actin, heat shock protein 70, heat shock protein 7c and prolactin-inducible protein have been identified as targets for deglutathionylation by GSTO1-1 [22]. In accordance with this are our results showing co-immunoprecipitation of β-actin with GSTO1.

Furthermore, our study showed a weak correlation between IL-1β/pro- IL-1β ratio, as a degree of IL-1β activation, and the level of GSTO1 expression in ccRCC tumor tissue. It might be speculated that this result reflects the established role of GSTO1-1 in modulation of IL-1β posttranslational processing [20]. However, for the potential assessment of stronger correlation, a larger study would be warranted.

The PI3K/Akt signaling pathway, involved in the regulation of proliferation, differentiation and survival of cancer cells, is highly activated in ccRCC [45]. It has been shown that the phosphorylation of Akt at S473 (Akt1 pS473), either by mTOR or by DNA-dependent protein kinase, promotes complete enzymatic activity of Akt [46]. Numerous downstream Akt effectors implicated in ccRCC progression include the mammalian target of rapamycin (mTOR), glycogen synthase kinase 3, Bcl-2-associated death promoter, NF-κB, as well as MAPK pathways signaling molecules, c-Jun NH2-terminal kinase (JNK) and extracellular signal-regulated kinase (ERK) [45]. Furthermore, among mTOR complex 1 (mTORC1) substrates involved in promoting cellular proliferation is ribosomal protein S6 kinase (S6K1/RSK1), which phosphorylates the ribosomal protein S6 (S6/RPS6) [46]. The results of this study demonstrated the increased expression of activated downstream effectors of PI3K/Akt/mTOR and Raf/MEK/ERK pathway in ccRCC tumor tissue compared to adjacent non-tumor tissue. These results confirmed constitutive activation of two important pro-survival pathways in ccRCC.

Further investigations were focused on the possible association of GSTO1 with analyzed signaling molecules. Based on data on co-immunoprecipitation of GSTO1 with Akt and several other downstream signaling molecules we assumed that those proteins might be the targets for GSTO1-mediated deglutathionylation. Indeed, a deglutathionylation modification was implicated in the activation of Akt and RSK1, downstream effector of mTOR pathway [8,47]. The possible regulation of Akt and RSK1 activity by GSTO1-1 might be of importance in different cellular processes, including survival, growth, proliferation and metabolism [46]. Interestingly, we did not find association of GSTO1 with ERK1/2.

Since there is no evidence that ERK1/2 can be regulated by glutathionylation, further investigations would be necessary.

Several molecular targets of the PI3K/Akt signaling cascade have been suggested in antitumor therapy [45]. Regarding metastatic ccRCC, several targeted therapies against VEGF have been approved, including sorafenib, sunitinib, pazopanib and axitinib [1]. Recently, it has been shown that some of these drugs also affect cellular redox homeostasis, beside their primary antitumor role [48]. In contrast to sorafenib, which shows prooxidant effects by a decrease in GSH level [49], sunitinib exhibits antioxidant effects via increase in GSH level and inhibition of neuronal nitric oxide synthase activity (NOS) [50]. Considering influence of those targeted therapies on redox state, research concerning GSTO1 inhibitors in cancers could be valuable. Several studies suggested promising results on antitumor effect of α-chloroacetamide-1, highly specific and highly sensitive GSTO1 inhibitors [51]. Namely, KT53 initiated a significant increase in cisplatin-induced cell death in the human breast cancer cell line [51]. Additionally, another member of this class of inhibitors, C1-27 showed potent antitumor activity in colorectal cancer cell lines and in vivo models of disease [52].

Further investigations clarifying relevance of GSTO1 and GSTO2 expression pattern during ccRCC progression could be valuable. Considering the relevance of investigated signaling pathways in progression of ccRCC, future research directions could be focused on determination of GSTO1 expression in metastatic disease, as well as its potential as a therapy target. In view of interaction between GSTO1 and investigated signaling molecules involved in cell survival, it would be of great importance to investigate effect of GSTO1 specific inhibitors on signaling pathways, as well as different cell death modalities on ccRCC cell lines. Beside the results on the effect of GSTO polymorphisms on overall survival, it would be beneficial to investigate its potential association with cancer specific survival in a larger cohort. Moreover, future studies on combined effect of several different GSTO1 polymorphisms on prognosis of ccRCC patients could be valuable.

4. Materials and Methods

4.1. Study Population

In this study, 239 patients (162 men, 77 women; average age 58.94 ± 11.64 years) from the Clinic of Urology, Clinical Center of Serbia, Belgrade, diagnosed with ccRCC were enrolled to investigate the prognostic significance of GSTO polymorphisms in ccRCC. Fuhrman nuclear grade and stage of each tumor was acquired by histopathological examination, according to Srigley et al. [53] and Tumor Node Metastais classification by Sobin et al. [54]. The follow-up information was available for 228 patients (154 men, 74 women; average age 59.19 ± 11.58). Thirty tumor and corresponding non-tumor tissue samples were obtained from patients that have undergone radical nephrectomy. The study was approved by the Institutional Ethical board (13 October 2011, approval number 29/X-3, Faculty of Medicine, University of Belgrade, Serbia and 6 July 2017, approval number 29/VII-14) and performed in accordance with ethical principles of the World Medical Association Declaration of Helsinki. Informed written consent was obtained from all patients.

4.2. Sample Preparation

Genomic DNA was isolated by QIAamp DNA Blood Mini Kit (Qiagen, Hilden, Germany) from 239 blood samples according to manufacturer's instructions. Cytosolic fractions of ccRCC and adjacent non-tumor tissue specimen were obtained after homogenization in lysis buffer (50 mmol/L Tris, 200 mmol/L NaCl, 1 mmol/L dithiothreitol, pH 7.8) supplemented with protease and phosphatase inhibitors (Sigma-Aldrich, St. Louis, MO, USA) for determination of protein expression and IL-1β level.

4.3. Genotyping

Genotyping of *GSTO1**C419A (rs4925), *GSTO2**A424G (rs156697) and *GSTO2**A183G (rs2297235) polymorphisms was achieved by quantitative polymerase chain reaction (qPCR) on Mastercycler ep

4.4. Western Blot and Immunoprecipitation

Equal amounts of proteins (30 µg) from acquired ccRCC and corresponding non-tumor cytosolic fractions were subjected to SDS-PAGE on Criterion™ TGX precast 26-well gels (4–15%) (Bio-Rad, Hercules, CA, USA) followed by the transfer of proteins onto nitrocellulose membrane. Immunodetection of proteins transferred to membrane was conducted by using primary antibodies against GSTO1 (mouse polyclonal Abcam, Cambridge, UK), GSTO2 (rabbit polyclonal, GeneTex, Irvine, CA, USA), Akt (Cell Signaling, Danvers, MA, USA), phospho-Akt (T308) (rabbit monoclonal, Cell Signaling, USA) and β-tubulin (mouse monoclonal, Sigma-Aldrich, USA). Akt/MAPK Signaling Pathway Antibody Cocktail was used for simultaneous detection of phosphorylated 90kDa ribosomal protein S6 kinase 1 (RSK1p90) phospho-S380, protein kinase B (Akt) phospho-S473, extracellular-signal-regulated kinase (ERK1 phospho-Y204)/ERK2 phospho-Y187) and ribosomal protein S6 (RPS6) phospho-S235/236 (rabbit, Abcam, UK). The next step was the incubation of membranes with appropriate HRP-conjugated secondary antibodies (anti-mouse developed in goat, Abcam, Cambridge, UK; anti-rabbit developed in donkey, GE Healthcare, UK). For visualization, Clarity™ Western ECL Substrate (Bio-Rad, USA) was used, followed by detection of chemiluminescence on ChemiDoc™ MP Imaging System (Bio-Rad, USA). ImageLab software (Bio-Rad, USA) was used for densitometric analysis of obtained blots.

Immunoprecipitation was performed using Catch and Release® v2.0 High Throughput (HT) Immunoprecipitation Assay Kit (Merck Millipore, Germany). ccRCC cytosolic fractions were incubated with the antibody against GSTO1 (Abcam, UK). Immunoprecipitated proteins were subjected to electrophoresis and Western blot analysis, as previously described.

4.5. Determination of IL-1β and pro- IL-1β Levels

The quantification of interleukin-1β (IL-1β) in ccRCC cytosolic fractions was assessed by Platinum ELISA (enzyme-linked immunosorbent assay) kit (Affimetrix, eBioscience, San Diego CA, USA), whereas the quantitative detection of pro-interleukin-1β (pro-IL-1β) was performed using Human pro-IL-1β ELISA kit (Elabscience Biotechnology Inc, Houston, TX, USA) according to the manufacturer's instructions.

4.6. Statistical Analysis

Statistical analysis was performed by Statistical Package for the Social Sciences (SPSS software version 17, SPSS Inc, Chicago, IL, USA). Kaplan-Meier analysis was used to evaluate the effect of GSTO genotypes on overall survival of ccRCC patients. Survival time was estimated as time from nephrectomy to the date of death or last follow-up (1 March 2018). The follow-up information was attainable for 228 ccRCC patients owing to the loss of 11 patients' contact information. Median follow-up was 67 months, ranging from 1 to 153 months. The long-rank test was used for the evaluation of differences in survival between different genotypes of each polymorphism. The prognostic value of investigated polymorphisms in overall mortality was estimated by the Cox regression analysis, adjusted by Fuhrman nuclear grade and pT stage, as established prognostic factors.

The difference in expression of investigated proteins in tumor compared to respective non-tumor tissue was evaluated by Wilcoxon test, whereas expression of GSTO1 and GSTO2 stratified by pT stage and Fuhrman nuclear grade was analyzed using Mann–Whitney rank-sum test and Kruskal-Wallis test, respectively. The association between GSTO1 expression and IL-1β/pro-IL1β ratio was determined using Spearman's coefficient of linear correlation.

A p value of ≤ 0.05 was considered to be statistically significant.

5. Conclusions

This study demonstrated a significant prognostic role of GSTO1 polymorphism in ccRCC. Furthermore, up-regulated GSTO1-1 and GSTO2-2 enzymes in ccRCC tumor tissue might contribute to aberrant redox homeostasis. The possible molecular mechanism underlying the role of GSTO1-1 in ccRCC progression might be partially explained by its deglutathionylase activity.

Supplementary Materials: The following are available online at http://www.mdpi.com/2072-6694/11/12/2038/s1, Figure S1: Whole Western blots with molecular weights, Table S1: Densitometry readings.

Author Contributions: Conceptualization, A.S.-R., T.S. and T.R.; methodology, T.R., V.C., T.D. and S.M.; software, Z.B. and T.R.; validation, Z.B.; formal analysis, Z.B. and T.R.; investigation, T.R., V.C., T.D., N.A., M.P.-E. and M.M.; resources, D.D. and Z.D.; data curation, T.R., V.C., D.D., Z.D., S.M. and Z.B.; writing—original draft preparation, T.R., M.P.-E., T.S. and A.S.-R.; writing—review and editing, T.R., M.P.-E., T.S. and A.S.-R.; visualization, T.R., T.D., M.M. and N.A.; supervision, A.S.-R.; project administration, T.S.; funding acquisition, T.S.

Funding: This work was supported by the Grant 175052 from the Serbian Ministry of Education, Science and Technological Development.

Conflicts of Interest: The authors declare no conflict of interest.

References

1. Hsieh, J.J.; Purdue, M.P.; Signoretti, S.; Swanton, C.; Albiges, L.; Schmidinger, M.; Heng, D.Y.; Larkin, J.; Ficarra, V. Renal cell carcinoma. *Nat. Rev. Dis. Primers* **2017**, *3*, 17009. [CrossRef] [PubMed]
2. Cancer Genome Atlas Research Network. Comprehensive molecular characterization of clear cell renal cell carcinoma. *Nature* **2013**, *499*, 43–49. [CrossRef] [PubMed]
3. Hsieh, J.J.; Manley, B.J.; Khan, N.; Gao, J.; Carlo, M.I.; Cheng, E.H. Overcome tumor heterogeneity-imposed therapeutic barriers through convergent genomic biomarker discovery: A braided cancer river model of kidney cancer. *Semin. Cell Dev. Biol.* **2017**, *64*, 98–106. [CrossRef] [PubMed]
4. Mehdi, A.; Riazalhosseini, Y. Epigenome Aberrations: Emerging Driving Factors of the Clear Cell Renal Cell Carcinoma. *Int. J. Mol. Sci.* **2017**, *18*, 1774. [CrossRef]
5. Sanchez, D.J.; Simon, M.C. Genetic and metabolic hallmarks of clear cell renal cell carcinoma. *Biochim. Biophys. Acta Rev. Cancer* **2018**, *1870*, 23–31. [CrossRef]
6. Kumar, A.; Kumari, N.; Gupta, V.; Prasad, R. Renal Cell Carcinoma: Molecular Aspects. *Indian J. Clin. Biochem.* **2018**, *33*, 246–254. [CrossRef]
7. Guo, H.; German, P.; Bai, S.; Barnes, S.; Guo, W.; Qi, X.; Lou, H.; Liang, J.; Jonasch, E.; Mills, G.B.; et al. The PI3K/AKT Pathway and Renal Cell Carcinoma. *J. Genet. Genomics* **2015**, *42*, 343–353. [CrossRef]
8. Liu, X.; Jann, J.; Xavier, C.; Wu, H. Glutaredoxin 1 (Grx1) Protects Human Retinal Pigment Epithelial Cells from Oxidative Damage by Preventing AKT Glutathionylation. *Investig. Ophthalmol. Vis. Sci.* **2015**, *56*, 2821. [CrossRef]
9. Tew, K.D.; Townsend, D.M. Glutathione-s-transferases as determinants of cell survival and death. *Antioxid. Redox Signal.* **2012**, *17*, 1728–1737. [CrossRef]
10. Pljesa-Ercegovac, M.; Savic-Radojevic, A.; Matic, M.; Coric, V.; Djukic, T.; Radic, T.; Simic, T. Glutathione Transferases: Potential Targets to Overcome Chemoresistance in Solid Tumors. *Int. J. Mol. Sci.* **2018**, *19*, 3785. [CrossRef]
11. Wu, B.; Dong, D. Human cytosolic glutathione transferases: Structure, function, and drug discovery. *Trends Pharmacol. Sci.* **2012**, *33*, 656–668. [CrossRef] [PubMed]
12. Abid, A.; Ajaz, S.; Khan, A.R.; Zehra, F.; Hasan, A.S.; Sultan, G.; Mohsin, R.; Hashmi, A.; Niamatullah, N.; Rizvi, S.A.-H.; et al. Analysis of the glutathione S-transferase genes polymorphisms in the risk and prognosis of renal cell carcinomas. Case-control and meta-analysis. *Urol. Oncol. Semin. Orig. Investig.* **2016**, *34*, 419.e1–419.e12. [CrossRef] [PubMed]
13. Board, P.G.; Menon, D. Glutathione transferases, regulators of cellular metabolism and physiology. *Biochim. Biophys. Acta Gen. Subj.* **2013**, *1830*, 3267–3288. [CrossRef] [PubMed]
14. Huang, W.; Shi, H.; Hou, Q.; Mo, Z.; Xie, X. GSTM1 and GSTT1 polymorphisms contribute to renal cell carcinoma risk: Evidence from an updated meta-analysis. *Sci. Rep.* **2015**, *5*, 17971. [CrossRef]

15. De Martino, M.; Klatte, T.; Schatzl, G.; Remzi, M.; Waldert, M.; Haitel, A.; Stancik, I.; Kramer, G.; Marberger, M. Renal cell carcinoma Fuhrman grade and histological subtype correlate with complete polymorphic deletion of glutathione S-transferase M1 gene. *J. Urol.* **2010**, *183*, 878–883. [CrossRef]
16. Coric, V.M.; Simic, T.P.; Pekmezovic, T.D.; Basta-Jovanovic, G.M.; Savic-Radojevic, A.R.; Radojevic-Skodric, S.M.; Matic, M.G.; Suvakov, S.R.; Dragicevic, D.P.; Radic, T.M.; et al. GSTM1 genotype is an independent prognostic factor in clear cell renal cell carcinoma. *Urol. Oncol.* **2017**, *35*, 409–417. [CrossRef]
17. Whitbread, A.K.; Masoumi, A.; Tetlow, N.; Schmuck, E.; Coggan, M.; Board, P.G. Characterization of the Omega Class of Glutathione Transferases. In *Methods in Enzymology*; Elsevier: Amsterdam, The Netherlands, 2005; Volume 401, pp. 78–99. ISBN 978-0-12-182806-6.
18. Board, P.G.; Menon, D. Structure, function and disease relevance of Omega-class glutathione transferases. *Arch. Toxicol.* **2016**, *90*, 1049–1067. [CrossRef]
19. Dulhunty, A.; Gage, P.; Curtis, S.; Chelvanayagam, G.; Board, P. The Glutathione Transferase Structural Family Includes a Nuclear Chloride Channel and a Ryanodine Receptor Calcium Release Channel Modulator. *J. Biol. Chem.* **2001**, *276*, 3319–3323. [CrossRef]
20. Laliberte, R.E.; Perregaux, D.G.; Hoth, L.R.; Rosner, P.J.; Jordan, C.K.; Peese, K.M.; Eggler, J.F.; Dombroski, M.A.; Geoghegan, K.F.; Gabel, C.A. Glutathione S-Transferase Omega 1-1 Is a Target of Cytokine Release Inhibitory Drugs and May Be Responsible for Their Effect on Interleukin-1β Posttranslational Processing. *J. Biol. Chem.* **2003**, *278*, 16567–16578. [CrossRef]
21. Zhou, H.; Brock, J.; Liu, D.; Board, P.G.; Oakley, A.J. Structural Insights into the Dehydroascorbate Reductase Activity of Human Omega-Class Glutathione Transferases. *J. Mol. Biol.* **2012**, *420*, 190–203. [CrossRef]
22. Menon, D.; Board, P.G. A Role for Glutathione Transferase Omega 1 (GSTO1-1) in the Glutathionylation Cycle. *J. Biol. Chem.* **2013**, *288*, 25769–25779. [CrossRef] [PubMed]
23. Piaggi, S.; Raggi, C.; Corti, A.; Pitzalis, E.; Mascherpa, M.C.; Saviozzi, M.; Pompella, A.; Casini, A.F. Glutathione transferase omega 1-1 (GSTO1-1) plays an anti-apoptotic role in cell resistance to cisplatin toxicity. *Carcinogenesis* **2010**, *31*, 804–811. [CrossRef] [PubMed]
24. Yan, X.; Pan, L.; Yuan, Y.; Lang, J.; Mao, N. Identification of Platinum-Resistance Associated Proteins through Proteomic Analysis of Human Ovarian Cancer Cells and Their Platinum-Resistant Sublines. *J. Proteome Res.* **2007**, *6*, 772–780. [CrossRef] [PubMed]
25. Lu, H.; Chen, I.; Shimoda, L.A.; Park, Y.; Zhang, C.; Tran, L.; Zhang, H.; Semenza, G.L. Chemotherapy-Induced Ca^{2+} Release Stimulates Breast Cancer Stem Cell Enrichment. *Cell Rep.* **2017**, *18*, 1946–1957. [CrossRef]
26. Allen, M.; Zou, F.; Chai, H.S.; Younkin, C.S.; Miles, R.; Nair, A.A.; Crook, J.E.; Pankratz, V.S.; Carrasquillo, M.M.; Rowley, C.N.; et al. Glutathione S-transferase omega genes in Alzheimer and Parkinson disease risk, age-at-diagnosis and brain gene expression: An association study with mechanistic implications. *Mol. Neurodegener.* **2012**, *7*, 13. [CrossRef]
27. Mukherjee, B.; Salavaggione, O.E.; Pelleymounter, L.L.; Moon, I.; Eckloff, B.W.; Schaid, D.J.; Wieben, E.D.; Weinshilboum, R.M. Glutathione S-transferase omega 1 and omega 2 pharmacogenomics. *Drug Metab. Dispos.* **2006**, *34*, 1237–1246. [CrossRef]
28. Djukic, T.I.; Savic-Radojevic, A.R.; Pekmezovic, T.D.; Matic, M.G.; Pljesa-Ercegovac, M.S.; Coric, V.M.; Radic, T.M.; Suvakov, S.R.; Krivic, B.N.; Dragicevic, D.P.; et al. Glutathione S-transferase T1, O1 and O2 polymorphisms are associated with survival in muscle invasive bladder cancer patients. *PLoS ONE* **2013**, *8*, e74724. [CrossRef]
29. Radic, T.M.; Coric, V.M.; Pljesa-Ercegovac, M.S.; Basta-Jovanovic, G.M.; Radojevic-Skodric, S.M.; Dragicevic, D.P.; Matic, M.G.; Bogdanovic, L.M.; Dzamic, Z.M.; Simic, T.P.; et al. Concomitance of Polymorphisms in Glutathione Transferase Omega Genes Is Associated with Risk of Clear Cell Renal Cell Carcinoma. *Tohoku J. Exp. Med.* **2018**, *246*, 35–44. [CrossRef]
30. Shin, J.Y.; Jung, H.J.; Moon, A. Molecular Markers in Sex Differences in Cancer. *Toxicol. Res.* **2019**, *35*, 331–341. [CrossRef]
31. Coll, R.C.; O'Neill, L.A.J. The Cytokine Release Inhibitory Drug CRID3 Targets ASC Oligomerisation in the NLRP3 and AIM2 Inflammasomes. *PLoS ONE* **2011**, *6*, e29539. [CrossRef]
32. Yoshida, N.; Ikemoto, S.; Narita, K.; Sugimura, K.; Wada, S.; Yasumoto, R.; Kishimoto, T.; Nakatani, T. Interleukin-6, tumour necrosis factor α and interleukin-1β in patients with renal cell carcinoma. *Br. J. Cancer* **2002**, *86*, 1396–1400. [CrossRef] [PubMed]

33. Petrella, B.L.; Vincenti, M.P. Interleukin-1β mediates metalloproteinase-dependent renal cell carcinoma tumor cell invasion through the activation of CCAAT enhancer binding protein β. *Cancer Med.* **2012**, *1*, 17–27. [CrossRef] [PubMed]
34. Dorak, M.T.; Karpuzoglu, E. Gender Differences in Cancer Susceptibility: An Inadequately Addressed Issue. *Front. Genet.* **2012**, *3*, 268. [CrossRef] [PubMed]
35. Djukic, T.; Simic, T.; Pljesa-Ercegovac, M.; Matic, M.; Suvakov, S.; Coric, V.; Dragicevic, D.; Savic-Radojevic, A. Upregulated glutathione transferase omega-1 correlates with progression of urinary bladder carcinoma. *Redox Rep.* **2017**, *22*, 486–492. [CrossRef] [PubMed]
36. Urzúa, U.; Roby, K.F.; Gangi, L.M.; Cherry, J.M.; Powell, J.I.; Munroe, D.J. Transcriptomic analysis of an in vitro murine model of ovarian carcinoma: Functional similarity to the human disease and identification of prospective tumoral markers and targets. *J. Cell. Physiol.* **2006**, *206*, 594–602. [CrossRef]
37. Li, Y.; Zhang, Q.; Peng, B.; Shao, Q.; Qian, W.; Zhang, J.-Y. Identification of glutathione S-transferase omega 1 (GSTO1) protein as a novel tumor-associated antigen and its autoantibody in human esophageal squamous cell carcinoma. *Tumor Biol.* **2014**, *35*, 10871–10877. [CrossRef]
38. Piaggi, S.; Marchi, S.; Ciancia, E.; DeBortoli, N.; Lazzarotti, A.; Saviozzi, M.; Raggi, C.; Fierabracci, V.; Visvikis, A.; Bisgaard, H.C.; et al. Nuclear translocation of glutathione transferase omega is a progression marker in Barrett's esophagus. *Oncol. Rep.* **2009**, *21*, 283–287. [CrossRef]
39. Lombardi, S.; Fuoco, I.; Di Fluri, G.; Costa, F.; Ricchiuti, A.; Biondi, G.; Nardini, V.; Scarpato, R. Genomic instability and cellular stress in organ biopsies and peripheral blood lymphocytes from patients with colorectal cancer and predisposing pathologies. *Oncotarget* **2015**, *6*, 14852–14864. [CrossRef]
40. Lusini, L.; Tripodi, S.A.; Rossi, R.; Giannerini, F.; Giustarini, D.; Del Vecchio, M.T.; Barbanti, G.; Cintorino, M.; Tosi, P.; Di Simplicio, P. Altered glutathione anti-oxidant metabolism during tumor progression in human renal-cell carcinoma. *Int. J. Cancer* **2001**, *91*, 55–59. [CrossRef]
41. Rodic, S.; Vincent, M.D. Reactive oxygen species (ROS) are a key determinant of cancer's metabolic phenotype: ROS are a key determinant of cancer's metabolic phenotype. *Int. J. Cancer* **2018**, *142*, 440–448. [CrossRef]
42. Pljesa-Ercegovac, M.; Mimic-Oka, J.; Dragicevic, D.; Savic-Radojevic, A.; Opacic, M.; Pljesa, S.; Radosavljevic, R.; Simic, T. Altered antioxidant capacity in human renal cell carcinoma: Role of glutathione associated enzymes. *Urol. Oncol.* **2008**, *26*, 175–181. [CrossRef] [PubMed]
43. Zhang, J.; Ye, Z.; Singh, S.; Townsend, D.M.; Tew, K.D. An evolving understanding of the S-glutathionylation cycle in pathways of redox regulation. *Free Radic. Biol. Med.* **2018**, *120*, 204–216. [CrossRef] [PubMed]
44. Scirè, A.; Cianfruglia, L.; Minnelli, C.; Bartolini, D.; Torquato, P.; Principato, G.; Galli, F.; Armeni, T. Glutathione compartmentalization and its role in glutathionylation and other regulatory processes of cellular pathways. *BioFactors* **2019**, *45*, 152–168. [CrossRef] [PubMed]
45. Wu, F.; Wu, S.; Tong, H.; He, W.; Gou, X. HOXA6 inhibits cell proliferation and induces apoptosis by suppressing the PI3K/Akt signaling pathway in clear cell renal cell carcinoma. *Int. J. Oncol.* **2019**, *54*, 2095–2105. [CrossRef]
46. Hemmings, B.A.; Restuccia, D.F. PI3K-PKB/Akt Pathway. *Cold Spring Harb. Perspect. Biol.* **2012**, *4*, a011189. [CrossRef]
47. Takata, T.; Tsuchiya, Y.; Watanabe, Y. 90-kDa ribosomal S6 kinase 1 is inhibited by S-glutathionylation of its active-site cysteine residue during oxidative stress. *FEBS Lett.* **2013**, *587*, 1681–1686. [CrossRef]
48. Teppo, H.-R.; Soini, Y.; Karihtala, P. Reactive Oxygen Species-Mediated Mechanisms of Action of Targeted Cancer Therapy. *Oxid. Med. Cell. Longev.* **2017**, *2017*, 1485283. [CrossRef]
49. Chiou, J.-F.; Tai, C.-J.; Wang, Y.-H.; Liu, T.-Z.; Jen, Y.-M.; Shiau, C.-Y. Sorafenib induces preferential apoptotic killing of a drug- and radio-resistant hep G2 cells through a mitochondria-dependent oxidative stress mechanism. *Cancer Biol. Ther.* **2009**, *8*, 1904–1913. [CrossRef]
50. Cui, W.; Zhang, Z.-J.; Hu, S.-Q.; Mak, S.-H.; Xu, D.-P.; Choi, C.-L.; Wang, Y.-Q.; Tsim, W.-K.; Lee, M.-Y.; Rong, J.-H.; et al. Sunitinib Produces Neuroprotective Effect Via Inhibiting Nitric Oxide Overproduction. *CNS Neurosci. Ther.* **2014**, *20*, 244–252. [CrossRef]
51. Tsuboi, K.; Bachovchin, D.A.; Speers, A.E.; Spicer, T.P.; Fernandez-Vega, V.; Hodder, P.; Rosen, H.; Cravatt, B.F. Potent and Selective Inhibitors of Glutathione S-transferase Omega 1 that Impair Cancer Drug Resistance. *J. Am. Chem. Soc.* **2011**, *133*, 16605–16616. [CrossRef]

52. Ramkumar, K.; Samanta, S.; Kyani, A.; Yang, S.; Tamura, S.; Ziemke, E.; Stuckey, J.A.; Li, S.; Chinnaswamy, K.; Otake, H.; et al. Mechanistic evaluation and transcriptional signature of a glutathione S-transferase omega 1 inhibitor. *Nat. Commun.* **2016**, *7*, 13084. [CrossRef] [PubMed]
53. Srigley, J.R.; Delahunt, B.; Eble, J.N.; Egevad, L.; Epstein, J.I.; Grignon, D.; Hes, O.; Moch, H.; Montironi, R.; Tickoo, S.K.; et al. The International Society of Urological Pathology (ISUP) Vancouver Classification of Renal Neoplasia. *Am. J. Surg. Pathol.* **2013**, *37*, 1469–1489. [CrossRef] [PubMed]
54. Sobin, L.H.; Gospodarowicz, M.K.; Wittekind, C.; International Union against Cancer (Eds.) *TNM Classification of Malignant Tumours*, 7th ed.; Wiley-Blackwell: Chichester, UK; Hoboken, NJ, USA, 2010; ISBN 978-1-4443-3241-4.

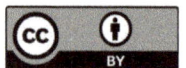

© 2019 by the authors. Licensee MDPI, Basel, Switzerland. This article is an open access article distributed under the terms and conditions of the Creative Commons Attribution (CC BY) license (http://creativecommons.org/licenses/by/4.0/).

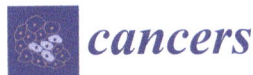

Article

MTA2 as a Potential Biomarker and Its Involvement in Metastatic Progression of Human Renal Cancer by miR-133b Targeting MMP-9

Yong-Syuan Chen [1,†], Tung-Wei Hung [2,3,†], Shih-Chi Su [4,5,†], Chia-Liang Lin [1], Shun-Fa Yang [6], Chu-Che Lee [7], Chang-Fang Yeh [1], Yi-Hsien Hsieh [1,8,9,*] and Jen-Pi Tsai [10,11,*]

1. Institute of Biochemistry, Microbiology and Immunology, Chung Shan Medical University, Taichung 40201, Taiwan; kevin810647@gmail.com (Y.-S.C.); hiking003@hotmail.com (C.-L.L.); yehchangfang@yahoo.com.tw (C.-F.Y.)
2. Division of Nephrology, Department of Medicine, Chung Shan Medical University Hospital, Taichung 40201, Taiwan; a6152000@ms34.hinet.net
3. School of Medicine, Chung Shan Medical University, Taichung 40201, Taiwan
4. Whole-Genome Research Core Laboratory of Human Diseases, Chang Gung Memorial Hospital, Keelung 20401, Taiwan; ssu1@cgmh.org.tw
5. Department of Dermatology, Drug Hypersensitivity Clinical and Research Center, Chang Gung Memorial Hospital, Linkou 24451, Taiwan
6. Institute of Medicine, Chung Shan Medical University, Taichung 40201, Taiwan; ysf@csmu.edu.tw
7. Department of Medicine Research, Buddhist Dalin Tzu Chi Hospital, Chiayi 62247, Taiwan; dm731849@tzuchi.com.tw
8. Department of Biochemistry, School of Medicine, Chung Shan Medical University, Taichung 40201, Taiwan
9. Clinical laboratory, Chung Shan Medical University Hospital, Taichung 40201, Taiwan
10. School of Medicine, Tzu Chi University, Hualien 97010, Taiwan
11. Division of Nephrology, Department of Internal Medicine, Dalin Tzu Chi Hospital, Buddhist Tzu Chi Medical Foundation, Chiayi 62247, Taiwan
* Correspondence: hyhsien@csmu.edu.tw (Y.-H.H.); tsaininimd1491@gmail.com (J.-P.T.); Tel.: +886-0424730022 (Y.-H.H.); +886-052648000 (J.-P.T.)
† These authors contributed equally to this work.

Received: 27 October 2019; Accepted: 21 November 2019; Published: 23 November 2019

Abstract: Metastasis-associated protein 2 (MTA2) was previously known as a requirement to maintain malignant potentials in several human cancers. However, the role of MTA2 in the progression of renal cell carcinoma (RCC) has not yet been delineated. In this study, MTA2 expression was significantly increased in RCC tissues and cell lines. Increased MTA2 expression was significantly associated with tumour grade ($p = 0.002$) and was an independent prognostic factor for overall survival with a high RCC tumour grade. MTA2 knockdown inhibited the migration, invasion, and in vivo metastasis of RCC cells without effects on cell proliferation. Regarding molecular mechanisms, MTA2 knockdown reduced the activity, protein level, and mRNA expression of matrix metalloproteinase-9 (MMP-9) in RCC cells. Further analyses demonstrated that patients with lower miR-133b expression had poorer survival rates than those with higher expression from The Cancer Genome Atlas database. Moreover, miR-133b modulated the 3'untranslated region (UTR) of MMP-9 promoter activities and subsequently the migratory and invasive abilities of these dysregulated expressions of MTA2 in RCC cells. The inhibition of MTA2 could contribute to human RCC metastasis by regulating the expression of miR-133b targeting MMP-9 expression.

Keywords: renal cell carcinoma; metastasis; MTA2; MMP-9; miR-133b

1. Introduction

Renal cell carcinoma (RCC), which accounts for more than 90% of new cases of kidney cancer, is the most lethal genitourinary cancer, with limited median survival time and overall survival when advanced or distant metastasis occurs [1,2]. According to molecular medicine, genetics and clinical response help to determine the cell type of RCC [3,4], and clear cell RCC (ccRCC) are the most common subtypes and account for the highest RCC mortality and incidence rates [5]. In recent years, tyrosine kinase inhibitors (TKI) towards the vascular endothelial growth factor (VEGF), the mammalian target of rapamycin (mTOR) inhibitor, clustered, regularly interspaced short palindromic repeats-Cas9 (CRISPR-Cas9), small molecule inhibitors, and immune checkpoint inhibitors have had promising clinical outcomes against advanced RCC [6–9]. Reports have shown that using adjuvant sunitinib in high-risk RCC patients after nephrectomy resulted in median disease-free survival [10]. Therefore, the development of potential and novel molecular targets for treating advanced or metastatic RCC has currently become a critical topic. Metastasis-associated protein 2 (MTA2) is a central component of the Mi-2/nucleosome remodeling and deacetylase (NuRD) complex and precisely controls cytoskeleton reorganisation at the transcriptional level; moreover, it is closely associated with tumour progression and metastasis [11]. MTA2 overexpression has been observed in several human cancers and is associated with tumour invasion capacity, metastasis, and poor prognosis [12]. In gastric cancer, MTA2 can be transcriptionally regulated by specificity protein 1 (Sp1), and MTA2 expression is closely related to tumour invasion, lymph node metastasis, and Tumor-Node-Metastasis (TNM) staging [13]. MTA2 is expressed in aggressive lung cancer, and its increased expression is correlated with poor prognosis [14]. In estrogen receptor-alpha–negative breast cancer, MTA2 expression is associated with poor prognosis and enhanced metastasis in vitro and in vivo through Rho pathway activation [15].

A family of zinc-dependent endopeptidases with matrix metalloproteinases (MMPs) are the most critical to targeting various extracellular matrix (ECM) or basement membrane components [16]. Malignant cells can destroy the intercellular connection, lyse the ECM, breach the basement membrane, invade the vasculature, and exhibit distant metastasis because of dysregulated MMP activity [17]. For example, studies on RCC have demonstrated that increased expression of matrix metalloproteinase-9 (MMP-9) or phosphorylated extracellular signal-regulated kinase (ERK) correspond to RCC severity, which is correlated with tumour size, TMN stage, invasion, distant metastasis, and cancer-specific survival [18,19]. Combination therapy and drug synergism for targeted glioma improved the antitumor activity of individual treatment approaches [20,21]. Dr. Tabouret et al., found that MMP2 and MMP9 can be used as biomarkers in predicting bevacizumab activity in high-grade glioma patients [22].

MicroRNAs (miRNA) are short noncoding RNAs containing 19–23 nucleotides. By binding partial sequence homology to the three prime untranslated region (3'-UTR) of target mRNAs, miRNAs can regulate gene expression at the posttranscriptional level and cause translational inhibition and mRNA degradation [23]. miR-133b belongs to a miRNA family which includes other miRNAs, such as miR-133a. Studies have indicated that miR-133b can regulate oncogenic transcripts of gastric, esophageal, or breast cancer by targeting Fascin Actin-Bundling Protein 1(FSCIN1)/Sp1 [24,25], the epidermal growth factor receptor (EGFR) [26] and SRY-Box Transcription Factor 9 (SOX9) [27], respectively. Moreover, aberrant miR-133b expression plays a role in RCC development by suppressing cell proliferation and migratory and invasive abilities by modulating MMP-9 expression [28], but the molecular mechanism of MTA2 regulating miR-133b involvement in RCC metastasis has not yet been elucidated. To the best of our knowledge, the potential modulation the progression roles of MTA2 and miR-133b in RCC remain unclear. This study investigates the clinicopathological implications of MTA2 and miR-133b by analysing RCC tissue data and examining the pathophysiological functions and underlying mechanisms of MTA2 regulation of miR-133b on human RCC cell progression.

2. Results

2.1. Expression and Effects of MTA2 in Human RCC and RCC Cells

MTA2 expression was examined through immunohistochemical (IHC) staining using a human kidney clear cell carcinoma tissue array procedure. As the tumour grade became severe, MTA2 expression was enhanced (Figure 1A). After staining, the correlation between MTA2 expression and clinicopathological parameters was analysed using data from 99 patients with RCC (Table 1). Patients diagnosed with grade 2 or 3 cancer had a significantly higher percentage of MTA2 expression compared with those diagnosed with grade 1 ($p = 0.002$). However, no significant association was observed between MTA2 expression and other parameters, such as tumour stage, age, or gender (Table 1). By using The Cancer Genome Atlas (TCGA) database, we observed higher mRNA expression of MTA2 in tumour tissues than in normal tissues (Figure 1B) and in higher tumour grades than in lower grades (Figure 1C). We further examined whether MTA2 expression was correlated with the postoperative survival of patients with RCC by using Kaplan–Meier survival analyses. Patients with RCC who had high MTA2 expression had a significantly lower survival rate compared with those with low MTA2 expression ($p = 0.014$, Figure 1D). Therefore, MTA2 expression level can serve as an independent prognostic factor for patients with RCC. Furthermore, western blot analysis and reverse transcription polymerase chain reactions (RT-PCR) were conducted to detect MTA2 expression in four RCC cell lines (A498, 786-O, Caki-1, and ACHN) and normal renal tubular cells (HK2 cells). RCC cell lines had a relatively high protein and mRNA expression of MTA2 compared with HK2 cells, (Figure 1E,F) indicating that the overexpression of MTA2 is involved in RCC.

Table 1. Correlation between metastasis-associated protein 2 (MTA2) expression and clinicopathological characteristics of renal cancer patients.

Characteristic	Number of Patients (%)		p Value
	MTA2 Staining		
	Negative	Positive	
Total Number of Patients	40 (40.4)	59 (59.5)	–
Age (Year)			
<59	20 (31.3)	26 (68.7)	0.580
≥59	20 (32.1)	33 (67.9)	
Gender			
Male	13 (43.3)	17 (56.7)	0.347
Female	27 (39.1)	42 (60.9)	
Tumor Grade			
1	29 (54.7)	24 (45.3)	0.002
2 + 3	11 (23.9)	35 (76.1)	
Tumor Stage			
I	27 (36.5)	47 (63.5)	0.129
II + III	2 (10)	18 (90)	

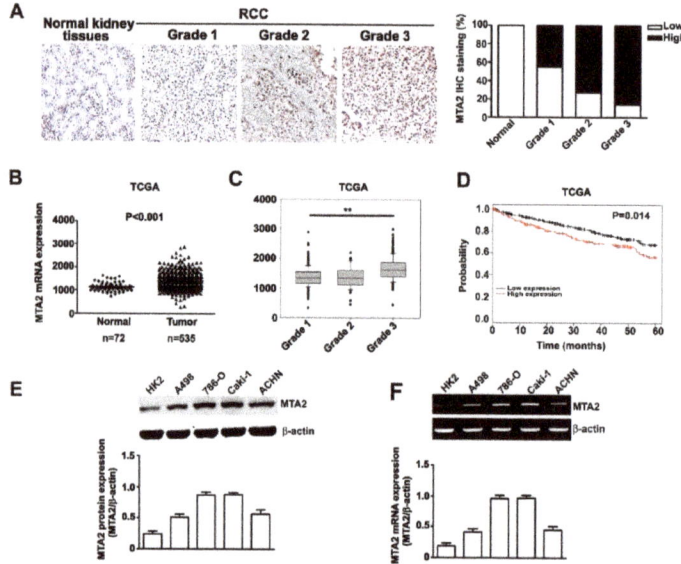

Figure 1. Expression and effects of metastasis-associated protein 2 (MTA2) in human renal cell carcinoma (RCC) and RCC cells. (**A**) Intensity of MTA2 expression in RCC grade 1, 2, and 3 and normal kidney tissues by using immunohistochemistry staining (×40). (**B**) MTA2 mRNA expression of RCC and normal tissue from The Cancer Genome Atlas (TCGA) datasets. (**C**) MTA2 mRNA expression in patients with RCC grade 1, 2, and 3. (**D**) Kaplan–Meier curve for overall survival of patients, categorised by low and high MTA2 expression. (**E**) Total lysates from HK2, A498, 786-O, Caki-1, and ACHN cells were isolated and analysed using western blotting to detect the individual expression of MTA2; β-actin was used as an internal control. (**F**) A reverse transcription polymerase chain reaction assay was applied to detect MTA2 mRNA expression. β-actin was used as an internal control for mRNA equal loading. Values are expressed as the mean ± SE of three independent experiments. ** $p < 0.01$ compared with normal kidney tissues.

2.2. Effect of MTA2 Knockdown on RCC Cell Proliferation

We examined the biological function of MTA2 in RCC cells by using a short hairpin RNA (shRNA) assay. MTA2 knockdown (shMTA2) inhibited MTA2 expression in three cell lines compared with short hairpin Luc (shLuc) cells in western blot analysis (Figure 2A). To further explore the influence of MTA2 on cell proliferation, we determined whether MTA2 knockdown had a cytotoxic effect on RCC cells using an (3-(4,5-Dimethylthiazol-2-yl)-2,5-diphenyltetrazolium bromide; MTT) MTT assay. We observed no difference in cell viability between shMTA2–RCC and shLuc–RCC cells (Figure 2B). Moreover, no differences in cell cycle distribution between shMTA2–RCC and shLuc–RCC cells were detected in the flow cytometry analysis (Figure 2C). Hence, MTA2 knockdown did not affect the proliferation of RCC cells.

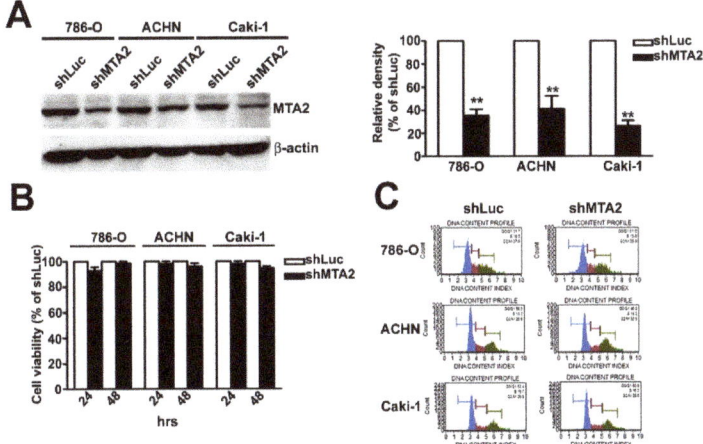

Figure 2. Metastasis-associated protein 2 (MTA2) knockdown did not influence viability or proliferation of renal cell carcinoma (RCC) cells. (**A**) MTA2 knockdown expression in shLuc or shMTA2 of 786-O, ACHN, and Caki-1 cells was verified using western blotting. (**B**) Cell viability of shLuc or shMTA2-786-O, ACHN, and Caki-1 cells was evaluated using an MTT assay after 24 and 48 h. (**C**) Flow cytometry analysis of shLuc–or shMTA2–786-O, ACHN, and Caki-1 cells. β-Actin was used as an internal control for protein equal loading. Values are expressed as the mean ± SE of three independent experiments. ** $p < 0.01$ compared with shLuc cells.

2.3. Effect of MTA2 Knockdown on RCC Cell Metastasis in Vitro and in Vivo

After MTA2 knockdown, RCC cells (786-O, Caki-1, and ACHN) exhibited significantly reduced MTA2 expression using western blot analysis (Figure 3A). The quantification analysis demonstrated that migratory and invasive abilities were markedly reduced in shMTA2–RCC cells compared with shLuc–RCC cells (Figure 3B). To examine the effects of MTA2 on the distant metastasis abilities of RCC in vivo, we injected shLuc– and shMTA2–786-O or Caki-1 cells into the tail vein of mice. The growth of tumours stained with hematoxylin and eosin (H&E) and the expression of Ki-67 in the shMTA2 groups by using IHC assay were markedly lower than those observed in the shLuc groups (Figure 3C). Lung nodules were counted after sacrificing these mice, and markedly fewer nodules were observed in the shMTA2–786-O and shMTA2–Caki-1 cells than in shLuc–786-O and shLuc–Caki-1 cells (Figure 3D). Thus, MTA2 played a central role in regulating distant metastasis in RCC.

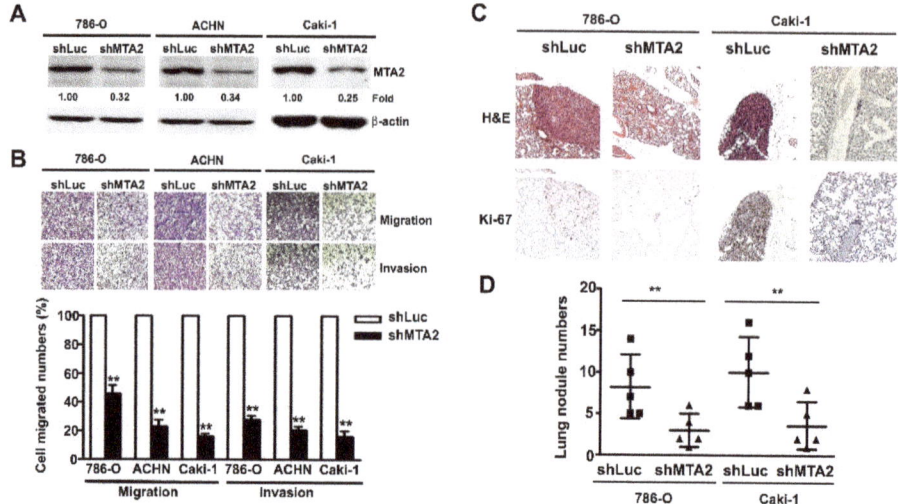

Figure 3. Metastasis-associated protein 2 (MTA2) knockdown inhibited migration and invasion of renal cell carcinoma cells and suppressed tumour metastasis in vivo. (**A**) MTA2 knockdown expression in 786-O, ACHN, and Caki-1 cells was verified using western blotting. (**B**) The migration and invasion abilities of shLuc and shMTA2-786-O, -ACHN, and –Caki-1 cells were determined using migration and Matrigel invasion assay. Cells in the lower surface of the Borden chamber were stained and photographed under a light microscope. The quantification of migrated cells are presented as a histogram. (**C**) Representative images of hematoxylin and eosin staining and Ki-67 expression in the shLuc and shMTA2 groups of 786-O and Caki-1 cells. (**D**) Considerably fewer metastatic lung colonies were observed in the shMTA2 group than in the shLuc group of 786-O and Caki-1 cells. Values are expressed as the mean ± standard error (SE) of three independent experiments. ** $p < 0.01$ compared with the shLuc cells.

2.4. Effect of MTA2 Knockdown on MMP-9 Expression in RCC Cells

To identify the molecular mechanism of MTA2 in the invasive behaviour of RCC, western blot analysis, quantitative reverse transcription-polymerase chain reaction (qRT-PCR) assay, and gelatin zymography demonstrated that MTA2 knockdown significantly decreased the protein, mRNA, and activity expression of MMP-9 in 786-O, Caki-1, and ACHN cells, but was not involved in MMP-2 (Figure 4A–C). The immunofluorescence assay results were similar (Figure 4D). Regarding the function of MTA2, we found that overexpressed MTA2 in HK2 cells was increased the protein and mRNA of MTA2 and MMP-9, compared with Neo-HK2 cells (Supplemental Figure S1A, S1B). Furthermore, migratory and invasive capacity in MTA2-overexpressing HK2 cells was significantly higher than that in Neo-HK2 cells (Supplemental Figure S1C). In addition, Kaplan–Meier survival and log rank analyses suggested that patients with RCC and high MMP-9 expression had lower survival rates compared with those with low MMP-9 expression ($p < 0.001$, Figure 4E). MMP-9 expression was also positively correlated with MTA2 expression in patients with RCC ($p < 0.001$, Figure 4F). Therefore, MTA2 played a main role in migration and invasion of RCC cells by inhibiting MMP-9 expression.

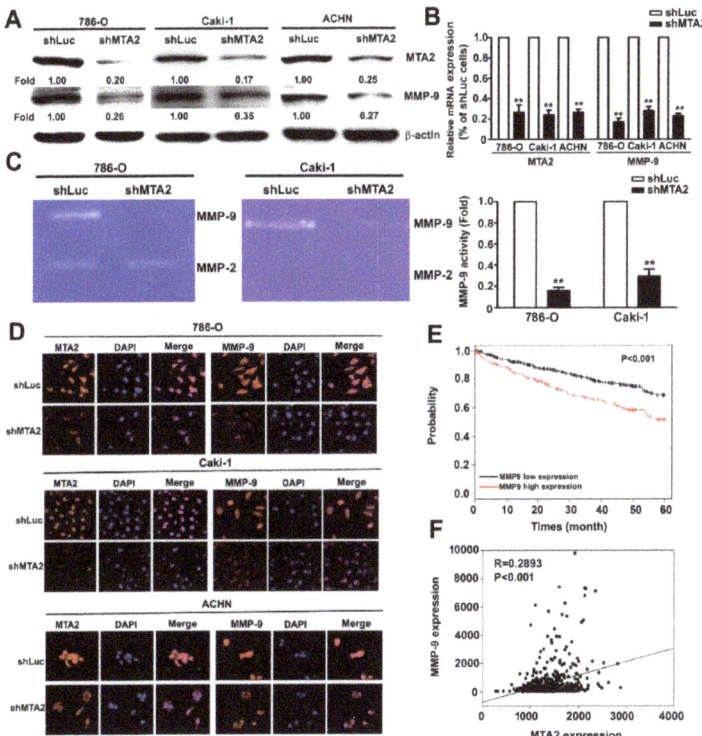

Figure 4. Metastasis-associated protein 2 (MTA2) knockdown inhibited the activity, expression, and mRNA levels of matrix metalloproteinase-9 (MMP-9) in renal cell carcinoma cells. (**A**, **B**) Total lysates and mRNA from shLuc– or shMTA2–786-O, Caki-1, and ACHN cells were isolated and analysed using western blotting and quantitative reverse transcription polymerase chain reaction assay to detect individual expression of MTA2 and MMP-9. β-Actin and GAPDH were used as internal controls. (**C**) Conditioned media were collected, and MMP-2 and MMP-9 activities were measured using gelatin zymography and quantified through densitometry. (**D**) shLuc- and shMTA2-786-O, -Caki-1, and -ACHN cells were stained with anti-MTA2 and anti-MMP-9 antibodies by using immunofluorescence staining, and cell nuclei (blue) were counterstained using 4′,6-diamidino-2-phenylindole (DAPI) reagent. (**E**) The Cancer Genome Atlas (TCGA) datasets was used to create the Kaplan–Meier curve portraying the overall survival of patients based on low or high MMP-9 expression. (**F**) Linear trend of the correlation between MTA2 and MMP-9 illustrated using the TCGA datasets. Values are expressed as the mean ± SE of three independent experiments. ** $p < 0.01$ compared with shLuc cells.

2.5. MMP-9 as the Target Gene of miR-133b and Association with Poor RCC Prognosis.

miR-133b target sites on the 3′-UTR regions of MMP-9 were identified using TargetScan, miRcode, and miRbase analytical programmes (Figure 5A). The MMP-9 3′-UTR promoter contained an miR-133b target sequence (Figure 5B). The quantitative polymerase chain reaction (qPCR) assay revealed a lower level of miR-133b in three RCC cells (786-O, Caki-1, A-498, and ACHN) than in HK2 cells (Figure 5C). In addition, miR-133b expression was increased in three shMTA2–RCC cells compared with in shLuc–RCC cells (Figure 5D). Using the TCGA database, we observed higher miR-133b expression in normal tissues compared with that in tumour tissues (Figure 5E). Kaplan–Meier survival analyses revealed that patients with RCC and low miR-133b expression had lower survival rates compared with those with high expression ($p = 0.0024$, Figure 5F). In summary, miR-133b could play a role in RCC development by regulating MMP-9 expression.

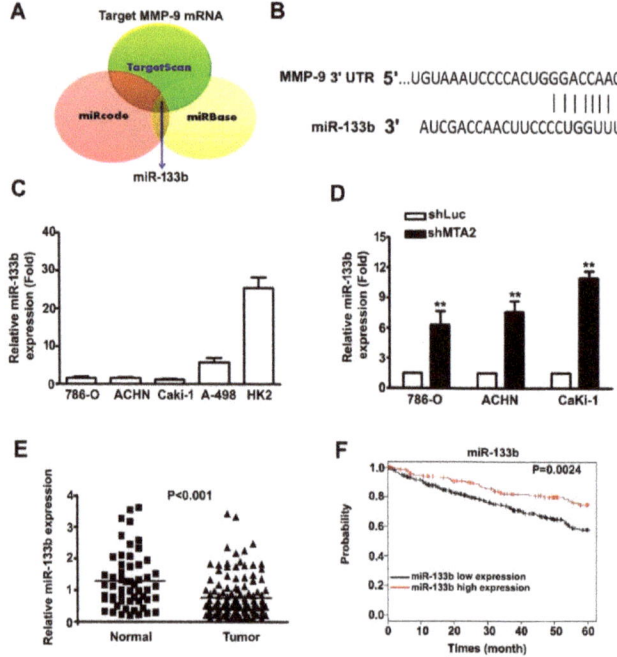

Figure 5. MMP-9 is the target for miR-133b and associated with poor renal cell carcinoma (RCC) prognosis. (**A**) Schematic of the proposed model depicting miR-133b targeting MMP-9 mRNA from three prediction datasets (TargetScan, miRcode, and miRBase). (**B**) Schematic of the predicted binding site of miR-133b at the 3′-UTR of MMP-9 promoter. (**C**) miR-133b expression in four RCC cells and normal kidney HK2 cells was measured using quantitative polymerase chain reaction (qPCR) assay. (**D**) miR-133b expression was detected in shLuc and shMTA2-RCC cells using qPCR. (**E**) miR-133b expression in tumour and normal tissues from The Cancer Genome Atlas RCC datasets. (**F**) Kaplan–Meier curve for the overall survival of patients with RCC categorised by low and high miR-133b expression. ** $p < 0.01$ compared with shLuc cells.

2.6. Effect of miR-133b on MMP-9 Expression Involved in Knockdown MTA2-Inhibiting RCC Cell Metastasis

To clarify the regulatory effects of miR-133b on RCC metastasis progression, we attempted to validate whether miR-133b could regulate the effects of MTA2 on modulating MMP-9 expression and metastasis ability in RCC cells. RT-qPCR, luciferase reporter assay, and western blotting were performed. Increased miR-133b expression in shMTA2 and shMTA2-NC-RCC cells that were treated with miR-133b antagomir significantly inhibited miR-133b expression in shMTA2-RCC cells (Figure 6A). In addition, shMTA2–RCC cells expressed lower MMP-9 3′-UTR promoter activity than shLuc–RCC cells. Treatment with miR-133b antagomir significantly inhibited miR-133b expression and reversed MMP-9 3′-UTR promoter activity induced by shMTA2 compared with those in shMTA2-NC cells (Figure 6B). Similar results were achieved with western blotting (Figure 6C). Moreover, transfection with miR-133b antagomir significantly increased migratory and invasive abilities in shMTA2–RCC cells compared with those in shMTA2-NC cells (Figure 6D). To further confirm the tumour-suppressing role of miR-133b, we transfected NC- or antagomir-133b into HK2 cells, which exhibited relatively high miR-133b expression among RCC cells. A western blotting assay revealed a significantly higher MMP-9 expression in antagomir-133b–transfected HK2 cells than in NC-transfected cells (Supplementary Figure S2A) and inhibition of endogenous miR-133b expression by using RT-qPCR assay (Supplementary Figure S2B). The in vitro migration and invasion assays suggested an increase in the migration and invasion ability of antagomir-133b-transfected HK2 cells compared with that of NC-transfected cells

(Supplementary Figure S2C). These studies indicated that MTA2 can affect RCC metastasis through miR-133b targeting of MMP-9 expression.

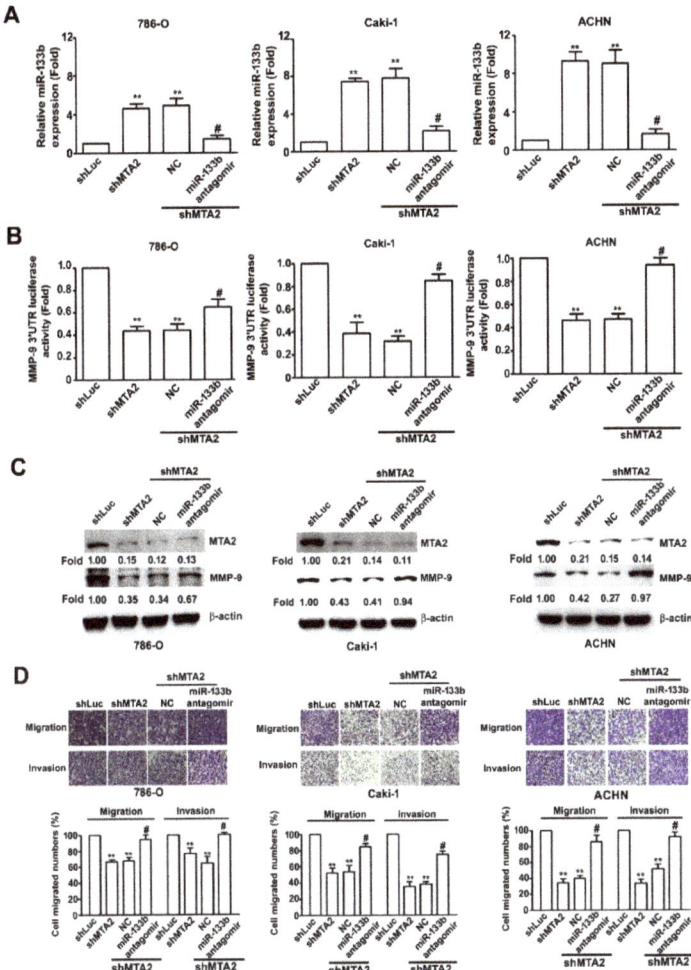

Figure 6. Effects of miR-133b on migratory and invasive ability in shMTA2-renal cell carcinoma (RCC) cells. (**A**) miR-133b expression in shMTA2–RCC cells after transfection with miR-133b antagomir or negative control (NC) were measured using RT-qPCR assays. (**B**) Luciferase activity assay. (**C**) Protein expressions of MTA2 and MMP-9 were detected using western blotting. β-Actin was used as an internal control. (**D**) Migration and invasion abilities of RCC cells were determined using migration and Matrigel invasion assays. Cells in the lower surface of the Borden chamber were stained and photographed under a light microscope at 400× magnification. Values are expressed as the mean ± SE of three independent experiments. ** $p < 0.01$ compared with the shLuc cells. # $p < 0.01$ compared with shMTA2. NC, miR-133b negative control.

3. Discussion

This study examined the hypothesis that the biological function and molecular mechanism of MTA2 induces miR-133b target MMP-9 expression in RCC metastasis progression. Our results indicated that (1) MTA2 expression was increased in RCC cells and was markedly correlated with high grade and poor survival rates of patients with RCC; (2) MTA2 did not affect RCC cell proliferation or cell cycle distribution; (3) MTA2 regulated the tumour metastasis of RCC cells and modulation of MMP-9 expression in vitro and in vivo; (4) miR-133b and MMP-9 expression in patients with RCC was negatively correlated with poor survival rates; (5) MTA2 knockdown inhibited RCC metastasis by targeting miR-133b and MMP-9 pathways. These results demonstrated the role of MTA2 in RCC metastasis, which is of tremendous help in creating new strategies against RCC metastasis at molecular translational levels.

MTA2 has been linked to tumour invasion depth, regional lymph node metastasis, distant metastasis, and poor long-term survival rates independent of age or gender in patients with esophageal squamous cell carcinoma [29], gastric cancer [13], non-small-cell lung cancer [30], and colorectal cancer [31]. Consistent with these studies, we observed higher MTA2 expression in tumour tissues compared with normal tissues and in all the RCC cell lines. Moreover, high MTA2 expression was markedly correlated with tumour grades and indicated low survival rates in accordance with the clinical pathologic data from our patients and TCGA database (Figure 1). Hence, we concluded that MTA2 overexpression has potential as an oncogenic factor for predicting the prognosis of patients with RCC.

Invasion and metastasis are characteristic features of cancer cells and a key impediment of effective prognosis [32]. In RCCs, overexpression of MMP-1, MMP-2, and MMP-9 is linked to tumour stage, histological grade, progression, invasion of microvasculature, and distant metastasis [33]. Targeting MTA2 with a short hairpin RNA could reduce cell proliferation and inhibit metastasis by downregulating MMP-2 or MMP-9 expression in breast cancer [34] and glioma cells [35]. Other reports have demonstrated that MTA2 overexpression could activate AKT and upregulate MMP-7 expression in nasopharyngeal carcinoma cells [36]. On the basis of these studies, we demonstrated that MTA2 knockdown could decrease the expression of MMP-9 and the invasive, migratory, and metastatic abilities of RCC cells. Therefore, MTA2 could influence the malignant factor that modulates MMP-9 expression for RCC.

Reports have demonstrated the downregulated expression of miR-133b, which is involved in the progression and in negative regulation of proliferation and metastasis in various tumours, such as glioma [37], breast cancer [27], prostate cancer [38], and bladder cancer [39]. In gastric cancer, miR-133b expression was negatively associated with lymph node metastasis, and miR-133b targeting Gli-1 markedly inhibited gastric cancer metastasis [40]. Kano et al. [24], revealed that miR-133b reduced proliferation and invasion of esophageal squamous cells by inhibiting FSCN1 expression. In ovarian cancer, the overexpression of miR-133b targeted EGFR and inhibited proliferation and invasion abilities by decreasing the phosphorylation of ERK1/2 and AKT pathways [41]. Overexpression of miR-133b induces RCC cell apoptosis by counteracting Janus kinase 2 (JAK2)/ Signal transducer and activator of transcription 3 (STAT3) pathway phosphorylation [42]. In addition to these studies, miR-133b inhibited RCC cell proliferation and metastasis by targeting MMP-9 [28]. However, the depth of the molecular mechanisms of MTA2 modulating miR-133b in RCC metastasis remains unclear. Consistent with the aforementioned results, MTA2 knockdown inhibited RCC metastasis by targeting MMP-9 expression. To explore the role of miR-133b in MTA2 regulating RCC metastasis, we used a miR-133b antagomir to restore MMP-9 expression in shMTA2 RCC cells. Similarly, inhibition of miR-133b in HK2 cells, which exhibit relatively high levels of miR-133b, significantly enhanced HK2 cell migration and invasion when treated with miR-133b antagomir. Therefore, miR-133b could modulate the effects of MTA2 on RCC cell invasion and migration abilities predominantly by targeting MMP-9 expression. At a clinical level, TCGA database analysis and Kaplan–Meier survival analyses revealed that patients with RCC with low miR-133b expression had lower survival rates compared with those with high expression, and miR-133b may be a prognostic marker of RCC. However, whether miR-133b is a predictor of clinical outcome in RCC cancer warrants further investigation.

In summary, our data suggested that MTA2 was overexpressed in RCC tissues and cells and positively correlated with tumour grade and MMP-9 expression in vitro and in vivo. Moreover, MTA2 knockdown inhibited RCC metastasis by regulating miR-133b targeting of MMP-9, and miR-133b was negatively correlated with RCC progression. Therefore, MTA2 regulation of miR-133b may be a novel diagnostic and therapeutic target for RCC treatment.

4. Materials and Methods

4.1. Materials and Reagents

MTT (tetrazolium dye, 3-(4,5-dimethylthiazol-2-yl)-2,5-diphenyltetrazolium bromide), Giemsa solution, and DAPI (4′-6-diamidino-2-phenylindole) were purchased from Sigma-Aldrich (St. Louis, MO). Dulbecco's Modified Eagle Medium: Nutrient Mixture F-12 (DMEM/F-12) medium powder was purchased from Gibco-Invitrogen Corporation (Gibco, Carlsbad, CA, USA), whereas the RPMI-1640 and minimum essential media (MEM) powder were purchased from HyClone (Pittsburgh, PA, USA). Fetal bovine serum (FBS), penicillin/streptomycin, and 0.25% trypsin were purchased from HyClone (Pittsburgh, PA, USA). The antibodies for western blotting and immunofluorescence assay against MTA2 (sc-55566) and β-actin (sc-69879) were purchased from Santa Cruz Biotechnology (Santa Cruz, CA, USA). Antibodies against MTA2 (ab171073) and MMP-9 (ab137867) were purchased from Abcam (Cambridge, UK). Antibodies against goat antirabbit immunoglobulin (IgG, AP132P) and goat antimouse IgG (AP124P) were purchased from Merck Millipore (Merck Millipore, Burlington, MA, USA). The human MTA2 plasmid was synthesized from the GENEWIZ company (Takeley, UK).

4.2. Human Kidney Clear Cell Carcinoma Tissue Array

Kidney clear cell carcinoma tissue array contained human kidney cancer specimens and normal kidney tissue (BC07115; US Biomax Inc., Rockville, MD, USA). Clinicopathological characteristics, such as gender, age, tumour grade, and tumour stage were obtained from medical records. Kidney clear cell carcinoma tissue arrays were detected using immunohistochemical (IHC) staining for MTA2 according to previous reports [43].

4.3. Cell Culture and shRNA Assay

Human renal cancer cell lines (786-O, Caki-1, A-498, and ACHN) and normal HK2 cells were purchased from the Bioresources Collection and Research Centre of the Food Industry Research and Development Institute (Hsinchu, Taiwan). The 786-O cell lines were cultured in RPMI-1640. A498, Caki-1, and ACHN cell lines were cultured in MEM. HK2 cell lines were cultured in DMEM-F12 media. All cell lines were supplemented with a medium containing 10% FBS (Gibco, USA) and 1% penicillin/streptomycin at a humidified atmosphere containing 5% CO_2 at 37 °C. For the shRNA assay, the shMTA2 (MTA2-shRNA-pLKO.1) and shLuc (Luc-shRNA-pLKO.1) plasmids were purchased from RNAi core of Academia Sinica (Taipei, Taiwan). The MTA2 target sequences were 5′-AGGGAGTGAGGAGTGAATTAA-3′, and the pLKO.1-Luc was a scrambled control. We used puromycin (2 μg/mL) to select stably transduced RCC cells as previously reported [44].

4.4. RNA Isolation, RT-PCR, and QRT-PCR

The total RNA was isolated from cells by using TRIzol (Invitrogen, Waltham, MA, USA). RNA samples (1 μg) were reverse transcribed to cDNA using GoScript Reverse Transcription Mix (Promega, Madison, WI, USA). RT-PCR was conducted using GoTaq Green Master Mix (Promega, USA). The PCR reaction conditions were 30 s at 95 °C, 30 cycles of 30 s at 95 °C for denaturation, 30 s at 52 °C for annealing, 90 s at 72 °C for extension, and 10 min at 72 °C for the final extension. mRNA levels were detected using the SYBR Green PCR Master Mix (Promega, USA) and analysed using Applied Biosystems Step One Plus Real-Time PCR System (Applied Biosystems, Waltham, MA, USA), as described by the manufacturer. The primers for the RT-PCR were MTA2 (forward: 5′-GTTCTGGCAATACGGCGAGT-3′, reverse: 5′-CTTCGGCTGAATGCACAAAGA-3′) and β-actin (forward: 5′-ACTGGAACGGTGAAGGTGAC-3′, reverse: 5′-AGAGAAGTGGGGTGGCTTTT-3′).

The primers for the qRT-PCR were MMP-9 (forward: 5′-ACGACGTCTTCCAGTACCGA-3′, reverse: 5′-TCATAGGTCACGTAGCCCAC-3′), and GAPDH (forward: 5′-CATCATCCCTGCCTCTACTG-3′, reverse; 5′-GCCTGCTTCACCACCTTC-3′). All reactions for RT-PCR and qRT-PCR were run in triplicate and normalised to the internal control products of β-actin and GAPDH.

4.5. Cell Viability Assay

The shLuc and shMTA2 cells were seeded into 24-well plates at a density of 2×10^4 cells/well and cultured for 24 and 48 h. MTT reagents were used to determine cell viability by following the manufacturer's protocol. Three wells were measured for cell viability in each treatment group. The absorbance value at a wavelength of 570 nm was used as an indicator of cell viability.

4.6. Cell Cycle Analysis

Cell cycle distribution was analysed using Muse Cell Analyser (Millipore, Hayward, CA, USA). The shLuc and shMTA2 cells were washed three times with ice-cold phosphate-buffered saline and fixed with 70% ethanol at −20 °C overnight. Then, cells were cultured in 50 μg/mL propidium iodide and 1 mg/mL RNase for 30 min at room temperature. Finally, the treated cells were analysed. At least 50,000 cells were acquired for each sample. The experiments were performed in triplicate.

4.7. In Vitro Cell Migration and Invasion Assays

In vitro migration assays were performed using Boyben chamber inserts containing an 8.0 μm polycarbonate membrane (Corning, New York, NY, USA). Membranes were coated with 5% Matrigel matrix (BD Biosciences, Bedford, MA, USA) to determine the tumour cell invasion. The shLuc and shMTA2 cells (2×10^4 cells/well) in 50 μL of serum-free media were added to the upper chamber, and 35 μL of medium/well with 10% FBS was added to the lower chamber. After 24 h of incubation at 37 °C, the cells remaining in the upper membrane were completely removed by gentle swabbing, whereas the migrated or invaded cells were attached to the lower part of the membrane insert. The lower surface of the membrane was fixed in 95% methanol for 10 min and stained with 0.5% crystal violet for 30 min. The cells were then counted under a microscope in five different fields. All experiments were performed in triplicate.

4.8. MiR-133b Antagomir and MTA2 Plasmid Transfection

The shLuc and shMTA2 cells were seeded into 6 cm dishes at a density of 2×10^5 cells/well for 24 h and transfected with the miR-133b antagomir and MTA2 plasmid by using the TurboFect transfection reagent (Thermo Fisher Scientific, Waltham, MA USA) as previously reported [45].

4.9. Western Blot Analysis

Total protein was extracted from the shLuc and shMTA2 cells. Protein concentration was determined using the Bradford method (Bio-Rad, Hercules, CA, USA). Primary antibodies, namely MTA2, MMP-9, and β-actin, were incubated overnight at 4 °C, washed twice, and then incubated with secondary antirabbit and antimouse IgG for 60 min. Immunoreactive bands were detected with a chemiluminescence kit (Millipore, Billerica, MA, USA) using the ImageQuant LAS 4000 mini according to the manufacturer's instructions.

4.10. Immunofluorescence Assay

After seeding 1×10^4 shLuc and shMTA2 cells/well in a Nunc Lab-Tek chambered cover glass (Thermo, USA) for 24 h, cells were washed twice with phosphate-buffered saline (PBS), fixed with 4% paraformaldehyde for 10 min, washed twice with PBS, permeabilised with PBS containing 0.1% Triton X-100 for 10 min, and blocked with 2% bovine serum albumin for 2 h. Primary antibodies against MTA2 and MMP-9 were incubated in 2% bovine serum albumin at 4 °C overnight, and second antibodies were incubated in 2% bovine serum albumin at room temperature for 2 h. DAPI was used as the counterstaining medium for the cell nucleus. The results were visualised using a Zeiss LSM 510 confocal microscope.

4.11. Gelatine Zymography

MMP activity in a serum-free medium after culturing with shLuc and shMTA2 cells in 786-O and Caki-1 was detected using 8% SDS-polyacrylamide gel electrophoresis (PAGE) containing 0.1% gelatin. After electrophoresis, the gel was washed with Tris-buffered saline containing 2.5% Triton X-100 and then incubated in a reaction buffer overnight. Finally, the gel was stained with Coomassie Brilliant Blue R-250.

4.12. TCGA Database and miRNA Prediction of Bioinformatic Analysis

Clinical mRNA expression data, such as overall survival status of patients with RCC, were downloaded from TCGA datasets. To identify the miR-133b target gene, we used miRBase (http://www.mirbase.org), miRcode (http://www.mircode.org/), and TargetScan (http://www.targetscan.org/) to surmise the miRNA binding site in the 3'-UTR of MMP-9.

4.13. Luciferase Reporter Assay

The shLuc and shMTA2 cells in 786-O, Caki-1, and ACHN cells were cotransfected with pGL4.13-MMP-9-3'UTR-wt/mut and pRL Renilla luciferase control reporter vectors by using the TurboFect transfection reagent. The 3'-UTR sequences of MMP-9 containing the miR-133b binding site were constructed in the pGL4.13 vector by using PCR assay. Luciferase activity was detected using the Dual-Luciferase Reporter Assay System (Promega, Madison, WI, USA). All experiment steps followed the protocol. The activity of pRL Renilla luciferase control reporter vectors was used as the internal control.

4.14. In Vivo Animal Model and Immunohistochemistry Analysis

Five-week-old C. B17 mice weighing approximately 20 g were obtained from the National Laboratory Animal Centre (Taipei, Taiwan). All animal experiments were conducted following the protocols approved by the Institutional Animal Care and Use Committee of Chung Shan Medical University (IACUC: 2120). The shLuc and shMTA2 cells (six mice/group) were injected into the tail veins at a density of 1×10^6 in 0.1 mL of saline. All mice were euthanised after 2 months, and lung tissues were resected. To investigate the metastasis ability of shLuc and shMTA2 cells, lung tissues were harvested, embedded with paraffin, fixed in formalin, and processed for IHC staining. The amount and size of shLuc and shMTA2 cells metastasised in the lungs were analysed using H&E and Ki-67 staining.

4.15. Statistical Analyses

Results are expressed as mean ± standard deviation. Differences between the two groups were analysed using Student's t-test or one-way analysis of variance followed by the Tukey post hoc test. The correlation between MTA2 and MMP-9 expression was measured using Spearman's correlation analysis. All statistical calculations were performed using SPSS 12.0. A *p*-value less than 0.05 or 0.01 was regarded as statistically significant.

5. Conclusions

This study is the first to demonstrate that MTA2 could serve as an indicator for predicting the prognosis of patients with RCC. Moreover, we highlighted that MTA2 could regulate the RCC process by modulating miR-133b targeting MMP-9 expression. Finally, we hypothesised that treatments for MTA2 or modulating the expression of miR-133b targeting MMP-9 are promising therapies in addition to current therapies for RCC.

Supplementary Materials: The following are available online at http://www.mdpi.com/2072-6694/11/12/1851/s1, Figure S1: MTA2 promote the migration and invasion of HK2 cells through modulating MMP-9 expression; Figure S2: MiR-133b influences cell migration/invasion and MMP-9 expression in HK2 cells.

Author Contributions: Conceptualization, Y.-S.C., C.-L.L., T.-W.H., C.-C.L., J.-P.T. and Y.-H.H.; methodology and statistical analysis, S.-F.Y., Y.-H.H., S.-C.S., C.-F.Y., J.-P.T.; Performed the experiments, Y.-S.C., C.-L.L., C.-F.Y., Y.-H.H.; Manuscript preparation: T.-W.H., S.-C.S., Y.-H.H., S.-C.S., J.-P.T. All authors read and approved the final manuscript.

Funding: This work was supported by grants from Dalin Tzu Chi Hospital, Buddhist Tzu Chi Medical Foundation (DTCRD104(2)-E-12) and the Ministry of Science and Technology (MOST 108-2314-B-040 -012-).

Conflicts of Interest: The authors declare that they have no competing interests.

References

1. Znaor, A.; Lortet-Tieulent, J.; Laversanne, M.; Jemal, A.; Bray, F. International variations and trends in renal cell carcinoma incidence and mortality. *Eur. Urol.* **2015**, *67*, 519–530. [CrossRef] [PubMed]
2. Chen, V.J.; Hernandez-Meza, G.; Agrawal, P.; Zhang, C.A.; Xie, L.; Gong, C.L.; Hoerner, C.R.; Srinivas, S.; Oermann, E.K.; Fan, A.C. Time on Therapy for at Least Three Months Correlates with Overall Survival in Metastatic Renal Cell Carcinoma. *Cancers (Basel)* **2019**, *11*, 1000. [CrossRef] [PubMed]
3. Ricketts, C.J.; De Cubas, A.A.; Fan, H.; Smith, C.C.; Lang, M.; Reznik, E.; Bowlby, R.; Gibb, E.A.; Akbani, R.; Beroukhim, R.; et al. The Cancer Genome Atlas Comprehensive Molecular Characterization of Renal Cell Carcinoma. *Cell. Rep.* **2018**, *23*, 313–326.e5. [CrossRef] [PubMed]
4. Huilgol, D.; Venkataramani, P.; Nandi, S.; Bhattacharjee, S. Transcription Factors That Govern Development and Disease: An Achilles Heel in Cancer. *Genes (Basel)* **2019**, *10*, 794. [CrossRef] [PubMed]
5. Hsieh, J.J.; Purdue, M.P.; Signoretti, S.; Swanton, C.; Albiges, L.; Schmidinger, M.; Heng, D.Y.; Larkin, J.; Ficarra, V. Renal cell carcinoma. *Nat. Rev. Dis. Primers* **2017**, *3*, 865–875. [CrossRef] [PubMed]
6. Hudes, G.; Carducci, M.; Tomczak, P.; Dutcher, J.; Figlin, R.; Kapoor, A.; Staroslawska, E.; Sosman, J.; McDermott, D.; Bodrogi, I.; et al. Temsirolimus, interferon alfa, or both for advanced renal-cell carcinoma. *N. Engl. J. Med.* **2007**, *356*, 2271–2281. [CrossRef]
7. Motzer, R.J.; Escudier, B.; McDermott, D.F.; George, S.; Hammers, H.J.; Srinivas, S.; Tykodi, S.S.; Sosman, J.A.; Procopio, G.; Plimack, E.R.; et al. Nivolumab versus Everolimus in Advanced Renal-Cell Carcinoma. *N. Engl. J. Med.* **2015**, *373*, 1803–1813. [CrossRef]
8. Ghosh, D.; Venkataramani, P.; Nandi, S.; Bhattacharjee, S. CRISPR-Cas9 a boon or bane: The bumpy road ahead to cancer therapeutics. *Cancer Cell. Int.* **2019**, *19*, 12. [CrossRef]
9. Bhattacharjee, S.; Nandi, S. Rare Genetic Diseases with Defects in DNA Repair: Opportunities and Challenges in Orphan Drug Development for Targeted Cancer Therapy. *Cancers (Basel)* **2018**, *10*, 298. [CrossRef]
10. Ravaud, A.; Motzer, R.J.; Pandha, H.S.; George, D.J.; Pantuck, A.J.; Patel, A.; Chang, Y.H.; Escudier, B.; Donskov, F.; Magheli, A.; et al. Adjuvant Sunitinib in High-Risk Renal-Cell Carcinoma after Nephrectomy. *N. Engl. J. Med.* **2016**, *375*, 2246–2254. [CrossRef]
11. Zhou, J.; Zhan, S.; Tan, W.; Cheng, R.; Gong, H.; Zhu, Q. P300 binds to and acetylates MTA2 to promote colorectal cancer cells growth. *Biochem. Biophys. Res. Commun.* **2014**, *444*, 387–390. [CrossRef] [PubMed]
12. Covington, K.R.; Fuqua, S.A. Role of MTA2 in human cancer. *Cancer Metastasis Rev.* **2014**, *33*, 921–928. [CrossRef] [PubMed]
13. Zhou, C.; Ji, J.; Cai, Q.; Shi, M.; Chen, X.; Yu, Y.; Liu, B.; Zhu, Z.; Zhang, J. MTA2 promotes gastric cancer cells invasion and is transcriptionally regulated by Sp1. *Mol. Cancer* **2013**, *12*, 102. [CrossRef] [PubMed]
14. Zhang, B.; Zhang, H.; Shen, G. Metastasis-associated protein 2 (MTA2) promotes the metastasis of non-small-cell lung cancer through the inhibition of the cell adhesion molecule Ep-CAM and E-cadherin. *Jpn. J. Clin. Oncol.* **2015**, *45*, 755–766. [CrossRef]
15. Covington, K.R.; Brusco, L.; Barone, I.; Tsimelzon, A.; Selever, J.; Corona-Rodriguez, A.; Brown, P.; Kumar, R.; Hilsenbeck, S.G.; Fuqua, S.A. Metastasis tumor-associated protein 2 enhances metastatic behavior and is associated with poor outcomes in estrogen receptor-negative breast cancer. *Breast Cancer Res. Treat.* **2013**, *141*, 375–384. [CrossRef]
16. Liotta, L.A.; Stetler-Stevenson, W.G. Tumor invasion and metastasis: An imbalance of positive and negative regulation. *Cancer Res.* **1991**, *51*, 5054s–5059s.

17. Gaffney, J.; Solomonov, I.; Zehorai, E.; Sagi, I. Multilevel regulation of matrix metalloproteinases in tissue homeostasis indicates their molecular specificity in vivo. *Matrix Biol.* **2015**, *44–46*, 191–199. [CrossRef]
18. Sato, A.; Nagase, H.; Obinata, D.; Fujiwara, K.; Fukuda, N.; Soma, M.; Yamaguchi, K.; Kawata, N.; Takahashi, S. Inhibition of MMP-9 using a pyrrole-imidazole polyamide reduces cell invasion in renal cell carcinoma. *Int. J. Oncol.* **2013**, *43*, 1441–1446. [CrossRef]
19. Cho, N.H.; Shim, H.S.; Rha, S.Y.; Kang, S.H.; Hong, S.H.; Choi, Y.D.; Hong, S.J.; Cho, S.H. Increased expression of matrix metalloproteinase 9 correlates with poor prognostic variables in renal cell carcinoma. *Eur. Urol.* **2003**, *44*, 560–566. [CrossRef]
20. Ghosh, D.; Nandi, S.; Bhattacharjee, S. Combination therapy to checkmate Glioblastoma: Clinical challenges and advances. *Clin. Transl. Med.* **2018**, *7*, 33. [CrossRef]
21. Omuro, A.; DeAngelis, L.M. Glioblastoma and other malignant gliomas: A clinical review. *JAMA* **2013**, *310*, 1842–1850. [CrossRef] [PubMed]
22. Tabouret, E.; Boudouresque, F.; Farina, P.; Barrie, M.; Bequet, C.; Sanson, M.; Chinot, O. MMP2 and MMP9 as candidate biomarkers to monitor bevacizumab therapy in high-grade glioma. *Neuro. Oncol.* **2015**, *17*, 1174–1176. [CrossRef] [PubMed]
23. Schickel, R.; Boyerinas, B.; Park, S.M.; Peter, M.E. MicroRNAs: Key players in the immune system, differentiation, tumorigenesis and cell death. *Oncogene* **2008**, *27*, 5959–5974. [CrossRef] [PubMed]
24. Kano, M.; Seki, N.; Kikkawa, N.; Fujimura, L.; Hoshino, I.; Akutsu, Y.; Chiyomaru, T.; Enokida, H.; Nakagawa, M.; Matsubara, H. miR-145, miR-133a and miR-133b: Tumor-suppressive miRNAs target FSCN1 in esophageal squamous cell carcinoma. *Int. J. Cancer* **2010**, *127*, 2804–2814. [CrossRef]
25. Qiu, T.; Zhou, X.; Wang, J.; Du, Y.; Xu, J.; Huang, Z.; Zhu, W.; Shu, Y.; Liu, P. MiR-145, miR-133a and miR-133b inhibit proliferation, migration, invasion and cell cycle progression via targeting transcription factor Sp1 in gastric cancer. *FEBS Lett.* **2014**, *588*, 1168–1177. [CrossRef]
26. Zeng, W.; Zhu, J.F.; Liu, J.Y.; Li, Y.L.; Dong, X.; Huang, H.; Shan, L. miR-133b inhibits cell proliferation, migration and invasion of esophageal squamous cell carcinoma by targeting EGFR. *Biomed. Pharmacother.* **2019**, *111*, 476–484. [CrossRef]
27. Wang, Q.Y.; Zhou, C.X.; Zhan, M.N.; Tang, J.; Wang, C.L.; Ma, C.N.; He, M.; Chen, G.Q.; He, J.R.; Zhao, Q. MiR-133b targets Sox9 to control pathogenesis and metastasis of breast cancer. *Cell Death Dis.* **2018**, *9*, 752. [CrossRef]
28. Wu, D.; Pan, H.; Zhou, Y.; Zhou, J.; Fan, Y.; Qu, P. microRNA-133b downregulation and inhibition of cell proliferation, migration and invasion by targeting matrix metallopeptidase-9 in renal cell carcinoma. *Mol. Med. Rep.* **2014**, *9*, 2491–2498. [CrossRef]
29. Liu, Y.P.; Shan, B.E.; Wang, X.L.; Ma, L. Correlation between MTA2 overexpression and tumour progression in esophageal squamous cell carcinoma. *Exp. Ther. Med.* **2012**, *3*, 745–749. [CrossRef]
30. Liu, S.L.; Han, Y.; Zhang, Y.; Xie, C.Y.; Wang, E.H.; Miao, Y.; Li, H.Y.; Xu, H.T.; Dai, S.D. Expression of metastasis-associated protein 2 (MTA2) might predict proliferation in non-small cell lung cancer. *Target. Oncol.* **2012**, *7*, 135–143. [CrossRef]
31. Ding, W.; Hu, W.; Yang, H.; Ying, T.; Tian, Y. Prognostic correlation between MTA2 expression level and colorectal cancer. *Int. J. Clin. Exp. Pathol.* **2015**, *8*, 7173–7180. [PubMed]
32. Deryugina, E.I.; Bourdon, M.A.; Reisfeld, R.A.; Strongin, A. Remodeling of collagen matrix by human tumor cells requires activation and cell surface association of matrix metalloproteinase-2. *Cancer Res.* **1998**, *58*, 3743–3750. [PubMed]
33. Narula, S.; Tandon, C.; Tandon, S. Role of Matrix Metalloproteinases in Degenerative Kidney Disorders. *Curr. Med. Chem.* **2018**, *25*, 1805–1816. [CrossRef] [PubMed]
34. Lu, J.; Jin, M.L. Short-hairpin RNA-mediated MTA2 silencing inhibits human breast cancer cell line MDA-MB231 proliferation and metastasis. *Asian Pac. J. Cancer Prev.* **2014**, *15*, 5577–5582. [CrossRef] [PubMed]
35. Cheng, C.Y.; Chou, Y.E.; Ko, C.P.; Yang, S.F.; Hsieh, S.C.; Lin, C.L.; Hsieh, Y.H.; Chen, K.C. Metastasis tumor-associated protein-2 knockdown suppresses the proliferation and invasion of human glioma cells in vitro and in vivo. *J. Neurooncol.* **2014**, *120*, 273–281. [CrossRef]
36. Wu, M.; Ye, X.; Deng, X.; Wu, Y.; Li, X.; Zhang, L. Upregulation of metastasis-associated gene 2 promotes cell proliferation and invasion in nasopharyngeal carcinoma. *OncoTargets Ther.* **2016**, *9*, 1647–1656. [CrossRef]

37. Zhang, Q.; Fan, X.; Xu, B.; Pang, Q.; Teng, L. miR-133b acts as a tumor suppressor and negatively regulates EMP2 in glioma. *Neoplasma* **2018**, *65*, 494–504. [CrossRef]
38. Huang, S.; Wa, Q.; Pan, J.; Peng, X.; Ren, D.; Li, Q.; Dai, Y.; Yang, Q.; Huang, Y.; Zhang, X.; et al. Transcriptional downregulation of miR-133b by REST promotes prostate cancer metastasis to bone via activating TGF-beta signaling. *Cell Death Dis.* **2018**, *9*, 779. [CrossRef]
39. Zhao, F.; Zhou, L.H.; Ge, Y.Z.; Ping, W.W.; Wu, X.; Xu, Z.L.; Wang, M.; Sha, Z.L.; Jia, R.P. MicroRNA-133b suppresses bladder cancer malignancy by targeting TAGLN2-mediated cell cycle. *J. Cell. Physiol.* **2019**, *234*, 4910–4923. [CrossRef]
40. Zhao, Y.; Huang, J.; Zhang, L.; Qu, Y.; Li, J.; Yu, B.; Yan, M.; Yu, Y.; Liu, B.; Zhu, Z. MiR-133b is frequently decreased in gastric cancer and its overexpression reduces the metastatic potential of gastric cancer cells. *BMC Cancer* **2014**, *14*, 34. [CrossRef]
41. Liu, X.; Li, G. MicroRNA-133b inhibits proliferation and invasion of ovarian cancer cells through Akt and Erk1/2 inactivation by targeting epidermal growth factor receptor. *Int. J. Clin. Exp. Pathol.* **2015**, *8*, 10605–10614. [PubMed]
42. Zhou, W.; Bi, X.; Gao, G.; Sun, L. miRNA-133b and miRNA-135a induce apoptosis via the JAK2/STAT3 signaling pathway in human renal carcinoma cells. *Biomed. Pharmacother.* **2016**, *84*, 722–729. [CrossRef] [PubMed]
43. Lai, C.Y.; Chen, C.M.; Hsu, W.H.; Hsieh, Y.H.; Liu, C.J. Overexpression of Endothelial Cell-Specific Molecule 1 Correlates with Gleason Score and Expression of Androgen Receptor in Prostate Carcinoma. *Int. J. Med. Sci.* **2017**, *14*, 1263–1267. [CrossRef] [PubMed]
44. Tseng, T.Y.; Chiou, H.L.; Lin, C.W.; Chen, Y.S.; Hsu, L.S.; Lee, C.H.; Hsieh, Y.H. Repression of metastasis-associated protein 2 for inhibiting metastasis of human oral cancer cells by promoting the p-cofilin-1/LC3-II expression. *J. Oral. Pathol. Med.* **2019**. [CrossRef] [PubMed]
45. Chiang, K.C.; Lai, C.Y.; Chiou, H.L.; Lin, C.L.; Chen, Y.S.; Kao, S.H.; Hsieh, Y.H. Timosaponin AIII inhibits metastasis of renal carcinoma cells through suppressing cathepsin C expression by AKT/miR-129-5p axis. *J. Cell. Physiol.* **2019**, *234*, 13332–13341. [CrossRef]

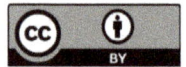

© 2019 by the authors. Licensee MDPI, Basel, Switzerland. This article is an open access article distributed under the terms and conditions of the Creative Commons Attribution (CC BY) license (http://creativecommons.org/licenses/by/4.0/).

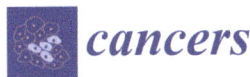

Article

MicroRNA-Mediated Metabolic Reprograming in Renal Cancer

Joanna Bogusławska [1], Piotr Popławski [1], Saleh Alseekh [2,3], Marta Koblowska [4,5], Roksana Iwanicka-Nowicka [4,5], Beata Rybicka [1], Hanna Kędzierska [1,†], Katarzyna Głuchowska [1], Karolina Hanusek [1], Zbigniew Tański [6], Alisdair R. Fernie [2,3] and Agnieszka Piekiełko-Witkowska [1,*]

1. Department of Biochemistry and Molecular Biology, Centre of Postgraduate Medical Education, ul. Marymoncka 99/103, 01-813 Warsaw, Poland; joanna.boguslawska@cmkp.edu.pl (J.B.); piotr.poplawski@cmkp.edu.pl (P.P.); beata.rybicka@cmkp.edu.pl (B.R.); h.kedzierska@cent.uw.edu.pl (H.K.); katarzyna.rodzik@cmkp.edu.pl (K.G.); karolina.hanusek@cmkp.edu.pl (K.H.)
2. Max-Planck Institute of Molecular Plant Physiology, 14476 Potsdam-Golm, Germany; Alseekh@mpimp-golm.mpg.de (S.A.); Fernie@mpimp-golm.mpg.de (A.R.F.)
3. Center for Plant Systems Biology and Biotechnology, 4000 Plovdiv, Bulgaria
4. Laboratory of Systems Biology, Faculty of Biology, University of Warsaw, 02-106 Warsaw, Poland; marta@ibb.waw.pl (M.K.); roxana@ibb.waw.pl (R.I.-N.)
5. Laboratory for Microarray Analysis, Institute of Biochemistry and Biophysics, Polish Academy of Sciences, 02-106 Warsaw, Poland
6. Masovian Specialist Hospital in Ostroleka, 07-410 Ostroleka, Poland; tanska@interia.pl
* Correspondence: apiekielko@cmkp.edu.pl; Tel.: +48-22-5693810
† Present affiliation of HK: Laboratory of Experimental Medicine, Centre of New Technologies, University of Warsaw, 02-097 Warsaw, Poland.

Received: 25 October 2019; Accepted: 15 November 2019; Published: 20 November 2019

Abstract: Metabolic reprogramming is one of the hallmarks of renal cell cancer (RCC). We hypothesized that altered metabolism of RCC cells results from dysregulation of microRNAs targeting metabolically relevant genes. Combined large-scale transcriptomic and metabolic analysis of RCC patients tissue samples revealed a group of microRNAs that contribute to metabolic reprogramming in RCC. miRNAs expressions correlated with their predicted target genes and with gas chromatography-mass spectrometry (GC-MS) metabolome profiles of RCC tumors. Assays performed in RCC-derived cell lines showed that miR-146a-5p and miR-155-5p targeted genes of PPP (the pentose phosphate pathway) (*G6PD* and *TKT*), the TCA (tricarboxylic acid cycle) cycle (*SUCLG2*), and arginine metabolism (*GATM*), respectively. miR-106b-5p and miR-122-5p regulated the NFAT5 osmoregulatory transcription factor. Altered expressions of G6PD, TKT, SUCLG2, GATM, miR-106b-5p, miR-155-5p, and miR-342-3p correlated with poor survival of RCC patients. miR-106b-5p, miR-146a-5p, and miR-342-3p stimulated proliferation of RCC cells. The analysis involving >6000 patients revealed that miR-34a-5p, miR-106b-5p, miR-146a-5p, and miR-155-5p are PanCancer metabomiRs possibly involved in global regulation of cancer metabolism. In conclusion, we found that microRNAs upregulated in renal cancer contribute to disturbed expression of key genes involved in the regulation of RCC metabolome. miR-146a-5p and miR-155-5p emerge as a key "metabomiRs" that target genes of crucial metabolic pathways (PPP (the pentose phosphate pathway), TCA cycle, and arginine metabolism).

Keywords: renal cell cancer; microRNA; metabolome; proliferation; PPP; pentose phosphate pathway; TCA cycle; miR-155-5p; miR-146a-5p; TCGA

1. Introduction

Renal cell cancer (RCC) is the most common subtype of kidney malignancies, affecting 300,000 people annually worldwide [1]. In approximately 25–30% of patients, metastasis is present at diagnosis, while a further 25% of patients develop metastases at later stages of the disease. Metastatic RCC (mRCC) is persistently difficult for treatment. Current therapeutic options include tyrosine kinase receptors inhibitors (TKIs), inhibitors of the mTOR (the mammalian target of rapamycin) pathway, or recently introduced inhibitors of immune checkpoints. All these treatments, however, prolong patients' life by only up to two years [2].

Recent studies provided strong evidence that aberrant cellular metabolism contributes to development and progression of RCC. Similar to all cancers, RCC is characterized by increased consumption of glucose with simultaneous enhanced production of lactate under normal oxygen supply (the Warburg effect). The other metabolic features of RCC include alterations in the TCA (the tricarboxylic acid cycle) cycle and the pentose-phosphate pathway (PPP) as well as the metabolism of amino acids and fatty acids [3]. In our previous study we found that disturbances in the metabolism of succinate, beta-alanine, purines, glucose, and *myo*-inositol are linked with poor survival of RCC patients [4]. Remarkably, apart from changes in levels of intracellular metabolites in RCC tumors, we found significant alterations in expressions of genes encoding key metabolic pathways. The causes of these alterations remain unknown.

In the current study, we hypothesized that disturbed expression of metabolic genes in RCC could be caused by microRNAs (miRs). These short, non-coding RNAs interact with microRNA response elements (MREs) located in 3'UTRs of target transcripts and either trigger their degradation or attenuate translation, thereby contributing to the regulation of gene expression. microRNAs influence cancer development and progression by changing the expressions of oncogenes and tumor suppressors as well as genes involved in key signaling pathways. Remarkably, one microRNA can regulate multiple target genes, while one gene can be commonly regulated by several microRNAs [5]. We and others showed that disturbed expression of microRNAs in renal cancer contributes to altered expression of genes regulating proliferation, migration, invasion, and apoptosis [6,7].

Here, we hypothesized that altered expression of genes involved in metabolic regulation in RCC could result from dysregulation of their targeting microRNAs. We verified our hypothesis by comprehensively analyzing expressions of nearly 100 microRNAs predicted to target altered metabolic genes in a large group of RCC patients, in order to identify and validate miRNAs that can act as regulators of the RCC metabolome. Remarkably, we show that metabolically relevant microRNAs affect proliferation of the RCC cells and contribute to the poor survival of RCC patients. To our knowledge, this is the first study addressing the role of microRNAs in global regulation of genes affecting renal cancer metabolome.

2. Results

2.1. The Expression of miRs Predicted to Target Metabolic Genes Is Altered in Renal Tumors

In our previous study, we identified a group of genes encoding metabolic enzymes for which altered expression was associated with changed metabolic profiles of RCC tumors [4]. Here, to validate the results of that study, we selected 20 genes based on their possible effects on patient survival, the number of predicted targeting miRNAs, and the fold changes in their expression (Table S1), and analyzed their expression in an independent group of 60 RCC-control tissue pairs (Figure 1A). This analysis confirmed altered expression of 19 genes encoding enzymes involved in the regulation of RCC metabolome (Table 1).

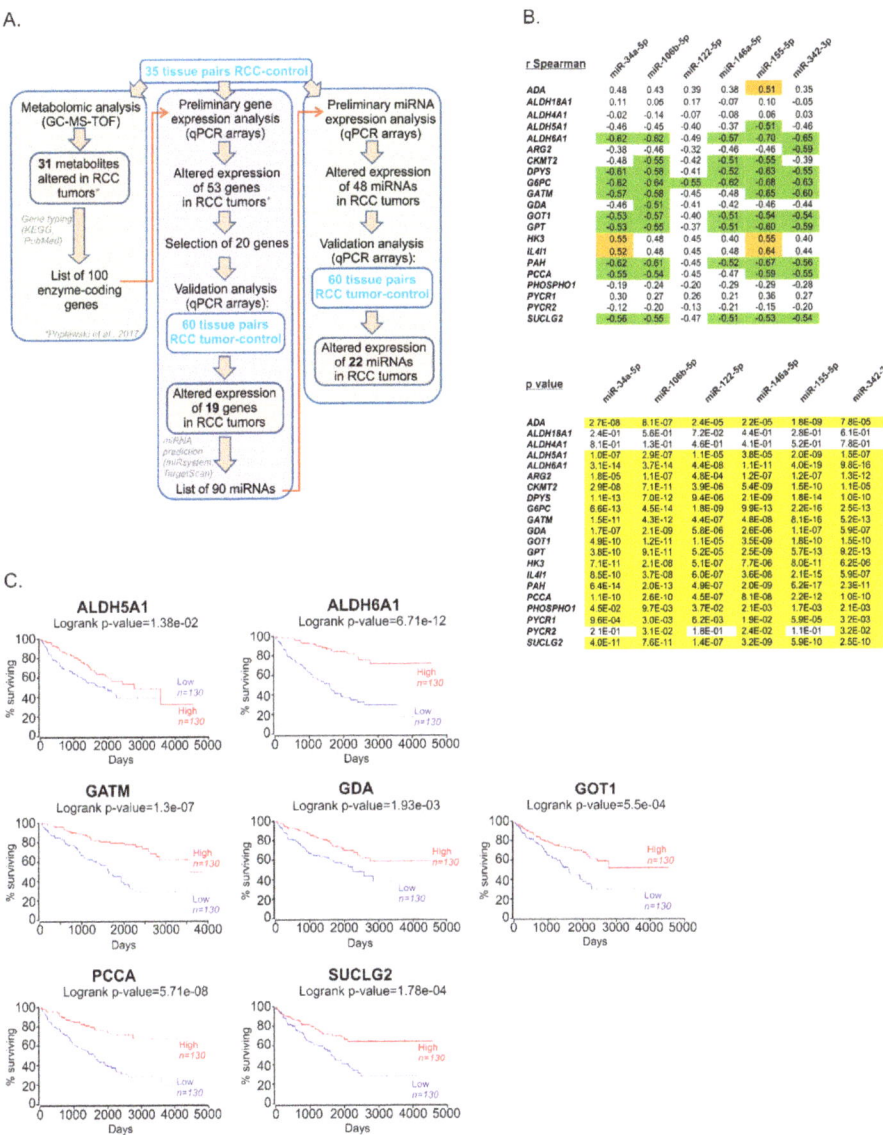

Figure 1. The expressions of microRNAs in relation to their predicted metabolically relevant gene targets. (**A**) The scheme of analysis of miRNAs predicted to regulated RCC metabolome. (**B**) Correlations between the expressions of metabolic genes and their predicted regulatory microRNAs, selected for functional analysis. Upper panel shows correlation coefficients. Green: r Spearman < −0.5; orange: r Spearman > 0.5. Lower panel: p values. Yellow: $p < 0.05$. Full data of correlation analysis are given in Table S3. $N = 60$ of RCC tumor samples and $n = 60$ of control tissue samples. (**C**) Altered expression of metabolic genes correlates with poor survival of RCC patients. Kaplan–Meier plots were generated using OncoLnc tool and KIRC (Kidney Renal Clear Cell Carcinoma) cohort of TCGA (The Cancer Genome Atlas) data. Patients were classified into Low and High expression groups basing on median mRNA expression (the expression profiles in two groups of patients are given in Figure S1). $N = 260$.

Based on the results of bioinformatic analysis and the selection criteria described in the Methods Section and File S1, we selected 90 microRNAs (Table S2) predicted to regulate 19 metabolic genes and analyzed their expression in 35 matched-pairs of ccRCC (clear cell Renal Cell Carcinoma) tumors and non-tumorous kidney samples. The expression of 48 microRNAs was statistically significantly different in RCC tumors when compared to controls ($p < 0.05$; threshold of expression change: 30%) (Table S2). Next, we performed validation analysis, using an independent group of 60 matched-pairs of ccRCC tumors and control samples, and confirmed altered expression of 22 microRNAs (Table 1). microRNAs for which expression was most increased included: miR-122-5p (+107.7-fold), miR-210-3p (+10.2-fold) and miR-34a-5p (+3.1-fold).

Table 1. The expressions of genes involved in the regulation of cell metabolism and their predicted regulatory miRNAs are altered in RCC tumor tissues.

A. Expression of Metabolic Genes in RCC		
Gene	FC	p Value
Increased expression in tumors		
1. ADA	+5.77	<0.0001
2. IL4I1	+4.20	<0.0001
3. HK3	+3.96	<0.0001
4. PYCR1	+1.56	<0.0001
Decreased expression in tumors		
5. PAH	−70.47	<0.0001
6. ALDH6A1	−21.41	<0.0001
7. CMKT2	−18.36	<0.0001
8. ALDH4A1	−14.72	<0.0001
9. GATM	−12.99	<0.0001
10. DPYS	−10.83	<0.0001
11. G6PC	−10.83	<0.0001
12. PCCA	−6.87	<0.0001
13. GPT	−6.62	<0.0001
14. GDA	−6.37	<0.0001
15. ALDH5A1	−5.54	<0.0001
16. SUCLG2	−5.35	<0.0001
17. ARG2	−4.45	<0.0001
18. GOT1	−3.68	<0.0001
19. PHOSPHO1	−1.35	=0.0215
B. Expression of miRNAs Predicted to Regulate Metabolic Genes in RCC		
MicroRNA	FC	p Value
Increased expression in tumors		
1. miR-122-5p	+107.7	<0.0001
2. miR-210-3p	+10.2	<0.0001
3. miR-155-5p	+8.3	<0.0001
4. miR-34a-5p	+3.1	<0.0001
5. miR-146a-5p	+2.1	<0.0001
6. miR-106b-5p	+2.1	<0.0001
7. miR-342-3p	+1.9	<0.0001
8. miR-454-3p	+1.6	<0.0001
9. miR-28-5p	+1.5	<0.0001
10. miR-126-3p	+1.5	<0.0001
11. miR-340-5p	+1.5	<0.0001
12. miR-20-5p	+1.4	<0.0001
Decreased expression in tumors		
13. miR-129-1-3p	−17.0	<0.0001
14. miR-129-2-3p	−6.6	<0.0001
15. miR-200b-3p	−4.3	<0.0001
16. miR-370-3p	−2.6	<0.0001
17. miR-20b-5p	−2.4	<0.0001
18. miR-133a-3p	−2.2	0.0262
19. miR-154-5p	−2.1	<0.0001
20. miR-135b-5p	−2.0	0.0003
21. miR-27b-3p	−1.6	<0.0001
22. miR-543	−1.5	0.0337

(**A**) The expression of metabolic genes. (**B**) The expressions of microRNAs predicted to target metabolic genes. FC: fold change (the ratio between median expressions in tumor and control tissue samples); threshold = 1.3. $n = 60$ (RCC tumor samples), $n = 60$ (paired-matched control samples). Statistical analysis was performed using Wilcoxon matched-pairs signed rank test. MicroRNAs selected for functional analysis are bolded.

Since the negative correlation between expression of miRNAs and target genes is a potential indicator of their functional association [8], we next checked whether the expressions of miRNAs correlated with the expressions of the metabolic genes. To this end, we constructed correlation matrix (Table S3) and searched for miRNAs of which expressions correlated with the highest number of target genes. This analysis revealed that top microRNAs for which expressions negatively correlated with genes expressions (r Spearman < −0.5, $p < 0.05$) included miR-34a-5p (9 correlating genes), miR-106b-5p (11 correlating genes), miR-146a-5p (8 correlating genes), miR-155-5p (11 correlating genes), and miR-342-3p (10 correlating genes). These five miRNAs were next selected for functional analysis of their impact on RCC cells. In addition, we also selected miR-122-5p, which was the top upregulated miRNA in RCC tumors. The correlations between miR-122-5p and metabolic genes were weaker, but still statistically significant (r Spearman = −0.35 to −0.49, $p < 0.05$) (Figure 1B). Remarkably, altered expression of all metabolic genes, predicted as targets of the selected miRNAs, correlated with poor survival of RCC patients, suggesting their potential link with the progression of the disease (Figure 1C).

Basing on the assumption that the miRNAs the most strongly correlating with metabolic genes could have the greatest impact on cellular metabolism, we next evaluated the effects of the five miRNAs (miR-34a-5p, miR-106b-5p, miR-122-5p, miR-146a-5p, and miR-155-5p) on mRNA expression of metabolic genes (Figure 2A) that were predicted as possible targets for specific miRNAs (Table S1). For each miRNA, we analyzed only the expression of transcripts of which 3′UTRs possessed potential binding sites for this specific miRNA as indicated by the bioinformatic analysis. Transfections of miRNA mimics in two RCC-derived cell lines resulted in downregulation of GATM mRNA by miR-155-5p, GDA by miR-106b-5p and miR-146a-5p, and SUCLG2 by miR-146a-5p and miR-155-5p. In addition, miR-155-5p statistically significantly suppressed the expressions of GDA and PCCA in only one of the analyzed cell lines. In Caki-2 cells, the expression of ALDH5A1 was stimulated by miR-122-5p and miR-146a-5p, while the expression of ALDH6A1 was stimulated by miR-106b-5p and miR-122-5p. miR-342-3p concomitantly increased the expression of PCCA in both analyzed cell lines (Figure 2A).

We subsequently evaluated the effects of miRNAs on protein expressions of metabolic genes. Firstly, we checked whether miRNAs could interact with sequences predicted as miRNA response elements (MREs) in target transcripts. To this end, the predicted binding sites were cloned into luciferase reporter system, which was co-transfected into RCC cells with miRNA mimics or non-targeting control oligonucleotides (Figure 2B). We found that miR-155-5p significantly suppressed luciferase activity under control of MREs cloned from *GATM* and *SUCLG2* sequences, while miR-106b-5p and miR-146a-5p decreased luciferase activity of two MREs cloned from *GDA*. Remarkably, no changes in luciferase activity were found when miRNA mimics were co-transfected with the reporter constructs with mutated MREs of *GATM*, *SUCLG2*, and *GDA* (Figure S2). We also observed miR-155-5p-mediated suppression of luciferase activity under control of MRE cloned from *PCCA*; however, this effect was not specific as indicated by experiments with mutated binding sequences (Figure S2). In accordance with the effect of miR-146a-5p on *ALDH5A1* mRNA (Figure 2A), luciferase activity was also increased when MRE cloned from *ALDH5A1* was treated with miR-146a-5p mimic (Figure 2B). However, miRNA mimics did not affect the activity of empty reporter vector (Figure S2).

Finally, we analyzed the effects of miRNA mimics on the endogenous expression of proteins encoded by metabolic genes (Figure 2C). The expression of GATM was dramatically reduced by transfection with miR-155-5p in Caki-2 cells but not in KIJ265T cells (Figure S3). The expressions of ALDH5A1, ALDH6A1, and GDA proteins were not changed by transfection of the miRNA mimics (Western blots for these proteins are shown in Figure S3). Antibodies against PCCA gave non-specific signals and were, therefore, discarded from the analysis (Figure S3).

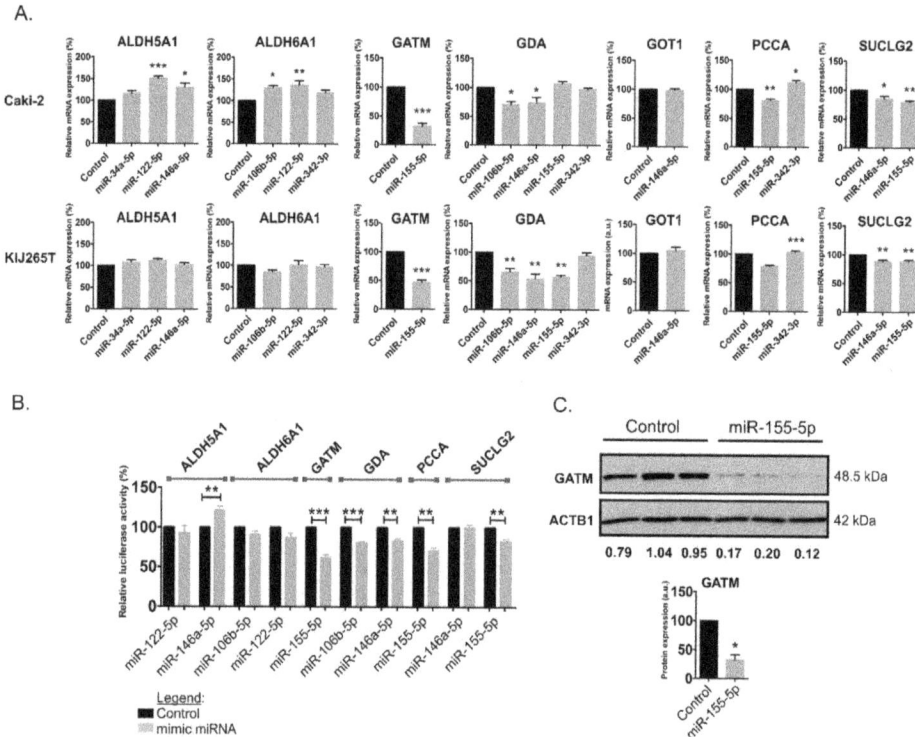

Figure 2. miRNA-mediated regulation of expressions of metabolically relevant genes. (**A**) The effects of miRNAs on mRNA expressions of metabolic genes predicted as potential miRNAs' targets. Caki-2 and KIJ265T cell lines were transfected using miRNA mimics or non-targeting scrambled control oligonucleotides and expression of target genes was evaluated using qPCR (quantitative real-time PCR). The plots show results of three independent biological experiments (exception: *GDA* expression in KIJ265T cells): for most miRNAs (except for miR-106b-5p) results of two independent experiments are shown; the expression of *GDA* in KIJ265T cell line was on the border of detection limit). Statistical analysis was performed using one-way ANOVA with Dunnett's Multiple Comparison Test, with exception of analysis of GATM and GOT1 for which t-test was used * $p < 0.05$, ** $p < 0.01$, *** $p < 0.001$. (**B**) The effects of miRNAs on the activity of luciferase reporter gene under control of cloned miRNA binding sites predicted in metabolic genes. Caki-2 cells were co-transfected with reporter plasmid bearing MRE (miRNA response element) for a given microRNA, and either microRNA mimic or non-targeting scrambled control oligonucleotides. The plots show results of three independent biological experiments. Statistical analysis was performed using Students t-test. (**C**) The effects of miR-155-5p on protein expressions of GATM in Caki-2 cells. Upper panel: Representative photographs of Western blots. Lower panel: Results of densitometric scanning of Western blots. The plot shows mean expression of GATM protein in three independent biological experiments performed in two-three replicates. * $p < 0.05$.

2.2. Metabolic miRNAs Affect Proliferation of RCC Cells and Correlate with Poor Survival of RCC Patients

Given the above-described findings, we next looked for potential associations between altered expression of miRNAs targeting metabolic genes and survival of RCC patients. Analysis of publicly available TCGA data revealed that high expression of miR-106b-5p, miR-155-5p, and miR-342-3p correlated with poor survival of RCC patients (Figure 3A). There was no statistically significant correlation between the expressions of miR-34a-5p, miR-122-5p, and miR-146a-5p and survival of patients. We subsequently analyzed the effects of metabolic miRNAs on the proliferation of RCC cells. Transfection of miR-106b-5p, miR-146a-5p, and miR-342-3p concomitantly stimulated proliferation in both analyzed RCC cell lines. The proliferation of cells transfected with miR-122-5p and miR-155-5p was also increased, although without statistical significance (Figure 3B).

These results indicate that altered expression of metabolically-relevant miRNAs could possibly contribute to cancer progression and shorten the survival time of RCC patients.

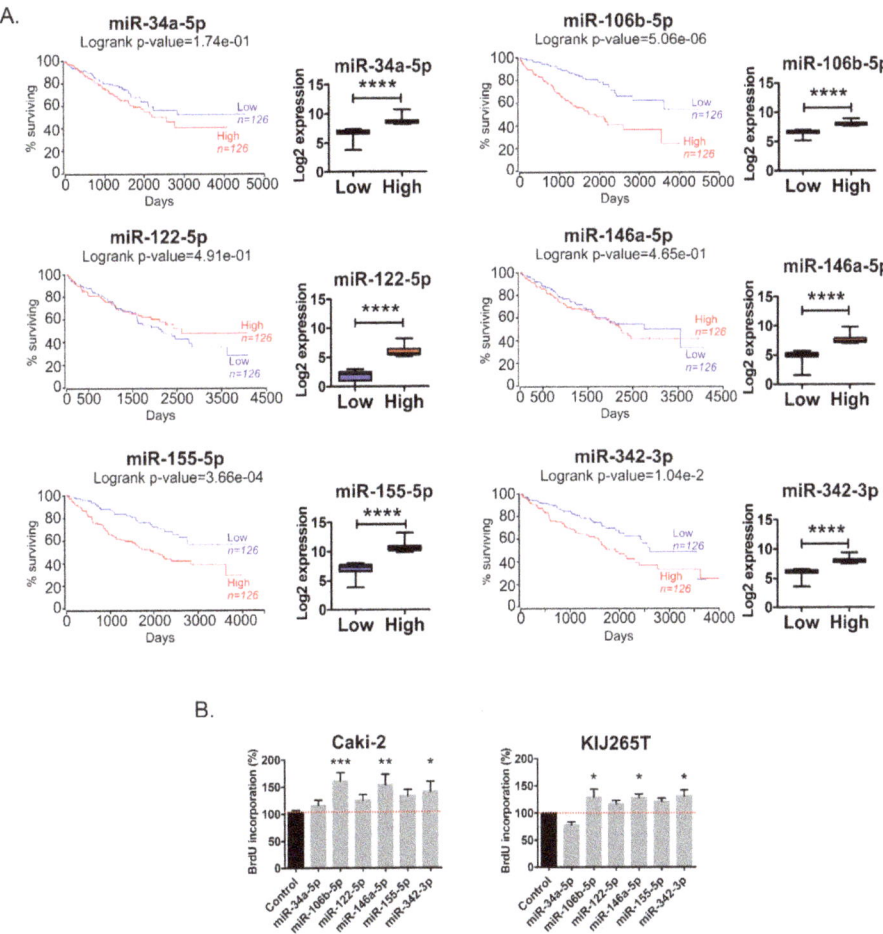

Figure 3. MicroRNAs effects on survival of RCC patients and proliferation of RCC cells. (**A**) Kaplan–Meier plots of RCC patients generated using OncoLnc tool and KIRC cohort of TCGA data. Patients were classified into Low and High expression groups basing on median miRNA expression data, which are shown on the graphs below the K-M plots. **** $p < 0.0001$; analysis was done using Mann–Whitney test. (**B**) The effects of microRNAs on proliferation of Caki-2 and KIJ265T cells. The plots show results of BrdU assay performed in three independent biological experiments. Statistical analysis was done using repeated measures ANOVA with Dunnett's Multiple Comparison post-test. * $p < 0.05$, ** $p < 0.01$, *** $p < 0.001$.

2.3. MiR-146a-5p is a Global Regulator of Key Metabolic Pathways in RCC

Next, we asked whether one specific miRNA could globally affect RCC metabolism. To answer this question, we implemented microarray analysis of RCC cells transfected with miR-146a-5p mimic or non-targeting control oligonucleotide. miR-146a-5p was selected for two reasons: firstly, it significantly stimulated proliferation of RCC cells (Figure 3B), indicating genuine reprogramming of cells functioning. Secondly, miR-146a-5p is the first miRNA for which functional interaction with TCA cycle was recently provided in vivo [9] and alterations of TCA cycle are a characteristic feature of RCC tumors [3]. The principal component analysis (PCA) and hierarchical clustering of RCC cells transfected with a miR-146a-5p mimic or non-targeting control oligonucleotide proved robustness of the obtained datasets and clear distinctiveness of compared groups (KIJ265T cell line transfected with miR-146a-5p mimic and transfected with non-targeting control oligonucleotide) (Figure 4A,B).

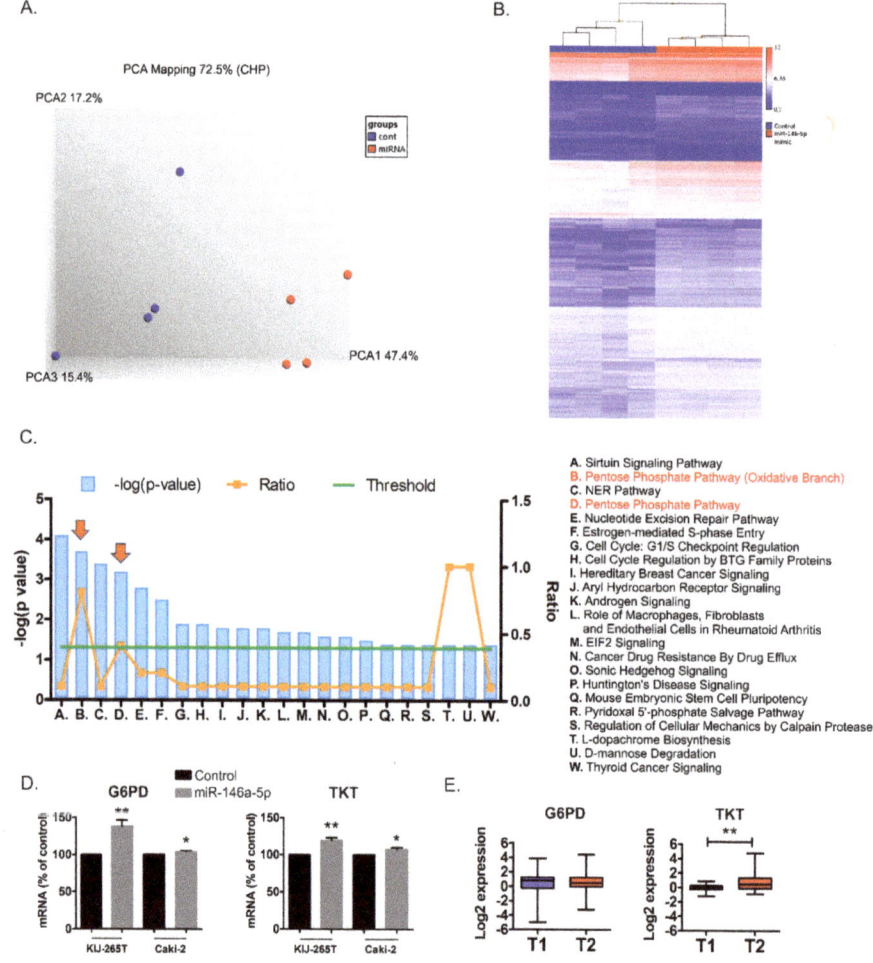

Figure 4. *Cont.*

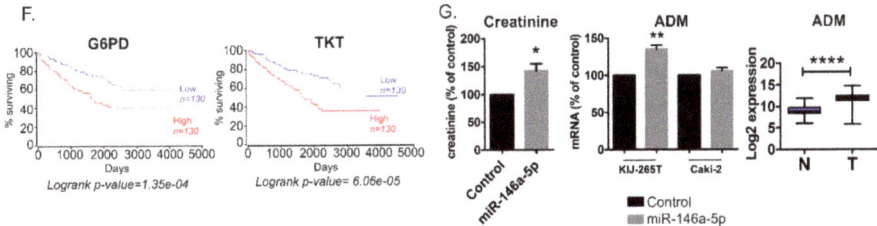

Figure 4. The effects of miR-146a-5p transfection in RCC cells. (**A**) Principal component analysis (PCA) of transcriptome data obtained from KIJ265T cell line transfected with miR-146a-5p mimic or non-targeting control oligonucleotide (Cont. (**B**) Hierarchical clustering based on differentially expressed genes generated using TAC 4.0. (**C**) Top pathways affected by miR-146a-5p transfection in RCC cells. The plot shows results of IPA Core Analysis performed on the genes affected by transfection of miR-146a-5p mimic (shown in Table S4). The overrepresented pathways are listed according to the –log (p value) (blue bars) (left y-axis). The threshold line (green) represents p value = 0.05. The ratio of the number of genes found in each pathway and the total number of genes in the pathway is shown in orange (right y-axis). PPP pathway is shown with arrows. (**D**) The expressions of genes involved in the pentose phosphate pathway (*G6PD*, *TKT*) are upregulated in RCC cells transfected with miR-146a-5p mimic. The effect of miR-146a-5p was analyzed in three independent biological experiments performed in triplicate. Statistical analysis was performed using t-test. * $p < 0.05$. ** $p < 0.01$. (**E**) The expression of *G6PD* and *TKT* in RCC tumors classified according to TNM system [1]. T1 ($n = 30$): tumors classified as Stages I and II (tumors limited to the kidney, with no signs of metastasis); T2 ($n = 30$): tumors classified as Stages III and IV (tumors which invade veins and neighboring structures as well as tumors with metastasis in lymph nodes or distant organs). Statistical analysis was performed using Mann–Whitney test. ** $p < 0.01$. (**F**) High expressions of *G6PD* and *TKT* correlate with poor survival of RCC patients. Kaplan–Meier plots of RCC patients were generated using OncoLnc tool and KIRC cohort of TCGA data. Patients were classified into Low and High expression groups basing on median gene expression data. (**G**) miR-146a-5p transfection increases creatinine levels in RCC cells. Left panel: The plot shows results of GC-MS analysis of RCC cells transfected with miR-146a-5p mimic or non-targeting control oligonucleotide. Middle panel: The expression of adrenomedullin (*ADM*) is increased in KIJ265T RCC cells transfected with miR-146a-5p mimic. Right panel: The expression of *ADM* is increased in RCC tumors (T, $n = 250$) when compared with control kidney samples (C, $n = 72$). The analysis was performed using publicly available transcriptomic data of TCGA consortium (KIRC cohort). Statistical analysis was performed using t-test. * $p < 0.05$. ** $p < 0.01$. **** $p < 0.0001$.

Transcriptome Analysis Console (TAC) software evaluation revealed the altered expression of 955 genes, including 810 up-regulated in 145-down-regulated transcripts (Table S4). TAC analysis revealed that miR-146a-5p affected the expressions of genes involved in the TCA cycle; the OXPHOS system in mitochondria; the pentose phosphate pathway (PPP); metabolism of amino acids, nucleotides, and glutathione; adipogenesis; fatty acids beta-oxidation; trans-sulfuration; and one-carbon metabolism (Table 2).

Both TAC (Table S5) and Ingenuity Pathway Analysis (Figure 4C) revealed that the pentose phosphate pathway was among the most altered metabolic pathways in miR-146a-5p transfected cells. qPCR validation confirmed that miR-146a-5p transfection induced expression of *G6PD* and *TKT*, two key genes encoding PPP enzymes (Figure 4D). The expression of *TKT* was higher in more advanced RCC tumors than in less advanced lesions. For *G6PD*, no statistically significant expression changes were observed (Figure 4E). Remarkably, high *TKT* and *G6PD* expressions in tumors significantly correlated with poor survival rates of RCC patients (Figure 4F), which may partially reflect the pro-proliferative effects of their stimulator, miR-146-5p. To analyze the impact of miR-146a-5p on metabolic profile of RCC cells, we performed GC-MS analysis of RCC cells transfected with the miR-146a-5p mimic. This analysis revealed increased levels of creatinine in KIJ265T cells transfected with miR-146a-5p when compared with those transfected with a non-targeting control oligonucleotide (Figure 4G). Interestingly, microarray analysis (Table S4) and qPCR validation in KIJ265T cells (Figure 4G) indicated that miR-146a-5p transfection caused upregulation of *ADM*, a gene encoding adrenomedullin which contributes to creatinine clearance [10–12], suggesting cellular response to increased creatinine levels. In Caki-2 cells, the expression of *ADM* was not statistically significantly changed following miR-146a-5p (Figure 4G). In accordance, GC-MS analysis revealed that creatinine levels were not statistically significantly changed in Caki-2 cells transfected with miR-146a-5p (not shown).

Table 2. miR-146a-5p affects expression of genes involved in key metabolic pathways. The table shows selected DEGs in RCC cells transfected with miR-146a-5p mimic, compared to cells transfected with non-targeting control oligonucleotide with functions in different metabolic pathways identified by biological pathway analysis with WikiPathways included in TAC 4.0.

Symbol	Entrez Gene Description	Metabolic Pathway	Fold Change	p-Value
ACO2	aconitase 2	TCA cycle, Amino acid metabolism, Metabolic reprogramming in colon cancer	1.53	3.40×10^{-3}
AHCY	Adenosylhomocysteinase	Trans-sulfuration pathway; Trans-sulfuration and one carbon metabolism	1.76	6.00×10^{-4}
ALDH1A1	aldehyde dehydrogenase 1 family member A1	Tryptophan metabolism	2.2	5.00×10^{-4}
CANT1	calcium activated nucleotidase 1	Pyrimidine metabolism	1.53	1.14×10^{-2}
CBS/CBSL	cystathionine-beta-synthase	Amino acid metabolism; Trans-sulfuration pathway; Trans-sulfuration and one carbon metabolism; One carbon metabolism and related pathways	1.57	2.00×10^{-4}
CEBPD	CCAAT enhancer binding protein delta	Adipogenesis	1.58	4.50×10^{-3}
CHDH	choline dehydrogenase	One carbon metabolism and related pathways	1.63	4.50×10^{-3}
CKB	creatine kinase B	Trans-sulfuration; Urea cycle and metabolism of amino groups	1.58	5.13×10^{-2}
CPT2	carnitine palmitoyltransferase 2	Fatty Acids Beta Oxidation	1.61	2.20×10^{-3}
DHODH	dihydroorotate dehydrogenase (quinone)	Pyrimidine metabolism	1.88	1.00×10^{-4}
DNMT3B	DNA methyltransferase 3 beta	Trans-sulfuration; Trans-sulfuration and one carbon metabolism; One carbon metabolism and related pathways	1.5	6.20×10^{-3}
E2F1	E2F transcription factor 1	Adipogenesis	1.82	9.00×10^{-4}
E2F4	E2F transcription factor 4	Adipogenesis	2.01	8.00×10^{-4}
ECHS1	enoyl-CoA hydratase, short chain 1	Fatty Acid Biosynthesis; Fatty Acid Beta oxidation; Tryptophan metabolism	1.55	1.29×10^{-2}
ECSIT	ECSIT signalling integrator	Mitochondrial complex I assembly model OXPHOS system	1.61	3.60×10^{-3}
ENTPD4	ectonucleoside triphosphate diphosphohydrolase 4	Pyrimidine metabolism	1.58	3.42×10^{-1}
ESRRA	estrogen related receptor alpha	Energy metabolism	1.69	1.00×10^{-4}
G6PD	glucose-6-phosphate dehydrogenase	Pentose Phosphate Pathway; Metabolic reprogramming in colon cancer; Glutathione metabolism	1.64	6.00×10^{-4}
GK	glycerol kinase	Fatty Acids Beta Oxidation	-1.75	4.30×10^{-3}
GPX4	glutathione peroxidase 4	One carbon metabolism and related pathways; Glutathion metabolism	1.82	3.40×10^{-3}
H6PD	hexose-6-phosphate dehydrogenase/glucose 1-dehydrogenase	Pentose Phosphate Pathway	1.72	4.40×10^{-3}
IDH2	isocitrate dehydrogenase (NADP (+)) 2, mitochondrial	TCA cycle; Metabolic reprogramming in colon cancer	1.91	9.25×10^{-5}
LMNA	lamin A/C	Adipogenesis	1.77	8.90×10^{-3}
LPIN3	lipin 3	Adipogenesis	2.13	2.30×10^{-3}
MEF2D	myocyte enhancer factor 2D	Adipogenesis; Energy metabolism	1.7	1.83×10^{-2}
MYBBP1A	MYB binding protein 1a	Energy metabolism	1.77	6.00×10^{-4}

Table 2. Cont.

Symbol	Entrez Gene Description	Metabolic Pathway	Fold Change	p-Value
NDUFAF8	NADH:ubiquinone oxidoreductase complex assembly factor 8	Electron Transport Chain (OXPHOS system in mitochondria)	1.55	8.00×10^{-4}
NDUFB7	NADH:ubiquinone oxidoreductase subunit B7	Electron Transport Chain (OXPHOS system in mitochondria); Mitochondrial complex I assembly model OXPHOS system	1.64	3.67×10^{-2}
NDUFS3	NADH:ubiquinone oxidoreductase core subunit S3	Electron Transport Chain (OXPHOS system in mitochondria); Mitochondrial complex I assembly model OXPHOS system	1.52	9.00×10^{-4}
PGAM5	PGAM family member 5, mitochondrial serine/threonine protein phosphatase	Metabolic reprogramming in colon cancer	1.52	1.20×10^{-2}
PGLS	6-phosphogluconolactonase	Pentose Phosphate Pathway	1.53	6.40×10^{-3}
PYCR2	pyrroline-5-carboxylate reductase 2	Metabolic reprogramming in colon cancer	1.5	6.00×10^{-3}
RAPGEF3	Rap guanine nucleotide exchange factor 3	Integration of energy metabolism	1.58	4.00×10^{-4}
SDHA	succinate dehydrogenase complex flavoprotein subunit A	Amino acid metablism; TCA cycle	1.52	2.60×10^{-2}
SEMA6B	semaphorin 6B	TCA cycle	1.5	1.60×10^{-3}
SHPK	sedoheptulokinase	Pentose Phosphate Pathway	1.63	4.00×10^{-4}
SOCS3	suppressor of cytokine signaling 3	Adipogenesis	1.53	1.28×10^{-2}
STK11	serine/threonine kinase 11	Integration of energy metabolism	1.69	6.00×10^{-4}
TKT	Transketolase	Pentose Phosphate Pathway; Metabolic reprogramming in colon cancer	1.56	2.00×10^{-3}

2.4. Metabolically-Relevant miRNAs Regulate the Expression of NFAT5

The fact that miR-146a-5p influenced the level of only one metabolite (creatinine) suggested that the combined action of several microRNAs may be required for reprogramming of cancer cell metabolism. In the search for such possible cooperative effects of miRNAs on RCC metabolism, we analyzed correlations between the expression of the 22 initially identified miRNAs and the levels of 54 metabolites in RCC tissue samples (Table S6). Strikingly, we found that miR-34a-5p, miR-106b-5, miR-122-5p, miR-146a-5p, and miR-155-5p were among the miRNAs with the highest number of correlating metabolites (Table S6). Furthermore, we found that expression of these microRNAs commonly correlated with similar metabolites. In particular, we found strong negative correlations (r Spearman ≤ -0.4, $p < 0.001$) between the expressions of all five microRNAs and the levels of *myo*-inositol (Figure 5A).

On the basis of these observations, we searched for the possible target genes that could mediate cooperative actions of miRNAs associated with metabolic changes in RCC tumors. To this end, we next selected miRNAs whose expression was most strongly negatively (r Spearman < -0.5) correlated with *myo*-inositol levels (Table S6), and searched for their potential target genes using the miRsystem platform that incorporates seven independent prediction algorithms [13]. Remarkably, we found *NFAT5* as the top gene, predicted to be commonly co-regulated by five out of seven analyzed microRNA: miR-106b-5p, miR-122-5p, miR-146a-5p, miR-155-5p, and miR-210-3p (Figure 5B and Table S7). Furthermore, we found that *NFAT5* expression in renal tumors is decreased (Figure 5C), which fits the profile of increased expression of the predicted targeting microRNAs. We also found strong negative correlations between the expression of *NFAT5* and the four predicted miRNAs in RCC tumor samples (Figure 5C) and other types of cancer (File S2). These results suggest that *NFAT5* could indeed be a common target of the miRNAs that affect *myo*-inositol levels in tumor tissues. Transfection with mimics of miR-106b-5p and miR-122-5p suppressed the expression of *NFAT5* in RCC cell line (Figure 5D). NFAT5 is an osmoprotective transcription factor that controls expression of genes that counteract signals inducing cell shrinkage during osmotic stress. The key NFAT5 targets are SLC5A3 (a *myo*-inositol transporter), SLC6A6 (a beta-alanine transporter), AKR1B1 (aldose reductase; catalyzes reduction of glucose to sorbitol), SLC14A2 (a urea transporter), and HSPA1B (a chaperone protecting cells against apoptosis induced by urea [14]. The expressions of most of these genes were decreased in renal tumors (Figure 5E). The only exception was *AKR1B1* for which expression was unaltered. Taken together, these results indicate that miRNA-mediated changes in NFAT5 expression could contribute to changed levels of osmolytes (e.g., *myo*-inositol) via altered expression of the proteins responsible for their transport in RCC cells.

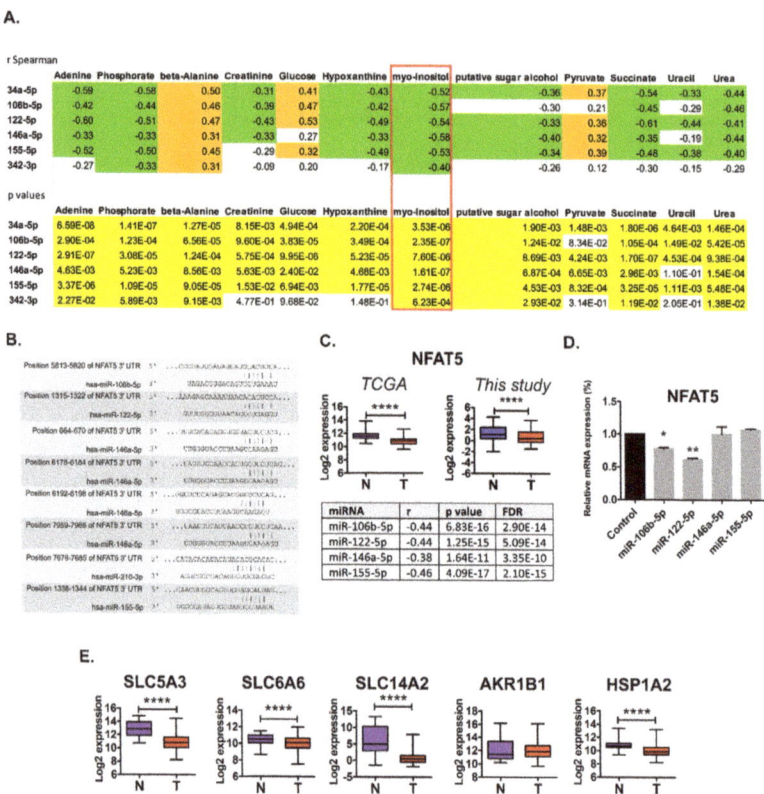

Figure 5. Osmoregulatory NFAT5 as a target of metabolically-relevant miRNAs in renal cancer. (**A**) Correlations between the expressions of microRNAs and metabolite levels in tissue samples from 70 control and RCC samples. Upper panel: Correlation coefficients. Orange: r Spearman > 0.3; green: r Spearman < −0.3. Lower panel: p values; yellow: $p < 0.05$. Full data of correlation analysis is given in Table S6. (**B**) The potential binding sites of miRNAs in *NFAT5* 3'UTR, predicted by TargetScan. (**C**) Upper panel: The expression of *NFAT5* is decreased in RCC tumors (TCGA cohort: T, $n = 250$; this study cohort: T, $n = 60$) when compared with control kidney samples (TCGA cohort: C, $n = 72$; this study cohort: C, $n = 60$). Statistical analysis was performed using t-test. **** < 0.0001. Lower panel: Negative correlations between the expressions of NFAT5 and the predicted microRNAs. Correlation analysis was performed using StarBase v2.0. on KIRC cohort of RCC patients ($n = 300$). For miR-210-3p, no data were available. (**D**) The expression of *NFAT5* mRNA is suppressed by miR-106b-5p and miR-122-5p in RCC cell line. Caki-2 cells were transfected with mimics of the respective microRNAs or non-targeting scrambled oligonucleotides. The plots show the results of three independent biological experiments. Statistical analysis was performed using repeated measures ANOVA with Dunnett's Multiple Comparison post-test. * $p < 0.05$, ** $p < 0.01$. (**E**) The expression of *NFAT5* target genes is decreased in RCC tumors (T, $n = 250$) when compared with control kidney samples (N, $n = 72$). The analysis was performed using publicly available transcriptomic data of TCGA consortium (KIRC cohort). Statistical analysis was performed using Students t-test. **** < 0.0001.

2.5. MiR-34a-5p, miR-106b-5p, miR-146a-5p and miR-155-5p Are PanCancer MetabomiRs

On the basis of the collected data presented above, we hypothesized that miRNAs identified in our study could be involved in global regulation of cancer metabolism. To this end, we searched for possible correlations between the expression of miR-34a-5p, miR-122-5p, miR-146a-5p, miR-155-5p, and miR-342-3p and their predicted target genes in the transcriptomes of 14 types of cancers in more than 6000 samples (Tables S8 and S9). Next, we selected miRNA targets of which expressions correlated in at least ten cancer types and performed PANTHER Functional Classification Test to find biological processes annotated to the analyzed genes (Figure 6A). Strikingly, "metabolic process" emerged at the top of annotated processes for most miRNAs targets. The only exception was miR-122-5p for which no gene targets were found which correlated in at least 10 cancer types. These results indicated that miR-34a-5p, miR-106b-5p, miR-146a-5p, and miR-155-5p could represent PanCancer metabo-miRs, involved in global regulation of cellular metabolism in cancer cells.

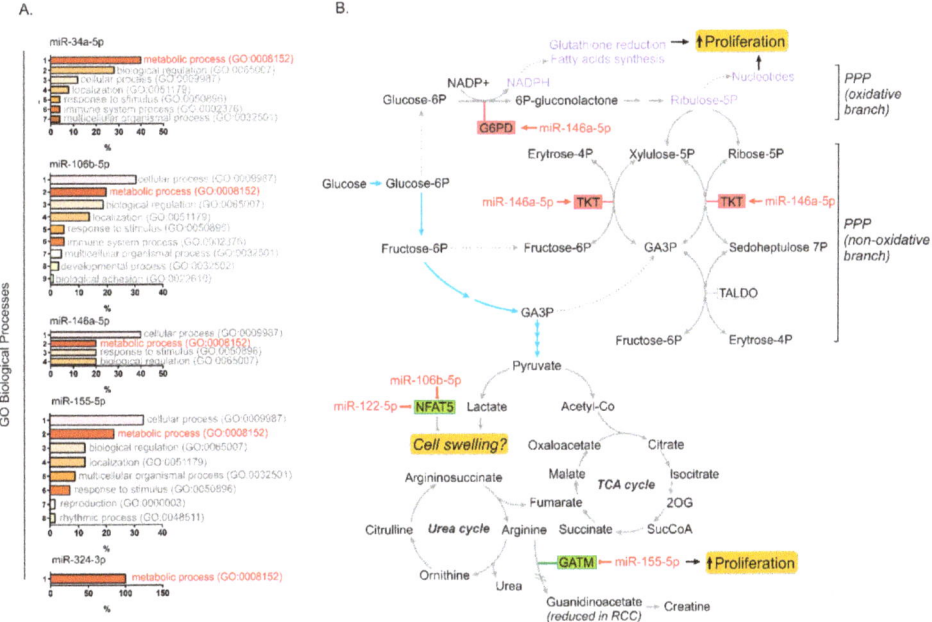

Figure 6. microRNA-mediated regulation of cancer metabolism. (**A**) Functional annotation of genes predicted as targets of microRNAs identified in our study in PanCancer analysis encompassing 14 cancer types and >6000 patients. Only genes for which expression correlated with a given microRNA in at least 10 cancer types were selected for the analysis. The list of genes is provided in Table S7. The plots show results of PANTHER Functional classification analysis according to GO Biological processes annotated to the predicted genes. (**B**) The model showing microRNAs affecting key metabolic pathways in RCC cells: miR-146a-5p upregulates key PPP genes (G6PD and TKT), thereby contributing to enhanced cancer cell proliferation; miR-155-5p suppresses the expressions of gene involved arginine metabolism (GATM); and miR-106b-5p and miR-122-5p may possibly counteract cell swelling induced by enhanced lactate production, by suppressing the expression of NFAT5, which governs the activity of genes encoding proteins transporting osmolytes (e.g., *myo*-inositol). Abbreviations: GA3P, glyceraldehyde-3-phosphate; 2OG, 2-oxoglutarate. Glycolysis is shown with blue arrows.

3. Discussion

In this paper, we present a group of microRNAs that regulate genes involved in key metabolic pathways and contribute to enhanced proliferation of renal cancer cells. We show that microRNAs can affect the RCC metabolome both directly (e.g., miR-155-5p targeting GATM) and indirectly, by cooperative regulation of the expression of NFAT5, a transcription factor governing the expression of transporters that control osmolality. We also show that miR-146a-5p globally affects the expression of genes involved in key metabolic pathways in RCC such as those associated with the PPP. Finally, the results of PanCancer analysis indicate that miR-34a-5p, miR-106b-5p, miR-146a-5p, miR-155-5p, and miR-342-3p may be involved in global regulation of metabolism in cancers of various origins.

Upregulation of the pentose phosphate pathway (PPP) is one of the key features of the dysregulated metabolism of RCC cells [15]. It enables efficient production of NADPH, utilized as a reducing agent contributing to redox homeostasis of cancer cells, and ribose-5-phosphate, required to support the high rates of nucleotide synthesis during intensive malignant proliferation [16] (Figure 6B). G6PD is a rate-limiting enzyme of the PPP and its inhibition attenuates survival of RCC cells [17]. We found that miR-146a-5p stimulated the expression of *G6PD* and *TKT*, the genes encoding two key enzymes of the oxidative and non-oxidative PPP branches, respectively. Interestingly, it was shown that transketolase (TKT) activity correlates with creatinine levels in uremic patients [18], which may possibly partially explain the observation that creatinine levels increased following miR-146a-5p transfection. Remarkably, other reports also demonstrated that creatinine concentrations can be affected by miRNAs [19,20]. Most metabolic genes affected by miR-146a-5p transfection exhibited upregulated gene expression (Table 2). This suggests that miR-146a-5p-mediated transcriptomic effects were not direct. Possible mediatory mechanisms may include activation of transcription regulators (e.g., E2F4 and NCOR2), mRNA processing factors or the suppression of inhibitory microRNAs (e.g., miR-29a) (Table S3). However, the exact mechanisms mediating miR-146a-5p-induced upregulation of gene expression remains to be delineated in the future.

GATM (*AGAT*) encodes glycine amidinotransferase, a mitochondrial enzyme that catalyzes the transfer of a guanido group from L-arginine to glycine, resulting in guanidinoacetic acid, which is a substrate for creatine synthesis. Suppressed expression of GATM in RCC tumors [4] is in line with recent findings of decreased excretion of guanidinoacetate (GAA) in RCC patients [21]. Interestingly, several studies have demonstrated that creatine inhibits growth of tumor cells both in vitro and in vivo [22–24]. The exact mechanism by which creatine attenuates cancer growth is unknown; however, possible mechanisms include inhibition of glycolysis or generation of acidosis [25]. It may thus be hypothesized that miR-155-5p-mediated downregulation of GATM in RCC cells may lead to a reduction of intracellular creatine pool, thereby preventing its anticancer activities. A possible tumor-suppressive role of GATM is supported by the fact that its low expression correlates with poor survival rates of RCC patients (Figure 1C). By contrast, high expression of miR-155-5p, which downregulates GATM, correlates with poor prognosis for RCC patients (Figure 3). We did not see the suppression of GATM protein by miR-155-5p in KIJ265T cells (Figure S3). This observation is in agreement with previous studies that showed that miR-155 regulates gene expression in a cell-type specific manner [26,27].

Intensive proliferation and metabolic activation of cells lead to osmotic stress which results from enhanced consumption of metabolites that function as intracellular osmolytes, such as *myo*-inositol or amino acids [28]. Our results suggest that enhanced expression of microRNAs, in particular miR-106b-5p and miR-122-5p, may contribute to osmotic stress by inhibiting the expression of *NFAT5*, a transcription factor that regulates gene expression in response to osmotic challenge [14,29]. Mammalian cells exposed to hypertonic environment respond by releasing water, and activating NFAT5, which in turn leads to accumulation of intracellular organic osmolytes, i.e., betaine, taurine, and *myo*-inositol [29]. NFAT5 is also involved in the regulation of cell survival, migration, proliferation and angiogenesis [29]. Furthermore, the possible role of NFAT5 in cancer is supported by the fact that genes encoding proteins involved in the transport of osmoregulators are markers of the cancer phenotype [30].

NFAT5 plays different functions during cancer development and progression. In melanoma cells, it stimulates invasion [31], while in thymoma it promotes T cells proliferation and activation [32]. In hepatocellular carcinoma, NFAT5 functions as a tumor suppressor and promotes apoptosis with concomitant inhibition of cell cycle progression [33]. *NFAT5* expression is regulated by multiple microRNAs, including miR-211 in melanoma [31]; miR-641 in glioma [34]; miR-1b, miR-106a, and miR-363-3p in differentiating Th17 cells [35]; miR-22 in colon cancer [36]; and miR-568 during Treg cells activation [37]. Furthermore, NFAT5 is a target of a group of osmoresponsive miRNAs that regulate its expression during osmoadaptation in mice [38]. During cell growth, NFAT5 regulates cell volume [28], which is influenced by constant changes in extracellular and intracellular osmolality. Changes in cell volume may affect concentrations of key signaling molecules, thereby influencing proliferation, migration, and cell death [39]. Persistent changes in cell volume can lead to necrotic volume increase (NVI) and finally to cell death [40]. The key molecular features of RCC pathology are metabolic reprogramming associated with enhanced lactate production and activation of hypoxia-induced signaling pathways [3]. Remarkably, both intracellular lactate accumulation and hypoxia can stimulate cell swelling [40–42]. Depletion of intracellular *myo*-inositol is a well-known mechanism that counteracts cell swelling [43,44]. Reduction of *myo*-inositol levels in the kidney may result from its reduced uptake by transporting proteins such as SLC5A3 [45]. It may thus be hypothesized that microRNA-induced changes in expression of NFAT5 and the resulting reduced expression of *myo*-inositol transporter may represent a mechanism which protects RCC cells against cell swelling-induced death.

Our study took advantage of the publicly available data of the PanCancer project [46]. This initiative of the TCGA consortium aims to analyze similarities and differences between different tumor types and tissue sites of origin. Since its launch in 2012, the PanCancer project has resulted in plethora of novel findings, including the importance of cell-of-origin in tumor pathology [47], development of clinical outcome endpoints recommended for 33 cancer types [48], new clustering of tumor types that may be implemented in future clinical trials [49], information on potential targets for new combinations therapies [50], and the collection of digitalized histopathological sections from more than 11,000 patients [51] that are already used for creation of new bioinformatic diagnostic tools. Since it was recently revealed that PanCancer metabolic profiling allows for prediction of responses to therapy [52], we hope that the results of our study will bring the basis for future research focused on finding better therapeutic options of RCC patients.

4. Materials and Methods

4.1. Tissue Samples

Ninety-five RCC tumor tissue samples and 95 matched-paired non-tumorous control kidney samples (190 tissue samples in total) were from the local Tissue Bank stored at $-80\,°C$ at the Department of Biochemistry and Molecular Biology, Centre of Postgraduate Medical Education. Collection of tissue samples was performed under approval of the Bioethical Committee of Centre of Postgraduate Medical Education (No. 18/PB/2012 and No. 75/PB-A/2014), with written informed consent obtained from patients.

4.2. Cell Lines

Caki-2 cell line was purchased from ATCC (Manassas, VA, USA). KIJ-265T cell line was a kind gift of Dr. John A. Copland and Mayo Foundation for Medical Education and Research (Rochester, MN, USA). Both cell lines were cultured in accordance with providers' instructions.

4.3. Transfections

The cells were seeded on 12-well, 6-well or 60-mm plates in complete medium and cultured for 24 h. Transfections were performed as described previously [6] using miRCURY LNA microRNA mimics/inhibitors or control oligonucleotides provided in Table S10.

4.4. Isolations of RNA and Proteins, Reverse Transcription

They were performed as previously described [6]. qPCR array analysis using Custom Panel (Roche Diagnostics, Mannheim, Germany) and Pick&Mix microRNA PCR Panels (Exiqon, Vedbaek, Denmark) were performed as previously [4,6]. Primers and probes for qPCR reactions are given in Tables S11 and S12. The expression of microRNAs in tissue samples was normalized against miR-103a-3p, for which stable expression was confirmed (Figure S4).

4.5. Cloning of miRNA Targets Sites and Luciferase Assays

They were performed using pmiRGLO reporter vector as provided in our previous study [6]. Sequences of oligonucleotides used for cloning of miRNA target sites are provided in Table S13.

4.6. Western Blots

WB were performed as in a previous study [53]. Details on antibodies and dilutions are given in Table S14.

4.7. Analysis of Proliferation

Proliferation of RCC cells was analyzed using BrdU assay (Roche Diagnostics, Mannheim, Germany) and an earlier described procedure [53].

4.8. Transcriptomic Analysis

For transcriptomic analysis, we used RNA isolated from four independent wells of a 12-well plate, transfected with miR-146a-5p mimic, and four independent wells of a 12-well plate, transfected with non-targeting control oligonucleotide. Microarray analysis was performed using Affymetrix Gene Atlas System according to the manufacturer's instructions. Briefly, 150 ng of total RNA that passed initial quality control screen (2100 Bioanalyzer, Agilent, Santa Clara, CA, USA) was used for target preparation using the GeneChip™ WT PLUS Reagent Kit (ThermoFisher Scientific, Waltham, MA, USA). Prepared samples were hybridized to the Affymetrix™ HuGene 2.1 ST Array Strips (Affymetrix, Santa Clara, CA, USA). Arrays after washing and staining, were scanned in Gene Atlas Imaging Station (Affymetrix) with .CEL files as data output. Data analysis was performed using Transcriptome Analysis Console (TAC) Software 4.0 (ThermoFisher) and Ingenuity Pathway Analysis Software (IPA, QIAGEN Bioinformatics, Hilden, Germany). After importing Human Gene 2.1 ST .CEL files into TAC 4.0, the array data were normalized by the RMA method. The probe summarization and the microarray quality control were done with TAC 4.0 according to the manufacturer's instructions. In the next step, TAC 4.0 one-way ANOVA was utilized to determine differentially expressed genes (DEGs) between treatment and control: KIJ265T cell line transfected with miR-146a-5p mimic or transfected with non-targeting control oligonucleotide, respectively. To minimize the variability originating from different sample preparation dates in a comparison analysis, TAC 4.0 batch effect was applied. The criteria for selecting DEGs were fold change ≤ -1.5 or fold change ≥ 1.5 and p value ≤ 0.05. Further bioinformatic analyses were performed with TAC 4.0 and Ingenuity Pathway Analysis Software (IPA, Qiagen Bioinformatics). The results of microarray analysis were validated using qPCR. To validate microarrays experiments, transfections with miR-146a-5p and non-targeting control oligonucleotides were repeated three times on independent days. Each day, transfections were performed using three wells of a 12-well plate for miR-146a-5p mimic and three wells of a 12-well plate for control oligonucleotide.

4.9. Metabolomic Analysis

Cells were cultured in medium without phenol red. Then, 72 h after transfection, cells were washed five times with PBS and metabolites were extracted with 1 mL of 1:3 methanol: MTBE extraction buffer containing internal standards (500 ng of 1,2-diheptadecanoyl-sn-glycero-3-phosphocholine (Avanti Polar Lipids, 850360P) and 500 ng of ^{13}C sorbitol. Metabolite profiling was performed using a gas chromatography mass spectrometer (GC-MS) as earlier described [4]. To measure cellular proteins, the cell residues were resuspended in 0.1 M NaOH containing 0.125% Triton X-100 [54].

4.10. Bioinformatics Analysis

Prediction of microRNAs targeting genes involved in metabolic pathways was performed using miRSystem (http://mirsystem.cgm.ntu.edu.tw/microrna.org [13]), TargetScan [55] and literature search according to the criteria described in File S1. miRsystem parameters were defined to include validated genes greater than or equal to 3 and O/E ratio greater than or equal to 2. Survival analysis was performed using OncoLnc tool (f http://www.oncolnc.org) [56] and SurvExpress (http://bioinformatica.mty.itesm.mx:8080/Biomatec/SurvivaX.jsp) [57] using KIRC cohorts of TCGA transcriptomic data. The expressions of ADM, NFAT5 and its target genes were analyzed using FireBrowse RESTful API visual interface (http://firebrowse.org/api/api-docs, api version: 1.1.38) on KIRC cohort data. Analysis of correlations between NFAT5 and miRNAs was performed using StarBase v2.0. on PanCancer data involving 14 types of cancer [58].

4.11. Statistical Analysis

Data distribution was analyzed using Shapiro–Wilk test. Statistical significance of two groups of data was analyzed using t-test, Wilcoxon matched-pairs signed rank test or Mann–Whitney test. Correlations were analyzed using Spearman r or Pearson r, depending on data distribution. Analysis of more than two groups of data was performed using one-way ANOVA with Dunnett's Multiple Comparison Test. $p < 0.05$ was considered statistically significant. Statistical analyses were done using GraphPad Prism 5.00 for Windows.

5. Conclusions

We found that increased expression of microRNAs in renal cancer contributes to disturbed expression of key genes involved in the regulation of RCC metabolome. The correlations between microRNAs expression and the profiles of RCC metabolites suggest that changes in expression of small non-coding microRNAs may contribute to the metabolic reprogramming and osmoregulation in renal tumors. In particular, miR-146a-5p and miR-155-5p emerge as a key "metabomiRs" that target genes of crucial metabolic pathways (PPP, TCA cycle, arginine metabolism) in RCC, while enhanced expression of miR-106b-5p may contribute to dysregulation of osmotic control in renal cancer cells. The fact that altered expressions of miR-106b-5p, miR-155-5p, and miR-342-3p correlate with poor survival of RCC patients strengthens their significance as oncogenic microRNAs in RCC. Finally, the results of our study indicate that miR-34a-5p, miR-106b-5p, miR-146a-5p, miR-155-5p, and miR-342-3p are PanCancer metabomiRs that may be involved in global regulation of cancer metabolism.

Supplementary Materials: The following are available online at http://www.mdpi.com/2072-6694/11/12/1825/s1: Table S1: Selection of 20 genes for validation analysis performed in this study. Table S2: Preliminary analysis of expression of 90 microRNAs predicted to target genes involved in metabolic pathways in RCC tumor tissues. Table S3: Analysis of correlations between the expressions of miRNAs and their predicted target genes. Table S4: The results of microarray analysis of KIJ265T cells transfected with miR-146a-5p mimic or non-targeting control oligonucleotide. (XLSX). Table S5: Pathways enriched in KIJ265T cells transfected with miR-146a-5p mimic compared to cells transfected with control oligonucleotide. Table S6: Analysis of correlations between the expressions of miRNAs and levels of metabolites in RCC tissue samples. Table S7: The search for genes commonly targeted by miRNAs for which expressions correlated with myo-inositol levels in RCC tissue samples. Table S8: PanCancer analysis of correlations between the expression of microRNAs and their target genes. Table S9: Analysis of correlations between the expressions of microRNAs and their predicted target genes. Table S10: microRNA mimics, inhibitors, and control oligonucleotides used for transfections. Table S11: qPCR primers. (DOCX). Table S12: microRNA LNA primers used in the study. Table S13: Oligonucleotides used for cloning of miRNA target sites. (DOCX). Table S14: Antibodies used in Western blots. (DOCX). Figure S1: The expression profiles of metabolically relevant genes predicted as targets for microRNAs in two groups of patients stratified into "Low" ($n = 130$) and "High" ($n = 130$) expression groups. Figure S2: The activity of luciferase reporter system under control of mutated MREs cloned from metabolic genes. Figure S3: Western blot analysis of proteins encoded by metabolic genes in RCC cells transfected with predicted miRNA mimics or scrambled non-targeting control oligonucleotide. Figure S4: The expression of miR-103a-3p in tissue samples. File S1: Criteria used for selection of miRNAs targeting genes involved in metabolic regulation. (DOCX). File S2: The expression of NFAT5 correlates with expression of the predicted regulatory miRNAs in cancers.

Author Contributions: Conceptualization, A.P.-W.; methodology, A.R.F. and M.K.; validation, J.B. and P.P.; formal analysis, A.P.-W., A.R.F., S.A., M.K., J.B., and P.P.; investigation, J.B., P.P., S.A., R.I.-N., M.K., B.R., H.K., K.G., and K.H.; resources, Z.T.; data curation, J.B., P.P., A.R.F., S.A., M.K., and A.P.-W.; writing—original draft preparation, A.P.-W.; writing—review and editing, all authors.; visualization, A.P.-W.; supervision, A.R.F., M.K., and A.P.-W.; project administration, A.P.-W.; and funding acquisition, J.B., A.R.F., and A.P.-W.

Funding: This research was funded by National Science Centre, Poland, grant number 2014/13/B/NZ5/00283 (to A.P.-W.) and The Polpharma Scientific Foundation's grant (to J.B.). S.A. and A.R.F. acknowledge funding of the PlantaSYST project by the European Union's Horizon 2020 research and innovation program (SGA-CSA Nos. 664621 and 739582 under FPA No. 664620).

Acknowledgments: The authors wish to thank John. A. Copland for providing KIJ265T cell line.

Conflicts of Interest: The authors declare no conflict of interest.

References

1. Ljungberg, B.; Bensalah, K.; Canfield, S.; Dabestani, S.; Hofmann, F.; Hora, M.; Kuczyk, M.A.; Lam, T.; Marconi, L.; Merseburger, A.S.; et al. EAU guidelines on renal cell carcinoma: 2014 update. *Eur. Urol.* **2015**, *67*, 913–924. [CrossRef] [PubMed]
2. Albiges, L.; Choueiri, T.; Escudier, B.; Galsky, M.; George, D.; Hofmann, F.; Lam, T.; Motzer, R.; Mulders, P.; Porta, C.; et al. A systematic review of sequencing and combinations of systemic therapy in metastatic renal cancer. *Eur. Urol.* **2015**, *67*, 100–110. [CrossRef] [PubMed]
3. Wettersten, H.I.; Aboud, O.A.; Lara, P.N., Jr.; Weiss, R.H. Metabolic reprogramming in clear cell renal cell carcinoma. *Nat. Rev. Nephrol.* **2017**, *13*, 410–419. [CrossRef] [PubMed]
4. Poplawski, P.; Tohge, T.; Boguslawska, J.; Rybicka, B.; Tanski, Z.; Trevino, V.; Fernie, A.R.; Piekielko-Witkowska, A. Integrated transcriptomic and metabolomic analysis shows that disturbances in metabolism of tumor cells contribute to poor survival of RCC patients. *Biochim. Biophys. Acta Mol. Basis Dis.* **2017**, *1863*, 744–752. [CrossRef] [PubMed]
5. Chandrasekaran, K.; Karolina, D.S.; Sepramaniam, S.; Armugam, A.; Wintour, E.M.; Bertram, J.F.; Jeyaseelan, K. Role of microRNAs in kidney homeostasis and disease. *Kidney Int.* **2012**, *81*, 617–627. [CrossRef] [PubMed]
6. Boguslawska, J.; Rodzik, K.; Poplawski, P.; Kedzierska, H.; Rybicka, B.; Sokol, E.; Tanski, Z.; Piekielko-Witkowska, A. TGF-beta1 targets a microRNA network that regulates cellular adhesion and migration in renal cancer. *Cancer Lett.* **2018**, *412*, 155–169. [CrossRef]
7. Morris, M.R.; Latif, F. The epigenetic landscape of renal cancer. *Nat. Rev. Nephrol.* **2017**, *13*, 47–60. [CrossRef]
8. Wang, Y.P.; Li, K.B. Correlation of expression profiles between microRNAs and mRNA targets using NCI-60 data. *BMC Genomics* **2009**, *10*, 218. [CrossRef]
9. Heggermont, W.A.; Papageorgiou, A.P.; Quaegebeur, A.; Deckx, S.; Carai, P.; Verhesen, W.; Eelen, G.; Schoors, S.; van Leeuwen, R.; Alekseev, S.; et al. Inhibition of MicroRNA-146a and Overexpression of Its Target Dihydrolipoyl Succinyltransferase Protect Against Pressure Overload-Induced Cardiac Hypertrophy and Dysfunction. *Circulation* **2017**, *136*, 747–761. [CrossRef]
10. Mori, Y.; Nishikimi, T.; Kobayashi, N.; Ono, H.; Kangawa, K.; Matsuoka, H. Long-term adrenomedullin infusion improves survival in malignant hypertensive rats. *Hypertension* **2002**, *40*, 107–113. [CrossRef]
11. Nishikimi, T.; Mori, Y.; Kobayashi, N.; Tadokoro, K.; Wang, X.; Akimoto, K.; Yoshihara, F.; Kangawa, K.; Matsuoka, H. Renoprotective effect of chronic adrenomedullin infusion in Dahl salt-sensitive rats. *Hypertension* **2002**, *39*, 1077–1082. [CrossRef] [PubMed]
12. Nishikimi, T.; Yoshihara, F.; Kanazawa, A.; Okano, I.; Horio, T.; Nagaya, N.; Yutani, C.; Matsuo, H.; Matsuoka, H.; Kangawa, K. Role of increased circulating and renal adrenomedullin in rats with malignant hypertension. *Am. J. Physiol. Regul. Integr. Comp. Physiol.* **2001**, *281*, R2079–R2087. [CrossRef] [PubMed]
13. Lu, T.P.; Lee, C.Y.; Tsai, M.H.; Chiu, Y.C.; Hsiao, C.K.; Lai, L.C.; Chuang, E.Y. miRSystem: An integrated system for characterizing enriched functions and pathways of microRNA targets. *PLoS ONE* **2012**, *7*, e42390. [CrossRef] [PubMed]
14. Ho, S.N. The role of NFAT5/TonEBP in establishing an optimal intracellular environment. *Arch Biochem. Biophys.* **2003**, *413*, 151–157. [CrossRef]

15. The Cancer Genome Atlas Research Network. Comprehensive molecular characterization of clear cell renal cell carcinoma. *Nature* **2013**, *499*, 43–49. [CrossRef] [PubMed]
16. Pinthus, J.H.; Whelan, K.F.; Gallino, D.; Lu, J.P.; Rothschild, N. Metabolic features of clear-cell renal cell carcinoma: Mechanisms and clinical implications. *Can. Urol. Assoc. J.* **2011**, *5*, 274–282. [CrossRef] [PubMed]
17. Lucarelli, G.; Galleggiante, V.; Rutigliano, M.; Sanguedolce, F.; Cagiano, S.; Bufo, P.; Lastilla, G.; Maiorano, E.; Ribatti, D.; Giglio, A.; et al. Metabolomic profile of glycolysis and the pentose phosphate pathway identifies the central role of glucose-6-phosphate dehydrogenase in clear cell-renal cell carcinoma. *Oncotarget* **2015**, *6*, 13371–13386. [CrossRef]
18. Markkanen, T.; Peltola, O.; Forsstrom, J.; Himanen, P. Pentose phosphate pathway of erythrocytes in uremia. *Acta Haematol.* **1972**, *48*, 269–277. [CrossRef]
19. Liu, L.; Pang, X.L.; Shang, W.J.; Xie, H.C.; Wang, J.X.; Feng, G.W. Over-expressed microRNA-181a reduces glomerular sclerosis and renal tubular epithelial injury in rats with chronic kidney disease via down-regulation of the TLR/NF-kappaB pathway by binding to CRY1. *Mol. Med.* **2018**, *24*, 49. [CrossRef]
20. Wei, Q.; Sun, H.; Song, S.; Liu, Y.; Liu, P.; Livingston, M.J.; Wang, J.; Liang, M.; Mi, Q.S.; Huo, Y.; et al. MicroRNA-668 represses MTP18 to preserve mitochondrial dynamics in ischemic acute kidney injury. *J. Clin. Invest* **2018**, *128*, 5448–5464. [CrossRef]
21. Monteiro, M.S.; Barros, A.S.; Pinto, J.; Carvalho, M.; Pires-Luis, A.S.; Henrique, R.; Jeronimo, C.; Bastos, M.L.; Gil, A.M.; Guedes de Pinho, P. Nuclear Magnetic Resonance metabolomics reveals an excretory metabolic signature of renal cell carcinoma. *Sci. Rep.* **2016**, *6*, 37245. [CrossRef] [PubMed]
22. Campos-Ferraz, P.L.; Gualano, B.; das Neves, W.; Andrade, I.T.; Hangai, I.; Pereira, R.T.; Bezerra, R.N.; Deminice, R.; Seelaender, M.; Lancha, A.H. Exploratory studies of the potential anti-cancer effects of creatine. *Amino Acids* **2016**, *48*, 1993–2001. [CrossRef] [PubMed]
23. Kristensen, C.A.; Askenasy, N.; Jain, R.K.; Koretsky, A.P. Creatine and cyclocreatine treatment of human colon adenocarcinoma xenografts: 31P and 1H magnetic resonance spectroscopic studies. *Br. J. Cancer* **1999**, *79*, 278–285. [CrossRef] [PubMed]
24. Miller, E.E.; Evans, A.E.; Cohn, M. Inhibition of rate of tumor growth by creatine and cyclocreatine. *Proc. Natl. Acad. Sci. USA* **1993**, *90*, 3304–3308. [CrossRef] [PubMed]
25. Patra, S.; Ghosh, A.; Roy, S.S.; Bera, S.; Das, M.; Talukdar, D.; Ray, S.; Wallimann, T.; Ray, M. A short review on creatine-creatine kinase system in relation to cancer and some experimental results on creatine as adjuvant in cancer therapy. *Amino Acids* **2012**, *42*, 2319–2330. [CrossRef]
26. Hsin, J.P.; Lu, Y.; Loeb, G.B.; Leslie, C.S.; Rudensky, A.Y. The effect of cellular context on miR-155-mediated gene regulation in four major immune cell types. *Nat. Immunol.* **2018**, *19*, 1137–1145. [CrossRef]
27. Nam, J.W.; Rissland, O.S.; Koppstein, D.; Abreu-Goodger, C.; Jan, C.H.; Agarwal, V.; Yildirim, M.A.; Rodriguez, A.; Bartel, D.P. Global analyses of the effect of different cellular contexts on microRNA targeting. *Mol. Cell* **2014**, *53*, 1031–1043. [CrossRef]
28. Ho, S.N. Intracellular water homeostasis and the mammalian cellular osmotic stress response. *J. Cell Physiol.* **2006**, *206*, 9–15. [CrossRef]
29. Halterman, J.A.; Kwon, H.M.; Wamhoff, B.R. Tonicity-independent regulation of the osmosensitive transcription factor TonEBP (NFAT5). *Am. J. Physiol. Cell Physiol.* **2012**, *302*, C1–C8. [CrossRef]
30. Shorthouse, D.; Riedel, A.; Kerr, E.; Pedro, L.; Bihary, D.; Samarajiwa, S.; Martins, C.P.; Shields, J.; Hall, B.A. Exploring the role of stromal osmoregulation in cancer and disease using executable modelling. *Nat. Commun.* **2018**, *9*, 3011. [CrossRef]
31. Levy, C.; Khaled, M.; Iliopoulos, D.; Janas, M.M.; Schubert, S.; Pinner, S.; Chen, P.H.; Li, S.; Fletcher, A.L.; Yokoyama, S.; et al. Intronic miR-211 assumes the tumor suppressive function of its host gene in melanoma. *Mol. Cell* **2010**, *40*, 841–849. [CrossRef] [PubMed]
32. Xin, Y.; Cai, H.; Lu, T.; Zhang, Y.; Yang, Y.; Cui, Y. miR-20b Inhibits T Cell Proliferation and Activation via NFAT Signaling Pathway in Thymoma-Associated Myasthenia Gravis. *Biomed. Res. Int.* **2016**, *2016*, 9595718. [CrossRef] [PubMed]
33. Qin, X.; Li, C.; Guo, T.; Chen, J.; Wang, H.T.; Wang, Y.T.; Xiao, Y.S.; Li, J.; Liu, P.; Liu, Z.S.; et al. Upregulation of DARS2 by HBV promotes hepatocarcinogenesis through the miR-30e-5p/MAPK/NFAT5 pathway. *J. Exp. Clin. Cancer Res.* **2017**, *36*, 148. [CrossRef] [PubMed]

34. Hinske, L.C.; Heyn, J.; Hubner, M.; Rink, J.; Hirschberger, S.; Kreth, S. Intronic miRNA-641 controls its host Gene's pathway PI3K/AKT and this relationship is dysfunctional in glioblastoma multiforme. *Biochem. Biophys. Res. Commun.* **2017**, *489*, 477–483. [CrossRef] [PubMed]
35. Kastle, M.; Bartel, S.; Geillinger-Kastle, K.; Irmler, M.; Beckers, J.; Ryffel, B.; Eickelberg, O.; Krauss-Etschmann, S. microRNA cluster 106a~363 is involved in T helper 17 cell differentiation. *Immunology* **2017**, *152*, 402–413. [CrossRef] [PubMed]
36. Alvarez-Diaz, S.; Valle, N.; Ferrer-Mayorga, G.; Lombardia, L.; Herrera, M.; Dominguez, O.; Segura, M.F.; Bonilla, F.; Hernando, E.; Munoz, A. MicroRNA-22 is induced by vitamin D and contributes to its antiproliferative, antimigratory and gene regulatory effects in colon cancer cells. *Hum. Mol. Genet.* **2012**, *21*, 2157–2165. [CrossRef]
37. Li, W.; Kong, L.B.; Li, J.T.; Guo, Z.Y.; Xue, Q.; Yang, T.; Meng, Y.L.; Jin, B.Q.; Wen, W.H.; Yang, A.G. MiR-568 inhibits the activation and function of CD4(+) T cells and Treg cells by targeting NFAT5. *Int. Immunol.* **2014**, *26*, 269–281. [CrossRef]
38. Luo, Y.; Liu, Y.; Liu, M.; Wei, J.; Zhang, Y.; Hou, J.; Huang, W.; Wang, T.; Li, X.; He, Y.; et al. Sfmbt2 10th intron-hosted miR-466(a/e)-3p are important epigenetic regulators of Nfat5 signaling, osmoregulation and urine concentration in mice. *Biochim. Biophys. Acta* **2014**, *1839*, 97–106. [CrossRef]
39. Pedersen, S.F.; Hoffmann, E.K.; Novak, I. Cell volume regulation in epithelial physiology and cancer. *Front Physiol.* **2013**, *4*, 233. [CrossRef]
40. Okada, Y.; Maeno, E.; Shimizu, T.; Manabe, K.; Mori, S.; Nabekura, T. Dual roles of plasmalemmal chloride channels in induction of cell death. *Pflugers Arch* **2004**, *448*, 287–295. [CrossRef]
41. Sforna, L.; Cenciarini, M.; Belia, S.; Michelucci, A.; Pessia, M.; Franciolini, F.; Catacuzzeno, L. Hypoxia Modulates the Swelling-Activated Cl Current in Human Glioblastoma Cells: Role in Volume Regulation and Cell Survival. *J. Cell Physiol.* **2017**, *232*, 91–100. [CrossRef] [PubMed]
42. Usher-Smith, J.A.; Fraser, J.A.; Bailey, P.S.; Griffin, J.L.; Huang, C.L. The influence of intracellular lactate and H+ on cell volume in amphibian skeletal muscle. *J. Physiol.* **2006**, *573*, 799–818. [CrossRef] [PubMed]
43. Heins, J.; Zwingmann, C. Organic osmolytes in hyponatremia and ammonia toxicity. *Metab. Brain Dis.* **2010**, *25*, 81–89. [CrossRef] [PubMed]
44. Lang, F. Effect of cell hydration on metabolism. *Nestle Nutr. Inst. Workshop Ser.* **2011**, *69*, 115–126; discussion 126–130. [CrossRef] [PubMed]
45. Chang, H.H.; Chao, H.N.; Walker, C.S.; Choong, S.Y.; Phillips, A.; Loomes, K.M. Renal depletion of myo-inositol is associated with its increased degradation in animal models of metabolic disease. *Am. J. Physiol. Renal Physiol.* **2015**, *309*, F755–F763. [CrossRef]
46. Cancer Genome Atlas Research Network; Weinstein, J.N.; Collisson, E.A.; Mills, G.B.; Shaw, K.R.; Ozenberger, B.A.; Ellrott, K.; Shmulevich, I.; Sander, C.; Stuart, J.M. The Cancer Genome Atlas Pan-Cancer analysis project. *Nat. Genet.* **2013**, *45*, 1113–1120. [CrossRef]
47. Hoadley, K.A.; Yau, C.; Hinoue, T.; Wolf, D.M.; Lazar, A.J.; Drill, E.; Shen, R.; Taylor, A.M.; Cherniack, A.D.; Thorsson, V.; et al. Cell-of-Origin Patterns Dominate the Molecular Classification of 10,000 Tumors from 33 Types of Cancer. *Cell* **2018**, *173*, 291–304.e6. [CrossRef]
48. Liu, J.; Lichtenberg, T.; Hoadley, K.A.; Poisson, L.M.; Lazar, A.J.; Cherniack, A.D.; Kovatich, A.J.; Benz, C.C.; Levine, D.A.; Lee, A.V.; et al. An Integrated TCGA Pan-Cancer Clinical Data Resource to Drive High-Quality Survival Outcome Analytics. *Cell* **2018**, *173*, 400–416.e11. [CrossRef]
49. Kruger, R. Charting a Course to a Cure. *Cell* **2018**, *173*, 277. [CrossRef]
50. Sanchez-Vega, F.; Mina, M.; Armenia, J.; Chatila, W.K.; Luna, A.; La, K.C.; Dimitriadoy, S.; Liu, D.L.; Kantheti, H.S.; Saghafinia, S.; et al. Oncogenic Signaling Pathways in The Cancer Genome Atlas. *Cell* **2018**, *173*, 321–337.e10. [CrossRef]
51. Cooper, L.A.; Demicco, E.G.; Saltz, J.H.; Powell, R.T.; Rao, A.; Lazar, A.J. PanCancer insights from The Cancer Genome Atlas: The pathologist's perspective. *J. Pathol.* **2018**, *244*, 512–524. [CrossRef] [PubMed]
52. Peng, X.; Chen, Z.; Farshidfar, F.; Xu, X.; Lorenzi, P.L.; Wang, Y.; Cheng, F.; Tan, L.; Mojumdar, K.; Du, D.; et al. Molecular Characterization and Clinical Relevance of Metabolic Expression Subtypes in Human Cancers. *Cell Rep.* **2018**, *23*, 255–269.e4. [CrossRef] [PubMed]
53. Boguslawska, J.; Kedzierska, H.; Poplawski, P.; Rybicka, B.; Tanski, Z.; Piekielko-Witkowska, A. Expression of Genes Involved in Cellular Adhesion and Extracellular Matrix Remodeling Correlates with Poor Survival of Patients with Renal Cancer. *J. Urol.* **2016**, *195*, 1892–1902. [CrossRef] [PubMed]

54. Usarek, M.; Jagielski, A.K.; Krempa, P.; Dylewska, A.; Kiersztan, A.; Drozak, J.; Girstun, A.; Derlacz, R.A.; Bryla, J. Proinsulin C-peptide potentiates the inhibitory action of insulin on glucose synthesis in primary cultured rabbit kidney-cortex tubules: Metabolic studies. *Biochem. Cell Biol.* **2014**, *92*, 1–8. [CrossRef] [PubMed]
55. Agarwal, V.; Bell, G.W.; Nam, J.W.; Bartel, D.P. Predicting effective microRNA target sites in mammalian mRNAs. *Elife* **2015**, *4*. [CrossRef] [PubMed]
56. Anaya, J. OncoLnc: Linking TCGA survival data to mRNAs, miRNAs, and lncRNAs. *Peerj. Comput. Sci.* **2016**, ARTN e6710.7717/peerj-cs.67. [CrossRef]
57. Aguirre-Gamboa, R.; Gomez-Rueda, H.; Martinez-Ledesma, E.; Martinez-Torteya, A.; Chacolla-Huaringa, R.; Rodriguez-Barrientos, A.; Tamez-Pena, J.G.; Trevino, V. SurvExpress: An online biomarker validation tool and database for cancer gene expression data using survival analysis. *PLoS ONE* **2013**, *8*, e74250. [CrossRef]
58. Li, J.H.; Liu, S.; Zhou, H.; Qu, L.H.; Yang, J.H. starBase v2.0: Decoding miRNA-ceRNA, miRNA-ncRNA and protein-RNA interaction networks from large-scale CLIP-Seq data. *Nucleic Acids Res.* **2014**, *42*, D92–D97. [CrossRef]

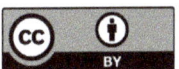

© 2019 by the authors. Licensee MDPI, Basel, Switzerland. This article is an open access article distributed under the terms and conditions of the Creative Commons Attribution (CC BY) license (http://creativecommons.org/licenses/by/4.0/).

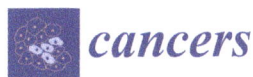

Article

Prognostic Implication of pAMPK Immunohistochemical Staining by Subcellular Location and Its Association with SMAD Protein Expression in Clear Cell Renal Cell Carcinoma

Minsun Jung [1], Jeong Hoon Lee [2], Cheol Lee [1], Jeong Hwan Park [3], Yu Rang Park [2] and Kyung Chul Moon [1,4,*]

[1] Department of Pathology, Seoul National University Hospital, Seoul 03080, Korea; jjunglammy@gmail.com (M.J.); fejhh@hanmail.net (C.L.)
[2] Department of Biomedical Systems Informatics, Yonsei University College of Medicine, Seoul 03722, Korea; sosal@snu.ac.kr (J.H.L.); YURANGPARK@yuhs.ac (Y.R.P.)
[3] Department of Pathology, SMG-SNU Boramae Medical Center, Seoul 07061, Korea; hopemd@hanmail.net
[4] Kidney Research Institute, Medical Research Center, Seoul National University College of Medicine, Seoul 03080, Korea
* Correspondence: blue7270@snu.ac.kr; Tel.: +82-2-740-8380

Received: 17 September 2019; Accepted: 19 October 2019; Published: 21 October 2019

Abstract: Although cytoplasmic AMP-activated protein kinase (AMPK) has been known as a tumor-suppressor protein, nuclear AMPK is suggested to support clear cell renal cell carcinoma (ccRCC). In addition, pAMPK interacts with TGF-β/SMAD, which is one of the frequently altered pathways in ccRCC. In this study, we investigated the prognostic significance of pAMPK with respect to subcellular location and investigated its interaction with TGF-β/SMAD in ccRCC. Immunohistochemical staining for pAMPK, pSMAD2 and SMAD4 was conducted on tissue microarray of 987 ccRCC specimens. Moreover, the levels of pSMAD2 were measured in Caki-1 cells treated with 5-aminoimidazole-4-carboxamide ribonucleotide. The relationship between *AMPK*/pAMPK and *TGFB1* expression was determined using the TCGA database. As a result, pAMPK positivity, either in the cytoplasm or nuclei, was independently associated with improved ccRCC prognosis, after adjusting for TNM stage and WHO grade. Furthermore, pAMPK-positive ccRCC displayed increased pSMAD2 and SMAD4 expression, while activation of pAMPK increased pSMAD2 in Caki-1 cells. However, *AMPK*/pAMPK expression was inversely correlated with *TGFB1* expression in the TCGA database. Therefore, pAMPK immunostaining, both in the cytoplasm and nuclei, is a useful prognostic biomarker for ccRCC. pAMPK targets TGF-β-independent phosphorylation of SMAD2 and activates pSMAD2/SMAD4, representing a novel anti-tumoral mechanism of pAMPK in ccRCC.

Keywords: clear cell renal cell carcinoma; AMP-activated protein kinases; immunohistochemistry; prognosis; SMAD proteins; transforming growth factor beta

1. Introduction

Clear cell renal cell carcinoma (ccRCC), the most common type of renal cell carcinoma, is characterized by genetic alterations that regulate cellular metabolism [1,2]. For example, accumulation of an oxygen-sensing protein, hypoxia-inducible factor (HIF)-α, by the mutational loss of the *VHL* tumor-suppressor gene supports ccRCC progression via angiogenesis and epithelial-mesenchymal transition (EMT) [2]. Another metabolic hallmark of ccRCC is a change in the glucose-sensing machinery caused by constitutive activation of the *PI3K/AKT/MTOR* pathway [1,2]. Activated mammalian target of rapamycin complex 1 (mTORC1) also stimulates development and progression of ccRCC, indicating that mTORC1 is a target for the treatment of metastatic ccRCC [1–3]. Furthermore, lipogenic metabolism is one of the important biologic signatures of ccRCC [2,4,5]. Consistent with these findings, altered expression of metabolism-associated molecules in ccRCC, including AMP-activated protein kinase (AMPK), has been reported to be significantly associated with clinical outcomes [1,6].

AMPK is an intracellular metabolic switch that increases catabolic processes upon activation by threonine (T172) phosphorylation; this phosphorylation is mediated by liver kinase B1 (LKB1) and is stimulated by an increased AMP:ATP ratio [7,8]. pAMPK has been highlighted for its roles as both a metabolic regulator and a tumor suppressor [7]. For example, the AMPK activator 5-aminoimidazole-4-carboxamide ribonucleotide (AICAR) has been shown to inhibit mTORC1 and thus negatively regulate proliferation and survival of multiple types of cancer cells, including ccRCC [7,9]. In agreement with these findings, increased AMPK/pAMPK expression is indicative of favorable survival in patients with carcinomas of the uterine cervix [10], ovary [11], and liver [12] whose tumor cells display cytoplasmic AMPK/pAMPK immunohistochemical (IHC) staining. Conversely, and paradoxically, nuclear pAMPK has been revealed to promote the survival, proliferation, and metastatic capacity of malignant cells under metabolic stress, likely through oncogene activation [13,14]. Recently, Liu et al. [14] demonstrated that nuclear pAMPK mediates the proliferation of glucose-deprived human renal cell carcinoma cells, by recruiting pyruvate kinase isozymes M2 and β-catenin. Although analysis from ccRCC tumor lysates revealed that increased AMPK mRNA and pAMPK are associated with favorable outcomes [1,6], the prognostic significance of pAMPK subcellular location has not yet been investigated in patients with ccRCC.

pAMPK has also been shown to attenuate signaling transduction via the transforming growth factor-β (TGF-β)/SMAD pathway in numerous non-neoplastic cells by inhibiting phosphorylation of SMAD2/SMAD3 or nuclear translocation of SMAD4 [15–19]. In cancer, the connection between pAMPK and TGF-β/SMAD has been poorly investigated, with the exception of one study in breast cancer cells which revealed that pAMPK decreased invasion via downregulation of TGF-β/SMAD-dependent EMT [20]. Upon receptor-regulated phosphorylation by TGF-β, pSMAD2/pSMAD3 forms a complex with SMAD4 and acts as a coactivator of numerous TGF-β target promoters in the nuclei that contributes to either tumorigenesis or tumor progression, depending on the context [21]. In light of the fact that nuclear SMAD2/SMAD3/SMAD4 expression was significantly associated with ccRCC prognosis [22], SMAD proteins may be targets of pAMPK in regulating the behavior of ccRCC. In this study, we aimed to clarify the prognostic significance of pAMPK with respect to the subcellular location in ccRCC, as revealed by IHC staining. In addition, we tried to determine whether the expression of SMAD proteins was governed by pAMPK in ccRCC.

2. Results

2.1. Patients and pAMPK IHC Staining

The demographic and clinicopathological characteristics of the discovery and validation of ccRCC patient cohorts are summarized in Table 1. In the discovery and validation cohorts, the male-to-female sex ratios were 2.8 and 3.0 and the median ages were 58 (range, 20–81) and 56 (range, 24–84) years, respectively.

IHC staining revealed cytoplasmic (Figure 1A,B) and nuclear (Figure 1B,C) pAMPK positivity in 250 (55.2%) and 228 (50.3%) samples, respectively, of the discovery cohort, and in 242 (45.3%) and 231 (43.3%) patients, respectively, of the validation cohort (Table 1). The results of this dichotomous assessment of cytoplasmic and nuclear pAMPK expression, described in detail in *Materials and Methods 4.3.*, showed high agreement between the tissue microarray (TMA) and matched whole-section slides from 10 randomly selected patients. Both cytoplasmic and nuclear pAMPK positivity was significantly associated with small tumor size ($p < 0.001$), low TNM stage ($p < 0.001$), and low WHO grade ($p < 0.001$) in the discovery cohort, which was verified in the validation cohort (Table 1).

Table 1. pAMPK expression and clinicopathological details of the discovery and validation cohorts.

Discovery Cohort	Cyt Pos [1]	Cyt Neg	p	Nuc Pos [1]	Nuc Neg	p	Total
Number	n = 250 (55.2%)	n = 203 (44.8%)		n = 228 (50.3%)	n = 225 (49.7%)		453
Age (year)			0.006			0.009	
≥58	118 (47.2%)	123 (60.6%)		107 (46.9%)	134 (59.6%)		241 (53.2%)
<58	132 (52.8%)	80 (39.4%)		121 (53.1%)	91 (40.4%)		212 (46.8%)
Sex			0.483			0.003	
Male	180 (72.0%)	153 (75.4%)		153 (67.1%)	180 (80.0%)		333 (73.5%)
Female	70 (28.0%)	50 (24.6%)		75 (32.9%)	45 (20.0%)		120 (26.5%)
Size (cm)[2]	3.0 [2.0–4.5]	5.0 [3.0–7.9]	<0.001 [3]	3.0 [2.0–4.7]	4.5 [3.0–7.5]	<0.001 [3]	3.5 [2.3–6.0]
TNM stage			<0.001			<0.001	
Low (I or II)	219 (87.6%)	138 (68.0%)		209 (91.7%)	148 (65.8%)		357 (78.8%)
High (III or IV)	31 (12.4%)	65 (32.0%)		19 (8.3%)	77 (34.2%)		96 (21.2%)
WHO grade			<0.001			<0.001	
Low (1 or 2)	141 (56.4%)	79 (38.9%)		155 (68.0%)	65 (28.9%)		220 (48.6%)
High (3 or 4)	109 (43.6%)	124 (61.1%)		73 (32.0%)	160 (71.1%)		233 (51.4%)
Validation cohort	**Cyt Pos [1]**	**Cyt Neg**	**p**	**Nuc Pos [1]**	**Nuc Neg**	**p**	**Total**
Number	n = 242 (45.3%)	n = 292 (54.7%)		n = 231 (43.3%)	n = 303 (56.7%)		534
Age (year)			0.078			0.045	
≥56	114 (47.1%)	161 (55.1%)		107 (46.3%)	168 (55.4%)		275 (51.5%)
<56	128 (52.9%)	131 (44.9%)		124 (53.7%)	135 (44.6%)		259 (48.5%)
Sex			0.737			0.001	
Male	183 (75.6%)	216 (74.0%)		156 (67.5%)	243 (80.2%)		399 (74.7%)
Female	59 (24.5%)	76 (26.0%)		75 (32.5%)	60 (19.8%)		135 (25.3%)
Size (cm)[2]	4.0 [3.0–6.0]	5.5 [3.8–8.8]	<0.001 [3]	4.0 [3.0–6.5]	5.3 [3.9–8.0]	<0.001 [3]	4.8 [3.2–7.5]
TNM stage			<0.001			<0.001	
Low (I or II)	204 (84.3%)	180 (61.6%)		191 (82.7%)	193 (63.7%)		384 (71.9%)
High (III or IV)	38 (15.7%)	112 (38.4%)		40 (17.3%)	110 (36.3%)		150 (28.1%)
WHO grade			0.085			<0.001	
Low (1 or 2)	140 (57.9%)	146 (50.0%)		155 (67.1%)	131 (43.2%)		286 (53.6%)
High (3 or 4)	102 (42.1%)	146 (50.0%)		76 (32.9%)	172 (56.8%)		248 (46.4%)

[1] pAMPK-positive tumor extent >10% [2] Median with 25–75% quartile [3] Mann–Whitney U test. The other p-values were calculated by Pearson's χ^2 test. Abbreviation: Cyt, cytoplasm; Pos, positive; Neg, negative; Nuc, nucleus.

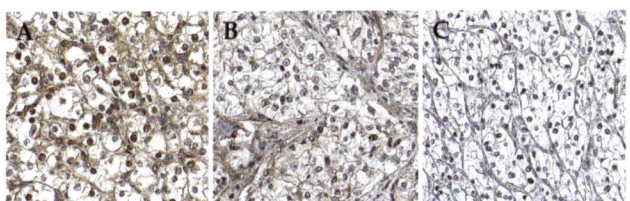

Figure 1. Immunohistochemical staining for pAMPK. (**A**) More than 50% of tumor cells expressed pAMPK both in the cytoplasm and nuclei; (**B**) More than 50% of tumor cells are stained for pAMPK in the cytoplasm but less than 10% of tumor cells show nuclear staining for pAMPK; (**C**) More than 50% of the tumor cells exhibits pAMPK only in the nuclei.

2.2. Positive IHC Staining for pAMPK Was Significantly Associated with Improved ccRCC Prognosis

The median follow-up periods from the discovery and validation cohorts were 121 (range, 1–178) and 102 (range, 2–288) months, respectively. The median overall survival (OS) was not reached in either cohort. Kaplan–Meier and log-rank tests showed that pAMPK-positive ccRCC, either in the cytoplasm or in the nuclei, was associated with longer progression-free survival (PFS) ($p < 0.001$), overall survival (OS) ($p < 0.001$), and cancer-specific survival (CSS) ($p < 0.001$) than pAMPK-negative ccRCC, both in the discovery and validation cohorts (Figure 2). Univariate Cox regression analysis showed that patients with pAMPK-positive ccRCC (with either a cytoplasmic or nuclear pattern) were less likely to experience disease progression ($p < 0.001$), death ($p < 0.001$), and disease-specific death ($p < 0.001$); these findings were true in both the discovery (Table 2) and validation (Table 3) cohorts. A multivariate analysis incorporating TNM stage and WHO grade showed that pAMPK positivity is an independent prognostic factor for favorable PFS (cytoplasmic, hazard ratio [HR] = 0.260, $p < 0.001$; nuclear, HR = 0.308, $p < 0.001$), OS (cytoplasmic, HR = 0.656, $p = 0.032$), and CSS (cytoplasmic, HR = 0.374, $p = 0.001$; nuclear, HR = 0.232, $p = 0.003$) in the discovery cohort (Table 2). The prognostic significance of cytoplasmic and nuclear pAMPK expression adjusted for TNM stage and WHO grade was confirmed in the validation cohort (Table 3).

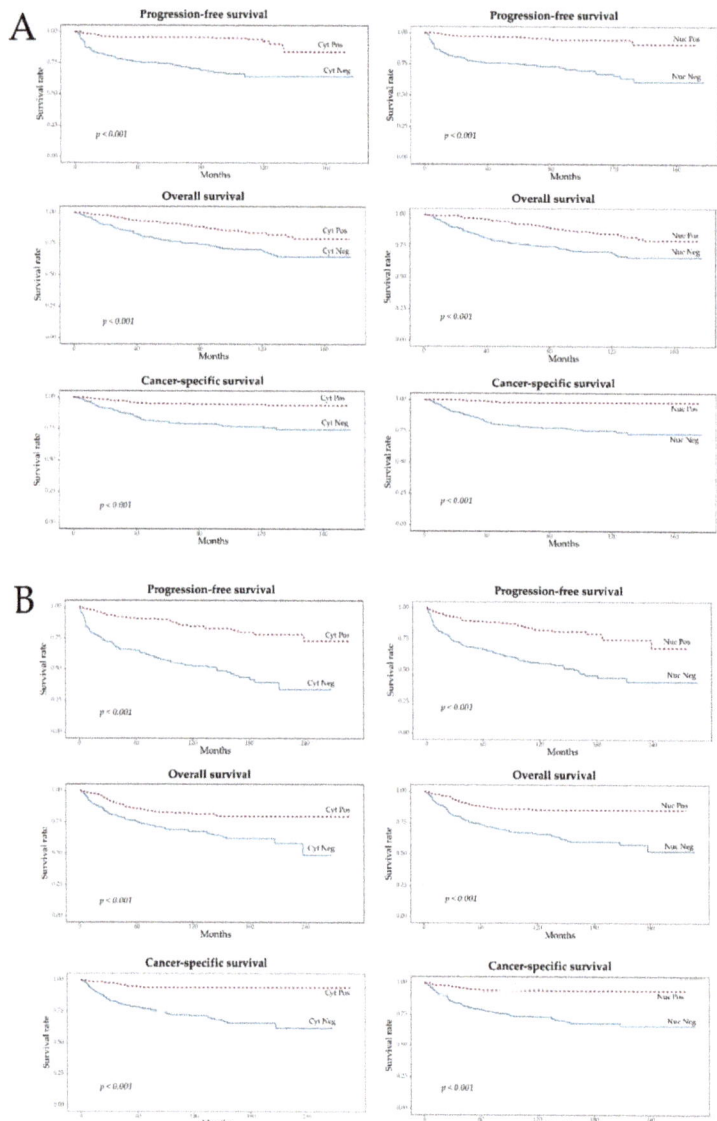

Figure 2. Survival analyses of pAMPK cytoplasmic and nuclear expression. (**A**) Discovery cohort; (**B**) Validation cohort. Cyt, cytoplasm; Pos, positive; Neg, negative; Nuc, nucleus.

Table 2. Cox regression analyses for pAMPK expression of the discovery cohort.

Analysis Detail	Progression-Free Survival		Overall Survival		Cancer-Specific Survival	
	HR (95% CI)	p	HR (95% CI)	p	HR (95% CI)	p
Univariate analysis						
pAMPK-C (Pos vs Neg)	0.190 (0.110–0.310)	<0.001	0.470 (0.320–0.680)	<0.001	0.200 (0.110–0.370)	<0.001
pAMPK-N (Pos vs Neg)	0.140 (0.080–0.260)	<0.001	0.440 (0.300–0.650)	<0.001	0.070 (0.030–0.19)	<0.001
TNM stage (≥III vs ≤II)	12.920 (8.150–20.490)	<0.001	5.480 (3.790–7.920)	<0.001	18.050 (10.100–32.270)	<0.001
WHO Grade (≥3 vs ≤2)	5.210 (2.980–9.120)	<0.001	2.770 (1.850–4.160)	<0.001	16.330 (5.930–44.950)	<0.001
Multivariate analysis						
pAMPK-C (Pos vs Neg)	0.260 (0.153–0.442)	<0.001	0.656 (0.446–0.965)	0.032	0.374 (0.205–0.681)	0.001
TNM stage (≥III vs ≤II)	8.644 (5.340–13.992)	<0.001	4.163 (2.806–6.178)	<0.001	9.535 (5.245–17.336)	<0.001
WHO Grade (≥3 vs ≤2)	2.601 (1.456–4.646)	0.001	1.774 (1.156–2.724)	0.009	7.163 (2.552–20.106)	<0.001
Multivariate analysis						
pAMPK-N (Pos vs Neg)	0.308 (0.159–0.595)	<0.001	0.767 (0.500–1.177)	0.225	0.232 (0.090–0.600)	0.003
TNM stage (≥III vs ≤II)	7.944 (4.868–12.965)	<0.001	4.250 (2.850–6.337)	<0.001	8.677 (4.754–15.837)	<0.001
WHO Grade (≥3 vs ≤2)	1.889 (1.024–3.487)	0.042	1.696 (1.082–2.660)	0.021	5.086 (1.777–14.556)	0.002

Abbreviation: HR, hazard ratio; CI, confidence interval; C, cytoplasm; Pos, positive; Neg, negative; N, nucleus.

Table 3. Cox regression analyses for pAMPK expression of the validation cohort.

Analysis Detail	Progression-Free Survival		Overall Survival		Cancer-Specific Survival	
	HR (95% CI)	p	HR (95% CI)	p	HR (95% CI)	p
Univariate analysis						
pAMPK-C (Pos vs Neg)	0.250 (0.180–0.360)	<0.001	0.480 (0.340–0.690)	<0.001	0.180 (0.100–0.310)	<0.001
pAMPK-N (Pos vs Neg)	0.300 (0.210–0.440)	<0.001	0.350 (0.230–0.510)	<0.001	0.180 (0.100–0.330)	<0.001
TNM stage (≥III vs ≤II)	6.430 (4.720–8.760)	<0.001	4.740 (3.390–6.620)	<0.001	10.340 (6.570–16.270)	<0.001
WHO Grade (≥3 vs ≤2)	3.010 (2.190–4.140)	<0.001	2.870 (2.020–4.080)	<0.001	4.640 (2.880–7.470)	<0.001
Multivariate analysis						
pAMPK-C (Pos vs Neg)	0.304 (0.210–0.441)	<0.001	0.629 (0.438–0.903)	0.012	0.256 (0.144–0.455)	<0.001
TNM stage (≥III vs ≤II)	4.630 (3.352–6.395)	<0.001	3.567 (2.505–5.079)	<0.001	6.446 (4.023–10.328)	<0.001
WHO Grade (≥3 vs ≤2)	2.244 (1.618–3.112)	<0.001	2.091 (1.453–3.010)	<0.001	2.935 (1.801–4.781)	<0.001
Multivariate analysis						
pAMPK-N (Pos vs Neg)	0.405 (0.280–0.585)	<0.001	0.471 (0.315–0.705)	<0.001	0.296 (0.164–0.536)	<0.001
TNM stage (≥III vs ≤II)	4.989 (3.617–6.883)	<0.001	3.601 (2.537–5.111)	<0.001	7.101 (4.434–11.371)	<0.001
WHO Grade (≥3 vs ≤2)	1.882 (1.350–2.623)	<0.001	1.844 (1.274–2.667)	0.001	2.344 (1.430–3.844)	<0.001

Abbreviation: HR, hazard ratio; CI, confidence interval; C, cytoplasm; Pos, positive; Neg, negative; N, nucleus.

2.3. pAMPK Induced Nuclear SMAD Protein Expression in ccRCC

We compared nuclear pSMAD2 and SMAD4 immunoreactivity of pAMPK-positive and pAMPK-negative tumors. The mean (± standard deviation) pSMAD2 expression was 57.0% (±26.2) and 30.4% (±19.7) ($p < 0.001$) in the cytoplasmic pAMPK-positive and pAMPK-negative ccRCC samples, respectively, and 52.5% (± 28.5) and 37.5% (± 23.0) ($p < 0.001$) in the nuclear pAMPK-positive and pAMPK-negative ccRCC specimens, respectively. Similarly, SMAD4 nuclear expression was observed in 20.0% (±22.6) and 2.6% (±5.9) ($p < 0.001$) of tumor cells with cytoplasmic pAMPK positivity and negativity, respectively, and in 19.0% (±23.2) and 5.4% (±10.5) ($p < 0.001$) of those with positive and negative nuclear pAMPK immunostaining, respectively (Figure 3B). We next sought to determine whether pAMPK positively regulates SMAD protein expression. AICAR treatment activated pAMPK and increased pSMAD2 expression in Caki-1 cells (Figure 3C,D).

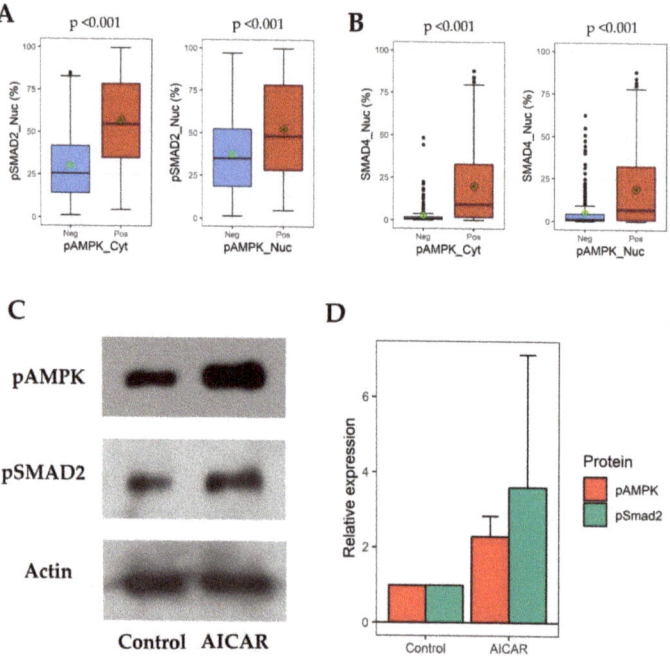

Figure 3. pSMAD2/SMAD4 upregulation by pAMPK in ccRCC. pAMPK-positive ccRCC, either in the cytoplasm or nuclei, shows higher nuclear expression levels of (**A**) pSMAD2 and (**B**) SMAD4 than pAMPK-negative ccRCC (Mann–Whitney U tests). Green square indicates the mean value; (**C**) AICAR activates pAMPK and induces pSMAD2 expression in Caki-1 cells; (**D**) The relative intensity of Western blot results before (control) and after AICAR treatment is shown as a mean (bar) with a standard deviation (line) (Rex 3.0.4, RexSoft Inc., Seoul, Korea).

Next, we asked whether the pAMPK-mediated SMAD induction was dependent on the TGF-β/SMAD pathway. To this end, we investigated the correlation between AMPK mRNA (*AMPKα1*, *AMPKα2*, *AMPKβ1*, *AMPKβ2*, *AMPKγ1*, and *AMPKγ2*) and phosphoprotein (T172) levels, and the mRNA expression levels of TGF-β (*TGFB1*) and SMAD (*SMAD2*, *SMAD4*) in the TCGA ccRCC database. Our analysis revealed that levels of AMPK mRNA and pAMPK were inversely correlated with *TGFB1* but were weakly and positively correlated with expression of *SMAD2* and *SMAD4* (Figure 4). Therefore, both cytoplasmic and nuclear pAMPK-positive ccRCC was enriched for nuclear pSMAD2 and SMAD4. Further, pAMPK induced phosphorylation of SMAD2 in a TGF-β-independent manner.

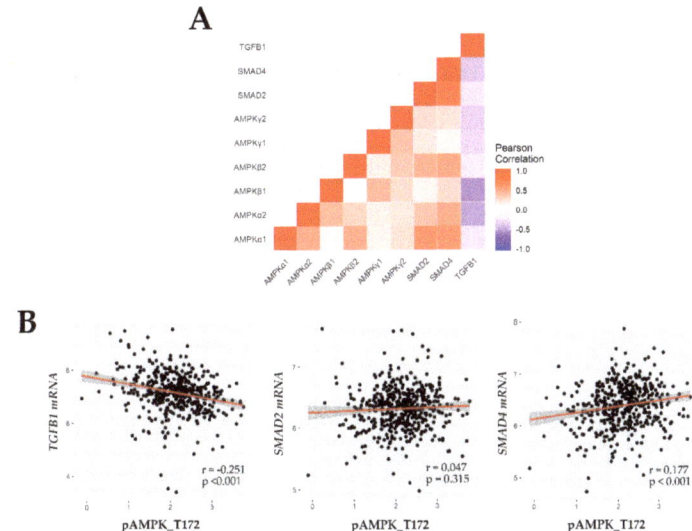

Figure 4. Correlation coefficient among *TGFB1*, *SMAD2*, *SMAD4*, and AMPK (mRNA and T172 phosphoprotein) analyzed from the TCGA ccRCC database. (**A**) *TGFB1* is inversely but *SMAD2* and *SMAD4* are positively correlated with AMPK mRNA in the TCGA mRNA database; (**B**) Similar trends are identified between *TGFB1/SMAD2/SMAD4* (TCGA mRNA database) and pAMPK^{T172} protein (TCGA reverse phase protein array data of the matched samples).

3. Discussion

Here, we have revealed the prognostic implication of IHC staining for pAMPK in large cohorts of ccRCC patients. pAMPK positivity was related to low-risk pathological traits of ccRCC, including small tumor size, early TNM stage, and low WHO grade, and was an independent favorable prognostic factor in ccRCC. These results were consistent across samples with cytoplasmic and/or nuclear pAMPK IHC staining, suggesting that IHC staining for pAMPK may be a useful prognostic biomarker for ccRCC. Furthermore, pAMPK-positive ccRCC showed higher levels of nuclear pSMAD2 and SMAD4 expression than those in pAMPK-negative tumors. Consistent with this result, Caki-1 cells treated with AICAR showed increased expression of pSMAD2. *SMAD2/SMAD4* mRNA also showed a modestly positive correlation with AMPK mRNA/phosphoprotein, whereas *TGFB1* showed an inverse correlation, suggesting that pAMPK activates SMAD expression through a non-TGF-β pathway.

pAMPK inhibits growth, invasion, EMT, and metastasis by modulating various signaling axes, including downregulation of mTORC1, HIF, and NF-κB and upregulation of Forkhead box class O (FoxO)3a and p53 [7,12,23–25]. In addition, pAMPK is responsible for restricting ATP-consumption by directly suppressing fatty acid synthesis enzymes, such as acetyl-CoA carboxylase and fatty acid synthase. In other words, pAMPK shifts metabolism away from the Warburg effect-like status, an environment that is supportive of ccRCC progression [1,6,7,24]. Our clinical results as well as previous preclinical data propose that AMPK activation may be useful as a ccRCC treatment strategy [25,26]. pAMPK expression may affect the treatment response to targeted agents in ccRCC. For example, rapamycin, an inhibitor to mammalian target of rapamycin, displayed additive counteraction against the invasion and growth of renal cell carcinoma when this was administered together with AICAR [25]. In addition, because pAMPK inhibits HIF-α activity and HIF-α stably upregulates vascular endothelial growth factor in ccRCC [2,25], the association between pAMPK expression and vascular endothelial growth factor receptor tyrosine kinase inhibitors might be worth investigating. However, the subcellular location-specific tumor-suppressive functions of AMPK have been controversial. For example, nuclear pAMPK increased transcription of pro-cancerous molecules, such as cyclin D1, c-myc, and Oct4, in cancer cells under metabolic stresses (e.g., in glucose-deprived conditions) [13,14]. The clinical significance of this nuclear pAMPK immunoreactivity has never been investigated in vivo because prior studies have reported that IHC staining for pAMPK is confined to the cytoplasm of normal and neoplastic human tissue [10–12,27,28]. In the ccRCC TCGA reports, the prognostic significance of pAMPK was demonstrated using protein array, without considering pAMPK subcellular localization [1,6]. We observed that both cytoplasmic and nuclear pAMPK is independently associated with favorable prognoses in ccRCC. Previous studies have revealed that nuclear pAMPK can function in either an inhibitory or a stimulatory manner in renal cell carcinoma, depending on context: the oncogenic function of nuclear AMPK is confined to glucose-deprived renal cell carcinoma cells, whereas regular tumor-suppressive functions predominate under usual conditions [14]. Therefore, it is reasonable to speculate that the hostile environments that encourage nuclear pAMPK to stimulate ccRCC progression were present in only a restricted number of patients in this study. In addition, it is noteworthy that glucose starvation can also lead to the activation of various signals other than AMPK, including Akt and ERK [23].

The TGF-β/SMAD signaling pathway, a major regulator of carcinogenesis and the progression of various tumor types [29], is frequently altered in ccRCC [1]. In fact, pAMPK has been shown to inhibit SMAD-mediated TGF-β signal transduction through various mechanisms, by which pAMPK exhibits anti-fibrogenic and anti-EMT functions [15–18,20]. For example, pAMPK prevented TGF-β-mediated phosphoactivation of SMAD2 and/or SMAD3 in vascular smooth muscle and breast cancer cells [17,20]. In mesenchymal cells, pAMPK also reduced the stability and nuclear localization of SMAD4 [18] and the interaction of SMAD3 with its coactivator, p300, without affecting the phosphorylation of SMAD2 or SMAD3 [16]. In contrast, we demonstrated that pAMPK-positive ccRCC showed higher levels of nuclear pSMAD2 and SMAD4 than those in pAMPK-negative tumors. We hypothesize that this positive relationship between pAMPK and pSMAD2/SMAD4 may be involved in an important, as-yet-unidentified mechanism that is critical to the inhibition of ccRCC. In addition, this may explain a previous report that ccRCC displaying nuclear SMAD2/SMAD3/SMAD4 protein expression had, for unknown reasons, favorable outcomes [22]. It is known that LKB1, kinase upstream of pAMPK, dictates phosphoactivation of AMPK, except on limited occasions when AMPK might be activated by calcium/calmodulin-dependent protein kinase kinase 2, TGF-β-activated kinase 1, or AMP through phosphorylation or allosteric modification [7,8]. AICAR is an AMP-mimetic that directly binds to AMPK and facilitates its phosphorylation by LKB1 [7,19]. Therefore, it is safe to say that LKB1 played a critical role in activating pAMPK in this study. LKB1 may directly increase TGF-β signaling in an AMPK-independent way, as suggested in other studies [30,31]. Nevertheless, we identified a negative correlation between *TGFB1* and both AMPK mRNA and pAMPK proteins in the TCGA ccRCC database, in agreement with a previous report [20]. Low *TGFB1* mRNA levels are likely attributable to an attenuated TGF-β/SMAD cascade [31]. The positive correlation between *SMAD2*/*SMAD4* mRNA levels and *AMPK*/pAMPK in the TCGA database was weak and inconsistent, compared to the tight correlation between pSMAD2/SMAD4 and pAMPK expression in our TMA and Western blot analyses. Therefore, we hypothesize that pAMPK post-transcriptionally or post-translationally activates pSMAD2/SMAD4 by phosphorylating SMAD2 via a TGF-β-independent mechanism. Furthermore, the results suggest that pAMPK probably conducts a tumor-suppressive function through pSMAD2/SMAD4 activation, at least in part. Upregulation of nuclear FoxO3a may connect the coactivation of pAMPK and SMAD. FoxO3 is also a good candidate for an interdependent molecule mediating the antitumoral functions of pAMPK and pSMAD2/SMAD4 in ccRCC. In ovarian cancer, FoxO3a interacted with a SMAD2/SMAD3/SMAD4 complex in the nucleus, which could maintain activated SMAD proteins at high levels, and this interaction in turn promoted the cell-cycle arrest synergistically [32,33]. In addition, previous studies showed that the activation of AMPK increased both the nuclear localization and stability of FoxO3a in cancer and enhanced the transcription of autophagy-associated genes, leading to cell death [23,34]. Taken together, this putative pAMPK/FoxO3/SMAD interaction may lead to favorable outcomes in pAMPK-positive ccRCC with high expression of SMAD proteins. Presumably, this is a novel biological function of pAMPK/pSMAD2/SMAD4 in ccRCC that warrants further studies. Secondly, given that AMPK is a kinase of diverse targets and the TGF-β/SMAD pathway engages in a reciprocal cross talk with various molecules [7,21], it is readily assumable that pAMPK might activate and cooperate with pSMAD2/SMAD4 to downregulate ccRCC, either directly or indirectly by way of modulating other pathways.

There are a few limitations in this study. Although it is well known that pSMAD2 and pSMAD3 are very similar proteins that can form a complex with SMAD4 to activate transcriptional responses [29], the interaction between pSMAD3 and pAMPK was not investigated in this study. Along with the positive correlation between pAMPK and nuclear pSMAD2/SMAD4 in IHC, the Western blot result puts forward the idea that pAMPK overexpression phosphorylates SMAD2 and subsequently activates pSMAD2/SMAD4 in ccRCC. However, more detailed in vitro studies adopting a constitutively active mutant of *AMPK* or depletion of pAMPK using compound C or siRNA to *AMPK* would profoundly improve the understanding of the causal relationship between pAMPK and pSMAD2/SMAD4 activation. In addition, despite the unequivocal overexpression of pSMAD2 and SMAD4 in pAMPK-positive tumors, it still remains uncertain whether pAMPK directly induces SMAD-mediated transcriptional activities in ccRCC. Previous reports demonstrated that SMAD activities were regulated by pAMPK at the transcriptional level in various conditions [15,16,20], which accompanied increased expression of the pAMPK and AMPKα2 subunit in the nuclei of human mesangial cells as well [15]. Although these results imply that pAMPK may directly associate with SMAD proteins and modulate their transcriptional function in the nuclei [15], this phenomenon has not been verified in ccRCC. Further investigation will be required to elucidate the detailed functional effects of pAMPK-induced activation of SMAD proteins, including SMAD-responsive transcription and the regulation of its downstream targets.

4. Materials and Methods

4.1. Patients' Cohorts

In total, 987 ccRCC samples were surgically resected at the Seoul National University Hospital between 1995 and 2008, and separated into discovery (n = 453; 2003–2008) and validation (n = 534; 1995-2004) cohorts. Of these samples, 294 cases of the discovery cohort and 493 cases of the validation cohort were radical nephrectomy specimens, while the others were partial nephrectomy specimens. Each tumor sample was reviewed for histologic type, TNM stage, and WHO grade. The TNM stage was reclassified according to the American Joint Committee on Cancer—Cancer Staging Manual, 8th edition [35]. Clinical data were obtained from medical records. Patients who received neoadjuvant treatment, displayed bilateral disease at the time of diagnosis, or who had Von Hippel–Lindau syndrome were excluded. This study was approved by the Institutional Review Board of Seoul National University Hospital (H-1810-150-983).

4.2. TMA Construction and IHC Staining

Two cores (2 mm in diameter) from each specimen were embedded in recipient paraffin blocks using a trephine apparatus (Superbiochips Laboratories, Seoul, Republic of Korea) for TMA construction. IHC staining was conducted on 4-μm-thick TMA sections using the Benchmark autostainer (Ventana, Tucson, AZ) according to the manufacturer's instructions. IHC staining was conducted using a rabbit monoclonal antibody against pAMPK^{T172} (1:100; Cat. #2535; Cell Signaling Technology, Danvers, MA), a rabbit polyclonal antibody against pSMAD2^{S467} (1:70; Cat. #ab53100; Abcam, Cambridge, UK), and a mouse monoclonal antibody against SMAD4 (1:100; Cat. #sc-7966; Santa Cruz Biotechnology). One TMA slide was stained without primary anti-pAMPK antibody as a negative control.

4.3. Establishment of Cut-Off Criteria for pAMPK IHC Staining Positivity

pAMPK expression was observed in the cytoplasm and the nuclei of tumor cells (Figure 1). Firstly, the extent of tumor cells in the discovery cohort displaying at least moderate immunoreactivity was assessed semiquantitatively as follows: <10%, 10–50%, and >50%. Based on both sample distribution and prognostic significance, 10% staining was defined as the best cut-off value for both cytoplasmic and nuclear pAMPK positivity (Figure S1). Next, the prognostic significance of pAMPK staining was confirmed in the validation cohort using the same cut-off criteria. Regarding discordant cases from duplicate TMA cores, the lower pAMPK expression level was used. To account for intratumoral heterogeneity, IHC staining for pAMPK was also conducted on whole sections from 10 randomly selected cases in the discovery cohort. The percentage of tumor cells (%) positive for nuclear pSMAD2 and SMAD4 was calculated from both TMA cores, using QuPath version 0.1.2 [36] on digitally scanned slides (Aperio AT2, Leica Biosystem, Wetzlar, Germany). The mean values of pSMAD2 and SMAD4 are shown.

4.4. Western Blot Analysis

A human ccRCC cell line, Caki-1, was obtained from the Korean Cell Line Bank (KCLB, Seoul, Republic of Korea) and was cultured in Dulbecco's Modified Eagle's Medium (DMEM) supplemented with 10% fetal bovine serum in a 5% CO_2 humidified incubator. To evaluate the AMPK/SMAD2 signaling pathway, we used the AMPK activator, AICAR (Sigma, St. Louis, MO, USA). Caki-1 cells were treated with 1 mM AICAR for 6 hours, and then, the cells were harvested for Western blot analysis. Cell lysates were electrophoretically resolved on a 10% polyacrylamide gel in a sodium dodecyl sulfate buffer and then transferred onto nitrocellulose membranes. Afterward, the blots were incubated with antibodies against pAMPK^{T172} (Cat. #2535, Cell Signaling Technology) and pSMAD2$^{S465/467}$ (Cat. #3108; Cell Signaling Technology). These experiments were conducted in triplicate and are presented as the mean ± standard deviation.

4.5. Characteristics of the TCGA ccRCC Dataset

ccRCC mRNA sequencing and reverse phase protein array data with clinicopathological information generated by the TCGA Research Network were obtained using the Broad Institute GDAC Firehose [37]. The mRNA sequencing dataset was generated from 552 primary ccRCC samples and quantified by RSEM (RNA-Seq by Expectation) [38]. The median age in this sample was 61 years (range, 26–90) and the male-to-female sex ratio was 1.8:1. Approximately, 60% (316/522) and 46% (236/514) of these patients had a low TNM stage (I or II) and low Furhman grade (1 or 2), respectively.

We next constructed a design matrix using the DGEList function in the EdgeR module. To filter out genes with low expression levels, we excluded those genes with counts per million (cpm) values <1 in at least half of the samples [39]. As a result of this filtering, *AMPKγ3* (*PRKAG3*) was omitted. RSEM read counts underwent Trimmed Mean of M-values (TMM) normalization and logCPM transformation using voom [40]. Of the patients whose samples were included in the mRNA dataset, 472 also had reverse phase protein array information, including pAMPK^{T172} protein expression levels. These data were analyzed to examine the correlation between *AMPK*/pAMPK^{T172} and *TGFB1*/*SMAD* mRNA expression.

4.6. Statistical Analysis

The interrelation between pAMPK IHC staining and clinicopathological characteristics was analyzed using Pearson's χ^2 test with Yates' correction for categorical variables and with the Mann–Whitney test for continuous variables. The PFS period was calculated as the interval between surgery and recurrence, progression, metastasis, or the last follow-up visit. The OS duration was defined as the period between surgery and death from any cause or the last follow-up. The CSS duration was defined as the interval between surgery and cancer-related death or the last follow-up visit. Kaplan–Meier analysis and the log-rank test were used to compare survival. A Cox proportional hazard regression model was used for univariate and multivariate survival analyses. The strength and direction of the linear relationships among *AMPK*/pAMPK, *TGFβ1*, and *SMAD2*/*SMAD4* expression was assessed using Pearson's r test. All statistical analyses were performed using SPSS Statistics 25 (IBM Co., Armonk, NY) or in R, with a 2-tailed $p < 0.05$ considered statistically significant.

5. Conclusions

Both cytoplasmic and nuclear pAMPK immunostaining are independently associated with favorable outcomes in ccRCC. pAMPK positivity is associated with nuclear overexpression of pSMAD2 and SMAD4, through stimulation of TGF-β-independent phosphorylation of SMAD2, which is a novel antitumoral mechanism for pAMPK in ccRCC. Understanding the interaction between pAMPK and SMAD proteins will facilitate the use of AMPK activation as a strategy for ccRCC treatment.

Supplementary Materials: The following are available online at http://www.mdpi.com/2072-6694/11/10/1602/s1, Figure S1: Establishment of the cut-off criteria for pAMPK positivity.

Author Contributions: Conceptualization, M.J. and K.C.M.; methodology, J.H.L. and K.C.M.; software, M.J. and J.H.L.; validation, M.J. and K.C.M.; formal analysis, M.J., J.H.L., and Y.R.P.; investigation, M.J., C.L., and J.H.P.; resources, K.C.M.; data curation, M.J., C.L., and J.H.P.; writing—original draft preparation, M.J.; writing—review and editing, M.J. and K.C.M.; visualization, M.J. and J.H.L.; supervision, K.C.M.; project administration, K.C.M.; funding acquisition, K.C.M.

Funding: This research was funded by Basic Science Research Program through the National Research Foundation of Korea (NRF) funded by the Ministry of Education (2018R1D1A1B07045763).

Conflicts of Interest: The authors declare no conflict of interest.

References

1. Cancer Genome Atlas Research Network. Comprehensive molecular characterization of clear cell renal cell carcinoma. *Nature* **2013**, *499*, 43–49. [CrossRef] [PubMed]
2. Massari, F.; Ciccarese, C.; Santoni, M.; Brunelli, M.; Piva, F.; Modena, A.; Bimbatti, D.; Fantinel, E.; Santini, D.; Cheng, L.; et al. Metabolic alterations in renal cell carcinoma. *Cancer Treat. Rev.* **2015**, *41*, 767–776. [CrossRef] [PubMed]
3. Bhaskar, P.T.; Hay, N. The two TORCs and Akt. *Dev. Cell* **2007**, *12*, 487–502. [CrossRef] [PubMed]
4. Park, J.H.; Jung, M.; Moon, K.C. The prognostic significance of nuclear expression of PHF2 and C/EBPalpha in clear cell renal cell carcinoma with consideration of adipogenic metabolic evolution. *Oncotarget* **2018**, *9*, 142–151. [CrossRef]
5. Jung, M.; Lee, C.; Park, J.H.; Moon, K.C. Prognostic significance of immunohistochemical staining for myoferlin in clear cell renal cell carcinoma and its association with epidermal growth factor receptor expression. *Urol. Oncol.* **2019**, in press. [CrossRef]
6. Ricketts, C.J.; De Cubas, A.A.; Fan, H.; Smith, C.C.; Lang, M.; Reznik, E.; Bowlby, R.; Gibb, E.A.; Akbani, R.; Beroukhim, R.; et al. The cancer genome atlas comprehensive molecular characterization of renal cell carcinoma. *Cell Rep.* **2018**, *23*, 313–326.e5. [CrossRef]
7. Shackelford, D.B.; Shaw, R.J. The LKB1-AMPK pathway: Metabolism and growth control in tumour suppression. *Nat. Rev. Cancer* **2009**, *9*, 563–575. [CrossRef]
8. Tamargo-Gomez, I.; Marino, G. AMPK: Regulation of metabolic dynamics in the context of autophagy. *Int. J. Mol. Sci.* **2018**, *19*, 3812. [CrossRef]
9. Woodard, J.; Joshi, S.; Viollet, B.; Hay, N.; Platanias, L.C. AMPK as a therapeutic target in renal cell carcinoma. *Cancer Biol. Ther.* **2010**, *10*, 1169–1178. [CrossRef]
10. Choi, C.H.; Chung, J.Y.; Cho, H.; Kitano, H.; Chang, E.; Ylaya, K.; Chung, E.J.; Kim, J.H.; Hewitt, S.M. Prognostic significance of AMP-dependent kinase alpha expression in cervical cancer. *Pathobiology* **2015**, *82*, 203–211. [CrossRef]
11. Li, C.L.; Liu, V.W.S.; Chiu, P.M.; Chan, D.W.; Ngan, H.Y.S. Over-expressions of AMPK subunits in ovarian carcinomas with significant clinical implications. *BMC Cancer* **2012**, *12*, 357. [CrossRef] [PubMed]
12. Zheng, L.; Yang, W.; Wu, F.; Wang, C.; Yu, L.; Tang, L.; Qiu, B.; Li, Y.; Guo, L.; Wu, M.; et al. Prognostic significance of AMPK activation and therapeutic effects of metformin in hepatocellular carcinoma. *Clin. Cancer Res.* **2013**, *19*, 5372–5380. [CrossRef] [PubMed]
13. Yang, Y.C.; Chien, M.H.; Liu, H.Y.; Chang, Y.C.; Chen, C.K.; Lee, W.J.; Kuo, T.C.; Hsiao, M.; Hua, K.T.; Cheng, T.Y. Nuclear translocation of PKM2/AMPK complex sustains cancer stem cell populations under glucose restriction stress. *Cancer Lett.* **2018**, *421*, 28–40. [CrossRef] [PubMed]

14. Liu, M.; Zhang, Z.; Wang, H.; Chen, X.; Jin, C. Activation of AMPK by metformin promotes renal cancer cell proliferation under glucose deprivation through its interaction with PKM2. *Int. J. Biol. Sci.* **2019**, *15*, 617–627. [CrossRef]
15. Mishra, R.; Cool, B.L.; Laderoute, K.R.; Foretz, M.; Viollet, B.; Simonson, M.S. AMP-activated protein kinase inhibits transforming growth factor-beta-induced Smad3-dependent transcription and myofibroblast transdifferentiation. *J. Biol. Chem.* **2008**, *283*, 10461–10469. [CrossRef]
16. Lim, J.Y.; Oh, M.A.; Kim, W.H.; Sohn, H.Y.; Park, S.I. AMP-activated protein kinase inhibits TGF-beta-induced fibrogenic responses of hepatic stellate cells by targeting transcriptional coactivator p300. *J. Cell. Physiol.* **2012**, *227*, 1081–1089. [CrossRef]
17. Stone, J.D.; Holt, A.W.; Vuncannon, J.R.; Brault, J.J.; Tulis, D.A. AMP-activated protein kinase inhibits transforming growth factor-beta-mediated vascular smooth muscle cell growth: Implications for a Smad-3-dependent mechanism. *Am. J. Physiol. Heart Circ. Physiol.* **2015**, *309*, H1251–H1259. [CrossRef]
18. Zhao, J.; Miyamoto, S.; You, Y.H.; Sharma, K. AMP-activated protein kinase (AMPK) activation inhibits nuclear translocation of Smad4 in mesangial cells and diabetic kidneys. *Am. J. Physiol. Ren. Physiol.* **2015**, *308*, F1167–F1177. [CrossRef]
19. Yadav, H.; Devalaraja, S.; Chung, S.T.; Rane, S.G. TGF-1/Smad3 pathway targets PP2A-AMPK-FoxO1 signaling to regulate hepatic gluconeogenesis. *J. Biol. Chem.* **2017**, *292*, 3420–3432. [CrossRef]
20. Li, N.S.; Zou, J.R.; Lin, H.; Ke, R.; He, X.L.; Xiao, L.; Huang, D.; Luo, L.; Lv, N.; Luo, Z. LKB1/AMPK inhibits TGF-beta1 production and the TGF-beta signaling pathway in breast cancer cells. *Tumour Biol.* **2016**, *37*, 8249–8258. [CrossRef]
21. Tang, J.; Gifford, C.C.; Samarakoon, R.; Higgins, P.J. Deregulation of negative controls on TGF-beta1 signaling in tumor progression. *Cancers* **2018**, *10*, 159. [CrossRef] [PubMed]
22. Park, J.H.; Lee, C.; Suh, J.H.; Chae, J.Y.; Moon, K.C. Nuclear expression of Smad proteins and its prognostic significance in clear cell renal cell carcinoma. *Hum. Pathol.* **2013**, *44*, 2047–2054. [CrossRef] [PubMed]
23. Chou, C.C.; Lee, K.H.; Lai, I.L.; Wang, D.; Mo, X.; Kulp, S.K.; Shapiro, C.L.; Chen, C.S. AMPK reverses the mesenchymal phenotype of cancer cells by targeting the Akt-MDM2-Foxo3a signaling axis. *Cancer Res.* **2014**, *74*, 4783–4795. [CrossRef] [PubMed]
24. Li, N.; Huang, D.; Lu, N.; Luo, L. Role of the LKB1/AMPK pathway in tumor invasion and metastasis of cancer cells (Review). *Oncol. Rep.* **2015**, *34*, 2821–2826. [CrossRef] [PubMed]
25. Liang, S.; Medina, E.A.; Li, B.; Habib, S.L. Preclinical evidence of the enhanced effectiveness of combined rapamycin and AICAR in reducing kidney cancer. *Mol. Oncol.* **2018**, *12*, 1917–1934. [CrossRef]
26. Zhang, Y.; Fan, Y.; Huang, S.; Wang, G.; Han, R.; Lei, F.; Luo, A.; Jing, X.; Zhao, L.; Gu, S.; et al. Thymoquinone inhibits the metastasis of renal cancer cells by inducing autophagy via AMPK/mTOR signaling pathway. *Cancer Sci.* **2018**, *109*, 3865–3873. [CrossRef]
27. Quentin, T.; Kitz, J.; Steinmetz, M.; Poppe, A.; Bar, K.; Kratzner, R. Different expression of the catalytic alpha subunits of the AMP activated protein kinase–an immunohistochemical study in human tissue. *Histol. Histopathol.* **2011**, *26*, 589–596. [CrossRef]
28. Vidal, A.P.; Andrade, B.M.; Vaisman, F.; Cazarin, J.; Pinto, L.F.R.; Breitenbach, M.M.D.; Corbo, R.; Caroli-Bottino, A.; Soares, F.; Vaisman, M.; et al. AMP-activated protein kinase signaling is upregulated in papillary thyroid cancer. *Eur. J. Endocrinol.* **2013**, *169*, 521–528. [CrossRef]
29. Matsuzaki, K. Smad phosphoisoform signaling specificity: The right place at the right time. *Carcinogenesis* **2011**, *32*, 1578–1588. [CrossRef]
30. Katajisto, P.; Vaahtomeri, K.; Ekman, N.; Ventela, E.; Ristimaki, A.; Bardeesy, N.; Feil, R.; DePinho, R.A.; Makela, T.P. LKB1 signaling in mesenchymal cells required for suppression of gastrointestinal polyposis. *Nat. Genet.* **2008**, *40*, 455–459. [CrossRef]
31. Vaahtomeri, K.; Ventela, E.; Laajanen, K.; Katajisto, P.; Wipff, P.J.; Hinz, B.; Vallenius, T.; Tiainen, M.; Makela, T.P. Lkb1 is required for TGFbeta-mediated myofibroblast differentiation. *J. Cell Sci.* **2008**, *121*, 3531–3540. [CrossRef]
32. Fu, G.; Peng, C. Nodal enhances the activity of FoxO3a and its synergistic interaction with Smads to regulate cyclin G2 transcription in ovarian cancer cells. *Oncogene* **2011**, *30*, 3953–3966. [CrossRef]
33. Gomis, R.R.; Alarcon, C.; He, W.; Wang, Q.; Seoane, J.; Lash, A.; Massague, J. A FoxO-smad synexpression group in human keratinocytes. *Proc. Natl. Acad. Sci. USA* **2006**, *103*, 12747–12752. [CrossRef]
34. Sridharan, S.; Jain, K.; Basu, A. Regulation of autophagy by kinases. *Cancers* **2011**, *3*, 2630–2654. [CrossRef]

35. Paner, G.P.; Stadler, W.M.; Hansel, D.E.; Montironi, R.; Lin, D.W.; Amin, M.B. Updates in the eighth edition of the tumor-node-metastasis staging classification for urologic cancers. *Eur. Urol.* **2018**, *73*, 560–569. [CrossRef]
36. Bankhead, P.; Loughrey, M.B.; Fernandez, J.A.; Dombrowski, Y.; McArt, D.G.; Dunne, P.D.; McQuaid, S.; Gray, R.T.; Murray, L.J.; Coleman, H.G.; et al. QuPath: Open source software for digital pathology image analysis. *Sci. Rep.* **2017**, *7*, 16878. [CrossRef]
37. Broad Institute GDAC Firehose. Available online: http://gdac.broadinstitute.org/ (accessed on 5 August 2019).
38. Li, B.; Dewey, C.N. RSEM: Accurate transcript quantification from RNA-Seq data with or without a reference genome. *BMC Bioinform.* **2011**, *12*, 323. [CrossRef]
39. Robinson, M.D.; McCarthy, D.J.; Smyth, G.K. edgeR: A Bioconductor package for differential expression analysis of digital gene expression data. *Bioinformatics* **2010**, *26*, 139–140. [CrossRef]
40. Ritchie, M.E.; Phipson, B.; Wu, D.; Hu, Y.; Law, C.W.; Shi, W.; Smyth, G.K. limma powers differential expression analyses for RNA-sequencing and microarray studies. *Nucleic Acids Res.* **2015**, *43*, e47. [CrossRef]

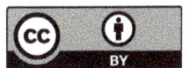 © 2019 by the authors. Licensee MDPI, Basel, Switzerland. This article is an open access article distributed under the terms and conditions of the Creative Commons Attribution (CC BY) license (http://creativecommons.org/licenses/by/4.0/).

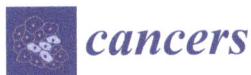

Article

Classic Chromophobe Renal Cell Carcinoma Incur a Larger Number of Chromosomal Losses Than Seen in the Eosinophilic Subtype

Riuko Ohashi [1,2,3], Peter Schraml [2], Silvia Angori [2], Aashil A. Batavia [2,4], Niels J. Rupp [2], Chisato Ohe [5], Yoshiro Otsuki [6], Takashi Kawasaki [7], Hiroshi Kobayashi [8], Kazuhiro Kobayashi [9], Tatsuhiko Miyazaki [9], Hiroyuki Shibuya [10], Hiroyuki Usuda [11], Hajime Umezu [12], Fumiyoshi Fujishima [13], Bungo Furusato [14,15], Mitsumasa Osakabe [16], Tamotsu Sugai [16], Naoto Kuroda [17], Toyonori Tsuzuki [18], Yoji Nagashima [19], Yoichi Ajioka [1,3] and Holger Moch [2,*]

1. Histopathology Core Facility, Faculty of Medicine, Niigata University, Niigata 951-8510, Japan; riuko@med.niigata-u.ac.jp (R.O.); ajioka@med.niigata-u.ac.jp (Y.A.)
2. Department of Pathology and Molecular Pathology, University and University Hospital Zurich, CH-8091 Zurich, Switzerland; Peter.Schraml@usz.ch (P.S.); Silvia.Angori@usz.ch (S.A.); Aashil.Batavia@usz.ch (A.A.B.); niels.rupp@usz.ch (N.R.)
3. Division of Molecular and Diagnostic Pathology, Graduate School of Medical and Dental Sciences, Niigata University, Niigata 951-8510, Japan
4. Department of Biosystems Science and Engineering, ETH Zurich, 4058 Basel, Switzerland
5. Department of Pathology and Laboratory Medicine, Kansai Medical University, Hirakata, Osaka 573-1010, Japan; ohec@hirakata.kmu.ac.jp
6. Department of Pathology, Seirei Hamamatsu General Hospital, Hamamatsu, Shizuoka 430-8558, Japan; otsuki@sis.seirei.or.jp
7. Department of Pathology, Niigata Cancer Center Hospital, Niigata 951-8566, Japan; takawa@niigata-cc.jp
8. Department of Pathology, Tachikawa General Hospital, Nagaoka, Niigata 940-8621, Japan; h-kobayashi15@tatikawa.or.jp
9. Department of Pathology, Gifu University Hospital, Gifu 501-1194, Japan; hern@live.jp (K.K.); tats_m@gifu-u.ac.jp (T.M.)
10. Department of Pathology, Niigata City General Hospital, Niigata 950-1197, Japan; shibuya2u@hosp.niigata.niigata.jp
11. Department of Diagnostic Pathology, Nagaoka Red Cross Hospital, Nagaoka, Niigata 940-2085, Japan; usuda@nagaoka.jrc.or.jp
12. Division of Pathology, Niigata University Medical & Dental Hospital, Niigata 951-8520, Japan; umezu@med.niigata-u.ac.jp
13. Department of Anatomic Pathology, Graduate School of Medicine, Tohoku University, Sendai, Miyagi 980-8575, Japan; ffujishima@patholo2.med.tohoku.ac.jp
14. Cancer Genomics Unit, Clinical Genomics Center, Nagasaki University Hospital, Nagasaki 852-8501, Japan; befurusato@me.com
15. Department of Pathology, Graduate School of Biomedical Sciences, Nagasaki University, Nagasaki 852-8501, Japan
16. Department of Molecular Diagnostic Pathology, School of Medicine, Iwate Medical University, Yahaba-cho, Shiwa-gun, Iwate 028-3695, Japan; mosakabe@iwate-med.ac.jp (M.O.); tsugai@iwate-med.ac.jp (T.S.)
17. Department of Diagnostic Pathology, Kochi Red Cross Hospital, Kochi 780-8562, Japan; kurochankochi@yahoo.co.jp
18. Department of Surgical Pathology, Aichi Medical University Hospital, Nagakute, Aichi 480-1195, Japan; tsuzuki@aichi-med-u.ac.jp
19. Department of Surgical Pathology, Tokyo Women's Medical University Hospital, Shinjuku-ku, Tokyo 162-8666, Japan; nagashima.yoji@twmu.ac.jp
* Correspondence: holger.moch@usz.ch; Tel.: +41-44-255-2500

Received: 8 August 2019; Accepted: 26 September 2019; Published: 3 October 2019

Abstract: Chromophobe renal cell carcinoma (chRCC) is a renal tumor subtype with a good prognosis, characterized by multiple chromosomal copy number variations (CNV). The World Health

Organization (WHO) chRCC classification guidelines define a classic and an eosinophilic variant. Large cells with reticular cytoplasm and prominent cell membranes (pale cells) are characteristic for classic chRCC. Classic and eosinophilic variants were defined in 42 Swiss chRCCs, 119 Japanese chRCCs and in whole-slide digital images of 66 chRCCs from the Cancer Genome Atlas (TCGA) kidney chromophobe (KICH) dataset. 32 of 42 (76.2%) Swiss chRCCs, 90 of 119 (75.6%) Japanese chRCCs and 53 of 66 (80.3%) TCGA-KICH were classic chRCCs. There was no survival difference between eosinophilic and classic chRCC in all three cohorts. To identify a genotype/phenotype correlation, we performed a genome-wide CNV analysis using Affymetrix OncoScan® CNV Assay (Affymetrix/Thermo Fisher Scientific, Waltham, MA, USA) in 33 Swiss chRCCs. TCGA-KICH subtypes were compared with TCGA CNV data. In the combined Swiss and TCGA-KICH cohorts, losses of chromosome 1, 2, 6, 10, 13, and 17 were significantly more frequent in classic chRCC ($p < 0.05$, each), suggesting that classic chRCC are characterized by higher chromosomal instability. This molecular difference justifies the definition of two chRCC variants. Absence of pale cells could be used as main histological criterion to define the eosinophilic variant of chRCC.

Keywords: chromophobe renal cell carcinoma; pale cell; eosinophilic variant; chromosomal loss; copy number analysis; renal cell carcinoma

1. Introduction

Chromophobe renal cell carcinoma (chRCC) is a distinct histological entity of renal cell carcinoma (RCC) described by Thoenes et al. [1] in 1985. chRCC accounts for approximately 5–7% of RCC [2–4]. Thoenes et al. used the term chromophobe cell for larger cells with reticular, but not clear cytoplasm and prominent cell membranes (plant cell-like) [1,2]. Three years later, these authors described eosinophilic cells with smaller size and with fine oxiphilic granularity as a second cell component of chRCC [3]. Crotty et al. used the term pale cell instead of the formerly used term chromophobe cell and considered pale cell and eosinophilic cell [5] as two main cell types in chRCC. Several ultrastructural studies showed that pale cells are characterized by numerous cytoplasmic microvesicles, a feature probably related to defective mitochondrial development, whereas mitochondria are abundant in eosinophilic cells [2,6–8].

Most chRCCs consist of both cell types, which are typically mixed, with eosinophilic cells usually arranged at the center and pale cells usually arranged at the periphery of the sheets or nests [2]. The 2016 World Health Organization (WHO) renal tumor classification acknowledges an eosinophilic variant of chRCC "that is sometimes difficult to distinguish from renal oncocytoma" [3–5,9,10] but there are no exact diagnostic criteria to classify an eosinophilic chRCC.

Previous studies have demonstrated losses of one copy in many chromosomes, especially in chromosomes 1, 2, 6, 10, 13, 17, 21 and sex chromosome in the majority of chRCCs (~71%). Losses of chromosome 1 and sex chromosome have been also reported in oncocytoma [4,9,11–15]. Recently, mutation of *TP53*, *PTEN*, *HNF1B* were observed in chRCCs [13,16,17]. Previous studies also disclosed frequent somatic mitochondrial DNA mutations in oncocytoma [13,18,19] and chRCCs [9,20], but a clear genotype/phenotype correlation has never been described in chRCC.

In this study, we analyzed the histopathological variants of chRCCs in 42 Swiss, 119 Japanese and in whole-slide digital images of 66 chRCCs from The Cancer Genome Atlas (TCGA) Kidney Chromophobe (KICH) dataset. Further, we utilized single-nucleotide polymorphism (SNP) arrays to assess genome-wide copy number variation (CNV) and correlated CNV to the histological variants in the Swiss and the TCGA-KICH data [13].

2. Results

2.1. Swiss Cohort

There were 22 of 33 (66.7%) classic chRCCs with typical voluminous pale cells in the Swiss cohort (Table 1). Tumors with and without pale cell are shown in Figure 1. There was no association between the chRCC subtypes with age, sex, and pT stage (Table 2). Molecular analysis using the OncoScan® CNV Assay (Affymetrix/Thermo Fisher Scientific, Waltham, MA, USA) revealed loss of part (>5% of gene loci) or the entirety of chromosome 1, 2, 6, 10, 13, 17, 21, and sex chromosome in the majority of cases (Figure 2 and Table 2). Among these chromosomal losses, chromosome 1 was most affected (32/33, 97.0%). Chromosome 2 (24/33, 72.7%), 6 (26/33, 78.8%), 10 (21/33, 63.6%), 13 (23/33, 69.7%), 17 (25/33, 75.8%), and 21 (17/33, 51.5%) were less frequently altered (Table 2).

Table 1. Demographic and clinical characteristics.

Characteristics	Swiss Cohort (Total)	TCGA-KICH	Japanese Cohort
Patient number	42	66	119
Age (years)			
Range	18–87	17–86	26–88
Median	59	50	60
Gender			
Female	13 (31.0%)	27 (40.9%)	69 (58.0%)
Male	29 (69.0%)	39 (59.1%)	50 (42.0%)
pT Stage or T stage, n (%) *			
1	25 (59.5%)	21 (31.8%)	85 (71.4%)
2	11 (26.2%)	25 (37.9%)	19 (16.0%)
3	6 (14.3%)	18 (27.3%)	14 (11.8%)
4	0 (0%)	2 (3.0%)	1 (0.8%)
Subtype			
classic	32 (76.2%)	53 (80.3%)	90 (75.6%)
eosinophilic	10 (23.8%)	13 (19.7%)	29 (24.4%)

* Swiss and Japanese cohort: pT stage, TCGA-KICH: T stage.

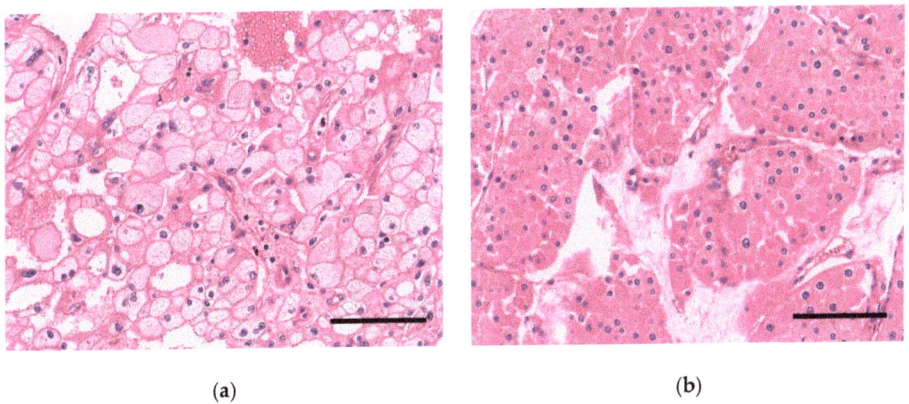

(a)　　　　　　　　　　　　(b)

Figure 1. Representative microscopic images of chromophobe renal cell carcinomas (chRCCs) in the Swiss cohort (hematoxylin and eosin staining, scale bar, 100 μm). (a) classic chRCC with pale cells. (b) eosinophilic chRCC without pale cells.

Table 2. Copy number variation (chromosomal losses) in classic and eosinophilic chromophobe renal cell carcinomas (chRCCs) (Chr. = chromosome) from 33 Swiss chRCCs (Affymetrix OncoScan® CNV Assay; Affymetrix/Thermo Fisher Scientific, Waltham, MA, USA) and combined Swiss/TCGA-KICH cohorts (The Cancer Genome Atlas copy number variation data).

Cohort	Swiss				Combined *			
Characteristics	n (%)	Classic chRCC [a] (%)	Eosinophilic chRCC [b] (%)	p-Value	n (%)	Classic chRCC [a] (%)	Eosinophilic chRCC [b] (%)	p-Value
Total	33	22 (66.7)	11 (33.3)		99	75 (75.8)	24 (24.2)	
Chr.1 status								
Loss	32 (97.0)	22 (100)	10 (90.9)	n.s.	87 (87.9)	70 (93.3)	17 (70.8)	<0.01
No loss	1 (3.0)	0 (0)	1 (9.1)		12 (12.1)	5 (6.7)	7 (29.2)	
Chr.2 status								
Loss	24 (72.7)	19 (86.4)	5 (45.5)	<0.05	73 (73.7)	63 (84.0)	10 (41.7)	<0.001
No loss	9 (27.3)	3 (13.6)	6 (54.5)		26 (26.3)	12 (16.0)	14 (58.3)	
Chr.6 status								
Loss	26 (78.8)	21 (95.5)	5 (45.5)	<0.01	78 (78.8)	68 (90.7)	10 (41.7)	<0.001
No loss	7 (21.2)	1 (4.5)	6 (54.5)		21 (21.2)	7 (9.3)	14 (58.3)	
Chr. 10 status								
Loss	21 (63.6)	16 (72.7)	5 (45.5)	n.s.	70 (70.7)	62 (82.7)	8 (33.3)	<0.001
No loss	12 (36.4)	6 (27.3)	6 (54.5)		29 (29.3)	13 (17.3)	16 (66.7)	
Chr.13 status								
Loss	23 (69.7)	17 (77.3)	6 (54.5)	n.s.	68 (68.7)	57 (76.0)	11 (45.8)	0.01
No loss	10 (30.3)	5 (22.7)	5 (45.5)		31 (31.3)	18 (24.0)	13 (54.2)	
Chr.17 status								
Loss	25 (75.8)	19 (86.4)	6 (54.5)	n.s.	75 (75.8)	64 (85.3)	11 (45.8)	<0.001
No loss	8 (24.2)	3 (13.6)	5 (45.5)		24 (24.2)	11 (14.7)	13 (54.2)	
Chr.21 status								
Loss	17 (51.5)	12 (54.5)	5 (45.5)	n.s.	52 (52.5)	42 (56.0)	10 (41.7)	n.s.
No loss	16 (48.5)	10 (45.5)	6 (54.5)		47 (47.5)	33 (44.0)	14 (58.3)	
Loss of any chromosome [c]								
present	29 (87.9)	21 (95.5)	8 (72.7)	n.s.	83 (83.8)	69 (92.0)	14 (58.3)	<0.001
absent	4 (12.1)	1 (4.5)	3 (27.3)		16 (16.2)	6 (8.0)	10 (41.7)	

[a] defined as the presence of pale cells, [b] defined as absence of pale cells, [c]: Loss of any: Loss of any chromosome among chr. 2, 6, 10, 13, 17, or 21, n.s.: not significant, * combined Swiss/TCGA-KICH cohorts.

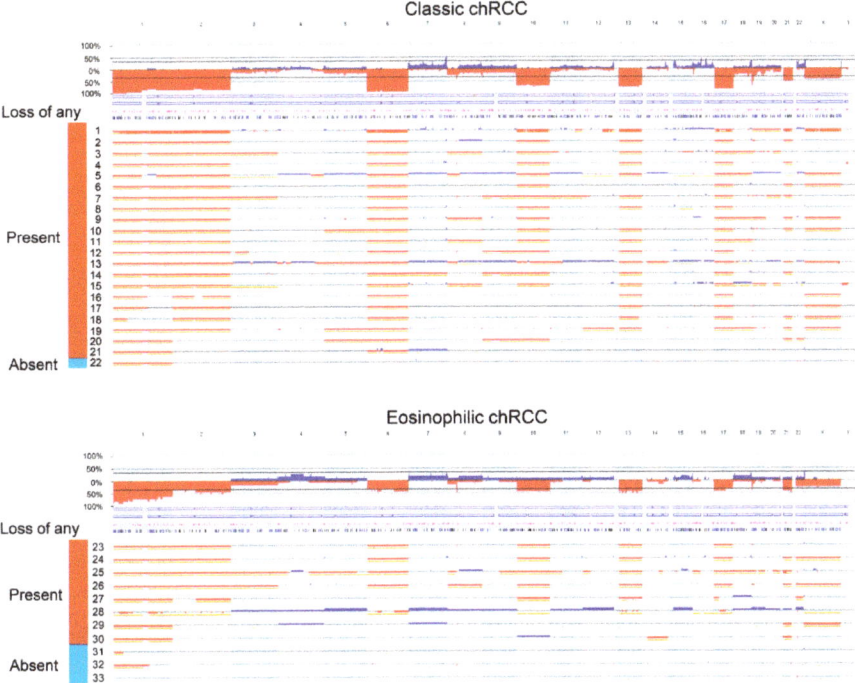

Figure 2. Copy number (CN) alterations and copy-neutral loss-of-heterozygosity detected by Affymetrix OncoScan® CNV Assay of 22 classic chromophobe renal cell carcinomas (chRCCs) (upper panel) and 11 eosinophilic chRCCs (lower panel) in the Swiss cohort. Red signal, blue signal, and yellow signal show copy-number loss, copy-number gain, and copy-neutral loss-of-heterozygosity, respectively. Loss of any: Loss of any chromosome among chromosome 2, 6, 10, 13, 17, or 21. Red: Present, Blue: Absent.

The Correlation between chromosomal losses and clinicopathological features of 33 chRCCs are summarized in Table 2. Classic chRCC showed significantly more chromosome 2 ($p < 0.05$), and chromosome 6 losses ($p < 0.01$) than eosinophilic RCC (Table 2). Among 22 classic chRCCs with pale cells, 19/22 (86.4%) showed chromosome 2 loss, 21/22 (95.5%) chromosome 6 loss, 16/22 (72.7%) chromosome 10 loss, 17/22 (77.3%) chromosome 13 loss, and 19/22 (86.4%) chromosome 17 loss.

2.2. TCGA Cohort

53 of 64 (80.3%) were classic chRCCs (Tables 1 and 2). Classic chRCCs from the Cancer Digital Slide Archive are shown in Figure 3. The publicly available copy number variation (CNV) analysis data of TCGA-KICH dataset revealed losses of chromosomes 1, 2, 6, 10, 13, 17, and 21 in the majority of chRCC as previously reported [13]. The CNV data are summarized in Table S1.

Classic chRCC showed significantly more chromosome 1, 2, 6, 10, 17 copy number (CN) losses ($p < 0.01$) and chromosome 13 CN loss ($p < 0.05$) (Table S1). When the Swiss and TCGA-KICH cohorts were combined, losses of chromosome 1, 2, 6, 10, 13 and 17 were significantly more frequent in classic chRCC with pale cells ($p < 0.05$, each) (Table 2).

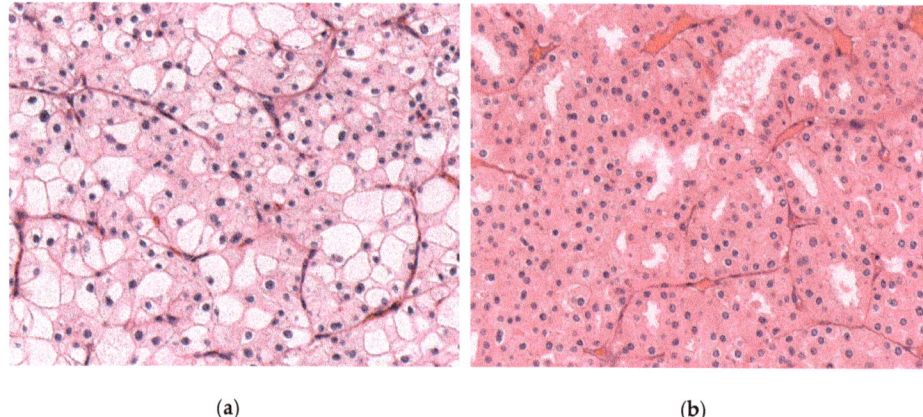

Figure 3. Representative microscopic images of chromophobe renal cell carcinomas (chRCCs) in the Cancer Genome Atlas Kidney Chromophobe (TCGA-KICH) cohort, whole-slide images from the Cancer Digital Slide Archive [21] (**a**) classic chRCC with pale cells (TCGA-KL-8345). (**b**) eosinophilic chRCC without pale cells (TCGA-KL-8326).

2.3. Chromophobe Renal Cancer Subtype and Survival

Higher pT stage (pT3–4 vs. pT1–2) and higher pN stage (pN1–2 vs. pN0) were significantly associated with worse survival by log-rank test (Figure 4a,b) and univariate Cox regression analysis (Table 3) in the Swiss-TCGA-Japanese cohort. There was no overall survival (OS) difference between classic and eosinophilic chRCC subtypes in the three independent cohorts of the Swiss (42 cases), TCGA-KICH (64 cases) and the Japanese (119 cases) nor in the Swiss-TCGA-Japanese combined cohort (Figure 4c). Multivariate Cox regression analysis, including pT stage (pT3–4 vs. pT1–2), pN stage (pN1–2 vs. pN0), WHO/ISUP grade (Grade 3/4 vs. Grade 2), and chRCC subtype showed that pT stage and pN stage were independent prognostic factors for OS, whereas no prognostic impact of the chRCC subtype or WHO/International Society of Urological Pathology (ISUP) grade was observed (Table 3).

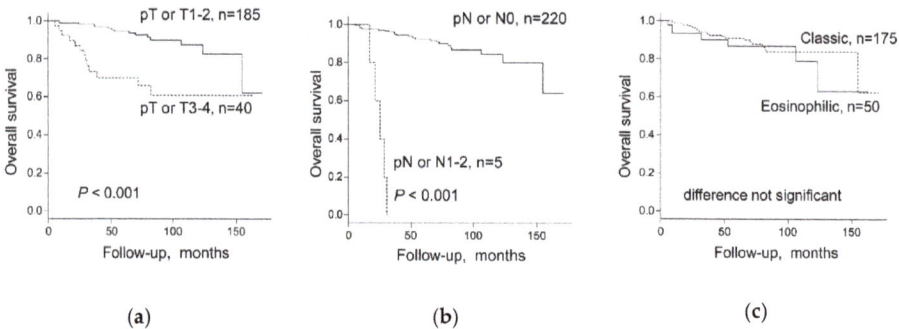

Figure 4. Overall survival stratified by (**a**) pT Stage or T stage (1–2 versus 3–4), (**b**) pN stage or N stage (pN1–2 versus pN0), and (**c**) chromophobe renal cell carcinoma (chRCC) subtype in all 225 chRCC patients combined from the Swiss, the Cancer Genome Atlas Kidney Chromophobe (TCGA-KICH), and Japanese cohorts. pT Stage or T stage: Swiss and Japanese cohorts, pT stage, and TCGA-KICH, T stage was used for the calculation. pN stage or N stage: Swiss and Japanese cohorts, pN stage, and TCGA-KICH, N stage was used for the calculation.

Table 3. Univariate and Multivariate Cox regression analysis on overall survival of 225 chRCC patients combined from Swiss, TCGA-KICH and Japanese cohorts.

Variables	Univariate		Multivariate	
	HR (95%CI)	p-Value	HR (95%CI)	p-Value
pT Stage or T stage * (3–4 vs. 1–2)	4.809 (2.275–10.16)	<0.001	3.177 (1.336–7.556)	<0.01
pN Stage or N stage * (1–2 vs. 0)	42.95 (13.16–140.1)	<0.001	21.140 (5.612–79.650)	<0.001
WHO/ISUP grade (Grade 3/4 vs. Grade 2) **	1.667 (0.502–5.537)	n.s.	2.010 (0.594–6.804)	n.s.
Subtype (classic vs. eosinophilic)	0.756 (0.321–1.782)	n.s.	0.520 (0.207–1.303)	n.s.

HR, hazard ratio, CI, confidence interval, n.s.: not significant. * Swiss and Japanese cohort: pT/pN stage, TCGA-KICH: T/N stage. ** WHO/ISUP grading system is not recommended for chRCC.

2.4. Chromosomal Copy Number Variation and Survival

Both, CN data and survival data were available from 30 Swiss chRCCs and 64 chRCCs from TCGA-KICH cohort. In the Swiss cohort, neither CN losses of each chromosome 1, 2, 6, 10, 13, 17, 21 in single analysis nor CN loss of any chromosome among chromosome 1, 2, 6, 10, 13, 17, 21 were associated with worse survival by log-rank test and univariate Cox regression analysis (Table 4). In the combined Swiss-TCGA cohort, only chromosome 21 CN loss was associated with shorter overall survival, whereas all other chromosomes were not associated with survival (Figure 5a and Table 4). Multivariate analysis showed that pT stage was the only independent prognostic factor for OS whereas no association was found between OS and CN loss of chromosome 21 or CN loss of any other chromosome among chromosome 1, 2, 6, 10, 13, 17, 21 (Table 5). Importantly, chRCCs without any CN loss of chromosome 1, 2, 6, 10, 13, 17, 21 groups revealed 100% survival in the combined Swiss/TCGA-KICH cohorts (Figure 5b and Table 4).

Table 4. Univariate survival analysis (Kaplan-Meier) with log-rank test (overall survival) of 94 chRCC patients combined from Swiss and TCGA-KICH cohorts (Chr. = chromosome).

Cohort	Swiss			Combined		
Characteristics	Cases, n (%)	Patient Death, n (%)	p-Value	Cases, n (%)	Patient Death, n (%)	p-Value
Total	30	5 (16.7)		94	14 (14.9)	
Chr.1 status						
Loss	30 (100)	5 (100)	n.s.	83 (88.3)	14 (100)	n.s.
No loss	0 (0)	0 (0)		11 (11.7)	0 (0)	
Chr.2 status						
Loss	22 (73.3)	4 (80.0)	n.s.	69 (73.4)	12 (85.7)	n.s.
No loss	8 (26.7)	1 (20.0)		25 (26.6)	2 (14.3)	
Chr.6 status						
Loss	25 (83.3)	4 (80.0)	n.s.	75 (79.8)	12 (85.7)	n.s.
No loss	5 (16.7)	1 (20.0)		19 (20.2)	2 (14.3)	
Chr. 10 status						
Loss	19 (63.3)	3 (60.0)	n.s.	67 (71.3)	12 (85.7)	n.s.
No loss	11 (36.7)	2 (40.0)		27 (28.7)	2 (14.3)	
Chr.13 status						
Loss	21 (70.0)	4 (80.0)	n.s.	64 (68.1)	11 (78.6)	n.s.
No loss	9 (30.0)	1 (20.0)		30 (31.9)	3 (21.4)	
Chr.17 status						
Loss	23 (76.7)	4 (80.0)	n.s.	71 (75.5)	11 (78.6)	n.s.
No loss	7 (23.3)	1 (20.0)		23 (24.5)	3 (21.4)	
Chr.21 status						
Loss	17 (56.7)	4 (80.0)	n.s.	50 (53.2)	12 (85.7)	<0.05
No loss	13 (43.3)	1 (20.0)		44 (46.8)	2 (14.3)	
Loss of any chromosome *						
present	30 (100)	5 (100)	n.s.	83 (88.3)	14 (100)	n.s.
absent	0 (0)	0 (0)		11 (11.7)	0 (0)	

* Loss of any chromosome: Loss of any chromosome among chr. 1, 2, 6, 10, 13, 17 or 21, n.s.: not significant.

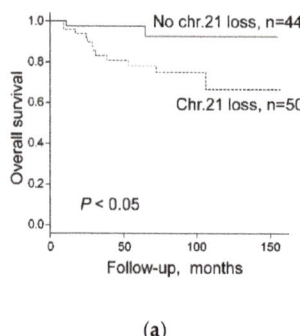 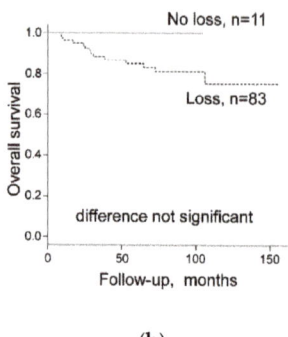

(a) (b)

Figure 5. Overall survival stratified by (**a**) chromosome 21 status (Chr.21 loss versus No chr.21 loss) and (**b**) Loss of any chromosome among chromosome 1, 2, 6, 10, 13, 17, or 21 (Loss versus No loss) in 94 chRCC patients combined from Swiss and the Cancer Genome Atlas Kidney Chromophobe (TCGA-KICH) cohorts.

Table 5. Univariate and Multivariate Cox regression analysis (overall survival) of 94 chRCC patients combined from Swiss and TCGA-KICH cohorts.

Variables	Univariate		Multivariate		Multivariate	
	HR (95%CI)	p-Value	HR (95%CI)	p-Value	HR (95%CI)	p-Value
pT Stage or T stage [a] (3–4 vs. 1–2)	6.323 (2.078–19.25)	0.001	5.505 (1.935–17.450)	<0.01	6.344 (2.010–20.03)	<0.01
Loss of any chromosome [b,c] (present vs. absent)	2.503 (0.331–320.637)	n.s.	1.319 (0.154–172.711)	n.s.		
Loss of chromosome 21 (present vs. absent)	4.684 (1.047–20.95)	<0.05			4.480 (1.000–20.08)	n.s.

HR, hazard ratio, CI, confidence interval, n.s.: not significant. a: Swiss and Japanese cohort: pT stage, [a] Swiss and Japanese cohort: pT stage, TCGA-KICH: T stage, [b] Loss of any: Loss of any chromosome of chromosome 1, 2, 6, 10, 13, 17, or 21, [c] Firth correction was used because of quasi-complete separation, there was no event in one of the subgroups.

3. Discussion

In our study, we used the absence of voluminous pale cells to define eosinophilic chRCC. Using this definition, classic chRCC is associated with significantly more frequent losses of chromosomes 1, 2, 6, 10, 13, and 17.

Various cytogenetic, comparative genomic hybridization, and recent molecular studies have confirmed the very unique and characteristic genotype with multiple chromosomal losses in chRCC [4,9,11–15]. However, previous attempts to correlate histological variants of chRCCs with a specific genotype have failed. More than 10 years ago, Brunelli et al. analyzed classic and eosinophilic chRCCs by fluorescence in situ hybridization, but they have not observed different frequencies of chromosomal 2, 6, 10, and 17 losses [11]. This is in contrast to our OncoScan results with more chromosomal CNV in classic than in eosinophilic chRCC. Our results are in line with a TCGA-KICH study by Davis et al., demonstrating in almost all classic chRCC there are characteristic chromosomal copy-number losses, whilst approximately 50% of all eosinophilic chRCC (9 of 19) experienced no chromosomal copy-number alterations [13]. Recently, Trpkov et al. proposed low-grade oncocytic tumors (LOT) as an emerging renal tumor entity [22]. They argue that LOT lacks multiple chromosomal losses and gains, and exhibits indolent clinical behavior. This tumor does not fit completely into either oncocytoma or eosinophilic chRCC, despite showing some similarities with both entities. Further studies are warranted to proof that LOT potentially represents a distinct type of tumor or if they should be regarded as variant of eosinophilic chRCC.

During our study design and the re-evaluation of histological slides for this study, we realized that there are no stringent diagnostic criteria to classify eosinophilic chRCC. The current 2016 WHO classification states that eosinophilic chRCC is almost purely composed of eosinophilic cells and that the majority of cells should be eosinophilic cells [2]. Given this lack of exact criteria, we decided to use the complete absence of pale cells as definition for eosinophilic chRCC, because pale cells are easily identifiable and can be clearly separated from eosinophilic cells.

As a consequence of this lack of stringent criteria for subtyping chRCC, distribution of chRCC variants varies extremely between different studies [2,3,10,11,23,24]. Davis et al. recently classified the TCGA-KICH tumors as classic and eosinophilic variants [13]. Our evaluation of TCGA-KICH digital whole slide images for chRCC only partially matched his classification of classical and eosinophilic variants, which can be explained by our more conservative cut-off to define eosinophilic chRCC (complete absence of pale cells).

Interestingly, there were no survival differences between eosinophilic and classic chRCC in 3 cohorts from TCGA, Japan and Europe. Given the morphological overlap between eosinophilic chRCC and benign oncocytoma, one could assume that eosinophilic chRCC have a better prognosis than classic chRCC. The prognostic similarity between eosinophilic and classic chRCC further underlines the importance to clearly separate eosinophilic chRCC from oncocytoma. Most importantly, classic chRCC had significantly more losses of chromosome 2 and 6 in the Swiss tumors and more losses of chromosome 1, 2, 6, 10, 13, and 17 in the TCGA dataset. Swiss classic chRCC showed only a trend to more chromosome 1, 10, 13, or 17 losses, probably due to the lower number of cases (Table 2). Almost all eosinophilic and all classic chRCC (91–100%) revealed chromosome 1 loss, suggesting that chromosome 1 loss may be an early event in chRCC tumorigenesis. Chromosome 1 losses have even been identified in oncocytoma [9,11,12,15]. This could be due to the misclassification of eosinophilic chRCCs as oncocytoma, but it is also tempting to speculate that there is a stepwise progression from oncocytoma to eosinophilic or classic chRCC with chromosome 1 loss as a genetic driver.

Treatment outcomes are poorly characterized in patients with metastatic chRCC. This is a consequence of rare metastasis of this subtype. Patients with metastatic chRCC can be treated with tyrosine kinase inhibitors. It has been recently shown that outcomes between metastatic chRCC and clear cell renal cell carcinoma (ccRCC) are similar when treated with conventional targeted therapies [25]. In addition, chRCC has to activate mutations in phosphatase and tensin homolog (PTEN)-phosphatidylinositol 3-kinase (PI3K)/Protein Kinase B (Akt)/mammalian target of the rapamycin (mTOR) pathway [13], which would result in an appropriate target for an mTOR inhibitor. Genomic instability, including whole-chromosome aneuploidy, is a hallmark of human cancer, but the level of chromosomal losses in chRCC is unique. We have recently identified $SF3B1$ on chromosome 2 as a Copy-number alterations Yielding Cancer Liabilities Owing to Partial losS (CYCLOPS) gene with a highly significant positive correlation to hypoxia-inducible factor-1α (HIF1α) [26]. It is therefore tempting to speculate that an Splicing factor 3B subunit 1 (SF3B1)/HIF1α pathway with potential therapeutical relevance exists in chRCC.

Due to the unique genomic background, chRCC should be enrolled in separate clinical trials to measure outcomes. However, chRCC is mostly included in clinical trials together with other non-clear cell RCCs. Accurate classification of metastatic lesions is therefore important as chRCC should be managed with different treatment algorithms. Kouba et al. have recently demonstrated that cytogenetics, showing multiple genetic losses is an additional tool in a metastatic RCC lesion for differential diagnosis of the primary [27]. Our own data show that chRCC without chromosomal losses have an indolent behavior. Therefore, analysis of chromosomal losses by fluorescence in situ hybridization (FISH) or other technologies could be used to assess the behavior of chRCC in organ-confined tumors or to better characterize metastatic lesions of RCC.

4. Materials and Methods

4.1. Swiss Patients

chRCC patients were identified from the files of the Department of Pathology and Molecular Pathology of the University Hospital Zurich between 1993 and 2013. Our retrospective study fulfilled the legal conditions according to Article 34 of the Swiss Law "Humanforschungsgesetz (HFG)", which, in exceptional cases, allows the use of biomaterial and patient data for research purposes without informed consent, if i) it is impossible or disproportionately difficult to obtain patient consent; ii) there is no documented refusal; iii) research interests prevail the individual interest of a patient. Law abidance of this study was reviewed and approved by the ethics commission of the Canton Zurich (KEK-ZH-Nr. 2014-0604 on 1st April 2015; PB_2016-00811 on 22nd February 2016). This study was conducted in accordance with the Declaration of Helsinki. The demographic and clinicopathological characteristics for 42 chRCCs with clinical data are summarized in Table 1.

All tumors were reviewed by two pathologists (R.O. and H.M.). At least two sections were observed for determination of the existence of pale cells in tumor tissue according to the standard international protocol for pathological examination of RCCs [28,29]. ChRCCs were defined according to the 2016 WHO classification as tumors composed of large polygonal cells with reticular, clear or eosinophilic cytoplasm showing distinct cell borders, sometimes perinuclear halo and irregular (raisinoid) nuclei.

Pale cells were described as being larger than eosinophilic cells, with voluminous pale, finely reticular, but not clear cytoplasm and with distinct cell borders. We used hematoxylin and eosin-stained sections and paid particular attention to the periphery of tumor cell sheet or nest, i.e., around the vascular septa and fibrous stroma in the tumor.

4.2. The Cancer Genome Atlas (TCGA) Dataset

Clinical information of TCGA-KICH was obtained from the National Cancer Institute Genomic Data Commons Data Portal [30]. In TCGA-KICH dataset, there were 66 primary chRCCs with matched copy number variation data [13]. The demographic and clinical characteristics for the selected 66 patients are summarized in Table 1. Detailed clinical data can be found in Table S2. For survival analysis, the patients with missing or with too short a follow-up (i.e., less than 30 days) were excluded from this study.

Digital whole slide images of TCGA cases were reviewed by using the Cancer Digital Slide Archive [21]. Publically available Level 3 TCGA data were downloaded from the FIREHOSE database [31], including GISTIC CN data.

4.3. Japanese Patients

chRCCs with available histological material was retrieved from the archives of 13 of the authors' institutions. The institutions are: Niigata University Medical & Dental Hospital (cases from 2002 to 2015), Kansai Medical University Hirakata Hospital (cases from 2007 to 2015), Seirei Hamamatsu General Hospital (cases from 2004 to 2015), Niigata Cancer Center Hospital (cases from 2002 to 2015), Tachikawa General Hospital (cases from 2007 to 2015), Gifu University Hospital (cases from 2005 to 2015), Niigata City General Hospital (cases from 2007 to 2015), Nagaoka Red Cross Hospital (cases from 2008 to 2015), Tohoku University Hospital (cases from 2008 to 2015), Nagasaki University Hospital (cases from 2014 to 2015), Iwate Medical University Hospital (cases from 2007 to 2015), Kochi Red Cross Hospital (cases from 2007 to 2015), and Aichi Medical University Hospital (cases from 2008 to 2015). The study did not include consultation cases. The study protocol was approved by the institutional review boards in all participating institutions. This study was a retrospective observational study, and an opt-out approach was used with the disclosure of this study on the website of each institution. The patients with missing or too short a follow-up (i.e., less than 30 days) were excluded from this study. All chRCCs were negative for vimentin except for focal sarcomatoid areas. The demographic and clinicopathological characteristics for the 119 chRCCs are summarized in Table 1.

4.4. OncoScan® CNV Assay of chRCCs

Tumor areas displaying >80% cancer cells without hemorrhage or necrosis were marked on the hematoxylin and eosin slides. DNA from FFPE tumor tissue samples was obtained by punching 4 to 6 tissue cylinders (diameter 0.6 mm) from each sample. DNA extraction from FFPE tissue was done as described [32]. The double-strand DNA concentration (dsDNA) was determined using the fluorescence-based Qubit dsDNA HS Assay Kit (Thermo Fisher Scientific, Waltham, MA, USA). Tumors with poor DNA quality were excluded from the study. Genome-wide DNA copy-number alterations and allelic imbalances of 33 chRCC were determined using the Affymetrix OncoScan® CNV Assay (Affymetrix/Thermo Fisher Scientific, Waltham, MA, USA) as previously described [33]. The demographic and clinicopathological characteristics for 33 Swiss chRCCs with clinical data are summarized in Table 1. Samples were further processed by IMGM Laboratories GmbH (Martinsried, Germany) for CNV (copy number variation) determination according to the Affymetrix OncoScan CNV Assay recommended protocol. The data were analyzed by the Nexus Copy Number 10.0 (Biodiscovery, Inc., El Segundo, CA, USA) software using Affymetrix TuScan algorithm. All array data were also manually reviewed for subtle alterations not automatically called by the software.

4.5. Statistical Analysis

All statistical analysis was done using R version 3.4.1 (R Foundation for Statistical Computing, Vienna, Austria) and EZR, Version 1.37 (Saitama Medical Center, Jichi Medical University, Saitama, Japan), which is a graphical user interface for R [34]. Fisher's exact test was used to assess the association between two categorical variables. A Kaplan–Meier analysis and the log-rank test were used to derive and compare survival curves. Univariate and multivariate regression analyses with the Cox proportional hazards model were used to identify prognostic factors. The significance threshold was set at a p-value of 0.05.

5. Conclusions

In conclusion, the molecular difference between classic and eosinophilic chRCCs justifies the definition of 2 chRCC variants. Using the absence of pale cells as a diagnostic criterion for the eosinophilic variant may improve the reproducibility of histopathological subtyping.

Supplementary Materials: The following are available online at http://www.mdpi.com/2072-6694/11/10/1492/s1, Table S1: Copy number variation (chromosomal losses) in classic and eosinophilic chromophobe renal cell carcinomas in TCGA-KICH cohort (Chr. = chromosome), Table S2: Clinicopathological and copy number variation data of 64 chRCC of TCGA-KICH cohort.

Author Contributions: Conceptualization, R.O., P.S. and H.M.; methodology, R.O., S.A., A.A.B. and H.M.; software, S.A. and A.A.B.; validation, R.O. and A.A.B.; formal analysis, R.O., S.A., A.A.B. and H.M.; investigation, R.O.; resources, R.O., P.S., N.J.R., C.O., Y.O., T.K., H.K., K.K., T.M., H.S., H.U. (Hiroyuki Usuda), H.U. (Hajime Umezu), F.F., B.F., M.O., T.S., N.K., T.T., Y.N., Y.A., and H.M.; data curation, R.O., P.S., N.J.R.; Writing—Original Draft preparation, R.O. and H.M.; Writing—Review and Editing, All authors; visualization, R.O. and A.A.B.; supervision, H.M.; project administration, P.S. and H.M.; funding acquisition, R.O. and H.M.

Funding: This work was supported in part by Niigata Foundation for the Promotion of Medicine (2015 to R.O.) and the Swiss National Science Foundation grant (No. S-87701-03-01 to H.M.).

Acknowledgments: The authors thank Susanne Dettwiler and Fabiola Prutek (Department of Pathology and Molecular Pathology, University Hospital Zurich), Kazue Kobayashi, Ayako Maruyama, Ayako Sato, Naoyuki Yamaguchi (Division of Molecular and Diagnostic Pathology, Niigata University Graduate School of Medical and Dental Sciences), Chikashi Ikegame, Kanae Takahashi, Yukie Kawaguchi and Chiaki Yokoyama (Division of Pathology, Niigata University Medical & Dental Hospital) for their outstanding technical assistance. They also thank Toshio Takagi (Department of Urology, Tokyo Women's Medical University) for insightful discussions on clinical aspects. The results published here are in part based upon data generated by the TCGA Research Network: https://www.cancer.gov/tcga.

Conflicts of Interest: The authors have no conflict of interest and nothing to disclose.

References

1. Thoenes, W.; Störkel, S.; Rumpelt, H.J. Human chromophobe cell renal carcinoma. *Virchows Arch. B* **1985**, *48*, 207–217. [CrossRef] [PubMed]
2. Paner, G.; Amin, M.B.; Moch, H.; Störkel, S. Chromophobe renal cell carcinoma. In *WHO Classification of Tumours of the Urinary System and Male Genital Organs*, 4th ed.; Moch, H., Humphrey, P.A., Ulbright, T.M., Reuter, V.E., Eds.; International Agency for Research on Cancer: Lyon, France, 2016; pp. 27–28.
3. Thoenes, W.; Störkel, S.; Rumpelt, H.J.; Moll, R.; Baum, H.P.; Werner, S. Chromophobe cell renal carcinoma and its variants—A report on 32 cases. *J. Pathol.* **1988**, *155*, 277–287. [CrossRef] [PubMed]
4. Yap, N.Y.; Rajandram, R.; Ng, K.L.; Pailoor, J.; Fadzli, A.; Gobe, G.C. Genetic and Chromosomal Aberrations and Their Clinical Significance in Renal Neoplasms. *Biomed. Res. Int.* **2015**, *2015*, 476508. [CrossRef]
5. Crotty, T.B.; Farrow, G.M.; Lieber, M.M. Chromophobe cell renal carcinoma: Clinicopathological features of 50 cases. *J. Urol.* **1995**, *154*, 964–967. [CrossRef]
6. Akhtar, M.; Kardar, H.; Linjawi, T.; McClintock, J.; Ali, M.A. Chromophobe cell carcinoma of the kidney. A clinicopathologic study of 21 cases. *Am. J. Surg. Pathol.* **1995**, *19*, 1245–1256. [CrossRef]
7. Latham, B.; Dickersin, G.R.; Oliva, E. Subtypes of chromophobe cell renal carcinoma: An ultrastructural and histochemical study of 13 cases. *Am. J. Surg. Pathol.* **1999**, *23*, 530–535. [CrossRef]
8. Tickoo, S.K.; Lee, M.W.; Eble, J.N.; Amin, M.; Christopherson, T.; Zarbo, R.J.; Amin, M.B. Ultrastructural observations on mitochondria and microvesicles in renal oncocytoma, chromophobe renal cell carcinoma, and eosinophilic variant of conventional (clear cell) renal cell carcinoma. *Am. J. Surg. Pathol.* **2000**, *24*, 1247–1256. [CrossRef]
9. Ng, K.L.; Rajandram, R.; Morais, C.; Yap, N.Y.; Samaratunga, H.; Gobe, G.C.; Wood, S.T. Differentiation of oncocytoma from chromophobe renal cell carcinoma (RCC): Can novel molecular biomarkers help solve an old problem? *J. Clin. Pathol.* **2014**, *67*, 97–104. [CrossRef]
10. Williamson, S.R.; Gadde, R.; Trpkov, K.; Hirsch, M.S.; Srigley, J.R.; Reuter, V.E.; Cheng, L.; Kunju, L.P.; Barod, R.; Rogers, C.G.; et al. Diagnostic criteria for oncocytic renal neoplasms: A survey of urologic pathologists. *Hum. Pathol.* **2017**, *63*, 149–156. [CrossRef]
11. Brunelli, M.; Eble, J.N.; Zhang, S.; Martignoni, G.; Delahunt, B.; Cheng, L. Eosinophilic and classic chromophobe renal cell carcinomas have similar frequent losses of multiple chromosomes from among chromosomes 1, 2, 6, 10 and 17, and this pattern of genetic abnormality is not present in renal oncocytoma. *Mod. Pathol.* **2005**, *18*, 161–169. [CrossRef]
12. Brunelli, M.; Delahunt, B.; Gobbo, S.; Tardanico, R.; Eccher, A.; Bersani, S.; Cossu-Rocca, P.; Parolini, C.; Balzarini, P.; Menestrina, F.; et al. Diagnostic usefulness of fluorescent cytogenetics in differentiating chromophobe renal cell carcinoma from renal oncocytoma: A validation study combining metaphase and interphase analyses. *Am. J. Clin. Pathol.* **2010**, *133*, 116–126. [CrossRef] [PubMed]
13. Davis, C.F.; Ricketts, C.J.; Wang, M.; Yang, L.; Cherniack, A.D.; Shen, H.; Buhay, C.; Kang, H.; Kim, S.C.; Fahey, C.C.; et al. The somatic genomic landscape of chromophobe renal cell carcinoma. *Cancer Cell* **2014**, *26*, 319–330. [CrossRef] [PubMed]
14. Paolella, B.R.; Gibson, W.J.; Urbanski, L.M.; Alberta, J.A.; Zack, T.I.; Bandopadhayay, P.; Nichols, C.A.; Agarwalla, P.K.; Brown, M.S.; Lamothe, R.; et al. Copy-number and gene dependency analysis reveals partial copy loss of wild-type SF3B1 as a novel cancer vulnerability. *Elife* **2017**, *6*, e23268. [CrossRef] [PubMed]
15. Quddus, M.B.; Pratt, N.; Nabi, G. Chromosomal aberrations in renal cell carcinoma: An overview with implications for clinical practice. *Urol. Ann.* **2019**, *11*, 6–14. [PubMed]
16. Bellanne-Chantelot, C.; Chauveau, D.; Gautier, J.F.; Dubois-Laforgue, D.; Clauin, S.; Beaufils, S.; Wilhelm, J.M.; Boitard, C.; Noël, L.H.; Velho, G.; et al. Clinical spectrum associated with hepatocyte nuclear factor-1beta mutations. *Ann. Intern. Med.* **2004**, *140*, 510–517. [CrossRef] [PubMed]

17. Sun, M.; Tong, P.; Kong, W.; Dong, B.; Huang, Y.; Park, I.Y.; Zhou, L.; Liu, X.D.; Ding, Z.; Zhang, X.; et al. HNF1B Loss Exacerbates the Development of Chromophobe Renal Cell Carcinomas. *Cancer Res.* **2017**, *77*, 5313–5326. [CrossRef]
18. Gasparre, G.; Hervouet, E.; de Laplanche, E.; Demont, J.; Pennisi, L.F.; Colombel, M.; Mège-Lechevallier, F.; Scoazec, J.Y.; Bonora, E.; Smeets, R.; et al. Clonal expansion of mutated mitochondrial DNA is associated with tumor formation and complex I deficiency in the benign renal oncocytoma. *Hum. Mol. Genet.* **2008**, *17*, 986–995. [CrossRef]
19. Lang, M.; Vocke, C.D.; Merino, M.J.; Schmidt, L.S.; Linehan, W.M. Mitochondrial DNA mutations distinguish bilateral multifocal renal oncocytomas from familial Birt-Hogg-Dubé tumors. *Mod. Pathol.* **2015**, *28*, 1458–1469. [CrossRef]
20. Nagy, A.; Wilhelm, M.; Sükösd, F.; Ljungberg, B.; Kovacs, G. Somatic mitochondrial DNA mutations in human chromophobe renal cell carcinomas. *Genes Chromosomes Cancer* **2002**, *35*, 256–260. [CrossRef]
21. Digital Slide Archive (DSA). Available online: https://cancer.digitalslidearchive.org/ (accessed on 9 May 2019).
22. Trpkov, K.; Williamson, S.R.; Gao, Y.; Martinek, P.; Cheng, L.; Sangoi, A.R.; Yilmaz, A.; Wang, C.; San Miguel Fraile, P.; Perez Montiel, D.M.; et al. Low-grade oncocytic tumour of kidney (CD117-negative, cytokeratin 7-positive): A distinct entity? *Histopathology* **2019**, *75*, 174–184. [CrossRef]
23. Amin, M.B.; Paner, G.P.; Alvarado-Cabrero, I.; Young, A.N.; Stricker, H.J.; Lyles, R.H.; Moch, H. Chromophobe renal cell carcinoma: Histomorphologic characteristics and evaluation of conventional pathologic prognostic parameters in 145 cases. *Am. J. Surg. Pathol.* **2008**, *32*, 1822–1834. [CrossRef]
24. Podduturi, V.; Yourshaw, C.J.; Zhang, H. Eosinophilic variant of chromophobe renal cell carcinoma. *Proc. Bayl. Univ. Med. Cent.* **2015**, *28*, 57–58. [CrossRef]
25. Yip, S.M.; Ruiz Morales, J.M.; Donskov, F.; Fraccon, A.; Basso, U.; Rini, B.I.; Lee, J.L.; Bjarnason, G.A.; Sim, H.W.; Beuselinck, B.; et al. Outcomes of Metastatic Chromophobe Renal Cell Carcinoma (chrRCC) in the Targeted Therapy Era: Results from the International Metastatic Renal Cell Cancer Database Consortium (IMDC). *Kidney Cancer* **2017**, *1*, 41–47. [CrossRef] [PubMed]
26. Ohashi, R.; Schraml, P.; Batavia, A.; Angori, S.; Simmler, P.; Rupp, N.; Ajioka, Y.; Oliva, E.; Moch, H. Allele Loss and Reduced Expression of CYCLOPS Genes is a Characteristic Feature of Chromophobe Renal Cell Carcinoma. *Transl. Oncol.* **2019**, *12*, 1131–1137. [CrossRef] [PubMed]
27. Kouba, E.J.; Eble, J.N.; Simper, N.; Grignon, D.J.; Wang, M.; Zhang, S.; Wang, L.; Martignoni, G.; Williamson, S.R.; Brunelli, M.; et al. High fidelity of driver chromosomal alterations among primary and metastatic renal cell carcinomas: Implications for tumor clonal evolution and treatment. *Mod. Pathol.* **2016**, *29*, 1347–1357. [CrossRef] [PubMed]
28. Algaba, F.; Delahunt, B.; Berney, D.M.; Camparo, P.; Compérat, E.; Griffiths, D.; Kristiansen, G.; Lopez-Beltran, A.; Martignoni, G.; Moch, H.; et al. Handling and reporting of nephrectomy specimens for adult renal tumours: A survey by the European Network of Uropathology. *J. Clin. Pathol.* **2012**, *65*, 106–113. [CrossRef] [PubMed]
29. Trpkov, K.; Grignon, D.J.; Bonsib, S.M.; Amin, M.B.; Billis, A.; Lopez-Beltran, A.; Samaratunga, H.; Tamboli, P.; Delahunt, B.; Egevad, L.; et al. Handling and staging of renal cell carcinoma: The International Society of Urological Pathology Consensus (ISUP) conference recommendations. *Am. J. Surg. Pathol.* **2013**, *37*, 1505–1517. [CrossRef]
30. GDC Data Portal-National Cancer Institute. Available online: https://portal.gdc.cancer.gov/ (accessed on 23 March 2019).
31. Broad GDAC Firehose-Broad Institute. Available online: http://gdac.broadinstitute.org/ (accessed on 21 February 2019).
32. Deml, K.F.; Schildhaus, H.U.; Compérat, E.; von Teichman, A.; Storz, M.; Schraml, P.; Bonventre, J.V.; Fend, F.; Fleige, B.; Nerlich, A.; et al. Clear cell papillary renal cell carcinoma and renal angiomyoadenomatous tumor: two variants of a morphologic, immunohistochemical, and genetic distinct entity of renal cell carcinoma. *Am. J. Surg. Pathol.* **2015**, *39*, 889–901. [CrossRef]

33. Noske, A.; Brandt, S.; Valtcheva, N.; Wagner, U.; Zhong, Q.; Bellini, E.; Fink, D.; Obermann, E.C.; Moch, H.; Wild, P.J. Detection of CCNE1/URI (19q12) amplification by in situ hybridisation is common in high grade and type II endometrial cancer. *Oncotarget* **2017**, *8*, 14794–14805. [CrossRef]
34. Kanda, Y. Investigation of the freely-available easy-to-use software "EZR" (Easy R) for medical statistics. *Bone Marrow Transplant.* **2013**, *48*, 452–458. [CrossRef]

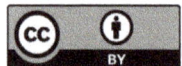

© 2019 by the authors. Licensee MDPI, Basel, Switzerland. This article is an open access article distributed under the terms and conditions of the Creative Commons Attribution (CC BY) license (http://creativecommons.org/licenses/by/4.0/).

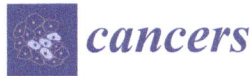

Article

Circular RNAs in Clear Cell Renal Cell Carcinoma: Their Microarray-Based Identification, Analytical Validation, and Potential Use in a Clinico-Genomic Model to Improve Prognostic Accuracy

Antonia Franz [1,2], Bernhard Ralla [1], Sabine Weickmann [1], Monika Jung [1], Hannah Rochow [1,2], Carsten Stephan [1,2], Andreas Erbersdobler [3], Ergin Kilic [4], Annika Fendler [1,2,5,†] and Klaus Jung [1,2,*,†]

1. Department of Urology, Charité—Universitätsmedizin Berlin, 10117 Berlin, Germany; antonia.franz@charite.de (A.F.); bernhard.ralla@charite.de (B.R.); sabine.weickmann@charite.de (S.W.); mchjung94@gmail.com (M.J.); hannah.rochow@charite.de (H.R.); carsten.stephan@charite.de (C.S.)
2. Berlin Institute for Urologic Research, 10115 Berlin, Germany
3. Institute of Pathology, University of Rostock, 18055 Rostock, Germany; andreas.erbersdobler@med.uni-rostock.de
4. Institute of Pathology, Hospital Leverkusen, 51375 Leverkusen, Germany; e.kilic@pathologie-leverkusen.de
5. Max Delbrueck Center for Molecular Medicine in the Helmholtz Association, Cancer Research Program, 13125 Berlin, Germany; annika.fendler@mdc-berlin.de
* Correspondence: klaus.jung@charite.de; Tel.: +49-450-515041
† These authors share senior authorship.

Received: 9 August 2019; Accepted: 23 September 2019; Published: 30 September 2019

Abstract: Circular RNAs (circRNAs) may act as novel cancer biomarkers. However, a genome-wide evaluation of circRNAs in clear cell renal cell carcinoma (ccRCC) has yet to be conducted. Therefore, the objective of this study was to identify and validate circRNAs in ccRCC tissue with a focus to evaluate their potential as prognostic biomarkers. A genome-wide identification of circRNAs in total RNA extracted from ccRCC tissue samples was performed using microarray analysis. Three relevant differentially expressed circRNAs were selected (circEGLN3, circNOX4, and circRHOBTB3), their circular nature was experimentally confirmed, and their expression—along with that of their linear counterparts—was measured in 99 malignant and 85 adjacent normal tissue samples using specifically established RT-qPCR assays. The capacity of circRNAs to discriminate between malignant and adjacent normal tissue samples and their prognostic potential (with the endpoints cancer-specific, recurrence-free, and overall survival) after surgery were estimated by C-statistics, Kaplan-Meier method, univariate and multivariate Cox regression analysis, decision curve analysis, and Akaike and Bayesian information criteria. CircEGLN3 discriminated malignant from normal tissue with 97% accuracy. We generated a prognostic for the three endpoints by multivariate Cox regression analysis that included circEGLN3, circRHOBT3 and linRHOBTB3. The predictive outcome accuracy of the clinical models based on clinicopathological factors was improved in combination with this circRNA-based signature. Bootstrapping as well as Akaike and Bayesian information criteria confirmed the statistical significance and robustness of the combined models. Limitations of this study include its retrospective nature and the lack of external validation. The study demonstrated the promising potential of circRNAs as diagnostic and particularly prognostic biomarkers in ccRCC patients.

Keywords: clear cell renal cell carcinoma; identification of circular RNAs; experimental validation of circular RNA; diagnostic and prognostic markers; circular RNAs in a clinico-genomic predictive model; cancer-specific survival; recurrence-free survival; overall survival

1. Introduction

Partial and radical nephrectomy is considered the standard of care for patients with localized clear cell renal cell carcinoma (ccRCC) [1]. Nevertheless, approximately 25% of patients experience recurrence after surgery with poor prognostic outcome within 5 years [2]. Consequently, precise stratification of recurrence risk after nephrectomy is necessary for personalized follow-up and treatment strategies. Existing prognostic models are based on conventional parameters such as tumor stage, grade, size, and resection status [1], all of which offer limited predictive accuracy for clinical outcomes [3]. Moreover, there is a broad consensus that molecular markers have, in addition to their diagnostic potential, the capacity to improve risk assessment when combined with clinicopathological factors [1,4]. At present, there are no recommended prognostic biomarkers in routine clinical use for ccRCC patients [1], though many have been evaluated experimentally [5–10].

In this regard, circular RNAs (circRNAs) are interesting potential novel biomarkers in ccRCC. CircRNAs are single-stranded, covalently closed RNA molecules without 3'- and 5'-ends and the poly(A) tail of linear RNA (linRNA). They were first identified in 2012 and are expressed widely throughout the human genome [11]; previously, they were regarded as transcriptional debris. Meanwhile, numerous studies identified their differential expression patterns in various cancers compared to normal tissue (reviewed in [12]). These expression patterns were found to be generally connected with their diagnostic, prognostic, and predictive potentials, highlighting a possible functional relevance in disease development [13,14].

Since circRNAs are a relatively new topic of scientific interest, the results of circRNA exploration in ccRCC remain limited [15–18]. Three recent reports focused on single circRNAs, which were mainly identified by database search for circRNAs fulfilling specific characteristics [15,16,18]. Only one report used three paired malignant and non-malignant kidney samples in a microarray screening for circRNAs [17]. However, with regard to the prognostic potential of circRNAs, subsequent analyses were restricted on overall survival and did not exceed the univariate Kaplan-Meier analysis. Thus, evaluation of the true prognostic potential of circRNAs in ccRCC based on genome-wide evaluation is of particular interest to apply circRNAs as biomarkers in clinical decision-making. Therefore, this study aimed to: (I) detect genome-wide differential expression patterns of circRNAs in ccRCC tissue using microarray analysis; (II) identify and validate promising circRNA candidates; and (III) evaluate the diagnostic and prognostic potentials of three circRNAs in 99 ccRCC samples and 85 adjacent normal tissue samples. Applying a combined model of both circRNA levels and clinical features, this study demonstrates the potential of circRNAs to improve prognostic value for cancer-specific (CSS), recurrence-free (RFS), and overall survival (OS).

2. Results

2.1. Patient Characteristics and Study Design

The study included ccRCC tumor samples from 99 patients and adjacent normal renal tissue samples from 85 patients undergoing radical or partial nephrectomy between 2003 and 2016 (Table 1). Samples were obtained retrospectively, and sample size was determined by a power-adapted calculation ($\alpha = 5\%$, power = 80%; Supplementary Information S1). The study was performed in three phases (Figure 1): (I) the discovery phase to identify differentially expressed circRNAs using a microarray screening approach; (II) the analytical validation phase to confirm the molecular characteristics of selected circRNAs and to establish "fit-for-purpose" RT-qPCR assays; and (III) the clinical assessment to evaluate the predictive value of these novel markers when applied alone and in combination with conventional clinicopathological factors.

Table 1. Characteristics of the ccRCC patients.

Characteristics	Total	ccRCC, Non-Metastatic [a]	ccRCC, Metastatic [a]	p-value [b]
Patients, no.	99	82	17	
Sex, female/male; n (%)	30/69	25/57 (30/70)	5/12 (29/70)	1
Age, yrs, median (range)	65 (36–87)	65 (36–87)	65 (37–78)	0.982
Pathological stage, no. (%)				
pT1	43	40 (49)	3 (18)	
pT2	8	8 (10)	0 (0)	0.004
pT3	47	34 (41)	13 (76)	
pT4	1	0 (0)	1 (6)	
TNM stage grouping, no. (%) [c]				
I	40	40	-	
II	8	8	-	
III	34	34	-	
IV	17	0	17	
Tumor size, median mm (range)	57 (20–220)	50 (20–220)	75 (35–150)	0.029
Surgical margin, no. (%)				
R0	85	73 (89)	12 (71)	
R1/2	11	7 (9)	4 (23)	0.138
Unclassified	3	2 (2)	1 (6)	
Fuhrman grade, no. (%)				
G1	9	8	1	
G2	68	60	8	0.025
G3	20	12	8	
G4	2	2	0	
Events during follow-up, n, (%)				
Metastasis	-	22 (27)	-	
Cancer-specific death	26 (26)	14 (17)	12 (71)	<0.0001
Overall death	42 (42)	30 (37)	12 (71)	0.014
Survival, months, median/mean (95% CI) [d]				
Cancer-specific	125 (111–139)	140 (127–153)	27.2 (14.1–40.4)	
Recurrence-free	-	127 (113–141)	-	
Overall	126 (90.4–166)	160 (103–160)	11.8 (8.2–39.9)	

Abbreviations: ccRCC, clear cell renal cell carcinoma; G, histopathological grading according to Fuhrman; pT, pathological tumor classification; R, surgical margin classification; CI, confidence interval. [a] Imaging was used to assess the presence/non-presence of metastases before surgery. [b] Calculated with Fisher's exact test, Chi-squared test or Mann-Whitney U test between the two groups. [c] TNM stage grouping according to UICC classification system. [d] Survival data obtained from the Kaplan-Meier analyses using the software MedCalc. The median survival (overall survival) corresponds to the time at which the survival probability reaches 50% or below. As the cancer-specific survival and recurrence-free survival did not reach this value in the non-metastatic cohort, the mean survival time was calculated (as area under the survival curve in the total follow-up interval) for both groups for comparison purposes.

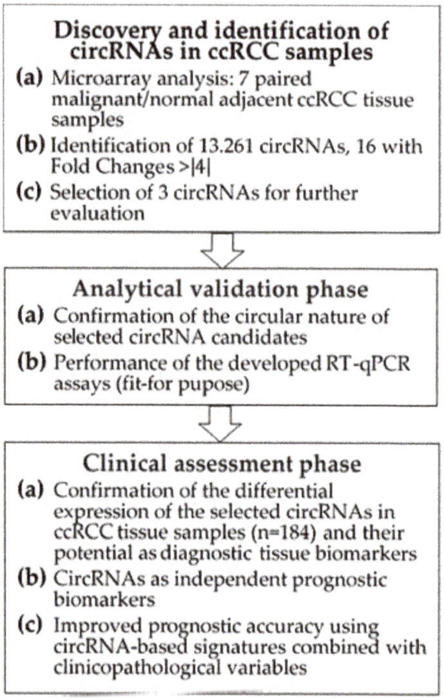

Figure 1. Flowchart of the study. Abbreviations: circRNA, circular RNA; ccRCC, clear cell renal cell carcinoma; RT-qPCR, reverse-transcription quantitative real-time polymerase chain reaction.

2.2. Discovery of circRNAs in ccRCC Tissue Using Microarray Analysis

2.2.1. Identification of Differentially Expressed circRNAs

A total of 13,261 circRNAs out of 13,617 distinct probes on the array were detected in seven matched ccRCC samples using the ArrayStar microarray approach (Supplemental Microarray Excel File). The number of circRNAs that derive from a single host gene forming multiple circRNA isoforms can vary [19]. Our microarray data revealed that approximately 50% of the detected circRNAs originated from ~75% of the 6271 host genes that produce only one or two circRNAs. However, some host genes accounted for up to 32 different circRNAs; approx. 15% of the detected circRNAs derived from host genes (3.8% of all host genes) that generate more than five circRNAs (Figure 2A). Exonic, intronic, antisense, and intergenic genomic regions can serve as sources for circRNAs. In ccRCC, 85% of the detected circRNAs derived from exonic gene sequences (Figure 2B) corresponding to data found in other human tissues [20]. Exonic circRNAs are generally assembled by one to five exons [20,21]. Analyzing the microarray data, we found 78 up-regulated and 91 down-regulated circRNAs with a higher than two-fold change ($p < 0.05$) in malignant compared to adjacent normal tissue samples (Figure 2C). This expression pattern resulted in a clear clustering of malignant vs. adjacent normal tissue using principal component analysis (Figure 2D).

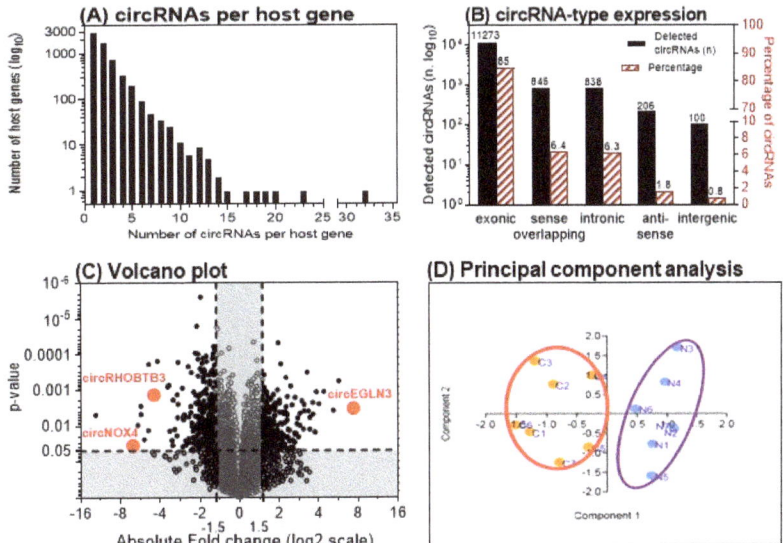

Figure 2. Microarray analysis results of matched clear cell renal cell carcinoma (ccRCC) tissue samples. (**A**) Number of circular RNAs (circRNAs) expressed per host gene in 7 matched ccRCC tissue samples. (**B**) Genomic origin of the detected circRNAs. (**C**) Volcano plot showing the up- and down-regulated circRNAs in malignant vs. adjacent normal tissue samples. Vertical and horizontal dashed lines indicate the thresholds of the 1.5-fold changes and the *p*-values of 0.05 in the *t*-test. The positions of the three detailed examined circRNAs in this study are marked. (**D**) Principal component analysis with the left cluster of tumor samples (C1–C7) and the right cluster with the paired adjacent normal tissue samples (N1–N7). (A and B adapted from [12]).

2.2.2. Selection of Three circRNAs for Further Evaluation

We further evaluated the differentially expressed circRNAs according to the following criteria: fold-change >4 with $p < 0.05$ and raw intensity above 500 on the microarray. Five up-regulated and eleven down-regulated circRNAs matched these ArrayStar microarray-related criteria. The nomenclature of circRNAs has not been standardized until now. In literature, different names occur depending on the reference database [12]. ArrayStar also uses its own designations. For the mentioned five up- and eleven down-regulated circRNAs, the circRNA IDs used in the databases ArrayStar and circBase [22] are summarized in Table 2. To identify circRNAs with a putative function in ccRCC initiation/progression, we selected circRNAs from host genes with putative roles in angiogenesis and hypoxia in ccRCC and other cancers including *EGLN3*, *NOX4*, and *RHOBTB3* [23–27]. Thus, corresponding circRNAs of the three host genes that are named according to the database circBase hsa_circ_0101692, hsa_circ_0023984, and hsa_circ_000744 were selected for further validation (Figure 2C). For greater clarity, the terms circEGLN3, circNOX4, and circRHOBTB3 are used hereafter for these circRNAs.

Table 2. List of circular RNAs (circRNAs) with at least a fourfold differential expression between the matched malignant vs. adjacent normal tissue samples ($n = 7$) in the microarray discovery study phase. The three circRNAs selected for further examination in this study are marked in bold letters.

circRNA in Manuscript	circRNA ID in ArrayStar [a,b]	circRNA ID in circBase [a,c]	Fold Change Expression in Tumor vs. Normal Tissue (p-value)	Best Transcript	Official Gene Symbol
Up-regulated circRNAs					
circEGLN3	**circRNA_405198**	**circ_0101692**	**7.32 (0.0033)**	**NM_022073**	**EGLN3**
-	circRNA_101202	circ_0029340	5.68 (0.0006)	NM_005505	SCARB1
-	circRNA_101341	circ_0031594	5.16 (0.0038)	NM_022073	EGLN3
-	circRNA_101803	circ_0003520	4.39 (0.0011)	NM_018092	NETO2
-	circRNA_103980	circ_0006528	4.01 (0.0024)	NM_138492	PRELID2
Down-regulated circRNAs					
-	circRNA_103093	circ_0060937	−12.3 (0.0049)	NM_000782	CYP24A1
-	circRNA_101120	circ_0027821	−6.73 (0.0342)	NR_024037	RMST
circNOX4	**circRNA_100933**	**circ_0023984**	**−6.44 (0.0475)**	**NM_016931**	**NOX4**
-	circRNA_100562	circ_0006577	−5.87 (0.0093)	NM_012425	RSU1
-	circRNA_031282	circ_0031282	−5.58 (0.0028)	NM_012244	SLC7A8
-	circRNA_103091	circ_0060927	−5.58 (0.0048)	NM_000782	CYP24A1
-	circRNA_023983	circ_0008350	−5.26 (0.0239)	NM_016931	NOX4
-	circRNA_1011001	circ_0025135	−4.89 (0.0132)	NM_001038	SCNN1A
-	circRNA_035435	circ_0035435	−4.84 (0.0002)	NM_032866	CGNL1
circRHOBTB3	**circRNA_007444**	**circ_0007444**	**−4.45 (0.0013)**	**NM_014899**	**RHOBTB3**
-	circRNA_101528	circ_0035436	−4.18 (0.0001)	NM_032866	CGNL1

[a] The obligatory prefix hsa_ was omitted to facilitate the readability. [b] More detailed annotations including source, chromosome localization, strand, circRNA type, and sequences are listed for all detected circRNAs in the Supplemental Microarray Excel File. [c] http://www.circbase.org and [22].

2.3. Analytical Validation of Selected circRNAs

2.3.1. Experimental Confirmation of the Circularity of Transcripts

We developed RT-qPCR assays for the three selected circRNAs and their linear counterparts on the basis of SYBRGreen I. The analytical specificity of all RT-qPCR products was verified by melting curve analysis and gel electrophoresis (with Supplemental Tables S1–S3 and Figure S1). Detection of circRNAs by sequencing or microarray analysis, as in our case, needs additional experimental confirmation of the circular nature of the identified transcripts to avoid false-positive results by measurement of non-circular RNA molecules with sequences similar to the specific backsplice junction [28]. Therefore, different molecular biology-based tests are recommended to validate circRNA-specific backsplice junctions [13,21,28,29]. Figure 3 summarizes our validation results based on the characteristics of circRNAs with regard to their resistance to the RNase R [13], their lack of a poly-A-tail [30], the amplification results in complementary DNA (cDNA) and genomic DNA (gDNA) using divergent and convergent primers, and the proof of the backsplice junctions by Sanger sequencing.

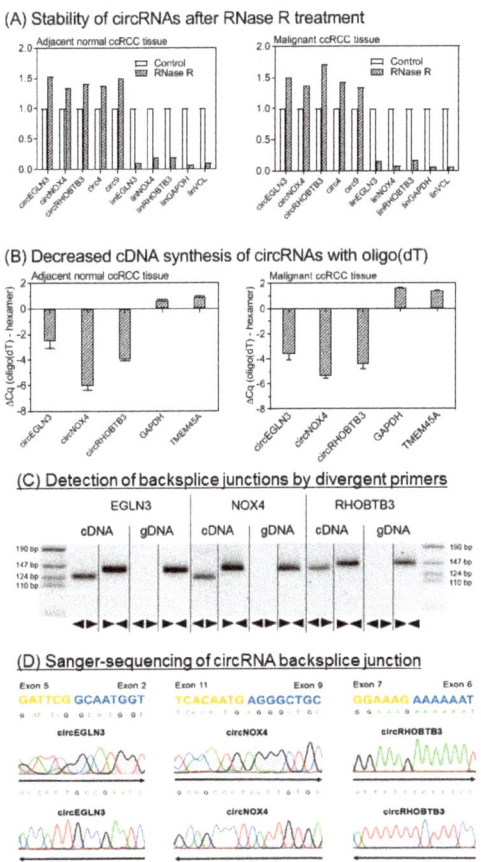

Figure 3. Analytical validation of the circular nature of circEGLN3, circNOX4, and circRHOBTB3. (**A**) Stability of circular RNAs (circRNAs) after RNase R treatment. CircRNAs are stable while linear mRNAs are degraded when treated with RNase R. Glyceraldehyde 3-phosphate dehydrogenase (GAPDH) mRNA (glyceraldehyde-3-phosphate dehydrogenase), VNL mRNA (vinculin), circ4, and circ9 were used as additional controls [13,31]. Data of triplicate experiments normalized to controls without RNase treatment are presented. (**B**) Random hexamer vs. oligo(dT) primers for cDNA synthesis. Random hexamer primers are used for amplification during cDNA synthesis of circRNAs as covalently closed structures of circRNAs lack a poly-A-tail. The binding capacity of oligo(dT) primers is therefore reduced without polyadenylated binding sites. In consequence, quantitation cycle (ΔCq) values in RT-qPCR are distinctly reduced when using random hexamer primers in comparison to oligo(dT) primers for circRNA cDNA synthesis. GAPDH and TMEM45A (transmembrane protein 45A) were used as mRNA controls. Significantly different mean values between the six circRNA samples and four mRNAs of GAPDH and TMEM45A as mRNA controls (mean values: −4.33 vs. 1.18, $p < 0.0001$) confirmed this characteristic feature of circRNAs. Different mean values of the circRNAs between the tissues were not observed ($p > 0.799$). (**C**) Gel electrophoresis of PCR products obtained from cDNA and genomic DNA (gDNA). Divergent (◀▶) primers used for circRNA measurements amplify sequences only in cDNA. Convergent (▶◀) primers show amplification of circRNA composing exons in cDNA and gDNA. (**D**) Base sequence of circRNA backsplice junction pictured by Sanger sequencing. Sanger sequencing was performed with forward (→) and reverse (←) primers. Methodical details for all here listed experiments are described in section "Material and Methods" and in Supplementary Information with Supplemental Table S4.

2.3.2. Analytical Performance of RT-qPCR Assays

In addition to the analytical specificity of the established assays, the repeatability (intra-assay variation) and reproducibility (inter-assay variation) of the measurements should be characterized as decisive indicator for the performance and robustness of quantitative tests. Data in Table 3 prove that the assays and measurements are suitable for "fit-for-purpose" RT-qPCR in first clinical studies.

Table 3. Repeatability and reproducibility of RT-qPCR measurements.

RNA	Repeatability [a]		Reproducibility [b]	
	Cq Value Mean (%RSD)	Concentration (AU) Mean (%RSD)	Cq Value Mean ± SD (%RSD)	Concentration (AU) Mean ± SD (%RSD)
circEGLN3	23.47 (0.284)	1.185 (4.51)	22.49 ± 0.138 (0.62)	2.132 ± 0.199 (9.33)
circNOX4	24.16 (0.493)	0.808 (9.35)	22.77 ± 0.108 (0.47)	1.118 ± 0.082 (7.30)
circRHOBTB3	25.64 (0.459)	0.0268 (9.27)	24.81 ± 0.190 (0.76)	0.036 ± 0.005 (14.2)
linEGLN3	20.83 (0.521)	32.72 (7.00)	23.93 ± 0.042 (0.18)	1.658 ± 0.046 (2.75)
linNOX4	27.65 (0.405)	0.204 (7.67)	25.50 ± 0.046 (0.18)	0.483 ± 0.015 (3.10)
linRHOBTB3	24.90 (0.214)	1.901 (3.43)	23.43 ± 0.147 (0.63)	3.791 ± 0.386 (10.2)
PPIA	19.33 (0.329)	32.01 (4.16)	19.18 ± 0.081 (0.42)	33.36 ± 1.745 (5.23)
TBP	25.18 (0.331)	2.330 (5.07)	24.99 ± 0.104 (0.42)	2.423 ± 0.156 (6.44)

Abbreviations: Cq, quantitation cycle; AU, arbitrary units; %RSD, percent relative standard deviation; SD, standard deviation; PPIA, peptidylprolyl isomerase A; TBP, TATA-box binding protein. PPIA and TBP served as reference genes [32]. [a] $n = 21$; %RSD was calculated from duplicate measurements using the root mean square method based on Cq values and calculated concentrations, respectively. [b] n = at least 8; %RSD (Cq) corresponds to the percent relative standard deviation calculated on the basis of the Cq values. %RSD (Concentration) corresponds to the percent relative standard deviation calculated on the basis of the normalized relative quantities (arbitrary units).

2.4. Clinical Assessment

2.4.1. Differential Expression of circRNAs in Relation to Clinicopathological Factors

In this first step of the clinical assessment phase, the expression data of the three circRNAs and their linear transcripts were measured and evaluated in all samples of the studied cohort. In Figure 4, the RT-qPCR normalized expression data of these three circRNAs and their corresponding linear transcripts (named in the following with the prefix "lin") in normal tissue and non-metastatic and metastatic primary tumor samples are shown. While the expression differences between tumor samples and adjacent normal tissue samples were significant for all circular and linear transcripts, no significant expression differences were found in primary tumors without (M0) and with (M1) metastasis.

The expression data of all three circRNAs and their linear transcripts in the tumor samples were not associated with age, sex, TNM stage, TNM-stage grouping, Fuhrman grade, surgical margin, tumor size, or metastatic status (Spearman rank correlation, Mann-Whitney U-test or Kruskal-Wallis test; $p > 0.10$; Supplementary Information with Table S5). Only *EGLN3* showed a significant progressive down-regulation from Fuhrman grade 1 to grade 4 for circEGLN3 (from 11.9 to 9.07, 7.76, and 0.742; $p = 0.006$, Kruskal-Wallis test with Jonckheere-Terpstra trend test) and for linEGLN3, respectively (from 6.47 to 5.25, 4.51, and 0.461; $p = 0.004$).

The expression levels of the circRNAs and their linear transcripts correlated closely with each other, showing similar correlation coefficients in both malignant and adjacent normal tissue samples (circEGLN3 and linEGLN3, $r_s = 0.742$ and 0.624; circNOX4 and linNOX4, $r_s = 0.849$ and 0.851; circRHOBTB3 and linRHOBTB3, $r_s = 0.749$ and 0.849; $p < 0.0001$ in all cases). However, the ratios of the circRNAs to their linear transcripts were significantly lower (Wilcoxon test with paired samples) in the adjacent normal tissue samples than in the tumor samples (median circEGLN3/linEGLN3 of 0.68 vs. 1.57, $p < 0.0001$; circNOX4/linNOX4 of 0.79 vs. 1.16, $p < 0.0001$; circRHOBTB3/linRHOBTB3 of 0.95 vs. 0.99, $p = 0.022$).

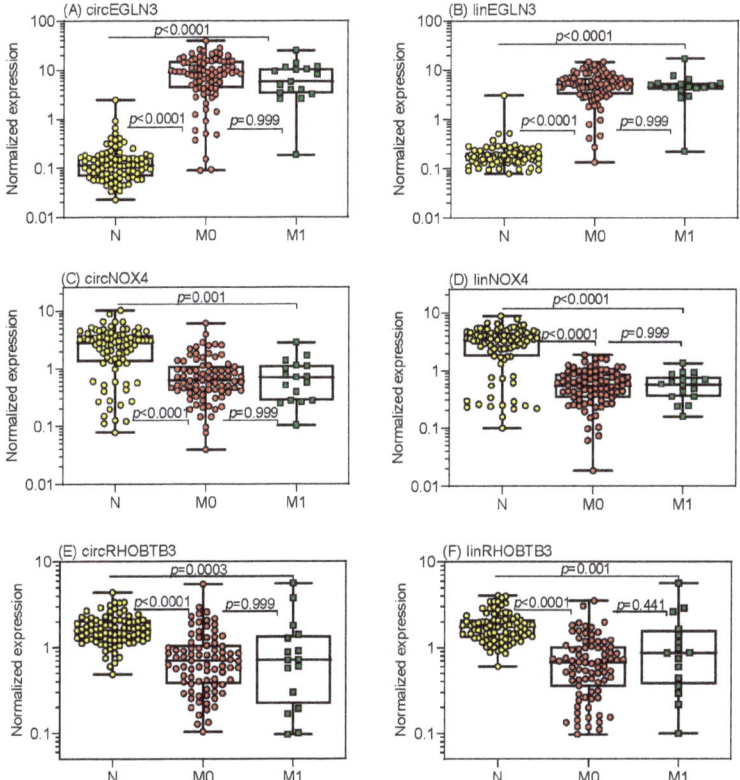

Figure 4. Expression of circular RNAs (circRNAs) and the linear transcripts of their host genes in tissue samples from patients suffering from clear cell renal cell carcinoma. Expression data of (**A**) circEGLN3, (**C**) circNOX4, and (**E**) circRHOBTB3 as well as the corresponding linear transcripts of the host genes (**B**) EGLN3, (**D**) NOX4, and (**F**) RHOBTB3 are shown in adjacent normal tissue distant from tumor ($n = 85$), in tissue from non-metastatic (M0, $n = 82$) and metastatic primary tumors (M1, $n = 17$) of patients with clear cell renal cell carcinoma at the time of surgery. CircRNA and linRNA expression ratios of M0 ($n = 60$) and M1 ($n = 16$) tissue samples in relation to their paired adjacent normal tissue samples did not statistically differ (p values between 0.302 to 0.712). PPIA (peptidylprolyl isomerase A) mRNA and TBP (TATA-box binding protein) mRNA were used as normalizers. Boxes in the box-and whisker plots represent the lower and upper quartiles with medians, whiskers illustrate the entire range of the samples. Significant differences between the study groups were estimated by the Kruskal-Wallis test with multiple comparisons corrected according to Holm-Sidak.

These ratio changes and numerous significantly different correlations for each of the circRNAs with the three linear transcripts (Table S6A–C) support the hypothesis of differential regulatory mechanisms in normal and cancer tissue. These data encouraged us to always include the corresponding linear transcripts in subsequent investigations.

Based on the expression data, receiver-operating characteristics curve (ROC) analysis was performed to test the discriminative ability of circRNAs and the linear transcripts in differentiating between malignant and adjacent normal ccRCC tissue (Table 4). The strong discriminative potential of both circEGLN3 and linEGLN3 with regard to sensitivity, specificity, and overall accurate classification of ~95% of tissues is remarkable.

Table 4. Receiver-operating characteristic curve analyses of circRNAs and their linear transcripts to discriminate between adjacent normal and malignant tissue.

RNAs	AUC (95% CI)	p-Value Different to AUC = 0.5	Differentiating Ability at the Youden Index [a]		% Overall Correct Classification
			Sensitivity (95% CI)	Specificity (95% CI)	
circEGLN3	0.98 (0.95–0.99)	<0.0001	95 (89–99)	95 (88–99)	94.6
circNOX4	0.81 (0.74–0.86)	<0.0001	91 (83–96)	71 (60–80)	80.4
circRHOBTB3	0.82 (0.76–0.87)	<0.0001	72 (62–80)	91 (82–96)	69.0
linEGLN3	0.98 (0.96–0.99)	<0.0001	96 (89–98)	99 (94–100)	95.7
linNOX4	0.85 (0.79–0.90)	<0.0001	99 (95–100)	78 (67–86)	88.0
linRHOBTB3	0.86 (081–0.91)	<0.0001	72 (62–80)	94 (87–98)	75.0
circEGLN3 +linEGLN3 [b]	0.99 (0.96–1.00)	<0.0001	95 (89–98)	99 (94–100)	95.7

Abbreviations: AUC, area under the receiver-operating characteristics curve; CI, confidence interval. [a] The Youden index as a measure of overall diagnostic effectiveness is calculated by [(sensitivity + specificity) − 1]. When equal weight is given to sensitivity and specificity of a test, the cutoff at the maximum value of this index, which graphically corresponds to the maximum vertical distance between the ROC curve and the diagonal line, is referred to as optimal criterion. [b] Calculated by binary logistic regression.

2.4.2. CircRNAs as Prognostic Markers and Elaboration of RNA Signatures

To assess the prognostic value of the new markers, we defined prediction accuracy of CSS as primary and RFS and OS as secondary endpoints. The endpoints were defined as the time from the surgery until the time of the corresponding event or the last follow-up.

Kaplan-Meier analysis was used to assess the association of the expression data of the three circRNAs and linear transcripts with the outcome endpoints. For that purpose, X-tile software [33] was applied to define optimized cutoff-points (Figure 5; Supplementary Information with Table S7 and Figure S2A,B).

For the primary CSS endpoint (Figure 5), increased expression values of both circEGLN3 and linEGLN3 were associated with better survival rates even though both transcripts were increased in malignant tissue in comparison to normal tissue (Figure 5A,B). Both circNOX4 and linNOX4 were not correlated to CSS (Figure 5C,D). Furthermore, circRHOBTB3 and linRHOBTB3 showed differing impacts on cancer-specific survival (Figure 5E,F). While high expression levels of circRHOBTB3 were associated with improved outcome, high levels of linRHOBTB3 were associated with reduced survival rates. The results were comparable using the two secondary endpoints (Figure S2A,B). The results for the linear transcripts were validated using the The Cancer Genome Atlas Kidney Renal Clear Cell Carcinoma (TCGA-KIRC) dataset, as this data collection does not contain circRNAs. Low expression of linEGLN3 and linNOX4 as well as high expression of linRHOBTB3 were associated with shorter overall survival of TCGA ccRCC specimens (Figure S3A–C).

In univariate Cox regression analysis, the hazard ratios of RNAs corresponded with the results from Kaplan-Meier curves (Table S7, Supplemental Figure S2A,B, and Figure 5). Subsequently, multivariate Cox regression analysis was performed including all circRNAs and linRNAs and a backward elimination approach (entry: $p < 0.05$, removal: $p > 0.100$) was used. Only circEGLN3, circRHOBTB3, and linRHOBTB3 remained in the reduced models for all three endpoints (Table 5).

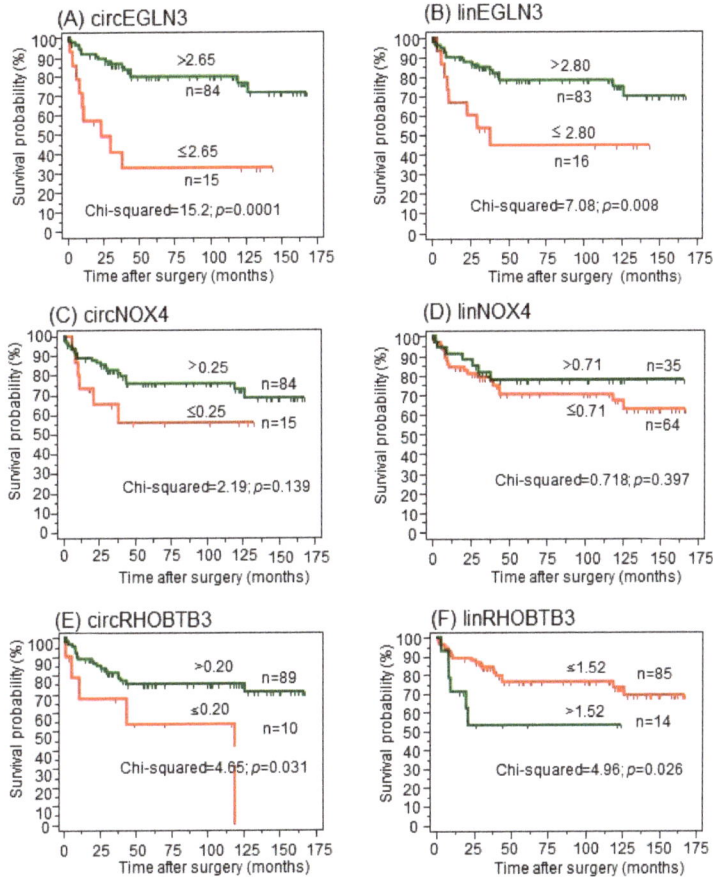

Figure 5. (A–F) Kaplan-Meier analysis of circular RNAs (circRNAs) and their linear transcripts with regard to cancer-specific survival after surgery. CircRNAs were dichotomized using the optimized cutoffs indicated by software X-tile [33] to discriminate between deceased and alive. Green curves represent patients with expression values above the cutoff; red curves represent patients with values equal or below the cutoff. The number of patients in the dichotomized groups and the cutoffs are indicated at the curves. The log-rank test was used to confirm significant differences between the survival probabilities.

C-statistics data for the models including all six RNA variables ("full model") compared with those obtained after backward elimination ("reduced model"), were not different (full vs. reduced model; CSS: 0.730 ± 0.060 vs. 0.726 ± 0.056, $p = 0.863$; RFS: 0.764 ± 0.057 vs. 0.735 ± 0.059, $p = 0.478$; OS: 0.741 ± 0.048 vs. 0.738 ± 0.046, $p = 0.897$; values given as AUC $\pm$ SE of the prognostic indices calculated in Cox regression analyses). We therefore used the reduced models with circEGLN3, circRHOBTB3, and linRHOBTB3 for the three outcome endpoints in the further evaluation and termed them "RNA signatures" (Table 5).

Table 5. Multivariate Cox Proportional Hazard Regression Analyses of Different Prediction Models for Outcome after ccRCC Nephrectomy [a].

Variable [b]	Cancer-Specific Survival		Recurrence-Free Survival		Overall Survival	
	HR (95% CI)	p-Value	HR (95% CI)	p-Value	HR (95% CI)	p-Value
RNA signature. [c,d,e]						
circEGLN3	0.24 (0.10–0.57)	0.001	0.53 (0.18–1.03)	0.074	0.49 (0.23–0.95)	0.037
circRHOBTB3	0.26 (0.09–0.73)	0.010	0.14 (0.04–0.49)	0.003	0.15 (0.05–0.49)	0.002
linRHOBTB3	2.57 (0.95–6.90)	0.062	11.1 (2.79–43.8)	0.001	4.46 (1.52–13.0)	0.006
Clinical model						
Tumor stage grouping (III+IV/I+II)	3.54 (1.16–10.8)	0.027	0.79 (0.25–2.48)	0.685	2.02 (0.95–4.27)	0.064
Fuhrman grading (3+4/1+2)	2.68 (1.03–7.02)	0.044	13.4 (4.06–44.3)	<0.0001	3.00 (1.32–6.82)	0.009
Surgical margin (R1/R0)	2.82 (1.05–7.59)	0.040	7.09 (1.75–28.7)	0.006	2.26 (0.91–5.59)	0.078
Tumor size (≥7 cm<)	1.10 (0.42–2.87)	0.838	1.03 (0.35–2.97)	0.963	0.99 (0.46–2.14)	0.988
Clinical model + RNA signature						
Tumor stage grouping (III+IV/I+II)	3.16 (0.93-10.8)	0.066	0.67 (0.19–2.37)	0.536	2.81 (1.23–6.42)	0.014
Fuhrman grading (3+4/1+2)	2.04 (0.73–5.74)	0.177	9.98 (2.99–33.4)	0.0002	2.25 (0.99–5.12)	0.053
Surgical margin (R1 vs. R0)	3.97 (1.28–12.3)	0.017	3.48 (0.76–15.9)	0.109	2.12 (0.87–5.18)	0.099
Tumor size (≥7 cm<)	1.16 (0.44–3.11)	0.762	1.22 (0.36–4.13)	0.746	0.76 (0.36–1.64)	0.490
circEGLN3	0.33 (0.13–0.79)	0.014	0.69 (0.22–2.19)	0.532	0.51 (0.24–1.09)	0.084
circRHOBTB3	0.25 (0.08–0.80)	0.019	0.21 (0.05–0.94)	0.041	0.16 (0.05–0.53)	0.003
linRHOBTB3	3.84 (1.35–10.9)	0.012	7.71 (1.55–38.3)	0.013	5.26 (1.74–15.9)	0.003
Clinical model + RNA signature after backward elimination						
Tumor stage grouping (III+IV/I+II)	3.98 (1.32–12.0)	0.014	–	–	2.89 (1.39–5.99)	0.005
Fuhrman grading (3+4/1+2)	–	–	8.53 (3.08–23.6)	<0.0001	2.52 (1.15–5.53)	0.021
Surgical margin (R1 vs. R0)	5.68 (2.09–15.4)	0.0007	3.54 (1.02–12.3)	0.047	–	–
Tumor size (≥7 cm<)	–	–	–	–	–	–
circEGLN3	0.28 (0.12–0.68)	0.005	–	–	0.50 (0.24–1.05)	0.067
circRHOBTB3	0.21 (0.07–0.65)	0.007	0.18 (0.04–0.75)	0.018	0.17 (0.05–0.56)	0.004
linRHOBTB3	3.59 (1.28–10.0)	0.015	8.19 (1.81–37.1)	0.006	5.37 (1.80–16.1)	0.003

Abbreviations: ccRCC, clear cell renal cell carcinoma; CI, confidence interval; G, histopathological grading according to Fuhrman; HR, hazard ratio; R, surgical margin classification. [a] The multivariate analysis included the RNA signature combination of circEGLN3, circRHOBTB3, and linRHOBTB3 after univariate analysis with a backward elimination approach of the six RNA and all clinicopathological factors of univariate analysis with p values < 0.05 (Supplementary Information 5, Supplemental Tables S7 and S8). [b] RNAs were dichotomized using the X-tile program [33] at the best threshold to discriminate between dead and alive in cancer-specific and overall survival, respectively as well as between recurrence and recurrence-free situation. These outcome-specific thresholds are indicated in the footnotes c, d, and e and correspond to those in the Kaplan-Meier curves. Clinicopathological variables are given with their categorized criteria in brackets. [c] Cutoffs for cancers-specific survival: circEGLN3 (2.65), circRHOBTB3 (0.20), and linRHOBTB3 (1.52). [d] Cutoffs for recurrence-free survival: circEGLN3 (2.10), circRHOBTB3 (0.50), and linRHOBTB3 (0.72). [e] Cutoffs for overall survival: circEGLN3 (2.73), circRHOBTB3 (0.27), and linRHOBTB3 (0.60).

2.4.3. A circRNA-Based Predictive Clinico-Genomic Model to Improve Prognostic Accuracy

Until now, clinicopathological variables are the basis to estimate the prediction of CSS, RFS, and OS after surgery and serve for benchmarking analysis of newly established tools. TNM-stage grouping including metastatic status, Fuhrman grading, tumor size, and surgical margin comprised significant clinicopathological predictors for all three outcome endpoints in Kaplan-Meier curves and univariate Cox regression analyses (Figure S4A–C, Table S8). These four variables were used combined in all outcome analyses and were called the "clinical model" (Table 5).

C-statistics data of the prognostic indices calculated in Cox regression analyses for the three endpoints using the "clinical model" and "RNA signature" were then compared and the results were not significantly different (Figure 6, legend: p values between 0.268 and 0.837). However, the results of the decision curve analysis show that the curves of the RNA-signature are always located above the curves of the "clinical model" and indicate a better accuracy. This is consistent with the recommendation that the decision curve analysis is the most informative metrics to demonstrate an incremental prognostic benefit [34]. Furthermore, the predictive outcome accuracy of the clinical models was improved upon combination with corresponding RNA signatures as shown by C-statistics and decision curve analysis (Figure 6).

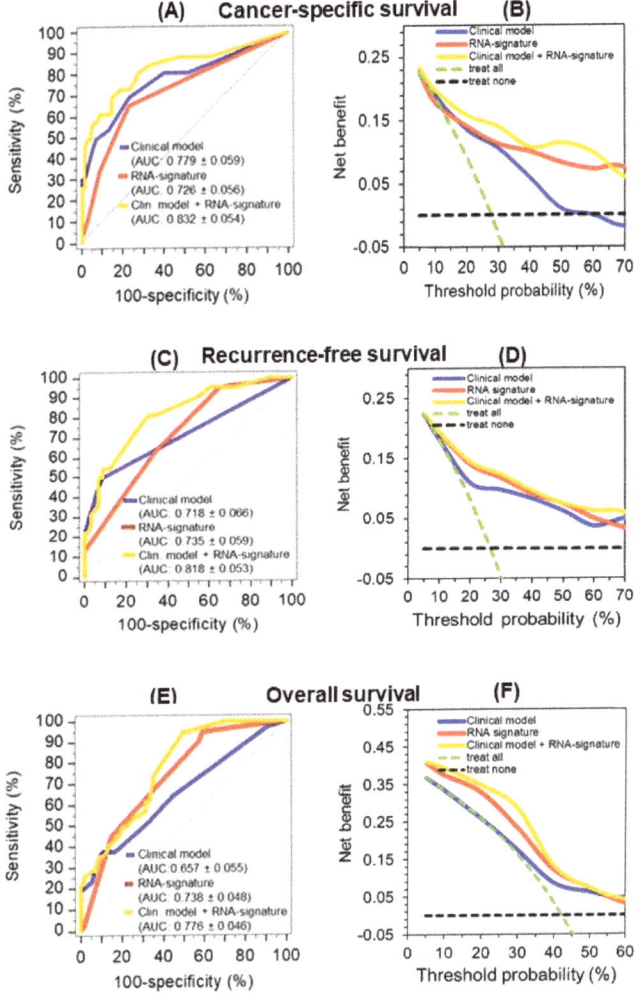

Figure 6. Improved predictive accuracy of cancer-specific (CSS), recurrence-free (RFS), and overall survival (OS) in a model with clinicopathological variables by including a circular RNA (circRNA) based signature. (**A**, **C**, and **E**) C-statistics curves of the prognostic indices of Cox regression analysis for the three endpoints using the models indicated in Table 5 ("clinical model", "RNA signature", and the combination of both ("clinical model + RNA signature") as well as (**B**, **D**, and **F**) the corresponding curves of decision curve analysis are shown here. The AUC values were not significantly different between the clinical model and the RNA signature for CSS ($p = 0.452$), RFS ($p = 0.837$), and OS ($p = 0.268$). The improved predictive accuracy of combining the "RNA signature" with the pure "clinical model" is shown by the increased AUC values indicated in parentheses next to the models in the subfigures. Curves in the decision curve analysis confirmed the benefit of combining the RNA signatures with the "clinical model.".

Furthermore, hazard ratios of the multivariate Cox regression analysis of the clinical model variables and those of the RNA signature confirmed that the RNA signature variables remained independent factors for the prediction of the corresponding outcomes in the full combined models, but also in the reduced models after backward elimination (Table 5). The robustness of this combined classifier was supported by the fact that backward elimination of the full model "clinical model + RNA signature" did not result in a loss of predictive accuracy (full vs. reduced model; CSS: 0.832 ± 0.054 vs. 0.821 ± 0.052 $p = 0.449$; RFS: 0.818 ± 0.053 vs. 0.816 ± 0.053, $p = 0.740$; OS: 0.776 ± 0.046 vs. 0.768 ± 0.047, $p = 0.529$; values given as AUC ± SE of the prognostic indices calculated in Cox regression analyses). Furthermore, internal bootstrapping validation confirmed the statistical significance and robustness of the combined models (Table S9). The improvement of the clinical model by including the corresponding RNA signatures was further demonstrated using the weight approach of the Akaike and Bayesian information criteria [35]. The final model including the four clinicopathological factors and the RNAs performed better than the "clinical model" with normalized probabilities of the Akaike and Bayesian criterion for CSS with 0.886 and 0.901, for RFS with 0.759 and 0.853, and for OS with 0.991 and 0.971, respectively.

2.5. In-silico Analysis of circRNA-miRNA-Gene Interaction

We identified potential miRNAs binding to the three circRNA candidates circEGLN3, circNOX4, and circRHOBTB3 with an algorithm provided by the CircInteractome tool [36], which is based on the database TargetScan [37]. MiRNAs were ranked according to the TargetScan context+ score. The five top-ranked miRNAs for each circRNA (all context + scores < −0.19) were chosen. Furthermore, potential gene interactions were identified for the miRNAs using the databases miRDB and TargetScan [37,38]. As cut-off values we chose a target score >90 (miRDB) and a total context++ score < −0.5. In Figure 7, only miRNA-gene interactions listed by both miRDB and TargetScan are shown.

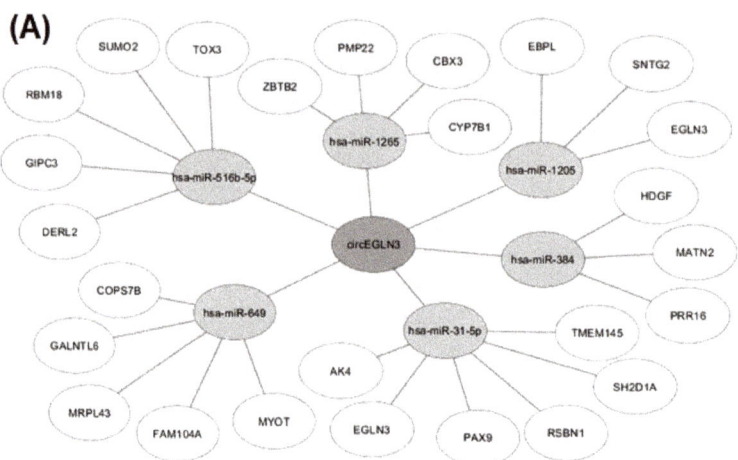

Figure 7. Cont.

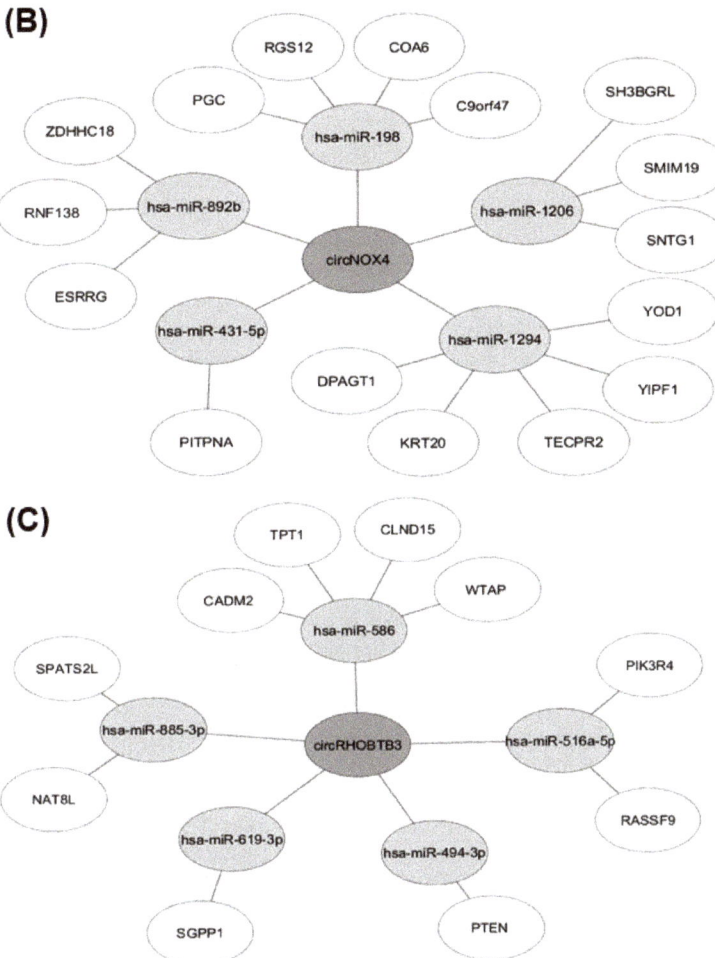

Figure 7. Results of in-silico analysis of circRNA-miRNA-gene interaction. MiRNAs with potential binding sites to (**A**) circEGLN3, (**B**) circNOX4, and (**C**) circRHOBTB3 were identified using CircInteractome [36] and subsequent miRNA-gene interactions were analyzed with the databases miRDB [38] and TargetScan [37].

3. Discussion

The current study represents hypothesis-generating research using a discovery-driven global approach [39]. We performed a genome-wide search for differentially expressed circRNAs in ccRCC tissue samples by microarray technology, the analytical and clinical validation of the three selected circRNAs circEGLN3, circNOX4, and circRHOBTB3 by RT-qPCR measurements, and successfully validated them as prognostic biomarkers in combination with conventional clinicopathological variables.

Numerous prognostic tools for ccRCC patients based exclusively on clinicopathological factors exist that have limited predictive accuracy of clinical outcome endpoints [40]. This supports the intention to include molecular markers to improve existing models [1,4]. Reports of various tools based on "omics"-markers alone or combined with clinicopathological variables have been published with promising results [1,3,4]. However, to the best of our knowledge, this study is the first to evaluate the prognostic potential of circRNAs in ccRCC tissue samples for the three clinically relevant survival endpoints of CSS, RFS, and OS.

In the discovery phase, we used microarray technology—considered to be more efficient in detecting circRNA molecules in comparison to RNA-sequencing methods [41]. The microarray contained 13 617 distinct probes, out of which 97.5% were detected in renal tissue and the principal component analysis of circRNAs clearly clustered between normal and tumor tissue. Differential expression analysis revealed 0.59% ($n = 78$) at least twofold up-regulated and 0.69% ($n = 91$) down-regulated circRNAs. These changes correspond to results observed in other solid tumors [20].

As briefly outlined in the Introduction, there have so far been few studies on circRNAs in ccRCC [15–18], which mostly focused on single circRNAs [15,16,18]. One working group investigated, based on database and literature searches, the effects of the androgen receptor and estrogen receptor beta via circHIAT1 and circATP2B1, respectively on the progression of ccRCC [15,16]. Another study examined the possible role of circABCB10 in ccRCC etiology [18]. These three circRNAs are not part of the up-/down-regulated circRNA list in our study obtained by microarray analysis. Although these studies provided interesting insights into functional aspects of circRNAs in ccRCC, their prognostic information was limited. A fourth study by Zhou al. [17] provided a list of the top 10 up- and down-regulated circRNAs based on a microarray search of three paired ccRCC tissue samples. Four of these 20 circRNAs are identical with four of the 17 top differentially expressed circRNAs, including the circEGLN3, listed in Table 2 (circBase ID: circ_0025135, circ_00331594, circ_0029340, and circ_0101692). However, circPCNXL2, which the authors reported as the circRNA with the highest up-regulation in the examined tissue samples, was not identified in our microarray analysis. This might be due to the different amount of tissue samples used for the microarray analysis or to a differing probe set on the microarray.

Despite the interesting details regarding differential expression and the ensuing discriminative potential between adjacent normal and malignant tissue (Table 4), our focus was directed at the prognostic potential of the three selected circRNAs from the circRNA profiles we obtained. In this context, the following expression particularities of the circRNAs and their linear transcripts are noteworthy: (I) we found no statistically different expression levels of circRNAs between the primary non-metastatic and metastatic tumors (Figure 4); (II) only Fuhrman grade as one relevant clinicopathological variable was associated with RNA expression (e.g., circEGLN3 and linEGLN3); and (III) we found differing and partly inverse correlations as well as changes in the abundance between circRNAs and their linear transcripts. Although the expression of most circRNAs is obviously in-line with the expression of their host genes [42], the host gene-independent expression of circRNAs, reflected in our study exemplarily in the inverse Kaplan-Meier curves of circRHOBTB3 and linRHOBTB3 (Figure 5) is of special interest. Similar findings have recently been reported also in prostate cancer and heart diseases [43,44]. We have considered these findings in the clinical assessment process by including the expression data of the linear transcripts from RNase R untreated total RNA samples in the analysis and clinical evaluation. This fact is also considered by the recently published MiOncoCirc database that includes circRNAs identified by a special capture exome RNA-sequencing protocol [45]. Using this sequencing protocol without RNase R pretreatment [46], the ratio between circular and the linear transcripts is preserved—comparable with the tissue sample—and allows a definite downstream analysis as mRNAs are not removed [45].

Thus, all these expression particularities and further the characteristics of uncorrelated differential expression in relation to conventional clinicopathological factors are specific for orthogonal biomarkers [47]. Consequently, new information can arise from the application of such biomarkers in clinical practice [48]. Indeed, multivariate Cox regression analysis showed that the RNA signatures developed with circEGLN3, circRHOBTB3, and linRHOBTB3 proved their hypothesized prognostic value for all three clinical endpoints (Table 5). Furthermore, in combination with the conventional risk factors of the clinical model, all three RNAs generally remained independent factors, also in the backward models (Table 5). Moreover, C-statistics and decision curve analysis data (Figure 6) as well as the Akaike and Bayesian information criteria and the internal bootstrap validation support the improved predictive accuracy of the combined model. We used bootstrapping for the internal validation as it is recommended as efficient method for internal validation of predictive models in favor of split-sample validation and cross-validation [49]. As already mentioned in the Results, we laid particular emphasis on the evaluation of the models using decision curve analysis as recently recommended standard to validate diagnostic/prognostic benefit [34]. Thus, the data allow us to consider circRNAs as potential prognostic biomarkers in the future to improve risk stratification of ccRCC patients after nephrectomy.

In addition to their role as promising new biomarkers in cancer and other diseases, circRNAs are also currently evaluated regarding their functional role in cancer initiation and progression (reviewed in [50]). In this context, miRNA sponging and consequential impact on the expression of cancer key genes is one of the most relevant features of circRNAs [14,51]. For example, elevated expression of circTP63 in lung squamous cell carcinoma was shown to be associated with accelerated tumor progression by sponging miR-873-3p and thus increased levels of FOXM1 [52]. In contrast, over-expression of circRNAs can also be protective against tumor progression as shown by the example of circSLCA1, which promotes the tumor suppressor PTEN via miR-130b/miR-494 sponging in bladder cancer [53]. With an in-silico analysis of the circRNA-miRNA-gene interactions of circEGLN3, circNOX4 and circRHOBTB3, we identified potential target genes of the circRNAs that might influence ccRCC development and progression (Figure 7). Interestingly, the in-silico analysis for circEGLN3 predicted a potential binding of miR-31-5p and miR-1205 to circEGLN3 and the corresponding linear RNA of EGLN3. EGLN3 is known to contribute to ccRCC initiation [25,26,54] by targeting HIF. The up-regulation of both circEGLN3 and linRNA of EGLN3 in ccRCC and the predicted interaction via miR-31-5p and miR-1205 could reflect a self-sustaining mechanism of the oncogene EGLN3. This hypothesis is supported by new reports that miRNA-31-5p acts as tumor suppressor and is down-regulated in renal cell carcinoma [55].

Furthermore, an interesting interaction was revealed for the down-regulated circRHOBTB3, which could be able to down-regulate the tumor-suppressor PTEN via absence of miR-494 sponging. The oncogenic effect of miR-494 up-regulation and subsequent PTEN inactivation is reported for many different cancers [53,56,57]. In our study, down-regulation of circRHOBTB3 is associated with poor survival outcome (Figure 6). This is especially interesting since the inverse survival outcome of circRHOBTB3 and linRHOBTB3 expression suggests a functional independency.

Nevertheless, the functional relevance of the interactions we identified based on in-silico data (Figure 7) remains to be experimentally confirmed, but this was beyond the scope of this hypothesis-generating study.

Despite the abovementioned statistical measures for bias-free analyses including the internal bootstrap-based validation and the confirmation by the Akaike and Bayesian information criteria, there are inherent limitations of this study. These include the retrospective nature of the study involving a limited number of patients selected solely based on available tissue samples, the focus on the application of biomarkers without exploring their possible molecular mechanisms, and the lack of external validation.

4. Materials and Methods

4.1. Patients and Tissue Samples

The study was approved by the local Ethics committee of the University Hospital Charité (Charité - Universitätsmedizin Berlin: EA1/134/12; approval date: 22nd June 2012) and an informed consent was obtained from patients. The study was carried out in accordance with the Declaration of Helsinki and considered the MIQE, REMARK, and STARD guidelines [58–60].

The study included ccRCC tumor samples from 99 patients and adjacent normal renal tissue samples from 85 patients undergoing radical or partial nephrectomy between 2003 and 2016 (Table 1). The patients were selected according to the availability of cryo-preserved tissue samples and the completeness of follow-up databased on the sample size calculation with $\alpha = 5\%$ and a power of 80% (Supplementary Information). Tumors were classified by two experienced uro-pathologists (A.E., E.K.) according to the 2010 TNM classification system and the Fuhrman grading system. In total, 17 patients exhibited metastases at the time of diagnosis and 22 developed metastases within the follow-up period until November 2018 (Table 1). None of the patients received systemic therapy prior to nephrectomy. Tissue specimens were sampled immediately after nephrectomy, either snap frozen in liquid nitrogen or immersed in RNAlater solution (Qiagen, Hilden, Germany), and stored at −80 °C until analysis as described in our previous publications [61–63].

4.2. Analytical Methods

4.2.1. Total RNA Samples and Their Characteristics

Total RNA was isolated from 30 to 98 mg tissue pieces. The isolation procedure from preserved tissue specimens using the miRNeasy Mini Kit (Qiagen) including an on-column DNA digestion step according to the producer's instructions, the spectrophotometric quantification (NanoDrop 1000 Spectrophotometer; NanoDrop Technologies, Wilmington, DE, USA), and the quality assessment of the total RNA samples (ratio of the absorbance at 260 nm to that at 280 nm and RNA integrity number on a Bioanalyzer 21000 (Agilent Technologies, Santa Clara, CA, USA) were detailed described in our previous publications [61–63]. The median ratio of 260 nm to 280 nm of the isolated RNA samples was 2.04 (95% CI, 2.03 to 2.04) and the median RNA integrity number was 7.70 (95% CI, 7.52 to 7.88). The median RNA concentration in the isolates of 30 μL nuclease-free water was 1118 (95% CI, 1029 to 1209) ng/μL. Isolated RNA samples were stored at −80 °C.

4.2.2. Microarray Detection of circRNAs

Microarray analyses were performed as custom order by ArrayStar Inc. (Rockville, MD, USA) using extracted total RNA from seven paired tissue samples of non-metastasized clear cell renal cell carcinomas (ccRCC: all patients with negative lymph nodes and negative surgical margin; 1× pT1 with Fuhrman grade 2, 1× pT2 with grade 2, 3× pT3 with grade 2, 2× pT3 with grade 3). The samples were treated with RNase R to digest linear RNAs and enrich circular RNAs. The circRNAs were amplified, transcribed, and fluorescently labelled on the 3'-end using Cy3. The prepared samples were hybridized on the ArrayStar Human Circular RNA Array that is designed to detect 13.617 circRNAs. Image scanning and analysis was performed with Agilent software (Agilent scanner model G2505C, Agilent Feature Extraction software version 11.0.1.1 and Agilent GeneSpring GX). Probe intensities were normalized with quantile normalization. Differential expression analysis was carried out with R Bioconductor 'limma' package by computing moderated t-statistics and Benjamini–Hochberg adjusted p values. All the data are compiled in the accompanying separate Excel file with all additional information and annotation details (Supplemental Microarray Excel File).

4.2.3. RT-qPCR Methodology and circRNA Validation Methods

RT-qPCR measurements were performed according to the recommendations of the MIQE guidelines [58]. The corresponding comments are listed in a checklist and apply for all assays (Supplementary Information with Supplemental Table S1). No template controls (NTC) and no reverse transcription controls (NRTC or no enzyme controls = NEC) were always performed and showed negative results. For cDNA synthesis, the Maxima First Strand cDNA Synthesis Kit for RT-qPCR (Thermo Fisher Scientific, Waltham, MA, USA; Cat.No. K1642) was used. All real-time qPCR runs were performed on the LightCycler 480 Instrument (Roche Molecular Diagnostics, Mannheim, Germany) in white 96-well plates (Cat.No. 04729692001) using at least technical duplicates and resulting mean values for further calculations. Maxima SYBR Green qPCR Master Mix (2X) (Thermo Fisher Scientific; Cat.No. K0252) was used. Primers were designed using the blasting tool provided by Primer3 [64] and synthesized by TIB MOLBIOL GmbH (Berlin, Germany). PPIA (peptidylprolyl isomerase A) and TBP (TATA-box binding protein) were used as normalizers [32]. Quantitative PCR data analysis was done using qbase + software, version 3.2 (Biogazelle, Zwijnaarde, Belgium). All analytical details (list of primers with their sequences, setups for all measurements, performance of RT-qPCR with melting curve analyses and agarose electrophoreses of RT-qPCR products) are compiled in Supplementary Information 2 with Supplemental Tables S2 and S3, and Supplemental Figure S1. The validation methods according for the three circRNAs based on the on the RNase R approach, the cDNA synthesis with random hexamer primers and oligo(dT) primers, the Sanger sequencing, and characterization of PCR products using divergent and convergent primers [13] are summarized in Supplementary Information 3.

4.3. Statistics and Data Analysis

SPSS Version 25 (IBM Corp., Armonk, NY, USA) with the bootstrap module, GraphPad Prism 8.1 (GraphPad Software, La Jolla, CA, USA), and MedCalc 19.0.6 (MedCalc Software, Ostend, Belgium) were used as statistical programs. $p < 0.05$ (two-sided) was considered statistically significant. Non-parametric tests (Mann-Whitney U-test, Kruskal-Wallis test, and Spearman rank correlation) for continuous data and Chi-squared or Fisher's exact tests for categorical data were applied. To obtain optimized cutoff-points of the circRNAs and linRNAs for the outcome assessments, the software X-tile was applied [33]. Kaplan-Meier and Cox proportional hazard regression analyses were used for survival analysis. C-statistics as ROCs with AUCs decision curve analysis [65,66] served to identify the discrimination/prediction capacity of the different variables and models. The Akaike and Bayesian information criteria were used for the model evaluation [35]. GPower 3.1.9.4 [67], GraphPad StatMate 2.0 (GraphPad Software), and MedCalc were used for sample size and power determinations. For the in-silico analysis of circRNAs, the prediction tool CircInteractome [36] was used and the subsequent miRNA-gene interactions for the predicted miRNAs were analyzed with the databases miRDB [38] and TargetScan [37]. TCGA-KIRC RNAseq data were downloaded and analyzed with R (version 3.6) using the "TCGA2stat" library and the "survival" library for Kaplan-Meier analysis.

5. Conclusions

This study was the first to identify differentially expressed circRNA candidates using a genome-wide approach that subsequently evaluated the candidates in terms of their prognostic potential in ccRCC patients. We showed that in combination with standard clinicopathological data, circRNA-based signatures improve prognostic accuracy when predicting CSS, RFS, and OS. Furthermore, we revealed potential functional relevance of circRNAs in ccRCC by exploring circRNA-miRNA-gene interactions. CircRNAs should be considered as potential prognostic biomarkers to improve risk stratification of ccRCC patients after nephrectomy. The further exploration of circRNA functions in ccRCC might lead to new findings regarding tumor biology and pathways.

Supplementary Materials: The following are available online at http://www.mdpi.com/2072-6694/11/10/1473/s1, Supplementary Information S1: Sample size and power calculations, Supplementary Information S2: RT-qPCR methodology, Supplementary Information S3: CircRNA validation methods, Supplementary Information S4: Associations between clinicopathological variables and circRNAs/linear transcripts, Supplementary Information S5: Cox regressions and Kaplan-Meier curves, Supplemental Microarray Excel File, Figure S1: Specificity of the circRNA RT-PCR products, Figure S2A,B: Kaplan-Meier curves of circRNAs and linRNAs, Figure S3A–C: Kaplan-Meier analysis using TCGA data, Figure S4A–C: Kaplan-Meier curves of clinicopathological factors, Table S1: MIQE checklist according to Bustin et al., Table S2: List of primers, Table S3: Characteristics of the PCR standard curves, Table S4: List of backsplice junctions and primers, Table S5: Associations of circRNAs and linear transcripts with clinicopathological variables, Table S6A: Correlation between circRNAs and linear transcripts in adjacent normal ccRCC tissue, Table S6B: Correlation between circRNAs and linear transcripts in malignant ccRCC samples, Table S6C: Significantly different correlation coefficients of circRNAs and linear transcripts between malignant and adjacent normal samples, Table S7: Univariate Cox regressions of circRNAs and linRNAs, Table S8: Univariate Cox regressions of clinicopathological factors, Table S9: Bootstrapping *p*-values of Cox regression analyses.

Author Contributions: Conceptualization, A.F. (Antonia Franz), A.F. (Annika Fendler) and K.J.; Data curation, A.F. (Antonia Franz), S.W. and K.J.; Formal analysis, A.F. (Antonia Franz), C.S. and A.F. (Annika Fendler); Funding acquisition, C.S., A.F. (Annika Fendler) and K.J.; Investigation, A.F. (Antonia Franz), S.W., M.J., H.R., A.E. and E.K.; Methodology, A.F., S.W., M.J. and K.J.; Project administration, B.R., S.W. and K.J.; Resources, B.R., C.S. and K.J.; Supervision, C.S., A.F. (Annika Fendler) and K.J.; Validation, S.W., M.J. and H.R.; Visualization, A.F. (Antonia Franz), S.W. and K.J.; Writing—original draft, A.F. (Antonia Franz), M.J., A.F. (Annika Fendler) and K.J.; Writing—review & editing, B.R., C.S., A.E., E.K. and A.F. (Annika Fendler).

Funding: This research was funded by Foundation of Urologic Research, Berlin, Germany by a research fellowship (grant number BFIU2017/18-AF) to Antonia Franz.

Acknowledgments: The authors would like to thank Dieter Beule und Andranik Ivanov (Berlin Institute of Health, Bioinformatics Core Unit) for interpretation of the microarray data and for helpful discussion and feedback on this manuscript. The support of the study through the Foundation of Urologic Research, Berlin, Germany by a research fellowship to cand. med. Antonia Franz is greatly acknowledged. The authors thank Siegrun Blauhut and Silke Rabenhorst for valuable technical assistance. The German Research Foundation (DFG) and the Open Access Publication Fund of Charité–Universitätsmedizin Berlin supported the Open Access publication of this article. The results here are in part based upon data generated by the TCGA Research Network: https://www.cancer.gov/tcga.

Conflicts of Interest: The authors declare no conflict of interest. The funders had no role in the design of the study; in the collection, analyses, or interpretation of data; in the writing of the manuscript, or in the decision to publish the results.

References

1. Ljungberg, B.; Albiges, L.; Abu-Ghanem, Y.; Bensalah, K.; Dabestani, S.; Fernández-Pello, S.; Giles, R.H.; Hofmann, F.; Hora, M.; Kuczyk, M.A.; et al. European Association of Urology Guidelines on Renal Cell Carcinoma: The 2019 Update. *Eur. Urol.* **2019**, *75*, 799–810. [CrossRef] [PubMed]
2. Dabestani, S.; Beisland, C.; Stewart, G.D.; Bensalah, K.; Gudmundsson, E.; Lam, T.B.; Gietzmann, W.; Zakikhani, P.; Marconi, L.; Fernández-Pello, S.; et al. Long-term Outcomes of Follow-up for Initially Localised Clear Cell Renal Cell Carcinoma: RECUR Database Analysis. *Eur. Urol. Focus* **2018**. [CrossRef] [PubMed]
3. Sun, M.; Shariat, S.F.; Cheng, C.; Ficarra, V.; Murai, M.; Oudard, S.; Pantuck, A.J.; Zigeuner, R.; Karakiewicz, P.I. Prognostic Factors and Predictive Models in Renal Cell Carcinoma: A Contemporary Review. *Eur. Urol.* **2011**, *60*, 644–661. [CrossRef] [PubMed]
4. Tan, P.H.; Cheng, L.; Rioux-Leclercq, N.; Merino, M.J.; Netto, G.; Reuter, V.E.; Shen, S.S.; Grignon, D.J.; Montironi, R.; Egevad, L.; et al. Renal tumors: Diagnostic and prognostic biomarkers. *Am. J. Surg. Pathol.* **2013**, *37*, 1518–1531. [CrossRef] [PubMed]
5. Klatte, T.; Seligson, D.B.; LaRochelle, J.; Shuch, B.; Said, J.W.; Riggs, S.B.; Zomorodian, N.; Kabbinavar, F.F.; Pantuck, A.J.; Belldegrun, A.S. Molecular Signatures of Localized Clear Cell Renal Cell Carcinoma to Predict Disease-Free Survival after Nephrectomy. *Cancer Epidemiol. Prev. Biomark.* **2009**, *18*, 894–900. [CrossRef] [PubMed]
6. Rini, B.; Goddard, A.; Knezevic, D.; Maddala, T.; Zhou, M.; Aydin, H.; Campbell, S.; Elson, P.; Koscielny, S.; Lopatin, M.; et al. A 16-gene assay to predict recurrence after surgery in localised renal cell carcinoma: Development and validation studies. *Lancet Oncol.* **2015**, *16*, 676–685. [CrossRef]
7. Shi, D.; Qu, Q.; Chang, Q.; Wang, Y.; Gui, Y.; Dong, D. A five-long non-coding RNA signature to improve prognosis prediction of clear cell renal cell carcinoma. *Oncotarget* **2017**, *8*, 58699–58708. [CrossRef]
8. Haddad, A.Q.; Luo, J.H.; Krabbe, L.M.; Darwish, O.; Gayed, B.; Youssef, R.; Kapur, P.; Rakheja, D.; Lotan, Y.; Sagalowsky, A.; et al. Prognostic value of tissue-based biomarker signature in clear cell renal cell carcinoma. *BJU Int.* **2017**, *119*, 741–747. [CrossRef]
9. Ghatalia, P.; Rathmell, W.K. Systematic Review: ClearCode 34—A Validated Prognostic Signature in Clear Cell Renal Cell Carcinoma (ccRCC). *Kidney Cancer* **2018**, *2*, 23–29. [CrossRef]
10. Zuo, S.; Wang, L.; Wen, Y.; Dai, G. Identification of a universal 6-lncRNA prognostic signature for three pathologic subtypes of renal cell carcinoma. *J. Cell. Biochem.* **2019**, *120*, 7375–7385. [CrossRef]
11. Salzman, J.; Gawad, C.; Wang, P.L.; Lacayo, N.; Brown, P.O. Circular RNAs Are the Predominant Transcript Isoform from Hundreds of Human Genes in Diverse Cell Types. *PLoS ONE* **2012**, *7*, e30733. [CrossRef] [PubMed]

12. Franz, A.; Rabien, A.; Stephan, C.; Ralla, B.; Fuchs, S.; Jung, K.; Fendler, A. Circular RNAs: A new class of biomarkers as a rising interest in laboratory medicine. *Clin. Chem. Lab. Med.* **2018**, *56*, 1992–2003. [CrossRef] [PubMed]
13. Memczak, S.; Jens, M.; Elefsinioti, A.; Torti, F.; Krueger, J.; Rybak, A.; Maier, L.; Mackowiak, S.D.; Gregersen, L.H.; Munschauer, M.; et al. Circular RNAs are a large class of animal RNAs with regulatory potency. *Nature* **2013**, *495*, 333–338. [CrossRef] [PubMed]
14. Hansen, T.B.; Jensen, T.I.; Clausen, B.H.; Bramsen, J.B.; Finsen, B.; Damgaard, C.K.; Kjems, J. Natural RNA circles function as efficient microRNA sponges. *Nature* **2013**, *495*, 384–388. [CrossRef] [PubMed]
15. Wang, K.; Sun, Y.; Tao, W.; Fei, X.; Chang, C. Androgen receptor (AR) promotes clear cell renal cell carcinoma (ccRCC) migration and invasion via altering the circHIAT1/miR-195-5p/29a-3p/29c-3p/CDC42 signals. *Cancer Lett.* **2017**, *394*, 1–12. [CrossRef] [PubMed]
16. Han, Z.; Zhang, Y.; Sun, Y.; Chen, J.; Chang, C.; Wang, X.; Yeh, S. ERβ-mediated alteration of circATP2B1 and miR-204-3p signaling promotes invasion of clear cell renal cell carcinoma. *Cancer Res.* **2018**, *78*, 2550–2563. [CrossRef]
17. Zhou, B.; Zheng, P.; Li, Z.; Li, H.; Wang, X.; Shi, Z.; Han, Q. CircPCNXL2 sponges miR-153 to promote the proliferation and invasion of renal cancer cells through upregulating ZEB2. *Cell Cycle* **2018**, *17*, 2644–2654. [CrossRef]
18. Huang, Y.; Zhang, Y.; Jia, L.; Liu, C.; Xu, F. Circular RNA ABCB10 promotes tumor progression and correlates with pejorative prognosis in clear cell renal cell carcinoma. *Int. J. Biol. Markers* **2019**, *34*, 176–183. [CrossRef]
19. Salzman, J.; Chen, R.E.; Olsen, M.N.; Wang, P.L.; Brown, P.O. Cell-Type Specific Features of Circular RNA Expression. *PLoS Genet.* **2013**, *9*, e1003777. [CrossRef]
20. Maass, P.G.; Glažar, P.; Memczak, S.; Dittmar, G.; Hollfinger, I.; Schreyer, L.; Sauer, A.V.; Toka, O.; Aiuti, A.; Luft, F.C.; et al. A map of human circular RNAs in clinically relevant tissues. *J. Mol. Med.* **2017**, *95*, 1179–1189. [CrossRef]
21. Szabo, L.; Salzman, J. Detecting circular RNAs: Bioinformatic and experimental challenges. *Nat. Rev. Genet.* **2016**, *17*, 679–692. [CrossRef] [PubMed]
22. Glažar, P.; Papavasileiou, P.; Rajewsky, N. circBase: A database for circular RNAs. *RNA* **2014**, *20*, 1666–1670. [CrossRef] [PubMed]
23. Campisano, S.; Bertran, E.; Caballero-Díaz, D.; La Colla, A.; Fabregat, I.; Chisari, A.N. Paradoxical role of the NADPH oxidase NOX4 in early preneoplastic stages of hepatocytes induced by amino acid deprivation. *Biochim. Biophys. Acta (BBA) Gen. Subj.* **2019**, *1863*, 714–722. [CrossRef] [PubMed]
24. Crosas-Molist, E.; Bertran, E.; Rodriguez-Hernandez, I.; Herraiz, C.; Cantelli, G.; Fabra, A.; Sanz-Moreno, V.; Fabregat, I. The NADPH oxidase NOX4 represses epithelial to amoeboid transition and efficient tumour dissemination. *Oncogene* **2017**, *36*, 3002–3014. [CrossRef] [PubMed]
25. Miikkulainen, P.; Högel, H.; Seyednasrollah, F.; Rantanen, K.; Elo, L.L.; Jaakkola, P.M. Hypoxia-inducible factor (HIF)-prolyl hydroxylase 3 (PHD3) maintains high HIF2A mRNA levels in clear cell renal cell carcinoma. *J. Biol. Chem.* **2019**, *294*, 3760–3771. [CrossRef]
26. Tanaka, T.; Torigoe, T.; Hirohashi, Y.; Sato, E.; Honma, I.; Kitamura, H.; Masumori, N.; Tsukamoto, T.; Sato, N. Hypoxia-inducible factor (HIF)-independent expression mechanism and novel function of HIF prolyl hydroxylase-3 in renal cell carcinoma. *J. Cancer Res. Clin. Oncol.* **2014**, *140*, 503–513. [CrossRef]
27. Zhang, C.S.; Liu, Q.; Li, M.; Lin, S.Y.; Peng, Y.; Wu, D.; Li, T.Y.; Fu, Q.; Jia, W.; Wang, X.; et al. RHOBTB3 promotes proteasomal degradation of HIFalpha through facilitating hydroxylation and suppresses the Warburg effect. *Cell Res.* **2015**, *25*, 1025–1042. [CrossRef]
28. Jeck, W.R.; Sharpless, N.E. Detecting and characterizing circular RNAs. *Nat. Biotechnol.* **2014**, *32*, 453–461. [CrossRef]
29. Starke, S.; Jost, I.; Rossbach, O.; Schneider, T.; Schreiner, S.; Hung, L.H.; Bindereif, A. Exon Circularization Requires Canonical Splice Signals. *Cell Rep.* **2015**, *10*, 103–111. [CrossRef]
30. Jeck, W.R.; Sorrentino, J.A.; Wang, K.; Slevin, M.K.; Burd, C.E.; Liu, J.; Marzluff, W.F.; Sharpless, N.E. Circular RNAs are abundant, conserved, and associated with ALU repeats. *RNA* **2013**, *19*, 141–157. [CrossRef]
31. Memczak, S.; Papavasileiou, P.; Peters, O.; Rajewsky, N. Identification and Characterization of Circular RNAs As a New Class of Putative Biomarkers in Human Blood. *PLoS ONE* **2015**, *10*, e0141214. [CrossRef] [PubMed]

32. Jung, M.; Ramankulov, A.; Roigas, J.; Johannsen, M.; Ringsdorf, M.; Kristiansen, G.; Jung, K. In search of suitable reference genes for gene expression studies of human renal cell carcinoma by real-time PCR. *BMC Mol. Biol.* **2007**, *8*, 47. [CrossRef] [PubMed]
33. Camp, R.L. X-Tile: A New Bio-Informatics Tool for Biomarker Assessment and Outcome-Based Cut-Point Optimization. *Clin. Cancer Res.* **2004**, *10*, 7252–7259. [CrossRef]
34. Steyerberg, E.W.; Pencina, M.J.; Lingsma, H.F.; Kattan, M.W.; Vickers, A.J.; Van, C.B. Assessing the incremental value of diagnostic and prognostic markers: A review and illustration. *Eur. J. Clin. Investig.* **2012**, *42*, 216–228. [CrossRef] [PubMed]
35. Wagenmakers, E.J.; Farrell, S. AIC model selection using Akaike weights. *Psychon. Bull. Rev.* **2004**, *11*, 192–196. [CrossRef] [PubMed]
36. Dudekula, D.B.; Panda, A.C.; Grammatikakis, I.; De, S.; Abdelmohsen, K.; Gorospe, M. CircInteractome: A web tool for exploring circular RNAs and their interacting proteins and microRNAs. *RNA Biol.* **2016**, *13*, 34–42. [CrossRef] [PubMed]
37. Agarwal, V.; Bell, G.W.; Nam, J.W.; Bartel, D.P. Predicting effective microRNA target sites in mammalian mRNAs. *eLife* **2015**, *4*, e05005. [CrossRef]
38. Wong, N.; Wang, X. miRDB: An online resource for microRNA target prediction and functional annotations. *Nucleic Acids Res.* **2015**, *43*, D146–D152. [CrossRef]
39. Littman, B.H.; Di, M.L.; Plebani, M.; Marincola, F.M. What's next in translational medicine? *Clin. Sci.* **2007**, *112*, 217–227. [CrossRef]
40. Klatte, T.; Rossi, S.H.; Stewart, G.D. Prognostic factors and prognostic models for renal cell carcinoma: A literature review. *World J. Urol.* **2018**, *36*, 1943–1952. [CrossRef]
41. Li, S.; Teng, S.; Xu, J.; Su, G.; Zhang, Y.; Zhao, J.; Zhang, S.; Wang, H.; Qin, W.; Lu, Z.J.; et al. Microarray is an efficient tool for circRNA profiling. *Brief. Bioinform.* **2018**. [CrossRef] [PubMed]
42. Tan, W.L.; Lim, B.T.; Anene-Nzelu, C.G.; Ackers-Johnson, M.; Dashi, A.; See, K.; Tiang, Z.; Lee, D.P.; Chua, W.W.; Luu, T.D.; et al. A landscape of circular RNA expression in the human heart. *Cardiovasc. Res.* **2017**, *113*, 298–309. [CrossRef] [PubMed]
43. Chen, S.; Huang, V.; Xu, X.; Livingstone, J.; Soares, F.; Jeon, J.; Zeng, Y.; Hua, J.T.; Petricca, J.; Guo, H.; et al. Widespread and Functional RNA Circularization in Localized Prostate Cancer. *Cell* **2019**, *176*, 831–843. [CrossRef] [PubMed]
44. Siede, D.; Rapti, K.; Gorska, A.; Katus, H.; Altmüller, J.; Boeckel, J.; Meder, B.; Maack, C.; Völkers, M.; Müller, O.; et al. Identification of circular RNAs with host gene-independent expression in human model systems for cardiac differentiation and disease. *J. Mol. Cell. Cardiol.* **2017**, *109*, 48–56. [CrossRef]
45. Vo, J.N.; Cieslik, M.; Zhang, Y.; Shukla, S.; Xiao, L.; Zhang, Y.; Wu, Y.M.; Dhanasekaran, S.M.; Engelke, C.G.; Cao, X.; et al. The Landscape of Circular RNA in Cancer. *Cell* **2019**, *176*, 869–881. [CrossRef]
46. Cieślik, M.; Chugh, R.; Wu, Y.M.; Wu, M.; Brennan, C.; Lonigro, R.; Su, F.; Wang, R.; Siddiqui, J.; Mehra, R.; et al. The use of exome capture RNA-seq for highly degraded RNA with application to clinical cancer sequencing. *Genome Res.* **2015**, *25*, 1372–1381. [CrossRef]
47. Gerszten, R.E.; Wang, T.J. The search for new cardiovascular biomarkers. *Nature* **2008**, *451*, 949–952. [CrossRef]
48. Ralla, B.; Busch, J.; Flörcken, A.; Westermann, J.; Zhao, Z.; Kilic, E.; Weickmann, S.; Jung, M.; Fendler, A.; Jung, K. miR-9-5p in Nephrectomy Specimens is a Potential Predictor of Primary Resistance to First-Line Treatment with Tyrosine Kinase Inhibitors in Patients with Metastatic Renal Cell Carcinoma. *Cancers* **2018**, *10*, 321. [CrossRef]
49. Steyerberg, E.W.; E Harrell, F.; Borsboom, G.J.; Eijkemans, M.J.; Vergouwe, Y.; Habbema, J.D. Internal validation of predictive models: Efficiency of some procedures for logistic regression analysis. *J. Clin. Epidemiol.* **2001**, *54*, 774–781. [CrossRef]
50. Meng, S.; Zhou, H.; Feng, Z.; Xu, Z.; Tang, Y.; Li, P.; Wu, M. CircRNA: Functions and properties of a novel potential biomarker for cancer. *Mol. Cancer* **2017**, *16*, 94. [CrossRef]
51. Hansen, T.B.; Kjems, J.; Damgaard, C.K. Circular RNA and miR-7 in cancer. *Cancer Res.* **2013**, *73*, 5609–5612. [CrossRef] [PubMed]
52. Cheng, Z.; Yu, C.; Cui, S.; Wang, H.; Jin, H.; Wang, C.; Li, B.; Qin, M.; Yang, C.; He, J.; et al. circTP63 functions as a ceRNA to promote lung squamous cell carcinoma progression by upregulating FOXM1. *Nat. Commun.* **2019**, *10*, 3200. [CrossRef] [PubMed]

53. Lu, Q.; Liu, T.; Feng, H.; Yang, R.; Zhao, X.; Chen, W.; Jiang, B.; Qin, H.; Guo, X.; Liu, M.; et al. Circular RNA circSLC8A1 acts as a sponge of miR-130b/miR-494 in suppressing bladder cancer progression via regulating PTEN. *Mol. Cancer* **2019**, *18*, 111. [CrossRef] [PubMed]
54. Högel, H.; Miikkulainen, P.; Bino, L.; Jaakkola, P.M. Hypoxia inducible prolyl hydroxylase PHD3 maintains carcinoma cell growth by decreasing the stability of p27. *Mol. Cancer* **2015**, *14*, 143. [CrossRef] [PubMed]
55. Li, Y.; Quan, J.; Chen, F.; Pan, X.; Zhuang, C.; Xiong, T.; Zhuang, C.; Li, J.; Huang, X.; Ye, J.; et al. MiR-31-5p acts as a tumor suppressor in renal cell carcinoma by targeting cyclin-dependent kinase 1 (CDK1). *Biomed. Pharmacother.* **2019**, *111*, 517–526. [CrossRef]
56. Lin, H.; Huang, Z.P.; Liu, J.; Qiu, Y.; Tao, Y.P.; Wang, M.C.; Yao, H.; Hou, K.Z.; Gu, F.M.; Xu, X.F. MiR-494-3p promotes PI3K/AKT pathway hyperactivation and human hepatocellular carcinoma progression by targeting PTEN. *Sci. Rep.* **2018**, *8*, 10461. [CrossRef]
57. Wang, J.; Chen, H.; Liao, Y.; Chen, N.; Liu, T.; Zhang, H.; Zhang, H. Expression and clinical evidence of miR-494 and PTEN in non-small cell lung cancer. *Tumor Biol.* **2015**, *36*, 6965–6972. [CrossRef]
58. Bustin, S.A.; Benes, V.; Garson, J.A.; Huggett, J.; Kubista, M.; Mueller, R.; Nolan, T.; Pfaffl, M.W.; Shipley, G.L.; Vandesompele, J.; et al. The MIQE Guidelines: Minimum Information for Publication of Quantitative Real-Time PCR Experiments. *Clin. Chem.* **2009**, *55*, 611–622. [CrossRef]
59. Altman, D.G.; McShane, L.M.; Sauerbrei, W.; Taube, S.E. Reporting Recommendations for Tumor Marker Prognostic Studies (REMARK): Explanation and elaboration. *PLoS Med.* **2012**, *9*, e1001216. [CrossRef]
60. Bossuyt, P.M.; Reitsma, J.B.; Bruns, D.E.; Gatsonis, C.A.; Glasziou, P.P.; Irwig, L.; Lijmer, J.G.; Moher, D.; Rennie, D.; De Vet, H.C.; et al. STARD 2015: An Updated List of Essential Items for Reporting Diagnostic Accuracy Studies. *Radiology* **2015**, *277*, 826–832. [CrossRef]
61. Jung, M.; Mollenkopf, H.J.; Grimm, C.; Wagner, I.; Albrecht, M.; Waller, T.; Pilarsky, C.; Johannsen, M.; Stephan, C.; Lehrach, H.; et al. MicroRNA profiling of clear cell renal cell cancer identifies a robust signature to define renal malignancy. *J. Cell. Mol. Med.* **2009**, *13*, 3918–3928. [CrossRef] [PubMed]
62. Wotschofsky, Z.; Meyer, H.A.; Jung, M.; Fendler, A.; Wagner, I.; Stephan, C.; Busch, J.; Erbersdobler, A.; Disch, A.C.; Mollenkopf, H.J.; et al. Reference genes for the relative quantification of microRNAs in renal cell carcinomas and their metastases. *Anal. Biochem.* **2011**, *417*, 233–241. [CrossRef] [PubMed]
63. Ralla, B.; Magheli, A.; Kempkensteffen, C.; Miller, K.; Jung, M.; Trujillo, E.; Wotschofsky, Z.; Kilic, E.; Fendler, A.; Jung, K.; et al. 773 Piwi-interacting RNAs as novel prognostic markers in clear cell renal cell carcinomas. *Eur. Urol. Suppl.* **2015**, *14*, e773. [CrossRef]
64. Untergasser, A.; Cutcutache, I.; Koressaar, T.; Ye, J.; Faircloth, B.C.; Remm, M.; Rozen, S.G. Primer3–new capabilities and interfaces. *Nucleic Acids Res.* **2012**, *40*, e115. [CrossRef]
65. Vickers, A.J.; Elkin, E.B. Decision curve analysis: A novel method for evaluating prediction models. *Med. Decis. Mak.* **2006**, *26*, 565–574. [CrossRef]
66. Stephan, C.; Jung, K.; Semjonow, A.; Schulze-Forster, K.; Cammann, H.; Hu, X.; Meyer, H.A.; Bogemann, M.; Miller, K.; Friedersdorff, F. Comparative assessment of urinary prostate cancer antigen 3 and TMPRSS2:ERG gene fusion with the serum [-2]proprostate-specific antigen-based prostate health index for detection of prostate cancer. *Clin. Chem.* **2013**, *59*, 280–288. [CrossRef]
67. Faul, F.; Erdfelder, E.; Lang, A.G.; Buchner, A. G*Power 3: A flexible statistical power analysis program for the social, behavioral, and biomedical sciences. *Behav. Res. Methods* **2007**, *39*, 175–191. [CrossRef]

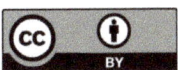

© 2019 by the authors. Licensee MDPI, Basel, Switzerland. This article is an open access article distributed under the terms and conditions of the Creative Commons Attribution (CC BY) license (http://creativecommons.org/licenses/by/4.0/).

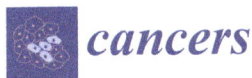

Article

Interleukin4Rα (IL4Rα) and IL13Rα1 Are Associated with the Progress of Renal Cell Carcinoma through Janus Kinase 2 (JAK2)/Forkhead Box O3 (FOXO3) Pathways

Mi-Ae Kang [1,†], Jongsung Lee [2,†], Sang Hoon Ha [3,†], Chang Min Lee [4], Kyoung Min Kim [5,6,7], Kyu Yun Jang [5,6,7,*] and See-Hyoung Park [4,*]

1. Department of Biological Science, Gachon University, Seongnam 13120, Korea; makang53@hanmail.net
2. Department of Integrative Biotechnology, Sungkyunkwan University, Suwon 16419, Korea; bioneer@skku.edu
3. Division of Biotechnology, Chonbuk National University, Iksan 54596, Korea; hasangpos@gmail.com
4. Department of Bio and Chemical Engineering, Hongik University, Sejong 30016, Korea; yycc456@naver.com
5. Department of Pathology, Chonbuk National University Medical School, Chonbuk National University, Jeonju 54896, Korea; kmkim@jbnu.ac.kr
6. Research Institute of Clinical Medicine, Chonbuk National University, Jeonju 54896, Korea
7. Biomedical Research Institute of Chonbuk National University Hospital, Chonbuk National University Hospital, Jeonju 54896, Korea
* Correspondence: kyjang@chonbuk.ac.kr (K.Y.J.); shpark74@hongik.ac.kr (S.-H.P.); Tel.: +82-63-270-3136 (K.Y.J.); +82-44-860-2126 (S.-H.P.)
† These authors contributed equally to this work.

Received: 2 September 2019; Accepted: 15 September 2019; Published: 18 September 2019

Abstract: Specific kinds of interleukin (IL) receptors are known to mediate lymphocyte proliferation and survival. However, recent reports have suggested that the high expression of IL4Rα and IL13Rα1 in tumor tissue might be associated with tumorigenesis in several kinds of tumor. We found that a significant association between mRNA level of IL4Rα or IL13Rα1 and the poor prognosis of renal cell carcinoma (RCC) from the public database (http://www.oncolnc.org/). Then, we evaluated the clinicopathological significance of the immunohistochemical expression of IL4Rα and IL13Rα1 in 199 clear cell RCC (CCRCC) patients. The individual and co-expression patterns of IL4Rα and IL13Rα1 were significantly associated with cancer-specific survival (CSS) and relapse-free survival (RFS) in univariate analysis. Multivariate analysis indicated IL4Rα-positivity and co-expression of IL4Rα and IL13Rα1 as the independent indicators of shorter CSS and RFS of CCRCC patients. For the in vitro evaluation of the oncogenic role of IL4Rα and IL13Rα1 in RCC, we knock-downed IL4Rα or IL13Rα1 and observed that the cell proliferation rate was decreased, and the apoptosis rate was increased in A498 and ACHN cells. Furthermore, we examined the possible role of Janus kinase 2 (JAK2), well-known down-stream tyrosine kinase under the heterodimeric receptor complex of IL4Rα and IL13Rα1. Interestingly, JAK2 interacted with Forkhead box O3 (FOXO3) to cause tyrosine-phosphorylation of FOXO3. Silencing IL4Rα or JAK2 in A498 and ACHN cells reduced the interaction between JAK2 and FOXO3. Moreover, pharmacological inhibition of JAK2 induced the nuclear localization of FOXO3, leading to increase apoptosis and decrease cell proliferation rate in A498 and ACHN cells. Taken together, these results suggest that IL4Rα and IL13Rα1 might be involved in the progression of RCC through JAK2/FOXO3 pathway, and their expression might be used as the novel prognostic factor and therapeutic target for RCC patients.

Keywords: IL4Rα; IL13Rα1; renal cell carcinoma; JAK2; FOXO3

1. Introduction

In 2018, about 65,000 Americans were diagnosed with kidney cancer. Among them, about 15,000 died of this disease [1]. Renal cell carcinoma (RCC) is the most common subtype (about 90%) of kidney cancer. Further, 80% of RCC are classified into clear cell renal cell carcinoma (CCRCC) [2,3]. At the time of initial diagnosis, more than 30% of the patients had metastasis and 20–40% of the patients had systemic metastasis after surgery [4]. Surgical resection is the first and effective treatment option for the early stage kidney cancer. However, there is still a high mortality rate in kidney cancer due to local or remote metastasis of cancer, which is usually highly resistant to the conventional chemotherapy and radiation therapy [5,6]. Thus, it is still needed to understand the detail molecular mechanism of RCC development for efficient care.

Interleukins (IL) are involved in mediating various biological function such as lymphocytes (T and B-cell) activation, proliferation, and differentiation [7–9]. Usually, each IL has different activity in the immune regulation process after binding to its receptor, but several kinds of ILs may have the common receptor on the cell membrane. IL4 and IL13 have not structurally nor functionally similar characteristics [10]. Both IL4 and IL13 can exert their function through binding to the IL4 receptor (IL4R). IL4Rα is one subunit of IL4R complex with a specific binding affinity for IL4. There are two types of IL4R complex, depending on the heterodimeric protein subunit components. Type I IL4R is composed of IL4Rα and γc subunit. Type II IL4R is composed of IL4Rα and IL13Rα1 subunit. After IL4 binds to IL4Rα, IL13 binds to IL13Rα1 to form a heterodimeric complex and combine the signal pathway [10–12]. Therefore, type II IL4R complex serves as a functional receptor for both IL4 and IL13 [13].

It has been reported that IL4 and IL13-mediated signaling pathways play an important role in tumor biology [14]. For example, IL4R complex is abnormally over-expressed in malignant ovarian, brain, lung, breast, pancreatic, colorectal, bladder, and other epithelial cell type tumors, suggesting that IL4R complex may be involved for tumor progression [14–19]. In addition, IL4 and IL13 could act as signaling molecules in the tumor microenvironment. Myeloid-derived suppressor cells (MDSCs) are known to be able to inhibit immune responses in the tumor microenvironment [20]. IL4 and IL13 can activate MDSCs to exert immunosuppression leading to promote tumor growth [21,22]. Furthermore, several studies have reported that single nucleotide polymorphisms (SNPs) in the IL4R gene are closely associated with tumor progression [23,24]. The possibility of treating tumors by blocking IL4Rα to reduce IL4 and IL13 signaling has been examined. Targeting IL4R signaling pathway for treating metastatic cancer has already been approved by the U.S. Food and Drug Administration (FDA) [25]. However, there is no direct study describing the possible oncogenic role of IL4R complex in RCC.

Janus kinase 2 (JAK2)/Signal transducer and activator of transcription 3 (STAT3) and PI3K/Akt are the main signaling pathways under IL4R complex [25–27]. It has been reported that the IL4R complex can promote the progress of lots of tumors by activating STAT6 and Akt. It seems that these pathways are closely related to each one to form a cross talking network. JAK2/STAT3 signaling pathway has been studied for the involvement in the development of lots of tumors [28]. STAT3 is an oncogenic transcriptional factor responsible for anti-apoptotic proteins such as Bcl2 and Bclxl [28]. STAT3 can be tyrosine-phosphorylated by JAK2 and the activated STAT3 translocates from cytoplasm into nucleus to induce the genes related to cell survival and proliferation. According to many recent studies, activated JAK2/STAT3 signaling has been observed in several kinds of tumors such as lung, prostate, and gastric cancers [29–31]. Thus, JAK2/STAT3 could serve as a potential target for cancer therapy. However, presently, there is no detailed study elucidating the relationship between IL4R complex and JAK2 in RCC.

Forkhead box O3 (FOXO3) belongs to the forkhead gene family and encodes FOXO3 transcriptional factor responsible for the regulation of genes associated with apoptosis, autophagy, and longevity [32–35]. FOXO3 is one of the well-known tumor-suppressive transcriptional factors [36]. For instance, in breast and leukemia cancer cells, anti-cancer drugs inhibit tumor development via upregulation of FOXO3 and B cell lymphoma 2 like 11 (Bim) expression [37–39]. Moreover, FOXO3 plays a pivotal role in cell cycle arrest through p27 upregulation and can induce G2/M phase cell cycle arrest in breast cancer cells [40,41]. In addition, FOXO3 has been studied for the downregulation of the oncogenic Myc transcriptional factor [42–44]. In RCC, the protein expression level of FOXO3 has been reported to be significantly downregulated. However, the mRNA expression level of FOXO3 was not much changed, implying that there might be the post-transcriptional regulation for FOXO3 protein in RCC [45].

In this study, we focus on the clinical outcomes, biological function, and molecular mechanisms of the expression of IL4Rα and IL13Rα1 in RCC progression. Upregulated IL4Rα and IL13Rα1 expression is sufficiently associated with clinical T stage and reduced overall survival of CCRCC patients and down-regulation of IL4Rα and IL13Rα1 expression induced the cell cycle arrest and apoptosis in A498 and ACHN cells. Mechanistically, IL4Rα and IL13Rα1 could increase JAK2 signaling pathway and suppress tumor-suppressive activity of FOXO3. Interestingly, JAK2 interacted with FOXO3 to cause tyrosine-phosphorylation of FOXO3. These results suggest that IL4Rα and IL13Rα1 might be involved in the progression of RCC through JAK2/FOXO3 pathway, and their expression might be used as the novel prognostic factor and promising therapeutic target for RCC patients.

2. Results

2.1. Immunohistochemical Expression of IL4Rα and IL13Rα1 Are Associated with Poor Prognosis of CCRCC Patients

When we searched OncoLnc public database, higher expression of mRNA of IL4Rα or IL13Rα1 was significantly associated with CCRCC patients (Log-rank, IL4Rα; $p < 0.001$, IL13Rα1; $p = 0.001$) (Figure S1). Similarly, high levels of IL4 and IL13 are detected in the tumor micro-environment, peripheral blood of prostate, bladder, and breast cancer patients. Therefore, the expression of IL4Rα and IL13Rα1 might be used as a new diagnostic and prognostic marker of CCRCC patients. In human CCRCC tissue, the expression of IL4Rα and IL13Rα1 were seen in both the cytoplasm and nuclei of tumor cells (Figure 1A). The cutoff points for immunohistochemical staining scores for IL4Rα and IL13Rα1 expression to classify negative- and positive-subgroups were six and seven, respectively (Figure 1B). At these cutoff points, 45.2% (90 of 199) and 37% (74/125) of CCRCC were subgrouped as IL4Rα-positive and IL13Rα1-positive groups, respectively (Table 1). In addition, there was a significant association between IL4Rα-positivity and IL13Rα1-positivity ($p < 0.001$). The IL13Rα1-positivity was significantly associated with higher tumor stage ($p = 0.019$) (Table 1). The factors significantly associated with both cancer-specific survival (CSS) and relapse-free survival (RFS) in univariate survival analysis, were sex, age of patients, tumor size, tumor stage, lymph node metastasis, and immunohistochemical expressions of IL4Rα and IL13Rα1 (Table 2). The IL4Rα-positivity had a 4.5-fold (95% confidence interval (95% CI); 1.848–11.250, $p < 0.001$) greater risk of death from CCRCC and a 2.8-fold (95% CI; 1.413–5.570, $p = 0.003$) greater risk of relapse or death from CCRCC. The IL13Rα1-positivity showed a 2.3-fold (95% CI; 1.076–4.961, $p = 0.032$) greater risk of death and a 2.2-fold (95% CI; 1.185–4.314, $p = 0.013$) greater risk of relapse or death of CCRCC patients (Table 2). The Kaplan-Meier survival curve for CSS and RFS, according to IL4Rα- and IL13Rα1-positivity are presented in Figure 1C. Furthermore, based on the molecular relationship between IL4Rα and IL13Rα1, we evaluated the clinicopathologic significance of co-expression pattern of IL4Rα and IL13Rα1 in CCRCCs. As shown in Figure 1D, co-expression pattern of IL4Rα and IL13Rα1 was significantly associated with CSS (Log-rank, overall $p < 0.001$) and RFS (Log-rank, overall $p < 0.001$). The 5-year- and 10-year-CSS of IL4Rα-/IL13Rα1- subgroup was 96% and 88%, respectively. The 5-year- and 10-year-CSS of IL4Rα+/IL13Rα1+ subgroup was 74% and 57%, respectively. However, despite the overall prognostic significance of four-subgroups of co-expression patterns of IL4Rα and IL13Rα1, the difference of survival between each subgroup was not significant (Figure 1D). Therefore, based on Kaplan-Meier survival curve for the four-subgroups of co-expression pattern of IL4Rα and IL13Rα1, we re-subgrouped to favorable (IL4Rα-/IL13Rα1-, IL4Rα-/IL13Rα1+, or IL4Rα+/IL13Rα1-) and poor prognostic (IL4Rα+/IL13Rα1+) subgroups (Figure 1E). This subgrouping for the co-expression patterns of IL4Rα and IL13Rα1 was significantly associated with age ($p = 0.007$), tumor size ($p = 0.029$), tumor stage ($p = 0.027$), and lymph node metastasis ($p = 0.017$) (Table 1), and significantly associated with CSS (Log-rank, $p < 0.001$) and RFS (Log-rank, $p < 0.001$) (Figure 1E). Especially, the 5-year- and 10-year-CSS of the favorable prognostic subgroup was 93% and 87%, respectively. In contrast, the 5-year- and 10-year-CSS of the poor prognostic subgroup was 74% and 57%, respectively (Figure 1E). The poor prognostic subgroup showed a 3.7-fold (95% CI; 1.771–7.933, $p < 0.001$) greater risk of death and a 3.4-fold (95% CI; 1.833–6.557, $p < 0.001$) greater risk of relapse or death of CCRCC patients (Table 2). When we performed multivariate analysis with sex, age, tumor stage, histologic nuclear grade, tumor necrosis, and the expression of IL4Rα and IL13Rα1, tumor stage (CSS; $p < 0.001$, RFS; $p < 0.001$) and IL4Rα expression (CSS; $p = 0.001$, RFS; $p = 0.004$) were the independent prognostic indicators for both CSS and RFS (Table 3, model 1). The IL4Rα-positivity had a 4.3-fold (95% CI; 1.753–10.713) greater risk of death and a 2.7-fold (95% CI; 1.372–5.422) greater risk of relapse or death of CCRCC patients (Table 3). When we performed multivariate analysis with inclusion of co-expression pattern of IL4Rα and IL13Rα1 instead of the expression of IL4Rα and IL13Rα1, co-expression pattern of IL4Rα and IL13Rα1 was an independent prognostic indicator for CSS (hazard ratio; 3.286, 95% CI; 1.542–7.000, $p = 0.002$) and RFS (hazard ratio; 3.158, 95% CI; 1.662–6.000, $p < 0.001$) (Table 3, model 2).

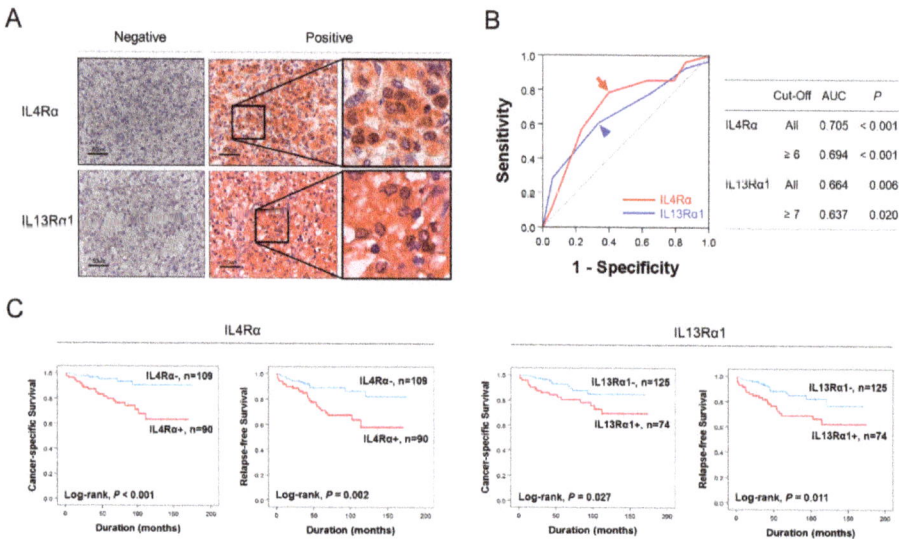

Figure 1. *Cont.*

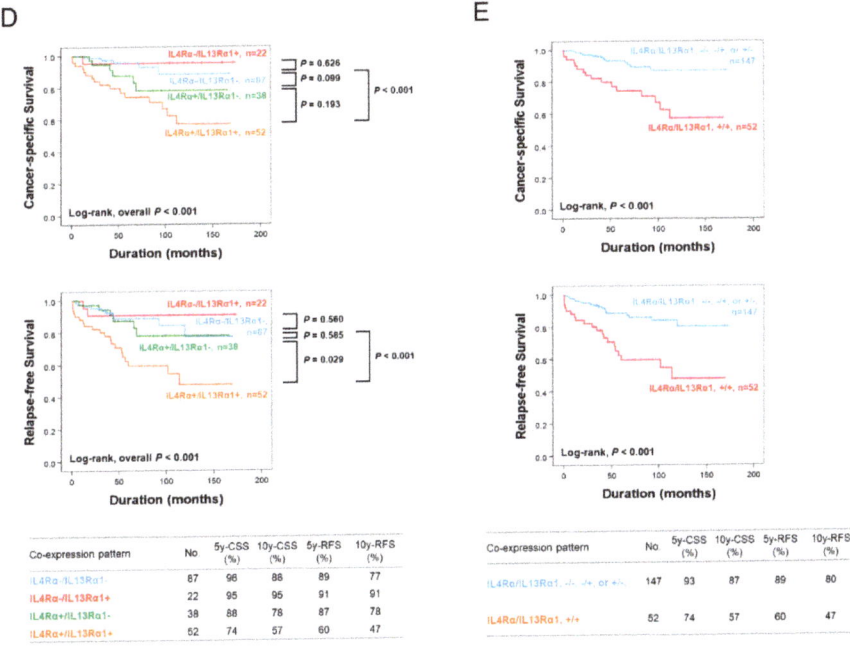

Figure 1. Immunohistochemical expression and survival analysis for the expression of interleukin4 receptor α (IL4Rα) and interleukin13 receptor α1 (IL13Rα1) in clear cell renal cell carcinoma (CCRCC). (**A**) Immunohistochemical expression of IL4Rα and IL13Rα1 in CCRCC tissue. Original magnification, ×400. (**B**) Analysis of sensitivity and specificity of the immunohistochemical staining score of IL4Rα and IL13Rα1 in CCRCC for the event of cancer-specific survival (death of the patient by CCRCC) by receiver operator characteristic curves. The cutoff points were determined at the highest area under the curve (AUC). Red arrow indicates a cutoff point for the IL4Rα immunostaining and blue arrowhead indicates a cut-off point for the IL13Rα1 immunostaining. (**C**) Kaplan-Meier survival analysis for cancer-specific survival and relapse-free survival according to the immunohistochemical positivity for IL4Rα and IL13Rα1 in 199 CCRCC. (**D**) Kaplan-Meier survival analysis in IL4Rα−/IL13Rα1−, IL4Rα−/IL13Rα1+, IL4Rα+/IL13Rα1−, and IL4Rα+/IL13Rα1+ subgroups according to the positivity for IL4Rα and IL13Rα1 expressions. (**E**) Kaplan-Meier survival analysis in two subgroups according to the co-expression patterns of IL4Rα and IL13Rα1; favorable (IL4Rα−/IL13Rα1−, IL4Rα−/IL13Rα1+, or IL4Rα+/IL13Rα1−) and poor prognostic (IL4Rα+/IL13Rα1+) subgroups. 5y-cancer-specific survival (CSS); 5-year cancer-specific survival rate, 10y-CSS; 10-year cancer-specific survival rate; 5y-RFS; five-year relapse-free survival rate, 10y- relapse-free survival (RFS); 10-year relapse-free survival rate.

Table 1. Clinicopathologic variables and the expression of interleukin4 receptor α (IL4Rα) and interleukin13 receptor α1 (IL13Rα1) in clear cell renal cell carcinoma (CCRCC) patients.

Characteristics		No.	IL4Rα Positive	p	IL13Rα Positive	p	IL4Rα/IL13Rα1 Pattern −/−, +/−, −/+	+/+	p
Sex	Male	140	67 (48%)	0.251	56 (40%)	0.206	101 (72%)	39 (28%)	0.393
	Female	59	23 (39%)		18 (31%)		46 (78%)	13 (22%)	
Age, y	≤55	81	30 (37%)	0.054	27 (33%)	0.352	68 (84%)	13 (16%)	0.007
	>55	118	60 (51%)		47 (40%)		79 (67%)	39 (33%)	
Tumor size, cm	≤7	168	73 (43%)	0.242	58 (35%)	0.070	129 (77%)	39 (23%)	0.029
	>7	31	17 (55%)		16 (52%)		18 (58%)	13 (42%)	
TNM stage	I	162	70 (43%)	0.232	54 (33%)	0.019	125 (77%)	37 (23%)	0.027
	II–IV	37	20 (54%)		20 (54%)		22 (59%)	15 (41%)	
LN metastasis	Absence	197	88 (45%)	0.118	72 (37%)	0.065	147 (75%)	50 (25%)	0.017
	Presence	2	2 (100%)		2 (100%)		0 (0%)	2 (100%)	

Table 1. Cont.

Characteristics		No.	IL4Rα Positive	p	IL13Rα Positive	p	IL4Rα/IL13Rα1 Pattern −/−, +/−, −/+	+/+	p
Nuclear grade	1	36	18 (50%)	0.055	10 (28%)	0.108	29 (81%)	7 (19%)	0.053
	2	121	47 (39%)		43 (36%)		93 (77%)	28 (23%)	
	3 and 4	42	25 (60%)		21 (50%)		25 (60%)	17 (40%)	
Necrosis	Absence	172	76 (44%)	0.457	61 (35%)	0.205	131 (76%)	41 (24%)	0.063
	Presence	27	14 (52%)		13 (48%)		16 (59%)	11 (41%)	
IL13Rα1	Negative	125	38 (30%)	<0.001					
	Positive	74	52 (70%)						

Table 2. Univariate Cox regression analysis of cancer-specific survival (CSS) and relapse-free survival (RFS) in clear cell renal cell carcinoma (CCRCC) patients.

Characteristics	No.	CSS HR	95% CI	p	RFS HR	95% CI	p
Sex, male (vs. female)	140	0.281	0.085–0.930	0.038	0.337	0.131–0.864	0.023
Age, year, >55 (vs. ≤55)	118	3.603	1.368–9.486	0.009	2.275	1.104–4.688	0.026
Tumor size, >7 cm (vs. ≤7 cm)	31	3.916	1.833–8.366	<0.001	4.755	2.495–9.065	<0.001
TNM stage, I (vs. II–IV)	37	4.044	1.922–8.509	<0.001	5.354	2.831–10.124	<0.001
LN metastasis, presence (vs. absence)	2	0.049	0–1.4 × 10^6	0.049	15.801	1.956–127.649	0.010
Nuclear grade, 1	36	1		0.095	1		0.012
2	121	1.223	0.352–4.257	0.751	1.296	0.441–3.808	0.638
3 and 4	42	2.761	0.759–10.047	0.123	3.337	1.097–10.148	0.034
Necrosis, presence (vs. absence)	27	2.502	1.062–5.894	0.036	1.598	0.703–3.631	0.263
IL4Rα positive (vs. negative)	90	4.560	1.848–11.250	<0.001	2.806	1.413–5.570	0.003
IL13Rα1 positive (vs. negative)	74	2.310	1.076–4.961	0.032	2.260	1.185–4.314	0.013
IL4Rα/IL13Rα1, +/+ (vs. −/−, −/+, or +/−)	52	3.748	1.771–7.933	<0.001	3.467	1.833–6.557	<0.001

HR: hazard ratio, CI: confidence interval, TNM: tumor-node-metastasis.

Table 3. Multivariate Cox regression analysis of CSS and RFS in CCRCC patients.

Characteristics	CSS HR	95% CI	p	RFS HR	95% CI	p
Model 1 *						
TNM stage, I (vs. I–IV)	3.603	1.706–7.607	<0.001	5.246	2.773–9.925	<0.001
Necrosis, presence (vs. absence)	2.407	1.003–5.777	0.049			
IL4Rα positive (vs. negative)	4.334	1.753–10.713	0.001	2.727	1.372–5.422	0.004
Model 2 **						
TNM stage, I (vs. II–IV)	3.507	1.656–7.423	0.001	4.961	2.617–9.404	<0.001
IL4Rα/IL13Rα1, +/+ (vs. −/−, −/+, or +/−)	3.286	1.542–7.000	0.002	3.158	1.662–6.000	<0.001

* The variables included in the multivariate analysis model 1 were sex, age, tumor stage, histologic nuclear grade, tumor necrosis, and the expression of IL4Rα and IL13Rα1. ** The variables included in the multivariate analysis model 2 were sex, age, tumor stage, histologic nuclear grade, tumor necrosis, and co-expression patterns of IL4Rα and IL13Rα1.

2.2. Silencing of IL4Rα or IL13Rα1 Decreases Cell Proliferation Rate and Increases Cell Cycle Arrest and Apoptosis in A498 and ACHN Cells

In human CCRCC tissue, we found a significant association between the expression IL4Rα and IL13Rα1 and poor prognostic properties. When we examined the protein expression level of IL4Rα in several kinds of RCC cell lines, we observed that ACHN and A498 cells showed relatively the higher protein expression level of IL4Rα than others (Figure S2). Therefore, we evaluated cell proliferation, arrest, and apoptosis after inducing knock-down of IL4Rα or IL13Rα1 in human RCC A498 and ACHN cells. In vitro cell assays (WST-1, cell counting, colony formation, cell cycle analysis, terminal deoxynucleotidyl transferase dUTP nick end labeling (TUNEL), and Annexin V staining assay) showed that knockdown of IL4Rα or IL13Rα1 with siRNA decreased cell proliferation rate and increased cell cycle arrest and apoptosis in A498 and ACHN cells (Figure 2A–F). In addition, western blotting analysis indicated that knockdown of IL4Rα or IL13Rα1 with siRNA increased cleaved poly [ADP-ribose] polymerase 1 (PARP1), cleaved caspase3, Bax, p21, p27, and FOXO3 expression but decreased Bcl2 expression (Figure 2G and Figure S4). Interestingly, knockdown of IL4R complex component caused the downregulation of each other. Then, we examined the phosphorylation level of JAK2 as one of down-stream kinases under the heterodimeric receptor complex of IL4Rα and IL13Rα1. The phosphorylation level of JAK2 was also downregulated by knockdown of IL4Rα or IL13Rα1 with siRNA. Collectively, these results suggest that knockdown of IL4Rα or IL13Rα1 with siRNA transfection is closely involved in proliferation, arrest, and apoptosis in A498 and ACHN cells as well as causing inhibition of JAK2 phosphorylation.

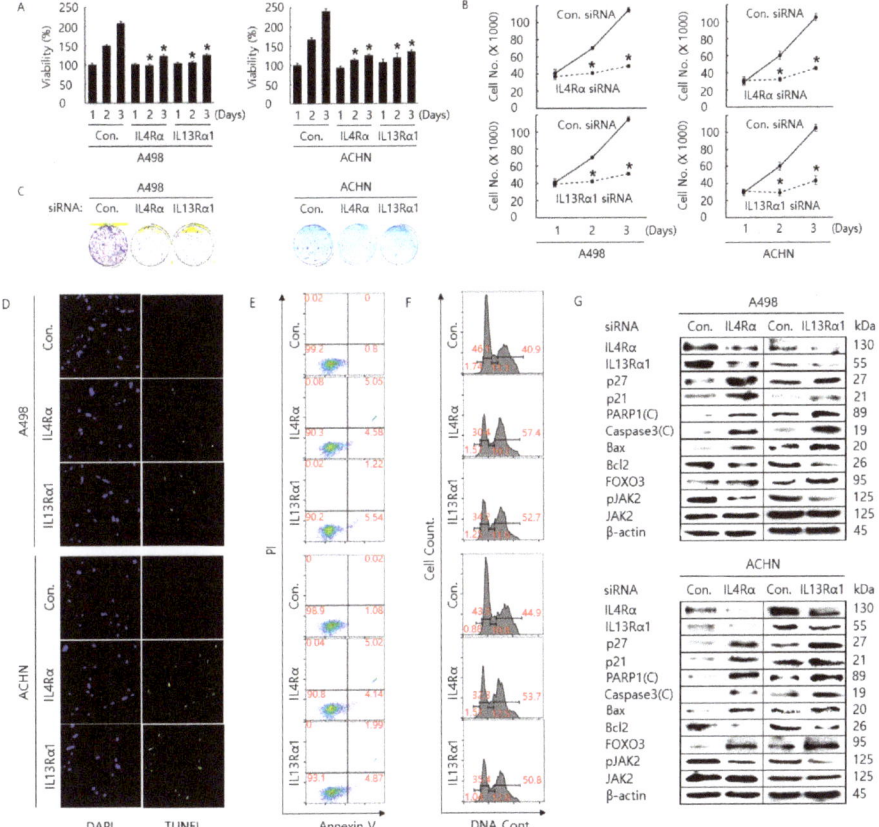

Figure 2. Anti-cancer effect by transfection of siRNA against IL4Rα or IL13Rα1 in A498 and ACHN cells. Time-dependent anti-cancer effect by transfection of siRNA against IL4Rα or IL13Rα1 in A498 and ACHN cells for 24, 48, and 72 h incubation after transfection. Cell viability and proliferation rate was determined by WST-1 assay (**A**) and cell counting assay (**B**), respectively. This result is representative data from three biological replicates, and the error bar indicates standard error (STE). * indicates the p-value < 0.05. (**C**) Anti-colony formation ability by transfection of siRNA against IL4Rα or IL13Rα1 in A498 and ACHN cells was determined by colony formation assay for 14 days after transfection. These results are representative data from three biological replicates. Apoptosis in A498 and ACHN cells transfected with siRNA against IL4Rα or IL13Rα1 for 48 h after transfection was determined by terminal deoxynucleotidyl transferase dUTP nick end labeling (TUNEL) assay (**D**) and Annexin V staining analysis (**E**). Cell cycle arrest was determined by cell cycle analysis (**F**). This result is representative data from three biological replicates. (**G**) Western blotting analysis of proteins related to apoptosis and cell cycle arrest in A498 and ACHN cells transfected with siRNA against IL4Rα or IL13Rα1 for 48 h after transfection. β-actin was used for a gel-loading control. Magnification for (**D**): ×20.

2.3. JAK2 Interacts with FOXO3 to Cause Tyrosine-Phosphorylation of FOXO3

When we examined the expression of FOXO3 in A498 and ACHN cells transfected with IL4Rα or IL13Rα1 siRNA, we found that the level of FOXO3 appeared to be inversely correlated with the phosphorylation (activation) status of JAK2. Therefore, we tested if JAK2 might interact with FOXO and contribute to a decrease in FOXO3 expression or not. As shown in Figure 3A, we observed that JAK2 protein interacted with FOXO3 protein where the protein interaction was weakened by the transfection of IL4Rα siRNA in A498 and ACHN cells. Then, we found that the expression level of FOXO3 was increased by the transfection of JAK2 siRNA or the treatment of AZD1480, one of the pharmacological inhibitors of JAK2 kinase, in A498 and ACHN cells (Figure 3B,C). To confirm whether JAK2 interacts with FOXO3, we performed co-immunoprecipitation with an antibody against Flag or FOXO3 followed by immunoblotting analysis with an antibody against HA or JAK2 in 293T cell co-transfected with over-expressing plasmid DNAs (pECE Flag-FOXO3 and pCMV3-C-HA-JAK2) (Figure 3D). Moreover, we performed a reciprocal co-immunoprecipitation with an antibody against HA or JAK2 followed by immunoblotting analysis with an antibody against an antibody against Flag or FOXO3. As shown in Figure 3D, protein interaction between JAK2 and FOXO3 was increased in 293T cell co-transfected with over-expressing plasmid DNAs (pECE Flag-FOXO3 and pCMV3-C-HA-JAK2) compared to 293T cell transfected with the control vectors. Also, we could observe that the tyrosine-phosphorylation level of FOXO3 increased in 293T cell co-transfected. These results implicate that JAK2 interacts with FOXO3 to cause tyrosine-phosphorylation of FOXO3 and regulate the protein level of FOXO3.

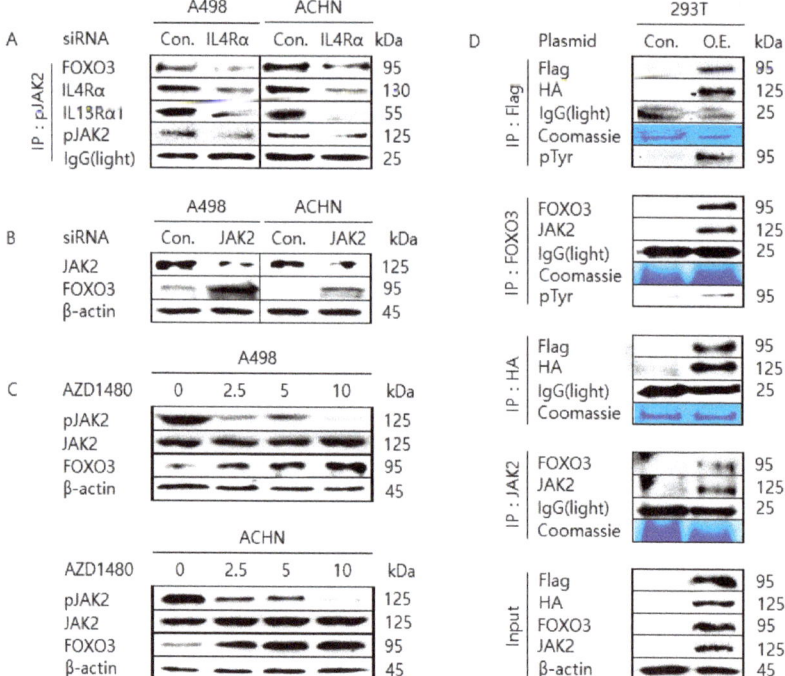

Figure 3. Interaction between Janus kinase 2 (JAK2) and Forkhead box O3 (FOXO3) protein in A498 and ACHN. (**A**) Silencing IL4Rα in A498 and ACHN cells reduced the interaction between JAK2 and FOXO3. Cells were transfected with control siRNA or siRNA against IL4Rα, and then cell lysates were immunoprecipitated with the anti-pJAK2 antibody. The immunoprecipitated proteins were resolved

on the sodium dodecyl sulfate polyacrylamide gel electrophoresis (SDS-PAGE) and immunoblotted by anti-IL4Rα, IL13Rα1, FOXO3, and pJAK2 antibody. The light chain of IgG was used for the loading control. (**B**) 293T cells were co-transfected with HA-JAK2 and Flag-FOXO3 (O.E.) or a control plasmid DNA (pCMV3-C-HA and pECE, Con.) as indicated. Then cell lysates were immunoprecipitated with anti-Flag, FOXO3, HA, JAK2, or pTyr antibody. The immunoprecipitated proteins were resolved on the SDS-PAGE and immunoblotted by the indicated antibody, respectively. The light chain of IgG and Coomassie Blue staining of SDS-PAGE were used for the loading control. (**C**) Silencing JAK2 in A498 and ACHN cells increased the expression of FOXO3. Cells were transfected with control siRNA or siRNA against JAK2, and then cell lysates were resolved on the SDS-PAGE and immunoblotted by anti-FOXO3 and JAK2 antibody. β-actin was used for the loading control. (**D**) Pharmacological inhibition of JAK2 in A498 and ACHN cells increased the expression of FOXO3. Cells were treated with dimethyl sulfoxide (DMSO) vehicle control or the indicated concentration of AZD1480, and then cell lysates were resolved on the SDS-PAGE and immunoblotted by anti-FOXO3, pJAK2, and JAK2 antibody. β-actin was used for the loading control.

2.4. Pharmacological Inhibition of JAK2 Induces the Nuclear Localization of FOXO3 and Increases FOXO3 Protein Stability

The half-life of FOXO3 protein is controlled by the proteasomal degradation after its phosphorylation [46–48]. Since we could find that FOXO3 protein interacts with JAK2 protein and the tyrosine-phosphorylation of FOXO3 was induced by JAK2, we tried to determine whether JAK2 affects the FOXO3 protein location, level, and ubiquitination status. As shown in Figure 4A, the cytoplasmic level of FOXO3 protein was decreased by AZD1480 treatment in A498 and ACHN cells, while the nuclear level of FOXO3 protein was significantly increased with a dose-dependent manner. Further, the cytoplasmic level of p27 protein was increased by AZD1480 treatment in a dose-dependent manner. These data were confirmed by the confocal analysis for staining FOXO3 protein in A498 and ACHN cells treated with AZD1480, which showed the nuclear accumulation of FOXO3 after treatment of AZD1480 (Figure 4B). These results suggest that AZD1480 could trigger the translocation of the FOXO3 protein from the cytoplasm into the nucleus in A498 and ACHN cells. Then, we found that the expression level of FOXO3 was decreased within 2 h in 293T cells co-transfected with over-expressing plasmid DNAs (pECE Flag-FOXO3 and pCMV3-C-HA-JAK2) but the expression level of FOXO3 was increased up to 4 h in the same 293T cells treated with AZD1480 with/out the treatment of CHX and MG132 (Figure 4C) suggesting that the proteasomal degradation of FOXO3 is controlled by AZD1480 treatment. Moreover, as shown in Figure 4D, immunoprecipitation analysis result with antibody against Flag after incubation of MG132 showed that poly-ubiquitination of FOXO3 was considerably weakened in 293T cells treated with AZD1480 compared to dimethyl sulfoxide (DMSO) vehicle control which is consistent with the above experimental results about the proteasomal degradation of FOXO3.

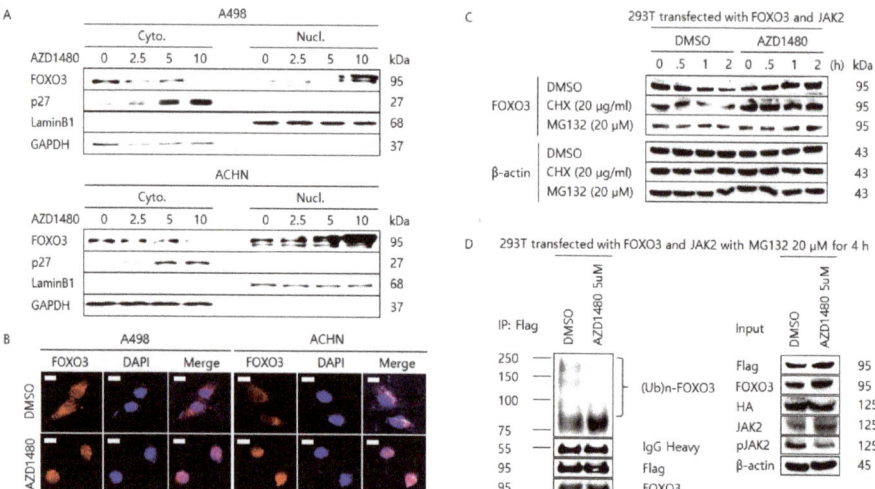

Figure 4. The nuclear localization of FOXO3 by inhibition of JAK2. (**A**) Cells were treated with DMSO vehicle control or the indicated concentration of AZD1480 (0, 2.5, 5, and 10 μM) for 48 h, washed with PBS, trypsinized, and lysed in the cytoplasmic fractional buffer. After separating the cytoplasmic fraction, the remaining pellet was washed with washing buffer and lysed with nuclear fractional buffer, and the supernatant was collected for the nuclear fraction. Glyceraldehyde 3-phosphate dehydrogenase (GAPDH) and Lamin B1 were used for a gel loading control for the cytoplasmic and nuclear protein fractions, respectively. (**B**) Pharmacological inhibition of JAK2 induces the nuclear localization of FOXO3 in A498 and ACHN. Cells were treated with DMSO vehicle control or AZD1480 (5 μM) for 2 h and then incubated with a primary antibody against FOXO3 followed by Alexa 594-conjugated anti-mouse secondary antibody. The nuclei were counterstained by 4′,6-diamidino-2-phenylindole (DAPI). Fluorescence images were captured with a confocal microscope. Scale bar: 5 μm (**C**) Pharmacological inhibition of JAK2 increases the protein stability of FOXO3 in 293T cells transfected with pECE Flag-FOXO3 and pCMV3-C-HA- JAK2 plasmid DNA via a proteasome-mediated pathway. Next, 293T cells were treated with DMSO (control vehicle), cycloheximide (CHX, 20 μg/mL), or MG-132 (20 μM) with/without AZD1480 (5 μM) for the indicated time and then cell lysates were resolved on the SDS-PAGE and immunoblotted by the anti-FOXO3 antibody. β-actin was used for the loading control. (**D**) Pharmacological inhibition of JAK2 decreases the ubiquitination of FOXO3 in 293T cells transfected with pECE Flag-FOXO3 and pCMV3-C-HA-JAK2 plasmid DNA. 293T cells were treated with DMSO (control vehicle) or MG132 (20 μM) with/without AZD1480 (5 μM) for the indicated time and then cell lysates were immunoprecipitated with anti-FOXO antibody and blotted with anti-ubiquitin, Flag, and FOXO3 antibody. The heavy chain of IgG was used for the loading control. For input analysis, cell lysates were resolved on the SDS-PAGE and immunoblotted by anti- JAK2, pJAK2, and FOXO3 antibody. β-actin was used for the loading control.

2.5. Pharmacological Inhibition of JAK2 Decreases Cell Proliferation Rate and Increases Cell Cycle Arrest and Apoptosis in A498 and ACHN Cells

To determine the anti-cancer effect of AZD1480 treatment, we performed cell proliferation, arrest, and apoptosis assays in A498 and ACHN cells treated with AZD1480. In vitro cell assays (WST-1, cell counting, colony formation, cell cycle analysis, TUNEL, and Annexin V staining assay) showed that AZD1480 treatment decreased cell proliferation rate and increased cell cycle arrest and apoptosis in A498 and ACHN cells with dose and time-dependent manner (Figure 5A–F). Furthermore, knockdown of JAK2 with siRNA also decreased cell proliferation rate in A498 and ACHN cells (Figure S3A–C). Western blotting analysis indicated that AZD1480 treatment significantly increased cleaved PARP1, cleaved caspase3, Bax, p21, p27, Bim(EL) and FOXO3 expression but decreased Bcl2 expression with dose and time-dependent manner (Figure 5G). Collectively, these results suggest that pharmacological inhibition by AZD1480 treatment is closely involved in proliferation, arrest, and apoptosis in A498 and ACHN cells through FOXO3 activation.

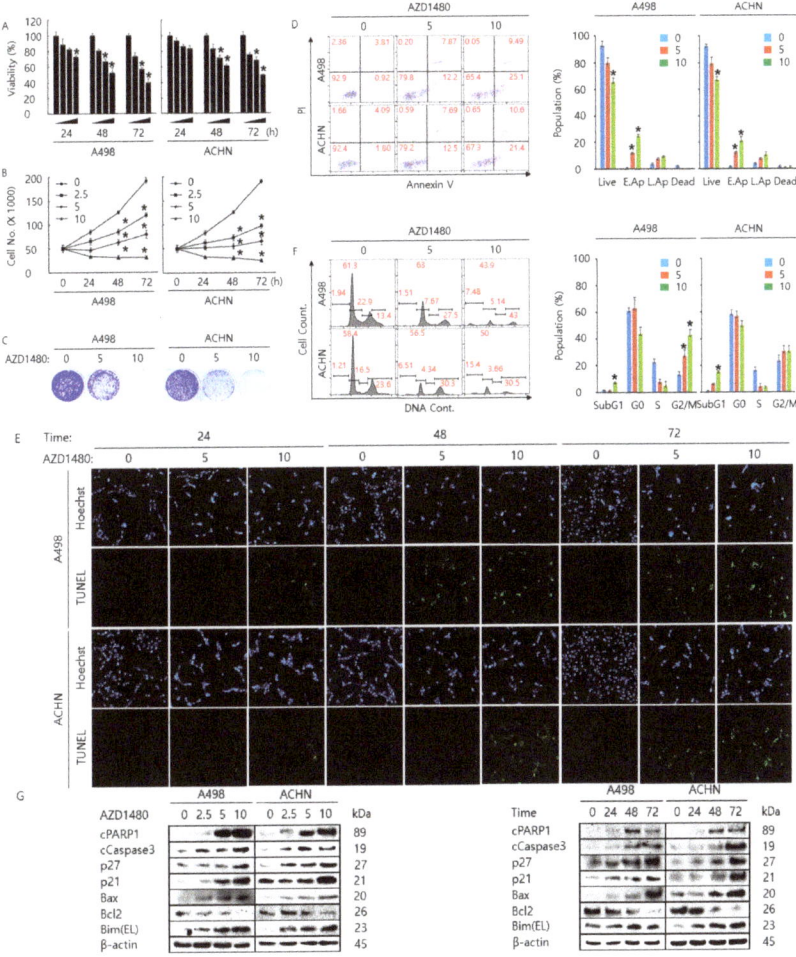

Figure 5. Anti-cancer effect by AZD1480 treatment in A498 and ACHN cells. (**A**) Dose and time-dependent anti-cancer effect by the indicated concentration of AZD1480 treatment in A498 and ACHN cells for 24, 48, and 72 h. Cell viability and proliferation rate was determined by WST-1 assay (**A**) and cell counting assay (**B**), respectively. This result is representative data from three biological replicates, and the error bar indicates standard error (STE). * indicates the p-value < 0.05. (**C**) Anti-colony formation ability by the indicated concentration of AZD1480 treatment in A498 and ACHN cells was determined by colony formation assay for 14 days. This result is representative data from three biological replicates. Apoptosis in A498 and ACHN cells treated by the indicated concentration of AZD1480 was determined by Annexin V staining analysis (**D**) and TUNEL assay (**E**). Live: live cells, E.Ap: early apoptotic cells, L.Ap: late apoptotic cells, and dead: dead cells. Cell cycle arrest was determined by cell cycle analysis (**F**). These results are representative data from three biological replicates. (**G**) Dose and time-dependent western blotting analysis of proteins related to apoptosis and cell cycle arrest in A498 and ACHN cells treated by the indicated concentration of AZD1480. β-actin was used for a gel-loading control. Magnification for (**E**): ×20.

3. Discussion

IL4 and IL13 are closely linked and expressed mono-allelically in Th2 cells [49]. IL4 and IL13 have many biological functions. One of them is to stimulate B and T-cell proliferation and differentiation of B-cell into plasma cell [50]. IL4 and IL13 share various biological functions [51]. They regulate immune responses under normal physiological conditions as well as in cancer [14]. IL4 and IL13 also play crucial roles in tumor biology and tumor immunology via activation of immune cells in the tumor microenvironment [14]. For example, it is reported that IL4 promoted tumor development via p21 mediated activation of STAT6 signaling pathways in IL4 downregulated melanoma models [52]. IL4 and IL13 bind to their receptors specifically, and both cytokines can have effects on cancer cells expressing appropriate receptors [53,54]. The receptor is made up of the heterodimer, IL4Rα, and IL13Rα1 chain [55]. IL4 and IL13 bind to IL4Rα and IL13Rα1 chains, forming functional structures in cancer cells [14]. It is reported that IL4Rα is overexpressed in human breast cancer and silencing of IL4Rα attenuated growth of metastatic breast cancer cells [56]. Moreover, IL4Ra expression activates colon tumor growth [57]. IL4Ra has also been recognized as a risk factor of pancreatic cancer [58]. IL4Rα activates directly mammary tumor metastasis [59]. IL4 and IL4Ra are related to the colorectal adenoma-carcinoma proliferation and the capacity of metastasis [24]. IL13Rα1 is an important to target of cancer therapy in human head and neck cancer animal models [60]. Overexpressed IL13Rα1 in tumor cells is closely related to patients with breast cancer [18]. Therefore, these receptors have been recognized as the main target of cancer treatment [61]. However, so far, there is no detailed research on the oncogenic role of IL4Rα and IL13Rα1 in RCC.

In this study, immunohistochemical expression of IL4Rα and IL13Rα1 was significantly associated with shorter CSS and RFS of CCRCC patients. Moreover, individual expression of IL4Rα and co-expression pattern of IL4Rα and IL13Rα1 were independent poor prognostic indicators of CCRCC patients by multivariate analysis. Especially, IL4Rα$^+$IL13Rα1$^+$ subgroup of CCRCC significantly associated with larger tumor size, higher tumor stage, and lymph node metastasis, and predicted a 3.2-fold greater risk of death of CCRCC patients compared with IL4Rα$^-$IL13Rα1$^-$/IL4Rα$^-$IL13Rα1$^+$/IL4Rα$^+$IL13Rα1$^-$ subgroups (Tables 1 and 3). These results suggest that the expression of IL4Rα and IL13Rα1 and their co-operative expression patterns are important in the progression of CCRCCs. As shown in Figure 1A, IL4Rα and IL13Rαl were detected in the cytoplasm and nuclei in CCRCC tissue samples. IL4Rα or IL13Rαl proteins are located in cell-membrane and composed of outer, inner, and cell membrane-integrated part. Outer part of IL4Rα or IL13Rαl protein recognizes IL4 or IL13. Inner part of IL4Rα or IL13Rαl protein binds to and activates the down-stream signaling proteins such as JAK2. Thus, we thought that not only the membrane expression but also the cytoplasmic expression of IL4Rα or IL13Rαl proteins might be detected by immunohistochemical staining analysis. Furthermore, the Human Protein Atlas public database (http://www.proteinatlas.org) indicates that both of IL4Rα and IL13Rα1 are expressed in the cytoplasmic membrane and nuclear of cells and the images from the Human Protein Atlas public database showed the cytoplasmic and nuclear expression of IL4Rα and IL13Rα1 as below captured. As shown in Figure 1D, IL4Rα−/IL13Rα1+ subgroup seems to lead to better prognosis than IL4Rα−/IL13Rα1− subgroup in terms of both of CSS and RFS rate. Type II IL4R is composed of IL4Rα and IL13Rαl subunit. Mechanistically, IL4 binds to IL4Rα and then IL13 binds to IL13Rαl to form a heterodimeric complex and combine the signal pathway [10–12]. Thus, we though that the reverse binding order (IL13 binds to IL13Rαl and then IL4 binds to IL4Rα) might cause abrogate the functional complex forming of type II IL4R, which lead to inhibit RCC development and prolong the survival rate of RCC patients.

Recent reports showed that IL4Rα and IL13Rα1 are overexpressed and activated in various types of epithelial tumor such as malignant glioma, ovarian, lung, pancreas, and colon carcinoma [17,62]. Therefore, IL4Rα and IL13Rα1 might be an effective therapeutic target of various human malignant tumors. Suppression of IL4 and IL13 as well as IL4Rα and IL13Rα1 might be tumor-suppressive especially in poor prognostic group of cancers expressing both IL4Rα and IL13Rα1 as like IL4Rα$^+$IL13Rα1$^+$ subgroup of CCRCC. RNA aptamer-mediated inhibition of IL4Rα induces apoptosis of MDSC and tumor-associated macrophage (TAM) which is associated with the tumoral immune escape [63]. Joshi et al. showed the higher expression of IL4Rα in anaplastic thyroid cancer (ATC), a highly aggressive thyroid cancer type than other types of thyroid cancer tissue from patients. They designed the IL4-Pseudomonas exotoxin (IL4-PE) conjugate and the treatment of IL4-PE decreased the colony formation ability of thyroid cancer cells and tumor growth in thyroid xenograft tumor model [64]. Furthermore, IL4R plays an essential role in regulating hepatocellular carcinoma (HCC) cell survival, proliferation, and metastasis and regulates the activation of JAK1/STAT6 and Jnk/Erk1/2 pathways [65]. As shown in the Figure 2G, interestingly, the knockdown of the IL4R complex component caused the downregulation of each other. Type II IL4R is composed of IL4Rα and IL13Rα1 subunit. We thought that if one of IL4R complex component is ablated by siRNA transfection, this might cause the protein degradation of each components to be accelerated since each component need to be physically interacted to form the functional complex of type II IL4R. We are planning to investigate if the half-life of IL4Rα or IL13Rα1 protein is controlled by the proteasomal degradation after transfection of siRNA against IL4Rα or IL13Rα1 into ACHN and A498 cells. In this study, knockdown of IL4R prohibited proliferation and induced apoptosis in HCC cells. Vadevoo et al. reported that they synthesized an IL4R-targeting peptide (IL4RPep-1-K) conjugated with the proapoptotic peptide (KLAKLAK)2 and demonstrated this peptide exerted the selective anti-cancer effect against IL4R-expressing tumor in vitro and in vivo (4T1 breast tumor-bearing mice model) [11]. In fact, our laboratory has been developing the novel drug delivery system using ultrasound and microbubble-liposome complex with IL4RPep-1-K to detect and treat IL4R-expressing tumor [66].

JAKs (JAK1, JAK2, JAK3, and Tyk) has seven domains called Janus homology domains (JH). Among these seven JHs, JH1 is the kinase domain responsible for a tyrosine kinase activity of JAKs and has the conserved tyrosine residues required for JAK activation (e.g., Y1007/Y1008 in JAK2). Phosphorylation of these dual tyrosines leads to the conformational changes in the JAK protein to facilitate the binding of the substrate [67]. JAK2 is a member of JAKs and a non-receptor tyrosine kinase. Compared with other JAKs, JAK2 lacks Src homology binding domains (SH2/SH3) [68]. JAK has been recognized as an important factor because it is closely related to various kinds of diseases [69–71]. Therefore, JAK inhibitor may play a crucial role in the treatment of diseases clinically. For instance, selective JAK2 inhibitor TG101348 attenuated myelofibrosis in a murine model of disease [69]. Furthermore, it was reported that JAK inhibitor had provided benefit to myeloproliferative neoplasms patients because it might reduce the production of pro-inflammatory cytokines [72]. FDA has approved several JAK inhibitors, such as Ruxolitinib, Tofacitinib, and Fedratinib [73,74]. Ruxolitinib, a small-molecule inhibitor of JAK1/2, was the first FDA approved drug for the treatment of myelofibrosis [75]. Recently, FDA approved Fedratinib, a small-molecule inhibitor of JAK2, for the treatment of myelofibrosis [76].

JAK2/STAT3 signaling pathway is known to be involved in a number of inflammatory, anti-inflammatory signaling pathways, and various pathological regulation processes [77]. It is reported that the expression of IL13Rα1 induced STAT3 activation by IL4 and IL13 in the stimulated human B cells [55]. JAK2/STAT3 signaling pathway plays a crucial role in the growth of breast cancer cells [78]. Inhibition of JAK2/STAT3 signaling pathway induces apoptosis in ovarian cancer cells [79,80]. Furthermore, inhibition of JAK2/STAT3 pathway suppresses the growth of gastric cancer in vitro and in vivo [81]. For treating RCC, JAK2/STAT3 has been recognized as an important target. A recent study showed that activation of JAK2/STAT3 signaling pathway promotes cell proliferation in CCRCC [82]. According to Xin et al, treatment of 786-O human renal cancer cells with AZD1480 showed only limited decrease in cell viability. They used 0, 0.5, and 1 μM of AZD1480 to perform MTS cell viability assay [83]. However, we used 0, 2.5, 5, and 10 μM of AZD1480 to perform WST-1 assay and we could observe the dose-and time dependent cell toxicity effect of AZD1480 in A498 and ACHN cells. When we tested the lower dose of AZD1480 (0.5 and 1 μM) for the cell viability assay, we also found the limited reduction of cell viability in A498 and ACHN cell. Thus, we thought that the range of AZD1480 dose might cause the different anti-cancer effect on the renal cancer cells. Moreover, Icaritin, a kind of flavonoid isolated from *Herba Epimedii*, suppressed JAK2/STAT3 signaling pathway, and proliferation of RCC [84]. Thus, it is important to find an effective reagent to inhibit JAK2/STAT3 signaling pathway in RCC. As described in the results section, we demonstrated that AZD1489, a kind of JAK2 inhibitor, decreased cell proliferation rate and increases cell cycle arrest and apoptosis in A498 and ACHN cells with dose and time-dependent manner. For the expansion of our research, now we are planning to develop a novel JAK2 inhibitor by screening FDA approved drug library to treat RCC.

Over the past decade, the relationship between FOXO3 and cancer cell development has been investigated. Down-regulation of FOXO3 is detected frequently in cancer development [85,86]. The relationship between FOXO3 and RCC also has been studied. Down-regulation of FOXO3 promotes tumor metastasis in RCC 786O cells [45]. Furthermore, FOXO3 upregulates the expression level of miR-30d, a kind of tumor-suppressive microRNAs, transcriptionally in RCC cell lines [87]. FOXO3 is one of the human FOXO transcription factors and know to be inhibited by the phosphorylation-dependent protein degradation in the cytoplasm [48,88]. A recent study demonstrated that Src kinases are required for the regulation of *Drosophila* FOXO3 (dFOXO) [89]. According to them, the introduction of Src42A, one of the constitutively active alleles, into the larval inhibited the starvation-mediated nuclear localization of dFOXO, and pharmacological inhibition of Src activity promoted the nuclear accumulation of dFOXO under the even high nutrient conditions. Src is one of the effector tyrosine kinase under the insulin or insulin-like growth factor (IGF) receptor signaling pathway. Thus far, the regulation of FOXO3 mediated by tyrosine phosphorylation has not been well-investigated. In this study, we also tried to show that JAK2 tyrosine kinase could phosphorylate FOXO3 and pharmacological inhibition of JAK2 induces the nuclear accumulation of FOXO3 in RCC cell lines. We also determined if tyrosine phosphorylation of FOXO3 by JAK2 affects the ubiquitination status of FOXO3. Ubiquitination pattern of FOXO3 protein was decreased significantly when FOXO3 and JAK2 were co-transfected in 293T cells with AZD1480, a kind of JAK2 inhibitor suggesting that ubiquitination of FOXO3 depends on inhibition of JAK2 activity. However, we still have the question which site of tyrosine in FOXO3 could be phosphorylated by JAK2 kinase and which E3 ligase is involved in this specific ubiquitination process. We are currently constructing several tyrosine mutants of FOXO3 to examine which tyrosine sites are phosphorylated by JAK2. Since JAK2/STAT3 and PI3K/Akt are the two kinds of main signaling pathways under IL4R complex, we might think about which signaling pathway plays more important in regulating the protein stability and ubiquitination status of FOXO3 among JAK2/STAT3 and PI3K/Akt. To examine this issue, we are seeking to perform the experiments for analyzing the protein stability and ubiquitination status of FOXO3 in the cells treated with JAK2 or Akt inhibitor as well as knock-downed or knock-outed JAK2 or Akt.

There have been a few reports describing the relationship between JAK2 and FOXO3. Ahn et al. demonstrated that enhanced reactive oxygen species (ROS) level and aberrant PI3K signaling decreased the nuclear localization of FOXO3 and catalase expression in JAK2V617F mutant positive cells. In addition, they showed that JAK2V617F-positive erythroblasts derived from myeloproliferative neoplasm patients also displayed the increased ROS level and reduced nuclear FOXO3 compared with the control erythroblasts [90]. Since JAK2 is known to phosphorylate and activate STATs in various kinds of cells, we might think about the possibility of the protein interaction between FOXO3 and STATs. Ma et al. reported that FOXO3 or FOXO1 binds to STAT3, leading to negatively regulate specificity protein 1 (SP1)-pro-opiomelanocortin (POMC) promoter complex [91]. In addition, Oh et al. showed that FOXO3 or FOXO1 interacts with STAT3 in the cytoplasm to regulates translocalization of FOXO3 or FOXO1 in CD4(+) T cells leading to control the inflammatory responses [92]. As described in the results section, we successfully showed that JAK2 interacts with FOXO3 to cause tyrosine-phosphorylation of FOXO3. Thus, we should consider what is the detailed relationship between JAK2, STAT3, and FOXO3 in cancer cells. For elucidating this issue, we are trying to investigate which phosphorylation step plays more important in RCC development by performing the protein binding experiments among these proteins.

4. Materials and Methods

4.1. Clear Cell Renal Cell Carcinoma Patients and Tissue Samples

The patients who performed the operation for the clear cell renal cell carcinoma (CCRCC) between July 1998 and August 2011 were evaluated in this study. Original histologic slides, tissue blocks, and medical records were available in 199 cases of CCRCC patients [93]. Clinical information was obtained by reviewing medical records. The histopathologic factors were reevaluated with original histologic slides according to the World Health Organization classification of the renal tumor [94]. Tumor stage was reevaluated according to the eighth edition of the staging system of the American Joint Committee on Cancer [95]. This study obtained institutional review board approval from Chonbuk National University Hospital (IRB No., CUH 2014-05-039-002) and was performed according to the Declaration of Helsinki. The approval contained a waiver for written informed consent based on the retrospective and anonymous character of this study.

4.2. Immunohistochemical Staining and Scoring

Immunohistochemical staining in CCRCC tissue sample for IL4Rα and IL13Rα1 were performed in histologic slides from tissue microarrays with one 3.0 mm cores per case. The tissue microarray core established from the tumor components with the highest histologic grade without any degeneration or necrosis. The paraffin-embedded histologic sections derived from the tissue microarray were deparaffinized, and antigen retrieval was performed by boiling in the microwave oven for 20 min in pH 6.0 antigen retrieval solution (DAKO, Glostrup, Denmark). Anti-IL4Rα (1:100, sc-165974, Santa Cruz Biotechnology, Santa Cruz, CA, USA) and anti-IL13Rα1 (1:100, sc-25849, Santa Cruz Biotechnology) antibodies were used as primary antibodies and visualized with the enzyme substrate 3-amino-9-ethylcarbazole. Scoring for the immunohistochemical staining slides was performed by two pathologists (Kyu Yun Jang and Kyoung Min Kim) with consensus by simultaneously observing in multi-viewing microscope without clinicopathologic information. The immunohistochemical staining score obtained by adding staining intensity point and staining area point. The staining intensity pointed from zero to three (0; no staining, 1; weak, 2; intermediate, 3; strong) and staining area pointed from zero to five (0; no staining, 1; 1%, 2; 2–10%, 3; 11–33%, 4; 34–66%, 5; 67–100%) [93,96,97]. Therefore, the score ranged from zero to eight.

4.3. Cell Culture

A498, ACHN, and 293T cells (ATCC, Manassas, VA, USA) were maintained in Dulbecco's modified Eagle's media (DMEM, Gibco, Waltham, MA, USA) media with 10% fetal bovine serum (FBS, Gibco, Waltham, MA, USA) and 1% streptomycin/penicillin at 37 °C in a humidified incubator containing 5% CO_2 in the air. Both cell lines were used at passages 4–10 for all experiments.

4.4. Chemical Reagents, Antibodies, and Plasmid DNAs

Mouse anti-β-actin, mouse anti-Flag, and mouse anti-HA antibody and the following chemicals and solvents (MG132, cycloheximide, dimethyl sulfoxide (DMSO), glycerol, glycine, sodium chloride, Trizma base, and Tween20) were from Sigma (St. Louis, MO, USA). AZD1480 was from Selleckchem (Houston, TX, USA). Rabbit anti-IL4Rα, rabbit anti-IL13Rα1, mouse anti-PARP1, rabbit anti-FOXO3, mouse anti-Lamin B1, and mouse anti-GAPDH antibodies were from Santa Cruz Biotechnology. Rabbit anti-JAK2, rabbit anti-pJAK2, rabbit anti-Tyr, rabbit anti-cleaved PARP1, rabbit anti-cleaved Caspase3, rabbit anti-Bax, rabbit anti-Bim, rabbit anti-Bcl2, rabbit anti-p21, and rabbit anti-p27 antibodies were from Cell Signaling (Danvers, MA, USA). Goat anti-rabbit (111-035-003) and goat anti-mouse (115-035-003) horseradish peroxidase-conjugated IgG were obtained from Jackson ImmunoResearch (West Grove, PA, USA). Enhanced chemiluminescence (ECL) reagents were obtained from Genedepot (Barker, TX, USA). pECE empty/Flag-FOXO3 and pCMV3-C-HA empty/HA-JAK2 plasmid DNA were from Addgene (Watertown, MA, USA) and Sino Biological (Wayne, PA, USA), respectively.

4.5. Water Soluble Tetrazolium Salts 1 (WST-1) Assay

Cells (1×10^3) were seeded in each well of a 96-well plate and incubated for 18 h at 37 °C in a humidified incubator containing 5% CO_2 in the air. After incubation, cells were treated with DMSO (0.1%) as a control vehicle and the indicated treatment for 24, 48, or 72 h. After incubation, 20 μL of WST-1 solution was added to each well for 4 h. Then, the visible absorbance at 460 nm of each well was quantified using a microplate reader.

4.6. Colony Formation Assay

Cells (5×10^2) were seeded in 6-cm dishes and incubated for 18 h at 37 °C in a humidified incubator containing 5% CO_2 in the air. After incubation, cells were treated with DMSO (0.1%) as a control vehicle or the indicated treatment for 14 days. The colonies were washed twice with PBS, fixed with 3.7% paraformaldehyde, and stained with 1% crystal violet solution in distilled water.

4.7. Western Blotting Analysis

Cells were washed with PBS and lysed in lysis buffer (50 mM Tris-HCl, 150 mM NaCl, 2 mM EDTA, 1% Triton X-100, 0.1% SDS, pH 8.0) with protease and phosphatase inhibitors. Cell lysates were centrifuged (10,000× g, 4 °C, 10 min), and the supernatants were separated on 10% SDS-PAGE gels and blotted onto nitrocellulose membranes (Bio-Rad Laboratories, Hercules, CA, USA). The membranes were blocked in 3% non-fat dry milk for 1 h at room temperature and probed with the appropriate antibodies. Membranes were then probed with HRP-tagged anti-mouse or anti-rabbit IgG antibodies diluted 1:5,000–1:20,000 in 3% non-fat dry milk for 1 h at room temperature. Chemiluminescence was detected using enhanced chemiluminescence (ECL).

4.8. Cytoplasmic and Nuclear Protein Fractionation

Cells were washed with PBS and lysed in cytoplasmic fractional buffer (10 mM HEPES, pH 8.0, 50 mM NaCl, 500 mM sucrose, 1 mM EDTA, 0.5 mM spermidine, 0.15 mM spermine, 0.2% Triton X-100, 1 mM DTT, 2 μM PMSF and 0.15 U/mL aprotinin) at 4 °C for 30 min. Cell lysates were centrifuged (10,000× g, 4 °C, 30 min), and the supernatant was collected for the cytoplasmic fraction. The pellet was washed twice the washing buffer (10 mM HEPES pH 8.0, 50 mM NaCl, 25% glycerol, 0.1 mM EDTA, 0.5 mM spermidine and 0.15 mM spermine) and lysed with nuclear fractional buffer (10 mM HEPES pH 8, 350 mM NaCl, 25% glycerol, 0.1 mM EDTA, 0.5 mM spermidine and 0.15 mM spermine) at 4 °C for 30 min. Lysates were centrifuged (10,000× g, 4 °C, 30 min), and the supernatant was collected for the nuclear fraction.

4.9. Immunofluorescence Analysis

Cells (5×10^5) were seeded in 6-cm dishes and incubated for 18 h at 37 °C in a humidified incubator containing 5% CO_2 in the air. After incubation, cells were treated with DMSO (0.1%) as a control vehicle and the indicated concentration of AZD1480 for 2 h. Cells were fixed with 4% paraformaldehyde solution, permeabilized with Triton X-100 (0.2%), blocked with bovine serum albumin (BSA, Gibco, Waltham, MA, USA) and incubated with a primary antibody against FOXO3 followed by Alexa 594-conjugated anti-mouse secondary antibody (Invitrogen, Carlsbad, CA USA). After counterstaining with DAPI, fluorescence images were captured with a confocal microscope (Zeiss LSM510 microscope, Carl Zeiss, Jena, Germany).

4.10. Immunoprecipitation Analysis

Cells were washed with PBS and lysed in lysis buffer (50 mM Tris-HCl, 150 mM NaCl, 2 mM EDTA, 1% Triton X-100, 0.1% SDS, pH 8.0) with protease and phosphatase inhibitors. Cell lysates were centrifuged (10,000× g, 4 °C, 10 min) and the supernatants were incubated with an antibody by rotating at 4 °C overnight followed by the addition of 20 μL of 50% protein A or G-agarose slurry and rotating for 1 h. Protein A or G-agaroses were collected and washed with lysis buffer. Immunoprecipitants were resolved by 10 or 12% SDS-PAGE and analyzed by Western blotting analysis.

4.11. TUNEL Assay

Cells (5×10^5) were seeded in 6-cm dishes and incubated for 18 h at 37 °C in a humidified incubator containing 5% CO_2 in the air. After incubation, cells were treated with DMSO (0.1%) as a control vehicle (or control siRNA) and the indicated treatment (or siRNA against IL4Rα or IL13Rα1) for 24, 48, or 72 h (or for 48 h). Cells were fixed with 4% paraformaldehyde solution and permeabilized with Triton X-100 (0.2%). Apoptosis was determined by enzymatic labeling of DNA strand breaks with a TUNEL assay kit (DeadEnd Fluorometric TUNEL System, Promega, Madison, WI, USA) according to the manufacturer's instructions. Nuclei were stained with DAPI.

4.12. Annexin V Staining Analysis

Cells (5×10^5) were seeded in 6-cm dishes and incubated for 18 h at 37 °C in a humidified incubator containing 5% CO_2 in the air. After incubation, cells were treated with DMSO (0.1%) as control vehicle (or control siRNA) and the indicated treatment (or siRNA against IL4Rα or IL13Rα1) for 48 h. Cells were washed with PBS, trypsinized, and resuspended in binding buffer. Cells were analyzed by using a FACSCalibur (BD Biosciences, San Jose, CA, USA), and the data were analyzed by FlowJo (De Novo Software, Glendale, CA, USA). Ten thousand events were collected in each run. The percentage of cells that are undergoing apoptosis was determined by using the FITC Annexin V Apoptosis Detection Kit I (BD PharMingen, San Jose, CA, USA) with propidium iodide (PI, Sigma, St. Louis, MO, USA) according to the manufacturer's instructions.

4.13. Cell Cycle Analysis

Cells (5×10^5) were seeded in 6-cm dishes and incubated for 18 h at 37 °C in a humidified incubator containing 5% CO_2 in the air. After incubation, cells were treated with DMSO (0.1%) as control vehicle (or control siRNA) and the indicated treatment (or siRNA against IL4Rα or IL13Rα1) for 48 h. Cells were washed with PBS, trypsinized, and fixed in ice-cold 70% ethanol overnight at −20°C. After fixation, the cells were centrifuged at 1350 rpm for 5 min and incubated with a PI solution for 30 min at 37 °C. Cell cycle distribution analysis was performed using flow cytometry (Beckman Coulter, Brea, CA, USA).

4.14. Transfection of siRNA and Plasmid DNA

Cells (5×10^5) were seeded in 6-cm dishes and incubated for 18 h at 37 °C in a humidified incubator containing 5% CO_2 in the air. After incubation, cells were transfected with siRNAs (control (Cat. No.: sc37007), IL4Rα (Cat. No.: sc-35661), IL13Rα1 (Cat. No.: sc-63337), or JAK2 (Cat. No.: sc-39099), 1 nM (Santa Cruz Biotechnology)) or plasmid DNAs (pECE empty/Flag-FOXO3 or pCMV3-C-HA empty/HA-JAK2 plasmid DNA, 1 μg) to 3 μL of Lipofectamine 2000 (Invitrogen) in 300 μL of serum-free media for 6 h at 37 °C in a humidified incubator containing 5% CO_2 in air. Then cell culture media was replaced with the fresh media containing 10% FBS, and cells were incubated for 18 h.

4.15. Statistical Analysis

The CCRCCs immunostained for IL4Rα and IL13Rα1 were grouped to negative and positive cases according to their expression with receiver operating characteristic curve analysis [93,97,98]. The cutoff points of IL4Rα and IL13Rα1 immunohistochemical staining were determined at the highest area under the curve to predict cancer-specific death of CCRCC patients. This study evaluated for cancer-specific survival (CSS) and relapse-free survival (RFS) of CCRCC patients through December 2012. The duration for CSS was calculated as the time from the date of diagnosis to the date of death from CCRCC or last contact. The death from CCRCC was considered an event for CCS analysis.

The death from other causes or alive of patients at last contact were treated as censored for CSS analysis. The duration for RFS was calculated as the time from the date of diagnosis to the date of relapse or death from CCRCC, or last contact. The relapse of CCRCC or death from CCRCC was an event in the RFS analysis. The patients who died from other causes or who were alive without relapse at last contact were treated as censored for RFS analysis. The prognostic significance of various clinicopathological factors in CCRCC patients was evaluated by univariate and multivariate Cox proportional hazards regression analyses, and Kaplan-Meier survival analysis. The associations between clinicopathologic factors and the expression of IL4Rα and IL13Rα1 were analyzed by Pearson's chi-square test. Data are expressed as the mean ± standard error (STE) of three independent experiments. Differences between groups were analyzed with one-way ANOVA when the variances were equal. SPSS software (version 20.0, IBM, palo alto, CA, USA) was used throughout. All statistical tests were two-sided, and p-values less than 0.05 were considered statistically significant.

5. Conclusions

Collectively, we investigated a biochemical mechanism to explain the relationship between IL4Rα and IL13Rα1 expressions, as well as the shorter survival see in CCRCC patients [99]. We demonstrated that IL4Rα and IL13Rα1 are associated with the proliferation of RCC cells and the protein stability of FOXO3 via JAK2. We showed a novel signaling pathway underlying the ubiquitination mediated degradation of FOXO3 protein depending on its tyrosine phosphorylation by JAK2, leading to contribute to RCC development. To the best of our knowledge, this is the first report that JAK2 is shown to regulate FOXO3 protein stability. Based on our findings, we proposed a schematic model for a novel role of JAK2 under IL4Rα and IL13Rα1 in regulating FOXO3 protein degradation and promoting RCC tumorigenesis (Figure 6). Our findings imply that IL4Rα and IL13Rα1 as a new prognostic marker. Further, the study implies that JAK2/FOXO3 are new therapeutic targets against RCC. Our findings support the notion that a unique oncogenic JAK2 mediates the degradation of FOXO3 protein and contributes to an understanding of the control of FOXO3 protein in the tumor.

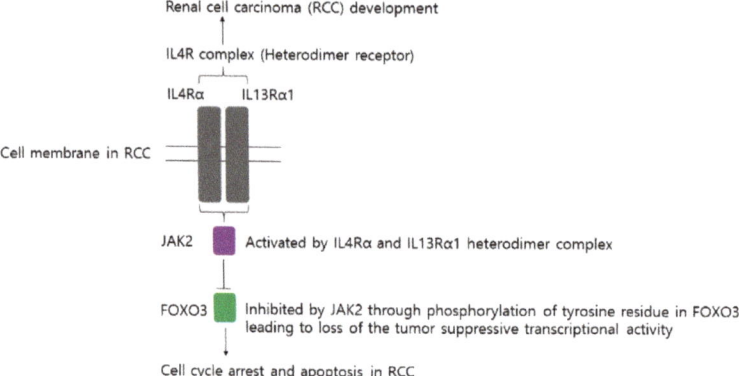

Figure 6. A diagram describes the role of IL4R complex (a heterodimeric complex of IL4Rα and IL13Rα1) in promoting RCC tumorigenesis via phosphorylation of tyrosine residue in FOXO3 by activation of JAK2 leading to loss of the tumor-suppressive transcriptional activity.

Supplementary Materials: The following are available online at http://www.mdpi.com/2072-6694/11/9/1394/s1, Figure S1: Higher expression of mRNA of both IL4Rα and IL13Rα1 are associated with shorter survival of clear cell renal cell carcinoma patients, Figure S2: Western blot analysis of IL4Rα expression in RCC cell lines, Figure S3: Anti-cancer effect by transfection of siRNA against JAK2 in A498 and ACHN cells. Figure S4: Western blot and densitometry analysis.

Author Contributions: M.-A.K., J.L., S.H.H., C.M.L., K.M.K., K.Y.J. and S.-H.P. conceived the presented idea, carried out the experiments, and wrote the manuscript. M.-A.K., J.L., S.H.H., C.M.L., K.M.K., K.Y.J. and S.-H.P. contributed to analysis and interpretation of the results. M.-A.K., J.L., S.H.H., C.M.L., K.M.K., K.Y.J. and S.-H.P. provided critical feedback, discussed the results, and contributed to writing the first draft and final manuscript. S.H.P sponsored the article processing charge.

Funding: This research was supported by the Basic Science Research Program (NRF-2014R1A6A3A04054307) through the National Research Foundation of Korea (NRF) funded by the Ministry of Science and ICT (MSIP). This research was supported by the Medical Research Center Program (NRF-2017R1A5A2015061) through the National Research Foundation of Korea (NRF) funded by the Ministry of Science and ICT (MSIP).

Acknowledgments: The authors appreciate other laboratory members for supporting this study.

Conflicts of Interest: The authors declare no conflict of interest. The funders had no role in the design of the study; in the collection, analyses, or interpretation of data; in the writing of the manuscript, or in the decision to publish the results.

References

1. Siegel, R.L.; Miller, K.D.; Jemal, A. Cancer statistics, 2018. *CA Cancer J. Clin.* **2018**, *68*, 7–30. [CrossRef]
2. Moch, H.; Gasser, T.; Amin, M.B.; Torhorst, J.; Sauter, G.; Mihatsch, M.J. Prognostic utility of the recently recommended histologic classification and revised TNM staging system of renal cell carcinoma: A Swiss experience with 588 tumors. *Cancer* **2000**, *89*, 604–614. [CrossRef]
3. Leibovich, B.C.; Lohse, C.M.; Crispen, P.L.; Boorjian, S.A.; Thompson, R.H.; Blute, M.L.; Cheville, J.C. Histological subtype is an independent predictor of outcome for patients with renal cell carcinoma. *J. Urol.* **2010**, *183*, 1309–1315. [CrossRef] [PubMed]
4. Wersall, P.J.; Blomgren, H.; Lax, I.; Kalkner, K.M.; Linder, C.; Lundell, G.; Nilsson, B.; Nilsson, S.; Naslund, I.; Pisa, P.; et al. Extracranial stereotactic radiotherapy for primary and metastatic renal cell carcinoma. *Radiother. Oncol.* **2005**, *77*, 88–95. [CrossRef] [PubMed]
5. Ljungberg, B.; Campbell, S.C.; Choi, H.Y.; Jacqmin, D.; Lee, J.E.; Weikert, S.; Kiemeney, L.A. The epidemiology of renal cell carcinoma. *Eur. Urol.* **2011**, *60*, 615–621. [CrossRef] [PubMed]
6. Escudier, B.; Szczylik, C.; Porta, C.; Gore, M. Treatment selection in metastatic renal cell carcinoma: Expert consensus. *Nat. Rev. Clin. Oncol.* **2012**, *9*, 327–337. [CrossRef] [PubMed]
7. Vignali, D.; Monti, P. Targeting homeostatic T cell proliferation to control beta-cell autoimmunity. *Curr. Diab. Rep.* **2016**, *16*, 40. [CrossRef] [PubMed]
8. Dinarello, C.A.; Mier, J.W. Interleukins. *Annu. Rev. Med.* **1986**, *37*, 173–178. [CrossRef] [PubMed]
9. Rosser, E.C.; Mauri, C. Regulatory B cells: Origin, phenotype, and function. *Immunity* **2015**, *42*, 607–612. [CrossRef] [PubMed]
10. McCormick, S.M.; Heller, N.M. Commentary: IL-4 and IL-13 receptors and signaling. *Cytokine* **2015**, *75*, 38–50. [CrossRef] [PubMed]
11. Vadevoo, S.M.P.; Kim, J.E.; Gunassekaran, G.R.; Jung, H.K.; Chi, L.; Kim, D.E.; Lee, S.H.; Im, S.H.; Lee, B. IL4 Receptor-Targeted Proapoptotic Peptide Blocks Tumor Growth and Metastasis by Enhancing Antitumor Immunity. *Mol. Cancer Ther.* **2017**, *16*, 2803–2816. [CrossRef] [PubMed]
12. LaPorte, S.L.; Juo, Z.S.; Vaclavikova, J.; Colf, L.A.; Qi, X.; Heller, N.M.; Keegan, A.D.; Garcia, K.C. Molecular and structural basis of cytokine receptor pleiotropy in the interleukin-4/13 system. *Cell* **2008**, *132*, 259–272. [CrossRef] [PubMed]
13. Hershey, G.K. IL-13 receptors and signaling pathways: An evolving web. *J. Allergy Clin. Immunol.* **2003**, *111*, 677–690. [CrossRef] [PubMed]
14. Suzuki, A.; Leland, P.; Joshi, B.H.; Puri, R.K. Targeting of IL-4 and IL-13 receptors for cancer therapy. *Cytokine* **2015**, *75*, 79–88. [CrossRef] [PubMed]
15. Todaro, M.; Perez Alea, M.; Scopelliti, A.; Medema, J.P.; Stassi, G. IL-4-mediated drug resistance in colon cancer stem cells. *Cell Cycle* **2008**, *7*, 309–313. [CrossRef] [PubMed]
16. Joshi, B.H.; Leland, P.; Lababidi, S.; Varrichio, F.; Puri, R.K. Interleukin-4 receptor alpha overexpression in human bladder cancer correlates with the pathological grade and stage of the disease. *Cancer Med.* **2014**, *3*, 1615–1628. [CrossRef] [PubMed]

17. Prokopchuk, O.; Liu, Y.; Henne-Bruns, D.; Kornmann, M. Interleukin-4 enhances proliferation of human pancreatic cancer cells: evidence for autocrine and paracrine actions. *Br. J. Cancer* **2005**, *92*, 921–928. [CrossRef]
18. Park, M.H.; Kwon, H.J.; Kim, J.R.; Lee, B.; Lee, S.J.; Bae, Y.K. Elevated Interleukin-13 Receptor Alpha 1 Expression in Tumor Cells Is Associated with Poor Prognosis in Patients with Invasive Breast Cancer. *Ann. Surg. Oncol.* **2017**, *24*, 3780–3787. [CrossRef]
19. Puri, S.; Joshi, B.H.; Sarkar, C.; Mahapatra, A.K.; Hussain, E.; Sinha, S. Expression and structure of interleukin 4 receptors in primary meningeal tumors. *Cancer* **2005**, *103*, 2132–2142. [CrossRef]
20. Malek, E.; de Lima, M.; Letterio, J.J.; Kim, B.G.; Finke, J.H.; Driscoll, J.J.; Giralt, S.A. Myeloid-derived suppressor cells: The green light for myeloma immune escape. *Blood Rev.* **2016**, *30*, 341–348. [CrossRef]
21. Wang, H.W.; Joyce, J.A. Alternative activation of tumor-associated macrophages by IL-4: priming for protumoral functions. *Cell Cycle* **2010**, *9*, 4824–4835. [CrossRef] [PubMed]
22. Ostrand-Rosenberg, S. Immune surveillance: A balance between protumor and antitumor immunity. *Curr. Opin. Genet. Dev.* **2008**, *18*, 11–18. [CrossRef] [PubMed]
23. Cho, Y.A.; Kim, J. Association of IL4, IL13, and IL4R polymorphisms with gastrointestinal cancer risk: A meta-analysis. *J. Epidemiol.* **2017**, *27*, 215–220. [CrossRef] [PubMed]
24. Landi, S.; Bottari, F.; Gemignani, F.; Gioia-Patricola, L.; Guino, E.; Osorio, A.; de Oca, J.; Capella, G.; Canzian, F.; Moreno, V.; et al. Interleukin-4 and interleukin-4 receptor polymorphisms and colorectal cancer risk. *Eur. J. Cancer* **2007**, *43*, 762–768. [CrossRef]
25. Bankaitis, K.V.; Fingleton, B. Targeting IL4/IL4R for the treatment of epithelial cancer metastasis. *Clin. Exp. Metastasis* **2015**, *32*, 847–856. [CrossRef] [PubMed]
26. Izuhara, K.; Harada, N. Interleukin-4 activates two distinct pathways of phosphatidylinositol-3 kinase in the same cells. *Biochem. Biophys. Res. Commun.* **1996**, *229*, 624–629. [CrossRef] [PubMed]
27. Ruckerl, D.; Jenkins, S.J.; Laqtom, N.N.; Gallagher, I.J.; Sutherland, T.E.; Duncan, S.; Buck, A.H.; Allen, J.F. Induction of IL-4Ralpha-dependent microRNAs identifies PI3K/Akt signaling as essential for IL-4-driven murine macrophage proliferation in vivo. *Blood* **2012**, *120*, 2307–2316. [CrossRef] [PubMed]
28. Mukthavaram, R.; Ouyang, X.; Saklecha, R.; Jiang, P.; Nomura, N.; Pingle, S.C.; Guo, F.; Makale, M.; Kesari, S. Effect of the JAK2/STAT3 inhibitor SAR317461 on human glioblastoma tumorspheres. *J. Transl. Med.* **2015**, *13*, 269. [CrossRef] [PubMed]
29. Wu, L.; Guo, L.; Liang, Y.; Liu, X.; Jiang, L.; Wang, L. Curcumin suppresses stem-like traits of lung cancer cells via inhibiting the JAK2/STAT3 signaling pathway. *Oncol. Rep.* **2015**, *34*, 3311–3317. [CrossRef]
30. Liu, Y.F.; Lu, Y.M.; Qu, G.Q.; Liu, Y.; Chen, W.X.; Liao, X.H.; Kong, W.M. Ponicidin induces apoptosis via JAK2 and STAT3 signaling pathways in gastric carcinoma. *Int. J. Mol. Sci.* **2015**, *16*, 1576–1589. [CrossRef]
31. Jorvig, J.E.; Chakraborty, A. Zerumbone inhibits growth of hormone refractory prostate cancer cells by inhibiting JAK2/STAT3 pathway and increases paclitaxel sensitivity. *Anticancer Drugs* **2015**, *26*, 160–166. [CrossRef] [PubMed]
32. Du, W.W.; Yang, W.; Chen, Y.; Wu, Z.K.; Foster, F.S.; Yang, Z.; Li, X.; Yang, B.B. Foxo3 circular RNA promotes cardiac senescence by modulating multiple factors associated with stress and senescence responses. *Eur. Heart J.* **2017**, *38*, 1402–1412. [CrossRef] [PubMed]
33. Hagenbuchner, J.; Lungkofler, L.; Kiechl-Kohlendorfer, U.; Viola, G.; Ferlin, M.G.; Ausserlechner, M.J.; Obexer, P. The tubulin inhibitor MG-2477 induces autophagy-regulated cell death, ROS accumulation and activation of FOXO3 in neuroblastoma. *Oncotarget* **2017**, *8*, 32009–32026. [CrossRef] [PubMed]
34. Kumazoe, M.; Takai, M.; Bae, J.; Hiroi, S.; Huang, Y.; Takamatsu, K.; Won, Y.; Yamashita, M.; Hidaka, S.; Yamashita, S.; et al. FOXO3 is essential for CD44 expression in pancreatic cancer cells. *Oncogene* **2017**, *36*, 2643–2654. [CrossRef] [PubMed]
35. Kumazoe, M.; Takai, M.; Hiroi, S.; Takeuchi, C.; Kadomatsu, M.; Nojiri, T.; Onda, H.; Bae, J.; Huang, Y.; Takamatsu, K.; et al. The FOXO3/PGC-1beta signaling axis is essential for cancer stem cell properties of pancreatic ductal adenocarcinoma. *J. Biol. Chem.* **2017**, *292*, 10813–10823. [CrossRef] [PubMed]
36. Coomans de Brachene, A.; Demoulin, J.B. FOXO transcription factors in cancer development and therapy. *Cell Mol. Life Sci.* **2016**, *73*, 1159–1172. [CrossRef] [PubMed]
37. Liang, R.; Ghaffari, S. Mitochondria and FOXO3 in stem cell homeostasis, a window into hematopoietic stem cell fate determination. *J. Bioenerg. Biomembr.* **2017**, *49*, 343–346. [CrossRef] [PubMed]

38. Natarajan, S.K.; Stringham, B.A.; Mohr, A.M.; Wehrkamp, C.J.; Lu, S.; Phillippi, M.A.; Harrison-Findik, D.; Mott, J.L. FoxO3 increases miR-34a to cause palmitate-induced cholangiocyte lipoapoptosis. *J. Lipid Res.* **2017**, *58*, 866–875. [CrossRef] [PubMed]
39. Peng, X.L.; So, K.K.; He, L.; Zhao, Y.; Zhou, J.; Li, Y.; Yao, M.; Xu, B.; Zhang, S.; Yao, H.; et al. MyoD- and FoxO3-mediated hotspot interaction orchestrates super-enhancer activity during myogenic differentiation. *Nucleic Acids Res.* **2017**, *45*, 8785–8805. [CrossRef] [PubMed]
40. Sang, T.; Cao, Q.; Wang, Y.; Liu, F.; Chen, S. Overexpression or silencing of FOXO3a affects proliferation of endothelial progenitor cells and expression of cell cycle regulatory proteins. *PLoS ONE* **2014**, *9*, e101703. [CrossRef] [PubMed]
41. Sunters, A.; Fernandez de Mattos, S.; Stahl, M.; Brosens, J.J.; Zoumpoulidou, G.; Saunders, C.A.; Coffer, P.J.; Medema, R.H.; Coombes, R.C.; Lam, E.W. FoxO3a transcriptional regulation of Bim controls apoptosis in paclitaxel-treated breast cancer cell lines. *J. Biol. Chem.* **2003**, *278*, 49795–49805. [CrossRef] [PubMed]
42. Park, S.H.; Chung, Y.M.; Ma, J.; Yang, Q.; Berek, J.S.; Hu, M.C. Pharmacological activation of FOXO3 suppresses triple-negative breast cancer in vitro and in vivo. *Oncotarget* **2016**, *7*, 42110–42125. [CrossRef] [PubMed]
43. Salcher, S.; Hagenbuchner, J.; Geiger, K.; Seiter, M.A.; Rainer, J.; Kofler, R.; Hermann, M.; Kiechl-Kohlendorfer, U.; Ausserlechner, M.J.; Obexer, P. C10ORF10/DEPP, a transcriptional target of FOXO3, regulates ROS-sensitivity in human neuroblastoma. *Mol. Cancer* **2014**, *13*, 224. [CrossRef] [PubMed]
44. Song, D.; Ma, J.; Chen, L.; Guo, C.; Zhang, Y.; Chen, T.; Zhang, S.; Zhu, Z.; Tian, L.; Niu, P. FOXO3 promoted mitophagy via nuclear retention induced by manganese chloride in SH-SY5Y cells. *Metallomics* **2017**, *9*, 1251–1259. [CrossRef] [PubMed]
45. Ni, D.; Ma, X.; Li, H.Z.; Gao, Y.; Li, X.T.; Zhang, Y.; Ai, Q.; Zhang, P.; Song, E.L.; Huang, Q.B.; et al. Downregulation of FOXO3a promotes tumor metastasis and is associated with metastasis-free survival of patients with clear cell renal cell carcinoma. *Clin. Cancer Res.* **2014**, *20*, 1779–1790. [CrossRef] [PubMed]
46. Greer, E.L.; Brunet, A. FOXO transcription factors at the interface between longevity and tumor suppression. *Oncogene* **2005**, *24*, 7410–7425. [CrossRef]
47. Vogt, P.K.; Jiang, H.; Aoki, M. Triple layer control: Phosphorylation, acetylation and ubiquitination of FOXO proteins. *Cell Cycle* **2005**, *4*, 908–913. [CrossRef]
48. Fu, Z.; Tindall, D.J. FOXOs, cancer and regulation of apoptosis. *Oncogene* **2008**, *27*, 2312–2319. [CrossRef]
49. Guo, L.; Hu-Li, J.; Paul, W.E. Probabilistic Regulation in TH2 Cells Accounts for Monoallelic Expression of IL-4 and IL-13. *Immunity* **2005**, *23*, 89–99. [CrossRef]
50. Junttila, I.S. Tuning the Cytokine Responses: An Update on Interleukin (IL)-4 and IL-13 Receptor Complexes. *Front. Immunol.* **2018**, *9*. [CrossRef]
51. Aversa, G.; Punnonen, J.; Cocks, B.G.; de Waal Malefyt, R.; Vega, F.; Zurawski, S.M.; Zurawski, G.; de Vries, J.E. An interleukin 4 (IL-4) mutant protein inhibits both IL-4 or IL-13-induced human immunoglobulin G4 (IgG4) and IgE synthesis and B cell proliferation: support for a common component shared by IL-4 and IL-13 receptors. *J. Exp. Med.* **1993**, *178*, 2213. [CrossRef] [PubMed]
52. Lee, H.L.; Park, M.H.; Song, J.K.; Jung, Y.Y.; Kim, Y.; Kim, K.B.; Hwang, D.Y.; Yoon, D.Y.; Song, M.J.; Han, S.B.; et al. Tumor growth suppressive effect of IL-4 through p21-mediated activation of STAT6 in IL-4Rα overexpressed melanoma models. *Oncotarget* **2016**, *7*, 23425–23438. [CrossRef] [PubMed]
53. Hallett, M.A.; Venmar, K.T.; Fingleton, B. Cytokine stimulation of epithelial cancer cells: The similar and divergent functions of IL-4 and IL-13. *Cancer Res.* **2012**, *72*, 6338–6343. [CrossRef] [PubMed]
54. Mueller, T.D.; Zhang, J.-L.; Sebald, W.; Duschl, A. Structure, binding, and antagonists in the IL-4/IL-13 receptor system. *BBA.-Mol. Cell Res.* **2002**, *1592*, 237–250. [CrossRef]
55. Umeshita-Suyama, R.; Sugimoto, R.; Akaiwa, M.; Arima, K.; Yu, B.; Wada, M.; Kuwano, M.; Nakajima, K.; Hamasaki, N.; Izuhara, K. Characterization of IL-4 and IL-13 signals dependent on the human IL-13 receptor α chain 1: redundancy of requirement of tyrosine residue for STAT3 activation. *Int. Immunol.* **2000**, *12*, 1499–1509. [CrossRef]
56. Venmar, K.T.; Carter, K.J.; Hwang, D.G.; Dozier, E.A.; Fingleton, B. IL4 receptor ILR4alpha regulates metastatic colonization by mammary tumors through multiple signaling pathways. *Cancer Res.* **2014**, *74*, 4329–4340. [CrossRef] [PubMed]
57. Koller, F.L.; Hwang, D.G.; Dozier, E.A.; Fingleton, B. Epithelial interleukin-4 receptor expression promotes colon tumor growth. *Carcinogenesis* **2010**, *31*, 1010–1017. [CrossRef]

58. Olson, S.H.; Orlow, I.; Simon, J.; Tommasi, D.; Roy, P.; Bayuga, S.; Ludwig, E.; Zauber, A.G.; Kurtz, R.C. Allergies, variants in IL-4 and IL-4Rα genes, and risk of pancreatic cancer. *Cancer Detect. Prev.* **2007**, *31*, 345–351. [CrossRef]
59. Venmar, K.T.; Fingleton, B. Lessons from immunology: IL4R directly promotes mammary tumor metastasis. *Oncoimmunology* **2014**, *3*, e955373. [CrossRef]
60. Kawakami, K.; Kawakami, M.; Joshi, B.H.; Puri, R.K. Interleukin-13 receptor-targeted cancer therapy in an immunodeficient animal model of human head and neck cancer. *Cancer Res.* **2001**, *61*, 6194–6200.
61. Shaik, A.P.; Shaik, A.S.; Majwal, A.A.; Faraj, A.A. Blocking interleukin-4 receptor α using polyethylene glycol functionalized superparamagnetic iron oxide nanocarriers to inhibit breast cancer cell proliferation. *Cancer Res. Treat.* **2017**, *49*, 322–329. [CrossRef] [PubMed]
62. Todaro, M.; Lombardo, Y.; Francipane, M.G.; Alea, M.P.; Cammareri, P.; Iovino, F.; Di Stefano, A.B.; Di Bernardo, C.; Agrusa, A.; Condorelli, G.; et al. Apoptosis resistance in epithelial tumors is mediated by tumor-cell-derived interleukin-4. *Cell Death Diff.* **2008**, *15*, 762–772. [CrossRef] [PubMed]
63. Roth, F.; De La Fuente, A.C.; Vella, J.L.; Zoso, A.; Inverardi, L.; Serafini, P. Aptamer-mediated blockade of IL4Ralpha triggers apoptosis of MDSCs and limits tumor progression. *Cancer Res.* **2012**, *72*, 1373–1383. [CrossRef] [PubMed]
64. Joshi, B.H.; Suzuki, A.; Fujisawa, T.; Leland, P.; Varrichio, F.; Lababidi, S.; Lloyd, R.; Kasperbauer, J.; Puri, R.K. Identification, characterization, and targeting of IL-4 receptor by IL-4-Pseudomonas exotoxin in mouse models of anaplastic thyroid cancer. *Discov. Med.* **2015**, *20*, 273–284. [PubMed]
65. Guo, C.; Ouyang, Y.; Cai, J.; Xiong, L.; Chen, Y.; Zeng, X.; Liu, A. High expression of IL-4R enhances proliferation and invasion of hepatocellular carcinoma cells. *Int. J. Biol. Markers* **2017**, *32*, 384–390. [CrossRef] [PubMed]
66. Park, S.H.; Yoon, Y.I.; Moon, H.; Lee, G.H.; Lee, B.H.; Yoon, T.J.; Lee, H.J. Development of a novel microbubble-liposome complex conjugated with peptide ligands targeting IL4R on brain tumor cells. *Oncol. Rep.* **2016**, *36*, 131–136. [CrossRef] [PubMed]
67. Kisseleva, T.; Bhattacharya, S.; Braunstein, J.; Schindler, C.W. Signaling through the JAK/STAT pathway, recent advances and future challenges. *Gene* **2002**, *285*, 1–24. [CrossRef]
68. Brooks, A.J.; Dai, W.; O'Mara, M.L.; Abankwa, D.; Chhabra, Y.; Pelekanos, R.A.; Gardon, O.; Tunny, K.A.; Blucher, K.M.; Morton, C.J.; et al. Mechanism of activation of protein kinase JAK2 by the growth hormone receptor. *Science* **2014**, *344*, 1249783. [CrossRef] [PubMed]
69. Wernig, G.; Kharas, M.G.; Okabe, R.; Moore, S.A.; Leeman, D.S.; Cullen, D.E.; Gozo, M.; McDowell, E.P.; Levine, R.L.; Doukas, J.; et al. Efficacy of TG101348, a selective JAK2 inhibitor, in treatment of a murine model of JAK2V617F-induced polycythemia vera. *Cancer Cell* **2008**, *13*, 311–320. [CrossRef] [PubMed]
70. Carobbio, A.; Finazzi, G.; Guerini, V.; Spinelli, O.; Delaini, F.; Marchioli, R.; Borrelli, G.; Rambaldi, A.; Barbui, T. Leukocytosis is a risk factor for thrombosis in essential thrombocythemia: interaction with treatment, standard risk factors, and Jak2 mutation status. *Blood* **2007**, *109*, 2310–2313. [CrossRef]
71. Tibes, R.; Bogenberger, J.M.; Geyer, H.L.; Mesa, R.A. JAK2 inhibitors in the treatment of myeloproliferative neoplasms. *Expert. Opin. Investig. Drugs* **2012**, *21*, 1755–1774. [CrossRef]
72. LaFave, L.M.; Levine, R.L. JAK2 the future: Therapeutic strategies for JAK-dependent malignancies. *Trends Pharmacol. Sci.* **2012**, *33*, 574–582. [CrossRef]
73. Mesa, R.A.; Yasothan, U.; Kirkpatrick, P. Ruxolitinib. *Nat. Rev. Drug Discov.* **2012**, *11*, 103. [CrossRef]
74. Wu, P.; Nielsen, T.E.; Clausen, M.H. FDA-approved small-molecule kinase inhibitors. *Trends Pharmacol. Sci.* **2015**, *36*, 422–439. [CrossRef]
75. Mascarenhas, J.; Hoffman, R. Ruxolitinib: The first FDA approved therapy for the treatment of myelofibrosis. *Clin. Cancer Res.* **2012**, *18*, 3008–3014. [CrossRef]
76. Menghrajani, K.; Boonstra, P.S.; Mercer, J.A.; Perkins, C.; Gowin, K.L.; Weber, A.A.; Mesa, R.; Gotlib, J.R.; Wang, L.; Singer, J.W.; et al. Predictive models for splenic response to JAK-inhibitor therapy in patients with myelofibrosis. *Leuk. Lymphoma* **2019**, *60*, 1036–1042. [CrossRef]
77. Rawlings, J.S.; Rosler, K.M.; Harrison, D.A. The JAK/STAT signaling pathway. *J. Cell Sci.* **2004**, *117*, 1281–1283. [CrossRef]

78. Marotta, L.L.; Almendro, V.; Marusyk, A.; Shipitsin, M.; Schemme, J.; Walker, S.R.; Bloushtain-Qimron, N.; Kim, J.J.; Choudhury, S.A.; Maruyama, R.; et al. The JAK2/STAT3 signaling pathway is required for growth of CD44(+)CD24(-) stem cell-like breast cancer cells in human tumors. *J. Clin. Investig.* **2011**, *121*, 2723–2735. [CrossRef]
79. Yoshikawa, T.; Miyamoto, M.; Aoyama, T.; Soyama, H.; Goto, T.; Hirata, J.; Suzuki, A.; Nagaoka, I.; Tsuda, H.; Furuya, K.; et al. JAK2/STAT3 pathway as a therapeutic target in ovarian cancers. *Oncol. Lett.* **2018**, *15*, 5772–5780. [CrossRef]
80. Kim, B.I.; Kim, J.H.; Sim, D.Y.; Nam, M.; Jung, J.H.; Shim, B.; Lee, J.; Kim, S.H. Inhibition of JAK2/STAT3 and activation of caspase9/3 are involved in KYS05090Sinduced apoptosis in ovarian cancer cells. *Int. J. Oncol.* **2019**, *55*, 203–210. [CrossRef]
81. Judd, L.M.; Menheniott, T.R.; Ling, H.; Jackson, C.B.; Howlett, M.; Kalantzis, A.; Priebe, W.; Giraud, A.S. Inhibition of the JAK2/STAT3 pathway reduces gastric cancer growth in vitro and in vivo. *PLoS ONE* **2014**, *9*, e95993. [CrossRef]
82. Wei, X.; Yu, L.; Li, Y. PBX1 promotes the cell proliferation via JAK2/STAT3 signaling in clear cell renal carcinoma. *Biochem. Biophys. Res. Commun.* **2018**, *500*, 650–657. [CrossRef]
83. Xin, H.; Herrmann, A.; Reckamp, K.; Zhang, W.; Pal, S.; Hedvat, M.; Zhang, C.; Liang, W.; Scuto, A.; Weng, S.; et al. Antiangiogenic and antimetastatic activity of JAK inhibitor AZD1480. *Cancer Res.* **2011**, *71*, 6601–6610. [CrossRef]
84. Li, S.; Priceman, S.J.; Xin, H.; Zhang, W.; Deng, J.; Liu, Y.; Huang, J.; Zhu, W.; Chen, M.; Hu, W.; et al. Icaritin inhibits JAK/STAT3 signaling and growth of renal cell carcinoma. *PLoS ONE* **2013**, *8*, e81657. [CrossRef]
85. Myatt, S.S.; Lam, E.W. The emerging roles of forkhead box (Fox) proteins in cancer. *Nat. Rev. Cancer* **2007**, *7*, 847–859. [CrossRef]
86. Cho, E.C.; Kuo, M.L.; Liu, X.; Yang, L.; Hsieh, Y.C.; Wang, J.; Cheng, Y.; Yen, Y. Tumor suppressor FOXO3 regulates ribonucleotide reductase subunit RRM2B and impacts on survival of cancer patients. *Oncotarget* **2014**, *5*, 4834–4844. [CrossRef]
87. Wu, C.; Jin, B.; Chen, L.; Zhuo, D.; Zhang, Z.; Gong, K.; Mao, Z. MiR-30d induces apoptosis and is regulated by the Akt/FOXO pathway in renal cell carcinoma. *Cell Signal* **2013**, *25*, 1212–1221. [CrossRef]
88. Hu, M.C.; Lee, D.F.; Xia, W.; Golfman, L.S.; Ou-Yang, F.; Yang, J.Y.; Zou, Y.; Bao, S.; Hanada, N.; Saso, H.; et al. IkappaB kinase promotes tumorigenesis through inhibition of forkhead FOXO3a. *Cell* **2004**, *117*, 225–237. [CrossRef]
89. Bulow, M.H.; Bulow, T.R.; Hoch, M.; Pankratz, M.J.; Junger, M.A. Src tyrosine kinase signaling antagonizes nuclear localization of FOXO and inhibits its transcription factor activity. *Sci. Rep.* **2014**, *4*, 4048. [CrossRef]
90. Ahn, J.S.; Li, J.; Chen, E.; Kent, D.G.; Park, H.J.; Green, A.R. JAK2V617F mediates resistance to DNA damage-induced apoptosis by modulating FOXO3A localization and Bcl-xL deamidation. *Oncogene* **2016**, *35*, 2235–2246. [CrossRef]
91. Ma, W.; Fuentes, G.; Shi, X.; Verma, C.; Radda, G.K.; Han, W. FoxO1 negatively regulates leptin-induced POMC transcription through its direct interaction with STAT3. *Biochem. J.* **2015**, *466*, 291–298. [CrossRef]
92. Oh, H.M.; Yu, C.R.; Dambuza, I.; Marrero, B.; Egwuagu, C.E. STAT3 protein interacts with Class O Forkhead transcription factors in the cytoplasm and regulates nuclear/cytoplasmic localization of FoxO1 and FoxO3a proteins in CD4(+) T cells. *J. Biol. Chem.* **2012**, *287*, 30436–30443. [CrossRef]
93. Kim, K.M.; Hussein, U.K.; Bae, J.S.; Park, S.H.; Kwon, K.S.; Ha, S.H.; Park, H.S.; Lee, H.; Chung, M.J.; Moon, W.S.; et al. The expression patterns of FAM83H and PANX2 are associated with shorter survival of clear cell renal cell carcinoma patients. *Front. Oncol.* **2019**, *9*, 14. [CrossRef]
94. Moch, H.; Humphrey, P.A.; Ulbright, T.M. *Who Classification of Tumours of the Urinaryt System and Male Genital Organs*, 4th ed.; World Health Organization: Washington, DC, USA, 2016.
95. Amin, M.B.; Edge, S.B.; Gress, D.M.; Meyer, L.R. *AJCC Cancer Staging Manual*, 8th ed.; American Joint Committee on Cancer, Springer: Chicago, IL, USA, 2017; p. e1024.
96. Allred, D.; Harvey, J.M.; Berardo, M.; Clark, G.M. Prognostic and predictive factors in breast cancer by immunohistochemical analysis. *Mod. Pathol.* **1998**, *11*, 155–168.
97. Kim, K.M.; Hussein, U.K.; Park, S.H.; Kang, M.A.; Moon, Y.J.; Zhang, Z.; Song, Y.; Park, H.S.; Bae, J.S.; Park, B.H.; et al. FAM83H is involved in stabilization of beta-catenin and progression of osteosarcomas. *J. Exp. Clin. Cancer Res.* **2019**, *38*, 267. [CrossRef]

98. Park, H.J.; Bae, J.S.; Kim, K.M.; Moon, Y.J.; Park, S.H.; Ha, S.H.; Hussein, U.K.; Zhang, Z.; Park, H.S.; Park, B.H.; et al. The PARP inhibitor olaparib potentiates the effect of the DNA damaging agent doxorubicin in osteosarcoma. *J. Exp. Clin. Cancer Res.* **2018**, *37*, 107. [CrossRef]
99. Anaya, J. OncoLnc: Linking TCGA survival data to mRNAs, miRNAs, and lncRNAs. *PeerJ Comp. Sci.* **2016**, *2*, e67. [CrossRef]

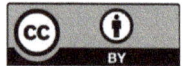

© 2019 by the authors. Licensee MDPI, Basel, Switzerland. This article is an open access article distributed under the terms and conditions of the Creative Commons Attribution (CC BY) license (http://creativecommons.org/licenses/by/4.0/).

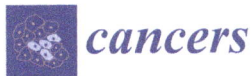

Article

Papillary Renal Cell Carcinomas Rewire Glutathione Metabolism and Are Deficient in Both Anabolic Glucose Synthesis and Oxidative Phosphorylation

Ayham Al Ahmad [1,2,3], Vanessa Paffrath [1,3], Rosanna Clima [4,5], Jonas Felix Busch [6], Anja Rabien [6], Ergin Kilic [7,8], Sonia Villegas [8], Bernd Timmermann [9], Marcella Attimonelli [4], Klaus Jung [3,6] and David Meierhofer [1,*]

1. Max Planck Institute for Molecular Genetics, Mass Spectrometry Facility, Ihnestrasse 63-73, 14195 Berlin, Germany
2. Fachbereich Biologie, Chemie, Pharmazie, Freie Universität Berlin, Takustraße 3, 14195 Berlin, Germany
3. Berlin Institute for Urologic Research, Charitéplatz 1, 10117 Berlin, Germany
4. Department of Biosciences, Biotechnology and Biopharmaceutics, University of Bari, Via E.Orabona, 470126 Bari, Italy
5. Department of Medical and Surgical Sciences-DIMEC, Medical Genetics Unit, University of Bologna, 40126 Bologna, Italy
6. Department of Urology, Charité—Universitätsmedizin Berlin, corporate member of Freie Universität Berlin, Humboldt-Universität zu Berlin, and Berlin Institute of Health, 10117 Berlin, Germany
7. Institut für Pathologie am Klinikum Leverkusen, Am Gesundheitspark 11, 51375 Leverkusen, Germany
8. Institute of Pathology, Charité—Universitätsmedizin Berlin, corporate member of Freie Universität Berlin, Humboldt-Universität zu Berlin, and Berlin Institute of Health, 10117 Berlin, Germany
9. Max Planck Institute for Molecular Genetics, Sequencing Core Facility, Ihnestrasse 63-73, 14195 Berlin, Germany
* Correspondence: meierhof@molgen.mpg.de; Tel.: +49-30-8413-1567; Fax: +49-30-8413-1960

Received: 26 July 2019; Accepted: 30 August 2019; Published: 3 September 2019

Abstract: Papillary renal cell carcinoma (pRCC) is a malignant kidney cancer with a prevalence of 7–20% of all renal tumors. Proteome and metabolome profiles of 19 pRCC and patient-matched healthy kidney controls were used to elucidate the regulation of metabolic pathways and the underlying molecular mechanisms. Glutathione (GSH), a main reactive oxygen species (ROS) scavenger, was highly increased and can be regarded as a new hallmark in this malignancy. Isotope tracing of pRCC derived cell lines revealed an increased de novo synthesis rate of GSH, based on glutamine consumption. Furthermore, profound downregulation of gluconeogenesis and oxidative phosphorylation was observed at the protein level. In contrast, analysis of the The Cancer Genome Atlas (TCGA) papillary RCC cohort revealed no significant change in transcripts encoding oxidative phosphorylation compared to normal kidney tissue, highlighting the importance of proteomic profiling. The molecular characteristics of pRCC are increased GSH synthesis to cope with ROS stress, deficient anabolic glucose synthesis, and compromised oxidative phosphorylation, which could potentially be exploited in innovative anti-cancer strategies.

Keywords: Papillary renal cell carcinoma (pRCC); proteome profiling; metabolome profiling; glutathione metabolism; metabolic reprogramming

1. Introduction

Papillary renal cell carcinoma (pRCC) is a heterogeneous disease, representing 7–20% of all renal cancers [1–3], subdivided into clinically and biologically distinct type I and type II entities [3]. Type I pRCC tumors consist of basophilic cells with papillae and tubular structures and small nucleoli, whereas pRCC type II tumors exhibit large cells with abundant eosinophilic cells and prominent nucleoli [3]. The cytogenetic differences are a trisomy 7 and 17 in pRCC type I and the loss of 1p and 3p in pRCC type II tumors [4,5]. Intra- and interchromosomal rearrangements are significantly increased in pRCC type II, leading frequently to a gene fusion involving the transcription factor *TFE3* [6], by which the promoter substitution appears to be the key molecular event, causing dysregulation of many signaling pathways already implicated in carcinogenesis [7]. Type I of this malignant tumor is characterized by frequent mutations in the *MET* oncogene, including alternative splice variants. Currently, the MET pathway is the most common target for developing new treatments for pRCC, such as the MET kinase inhibitor Savolitinib, which interrupts angiogenesis [8]. Type II has more likely mutations such as *SETD2*, *NF2*, and the inactivation of *CDKN2A* by mutation, deletion, or CpG island hypermethylation [5,9]. Structural variants were observed in sporadic events, including duplications in *EGFR* and *HIF1A*, and deletions in *SDHB*, *DNMT3A*, and *STAG2* [10]. These genes and several more, which can be found mutated in both tumor types, play a pivotal role in epigenetic regulation, signaling, and proliferation regulation, such as in PI3K/AKT/mTOR, NRF2-ARE, and the Hippo pathways. Furthermore, type II pRCC was subdivided into three subtypes, based on distinct molecular and phenotypic features. pRCC type II tumors are more likely to metastasize [4], and *FH* mutations and DNA hypermethylation were found to be correlate with inferior prognosis [5,9]. Hence, the hypermethylation group was termed "CpG island methylation phenotype" (CIMP), which additionally featured a metabolic shift known as the Warburg effect [5].

Many studies have been performed recently at the transcript level in pRCC to better understand its classification and subclassification and to elucidate pathway remodeling in these cancer [5,11] studies. Based on all these findings, a new classification system was proposed. Compared with the current model where the organ of origin determines the tumor type, a system was proposed based solely on molecular features which could be considered more relevant for tumor classification [12].

Nephrectomy or partial nephrectomy and in the presence of metastases, and treatment with vascular endothelial growth factor (VEGF) and mammalian target of rapamycin (mTOR) inhibitors are currently considered the standard treatments. Furthermore, resection or irradiation of metastases can be a useful palliative treatment for patients with brain metastases or osseous metastases that are painful or increase the risk of fracture [13].

Besides transcript data, little is known in pRCC about its regulation at the protein- and metabolome level, the underlying molecular mechanisms, the alterations of metabolic pathways, and how well these "omics" data correlate with each other. One study compared metabolomic/lipidomic profiles of clear cell RCC (ccRCC), chromophobe RCC (chRCC), and pRCC, and determined that RCC subtypes clustered into two groups separating ccRCC and pRCC from chRCC, which mainly reflected the different cells of origin [14].

To fill in the aforesaid knowledge gaps, we undertook a multi-'omics' survey to compare seven type I, seven type II, and five metastatic type II pRCCs with patient-matched adjacent healthy kidney tissues. To confirm the main findings obtained by profiling, the dysregulated pathways were validated by either enzymatic measurements or isotope tracing experiments.

2. Results

2.1. Proteome Profiling of pRCC

Malignant and non-malignant tissues from 19 nephrectomies representing papillary RCC of type I, II, and IIM (with metastases) were investigated; clinical parameters are shown in Table 1. Proteome profiling revealed a total of 8554 protein groups, consisting of 1,330,129 identified peptides in all 19 pRCC samples and adjacent healthy kidney tissues, both at a false discovery rate (FDR) of 1% (Table S1). 3785, 3838, and 4200 protein groups could be quantified by label-free quantification in type I, II, and IIM, respectively.

Table 1. Clinical and pathologic features of the pRCC cohort.

Case ID	Age at Surgery	Gender	Pathologic T Grade	Fuhrman Grade	Tumor Size (cm)
C1 type I	68	Male	pT3a	3	5
C2 type I	83	Male	pT1b	1	6.5
C3 type I	60	Male	pT1a	2	3.9
C4 type I	74	Male	pT1b	2	6
C5 type I	35	Male	pT3a	2	3.5
C6 type I	49	Male	pT1b	2	4.2
C7 type I	59	Male	pT1b	2	4.5
C1 type II	54	Male	pT3b	3	16
C2 type II	70	Male	pT1a	2	2.5
C3 type II	57	Male	pT2b	3	12.5
C4 type II	80	Female	pT1b	2	6.2
C5 type II	77	Male	pT3b	2	6
C6 type II	81	Female	pT3a	3	8.5
C7 type II	71	Male	pT2a	3	7.5
C1 type IIM	42	Male	pT3a	3	6.5
C2 type IIM	72	Male	pT3a	3	17
C3 type IIM	67	Female	pT3a	3	5.5
C4 type IIM	80	Male	pT2b	3	11
C5 type IIM	32	Male	pT3a	3	10.3

Pearson correlation ranged from 0.597 to 0.951 for controls and 0.631 to 0.938 for all pRCC specimens for the least to the most similar individuals. Furthermore, proteome profiling revealed pRCC I, II, and IIM versus healthy adjacent kidney tissues as distinct groups in a principal component analysis (Figure 1A–C).

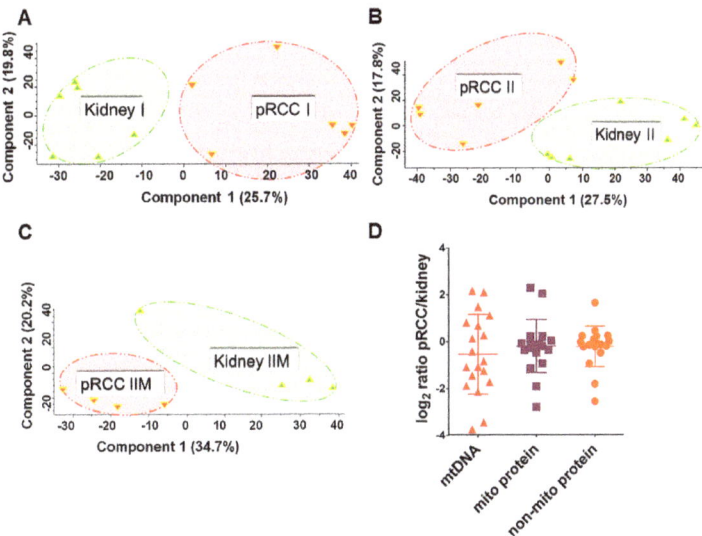

Figure 1. Principal component analysis (PCA) and evaluation of the mitochondrial DNA (mtDNA) and mitochondrial protein content in papillary renal cell carcinoma (pRCC). PCA analysis in (**A**) pRCC type I ($n = 6$), (**B**) pRCC type II ($n = 6$), and (**C**) pRCC type IIM ($n = 4$) revealed spatial separation for the proteome profiles. (**D**) $\log_2$ ratios of the mtDNA (mean -0.55 ± 1.7 standard deviation (SD)) based on whole-exome sequencing (WES) read depths, the mitochondrial- (mean -0.19 ± 1.13 SD) and non-mitochondrial proteome (-0.22 ± 0.86 SD) in pRCC versus controls, ($n = 19$).

Significantly regulated proteins were identified by a *t*-test and volcano plots are shown for pRCC type I, II, and IIM (Table S2, Figure S1A–C).

2.2. mtDNA Mutations in pRCC Did Not Reveal Any Major Impact on the Respiratory Chain

The assembly of mitochondrial whole-exome sequencing (WES) reads derived from 19 patients with pRCC and matched with adjacent healthy kidney tissues showed adequate coverage and quality for reliable mtDNA reconstruction and variant calling (Table S3). Mitochondrial mean coverage read depth and mitochondrial assembled bases in the WES dataset ranged from 12.42X to 371.41X and from 91.21% to 100%, respectively. The mtDNA content was 46% reduced (Figure 1D), based on $\log_2$ ratios of the mtDNA WES read depths between pRCC and matching controls, which is in line with a previous observation in RCC by Southern blot [15]. Furthermore, the abundance of proteins located within the mitochondrion versus all non-mitochondrial proteins showed no difference (Figure 1D).

A total of 260 somatic mtDNA mutations were detected in pRCC samples. Altogether 86 mutations were located within the protein-coding genes, divided into 44 synonymous, 40 non-synonymous and two nonsense mutations. Among the non-synonymous variants, 25 showed a disease score higher than the threshold (>0.7) and a nucleotide variability that was lower than the nucleotide variability cutoff (0.0026). A total of 197 germline mutations were detected, but only one of the seven non-synonymous germline variants were shown to be potentially pathogenic (Table S4).

Although 25 somatic non-synonymous and potentially pathogenic events were identified, it was not possible to infer a strong relationship with pRCC, considering that all mutations were found in only ten of the 19 tumors. None of the somatic mutations were shared between the different subjects and homoplasmic rates were generally very low (Table S4), however, the number of studied cases was too low to draw any final conclusions.

An analysis of copy number variations (CNV) revealed a fragmented pattern of chromosomal gains and losses spread over all chromosomes in all pRCC types (Figure S2), but no clear chromosomal patterns were identified.

2.3. Significantly Decreased Enzymatic Activity of the Respiratory Chain in pRCC

A gene set enrichment analysis (GSEA) was conducted to identify significantly rewired metabolic pathways in the tumor. Significant decreases in all three investigated pRCC types were found in the Kyoto Encyclopedia of Genes and Genomes (KEGG) pathways for oxidative phosphorylation, thetricarboxylic acid cycle (TCA), branched-chain amino acids, cytochrome P450 drug metabolism, peroxisomes, fatty acid metabolism, and several amino acid metabolism pathways. (Figure 2A, Figure S3, Table S5). The OXPHOS system was the most severely reduced in all pRCC types. Interestingly, there was no obviously different regulation between the three types of pRCC that was detectable at the protein pathway level. The three most significantly increased KEGG pathways in all pRCCs were the spliceosome, the ribosome and the cell cycle (Figure 2A; Figure S3, Table S5). An aberrantly increased rate of ribosome biogenesis has been recognized as a hallmark of many cancers, caused by hyperactivation of RNA polymerase I transcription and ribosome biogenesis factors, reviewed in [16,17].

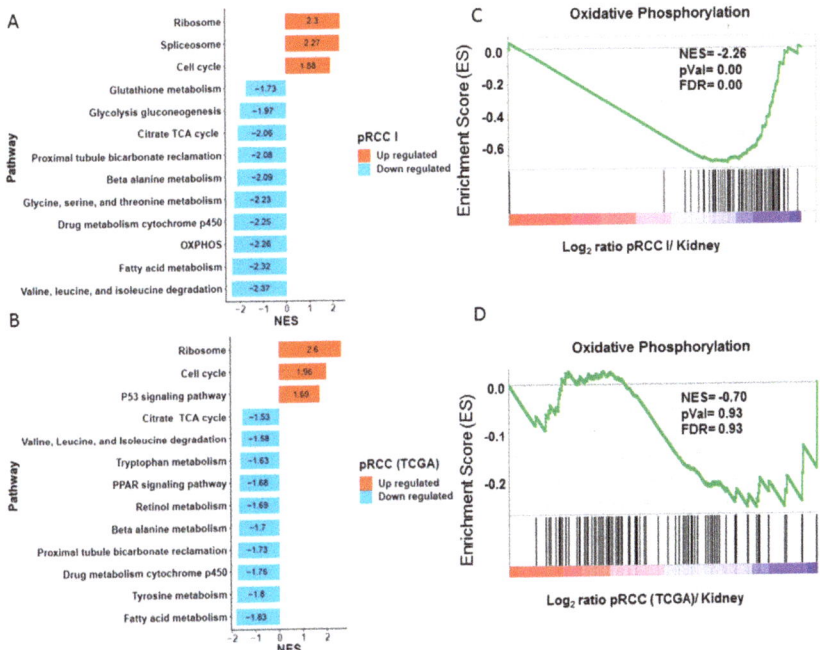

Figure 2. Significantly regulated Kyoto Encyclopedia of Genes and Genomes (KEGG) pathways between the proteomes of (**A**) papillary renal cell carcinoma (pRCC) type I and healthy kidneys and (**B**) of the transcriptome data retrieved from The Cancer Genome Atlas (TCGA). Shown is a collapsed list, the applied cutoff is $p \leq 0.05$ and $q \leq 0.1$. Specific enrichment plots for the KEGG pathway "oxidative phosphorylation" are shown for (**C**) the proteome and (**D**) the transcript data from TCGA. The Vacuolar-type H ± ATPases (V-ATPases) were removed from the pathway "oxidative phosphorylation" displayed in C and D, as they are wrongly assigned in this KEGG pathway. Normalized enrichment score, NES; Size, number of proteins/genes identified within a pathway.

In order to investigate the regulation of the respiratory chain between pRCC and controls in more detail, separate gene sets for all five OXPHOS complexes were created, including the assembly factors. This revealed a reduction in protein abundance for all complexes with the highest observed for complex I (CI) in pRCC, exemplarily shown for type I tumors (Figure 3A, Figure S4). Only assembly factors, that weren't part of the final complexes, were not decreased.

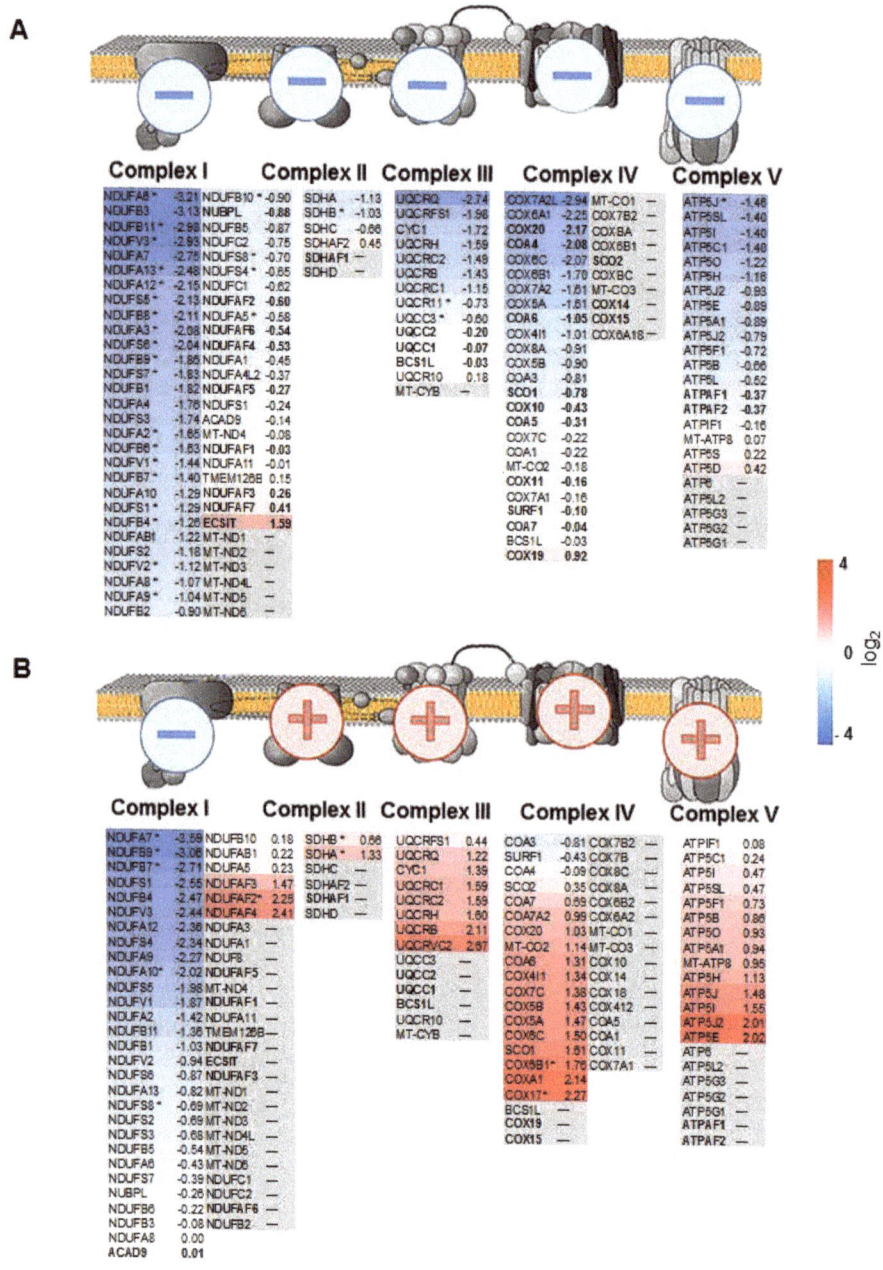

Figure 3. Protein abundance ratios for all individual complexes of the respiratory chain, shown for (**A**) papillary renal cell carcinoma (pRCC) type I and (**B**) renal oncocytomas. Illustrated are schemes of the four OXPHOS complexes and the F_0F_1ATPase, including subunits and assembly factors and the according $\log_2$ fold change between pRCC or renal oncocytomas versus kidney samples. The color gradient intensity in the subunit expresses the low (blue) or high (red) abundance of this protein in the tumor. Assembly factors, not part of the final complexes are shown in bold. * indicates significantly regulated proteins.

2.4. Anti-Correlation of Transcripts and Proteins of the Respiratory Chain in pRCC

Altogether, 291 existing pRCC and 32 control transcriptome data retrieved from TCGA (ID: KIRP) [5] were used to clarify the correlation between the abundance of proteins and the expression of transcripts in pRCC versus controls (Table S6). GSEA was performed and identified that most of the significantly regulated pathways (Figure 2B, Figure S3, Table S7) were very similarly regulated for our proteome study. The ribosome and cell cycle were significantly increased in both omics datasets, whereas the TCA cycle, drug metabolism, fatty acid metabolism, and the pathways involved in amino acid metabolism were all significantly decreased (Figure 2A,B; Figure S3A,B, Tables S5 and S7). The only striking differences were the "spliceosome" pathway, which was significantly up-regulated only in the pRCC proteomes and the "oxidative phosphorylation" pathway, which was the most decreased pathway at the protein level (Figure 2C, Figure S3C,D), but that was unchanged at the transcript level (Figure 2D). Since this KEGG pathway also includes the vacuolar-type $H \pm$ ATPases (V-ATPases), which are not part of the respiratory chain, we manually removed them from the analysis. The enzymatic activities of the individual respiratory chain complexes and citrate synthase (CS) were measured for pRCC and the adjacent matching healthy tissues. This revealed a significant reduction in all enzymatic activities of the respiratory chain, the F_0F_1 ATPase, and CS in pRCC (Figure 4A–F). Thus, the regulation of the respiratory chain was not determined by the abundance of the respective transcripts but was correlated with the abundance and enzymatic activity of the OXPHOS complexes.

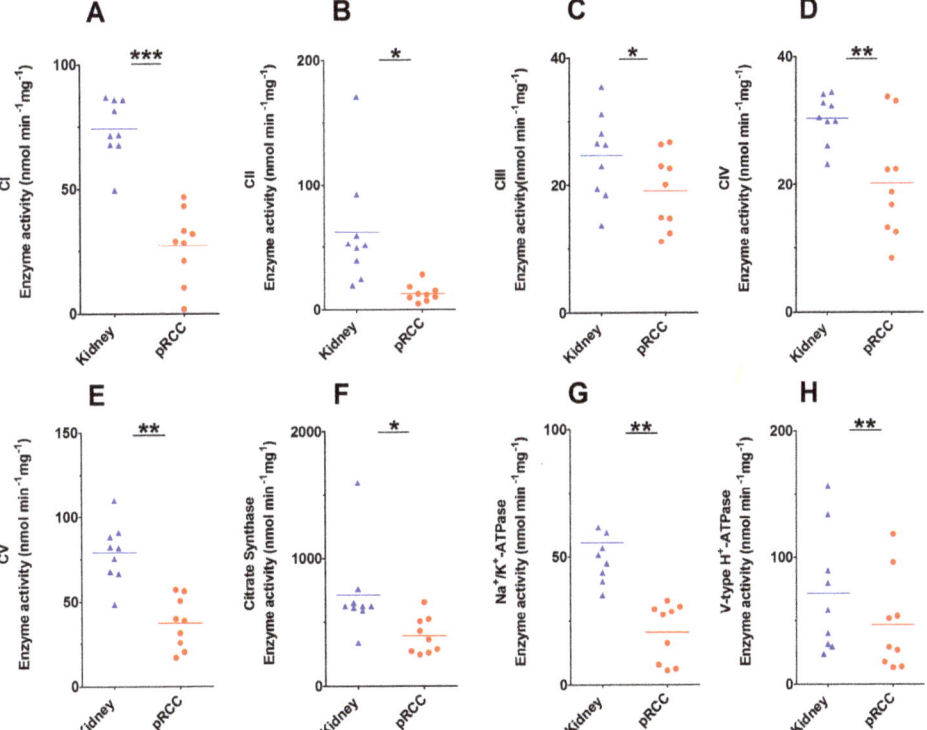

Figure 4. Enzymatic activities of the respiratory chain, F_0F_1 ATPases, citrate synthase, and the P- and V- ATPases in papillary renal cell carcinoma (pRCC) versus kidney control tissues. (**A**) Complex I (CI), (**B**) Complex II (CII), (**C**) Complex III (CIII), (**D**) Complex IV (CIV), (**E**) F_0F_1 ATPase (CV), (**F**) Citrate synthase (CS), (**G**) P-ATPases, (**H**) V-ATPases. *p*-values are: * $p < 0.05$, ** $p < 0.01$, and *** $p < 0.001$ by a paired *t*-test; nmol min/mg protein. $n = 3$ for each type I, II, and IIM.

2.5. Comparison of the Abundance of Proteins Involved in the Respiratory Chain between Malignant pRCC and Benign Renal Oncocytomas

In our previous study on renal oncocytomas, we identified a coordinated up-regulation of proteins of the OXPHOS complexes II-V and the mtDNA, but a striking reduction in the abundance of CI proteins (Figure 3A) [18]. This was explained by several specific low-level heteroplasmic mtDNA mutations of the CI genes in renal oncocytomas. In contrast, all pRCC tumor types featured a general reduction in all OXPHOS complexes (Figure 3B, Figure S4) where mtDNA mutations seemed to play no major role, but where the number of mtDNA molecules correlated with respiratory chain protein abundances between these tumor entities.

2.6. pRCCs have Significantly Decreased Levels of V- and P-ATPases

Vacuolar-type H^+-ATPases (V-ATPase) acidify a wide array of intracellular organelles and pump protons via ATP hydrolysis across intracellular and plasma membranes. Acidity is one of the main features of tumors, V-ATPases control their microenvironment by proton extrusion into the extracellular medium [19]. This allows secreted lysosomal enzymes to work more efficiently to degrade the extracellular matrix and promote cellular invasion. In contrast to almost all other cancer types, the V-ATPases were found to be down-regulated in pRCC: This specifically applies to the V-type proton ATPase subunit B, kidney isoform (ATP6V1B1), 21-, 14-, 13-fold (fold changes are shown sequentially for type I, II, IIM, respectively) and others such as ATP6V1H, 3-, 4-, 4-fold; ATP6F1, 3-, 3-, 2-fold; ATP6V1E1, 3-, 3-, 4-fold; and ATP6V1A, 2-, 2-, 2-fold; (Table S2). This seems to be a specific feature of pRCC and might play a key role in malignancy.

Similar to the V-ATPases, P-type cation transport ATPases, and the subfamily of Na^+/K^+ ATPases were decreased in pRCC (ATP1A1, 4-, 4-, 5-fold; ATP1B1, 4-, 6-, 5-fold; Table S2). These ATPases are an integral part of the membrane proteins responsible for establishing and maintaining the electrochemical gradients of Na^+ and K^+ ions across the plasma membrane. They are also important for osmoregulation, sodium-coupled transport of several organic and inorganic molecules, and the electrical excitability of nerve and muscle. The enzymatic activities of V- and P- ATPase types were evaluated and showed a significantly reduced activity in pRCC tissues (Figure 4G,H), which correlated to the observed protein abundances.

2.7. Anabolic Glucose Synthesis Was Abated in pRCC

The KEGG pathway "glycolysis and gluconeogenesis" was significantly reduced in pRCC (Table S5). This pathway describes two opposing functions: the metabolic generation of pyruvate from glucose and the anabolic synthesis of glucose from different substrates, such as glycerol, lactate, pyruvate, propionate, and gluconeogenic amino acids. A more detailed view of each metabolic pathway showed that the abundance of all glycolytic enzymes was either unchanged or increased, whereas all enzymes solely involved in gluconeogenesis were significantly reduced in most pRCCs, such as for pyruvate carboxylase (PC) (17-, 16-, 7-fold), phosphoenolpyruvate carboxykinase 1 (PCK1) (124-, 136-, 388-fold), phosphoenolpyruvate carboxykinase 2 (PCK2) (12-, 11-, 45-fold), fructose-bisphosphate aldolase B (ALDOB)(100-, 208-, 145-fold), fructose-1,6-bisphosphatase 1 (FBP1) (5-, 12-, 49-fold), and fructose-1,6-bisphosphatase 2 (FBP2) (not detected (nd), nd, 53-fold) (Figure 5A–C, Table S2). Interestingly, the two fructose-bisphosphate aldolase isoforms A (2-, 2-, 5-fold) and C (1-, 1-, 4-fold) were instead increased or unchanged in pRCC (Figure 5D).

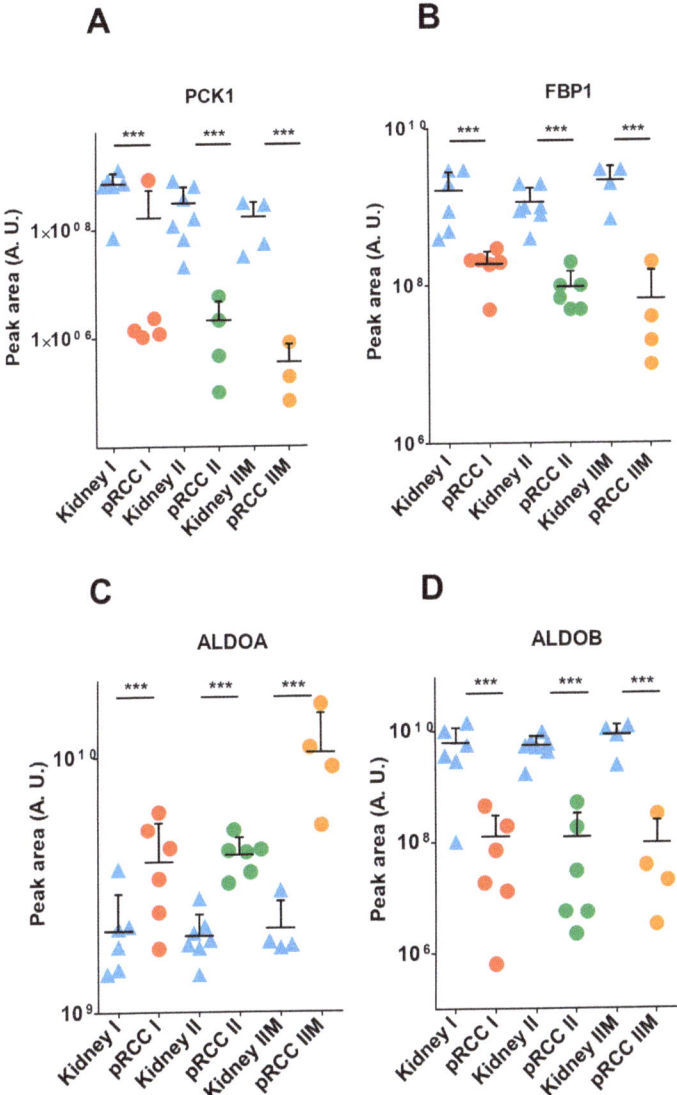

Figure 5. Protein abundances of gluconeogenic enzymes in papillary renal cell carcinoma (pRCC) and normal kidney tissues. (**A**) PCK1, phosphoenolpyruvate carboxykinase 1; (**B**) FBP1, fructose-1,6-bisphosphatase; (**C**) ALDOA, fructose-bisphosphate aldolase A; (**D**) and ALDOB. *p*-value is: *** $p < 0.001$ by a two-tailed Student's *t*-test.

These isoforms have a high affinity for fructose-bisphosphate (FDP) to foster glycolysis, whereas the highly diminished isoform B has a low affinity for FDP and hence converts the back-reaction from glyceraldehyde-3-phosphate to FDP during gluconeogenesis [20,21]. A similar decrease in the respective transcripts was found in the TCGA data, where *ALDOB* was 600-fold and *ALDOC* 2-fold decreased and *ALDOA* 2-fold increased.

A specific and regulated interaction between ALDOB and the rate-limiting gluconeogenic enzyme fructose-1, 6-bisphosphatase 1 (FBP1) has been shown. This result confirms the view that ALDOA and

ALDOB play different roles in glucose metabolism [22]. The shut-down of the gluconeogenic pathway was thus one of the most relevant metabolic changes observed and can be regarded as a metabolic hallmark in pRCC.

2.8. Dramatically Increased Glutathione Levels in pRCC Are Based on Glutamine Consumption

Metabolome profiling revealed a highly significant increase in reduced glutathione (GSH, 47-, 68-, 219-fold; fold changes are shown sequentially for type I, II, IIM, respectively) and oxidized glutathione (GSSG, 871-, 847-, 6,707-fold) in pRCC types, Figure 6A–F, Table S8). A case by case specific GSH/GSSG ratio was calculated (Figure 6F) and revealed that there was a 10-fold average increase in oxidative stress burden in the tumor.

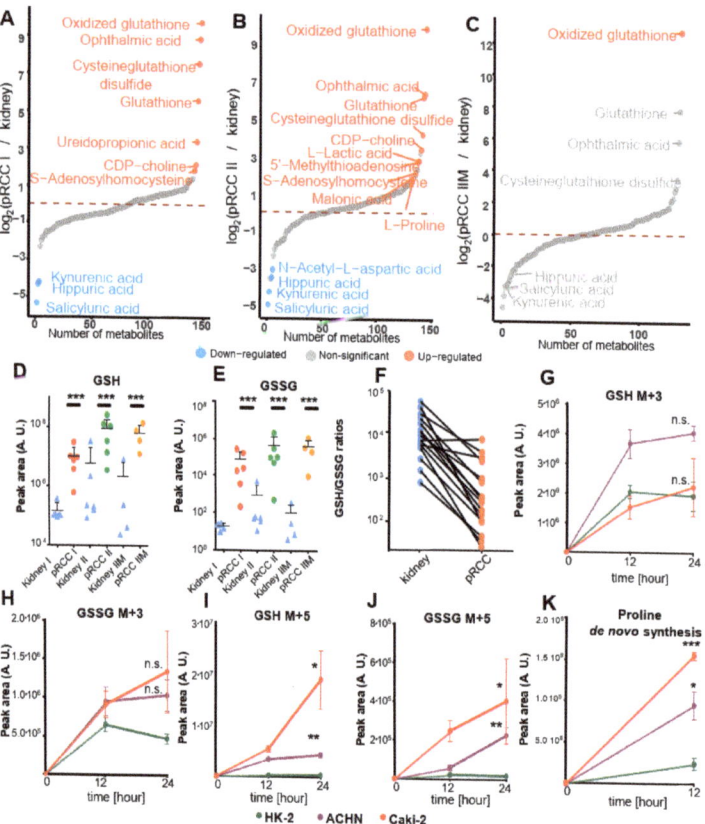

Figure 6. Metabolome profiling, specific abundancies of reduced and oxidized glutathione in tissues, and de novo synthesis of glutathione in papillary renal cell carcinoma (pRCC) Metabolome profile of (**A**) pRCC type I ($n = 6$), (**B**) pRCC type II ($n = 6$), and (**C**) pRCC type IIM ($n = 4$) versus kidney tissues. Significantly (FDR < 0.05) up- and down-regulated metabolites are shown in red and blue, respectively. (**D**) Relative abundance of glutathione (GSH) and (**E**) of oxidized glutathione (GSSG) in the tissues and (**F**) the according case-specific GSH/GSSG ratios. Metabolic tracing of (**G,H**) $^{13}C_6$ glucose and of (**I,J**) $^{13}C_5{}^{15}N$ glutamic acid to monitor GSH (**G,I**) de novo synthesis and its oxidation product GSSG (**H,J**) in the pRCC cell lines Caki-2 and ACHN compared to HK-2 control cells. (**K**) Proline de novo synthesis based on $^{13}C_5{}^{15}N$ glutamic acid in the same cell lines. Mean ± SD, $n = 3$ cell culture replicates, p-values: * $p < 0.05$, ** $p < 0.01$, and *** $p < 0.001$ by a paired t-test.

Glutathione functions as a cellular redox buffer for detoxification and can be either synthesized de-novo or imported via the glutathione salvage pathway, where extracellular GSH is cleaved by γ-glutamyltranspeptidases (GGTs) [23]. Furthermore, ophthalmic acid, a tripeptide analog of glutathione, was increased (468-, 77-, 58-fold) in pRCC. It was described as a byproduct of glutathione synthetase (GS) and γ-glutamylcysteine synthetase (GCS) and as a new biomarker of oxidative stress [24].

Remarkably, even though metabolites involved in glutathione metabolism were significantly increased in pRCC, the abundance of glutathione synthetase (GSS) was unchanged (1-, 1-, 1-fold; Table S2). Glutamate cysteine ligase (GCL) is the rate-limiting step in GSH biosynthesis. Only the pRCC type IIM had significantly elevated levels of glutamate cysteine ligase regulatory subunit (GCLM) (1-, 2-, 10-fold), the regulatory subunit of this enzyme alleviates the feedback inhibition of GSH together with the catalytic subunit GCLC [25].

Cysteineglutathione disulfide, which can react with protein thiol groups, causing the reversible post-translational modification S-glutathionylation for transducing oxidant signals [26] was (187-, 17-, 11-fold) elevated. In contrast, the glutathione S-transferase A2 (GSTA2, 146-, 36-, 85-fold), microsomal glutathione S-transferase 1 (MGST1, 5-, 1-, nd-fold), and glutathione S-transferase Mu 2 and 3 (GSTM2, 5-, 5-, 3-fold; GSTM3, 8-, 10-, 5-fold), which conjugate reduced glutathione to a wide number of exogenous and endogenous hydrophobic electrophiles, were reduced in pRCC, but other enzymes were unchanged, such as glutathione S-transferase theta-1 (GSTT1), glutathione S-transferase P (GSTP1), glutathione S-transferase kappa 1 (GSTK1), and glutathione S-transferase omega-1 (GSTO1). Glutathione peroxidase 3, which protects cells and enzymes from oxidative damage by catalyzing the reduction of hydrogen peroxide, lipid peroxides, and organic hydroperoxide was also significantly reduced in pRCC (GPX3, 6-, 5-, 6-fold).

The two identified glutathione transferases, which catalyze the conjugation of GSH to xenobiotic substrates for detoxification, were also strongly reduced in pRCC, e.g., glutathione hydrolase 1 proenzyme GGT1 (3-, 4-, 4-fold) and GGT5 (20-, 8-, 17-fold). They cleave the gamma-glutamyl peptide bond of glutathione conjugates, the only one identified was gamma-glutamyl lysine, which was increased (2-, 3-, 3-fold) in pRCC. γ-Glutamyl amino acids can be further metabolized by γ-glutamyl cyclotransferase (GGACT) [27], whose level was decreased (13-, 45-, 108-fold) to produce pyroglutamic acid (5-oxoproline), which was not significantly regulated (2-, 2-, -2-fold) as well as other amino acids.

These data show a notable rewiring of the entire process of glutathione metabolism in pRCC, however, metabolite and protein abundances do not necessarily reflect the metabolic flux. To address the question, as to whether GSH is continuously made by de novo synthesis and which substrates significantly contribute to its synthesis, two isotope tracing experiments were performed in the pRCC derived cell lines Caki-2 and ACHN and the kidney control cell line HK-2 at time points 0, 12, and 24 h. The first experiment employed $^{13}C_6$ labeled glucose, the second $^{13}C_5{}^{15}N$ glutamic acid as a tracer, a generalized labeling scheme for both is depicted in Figure 7.

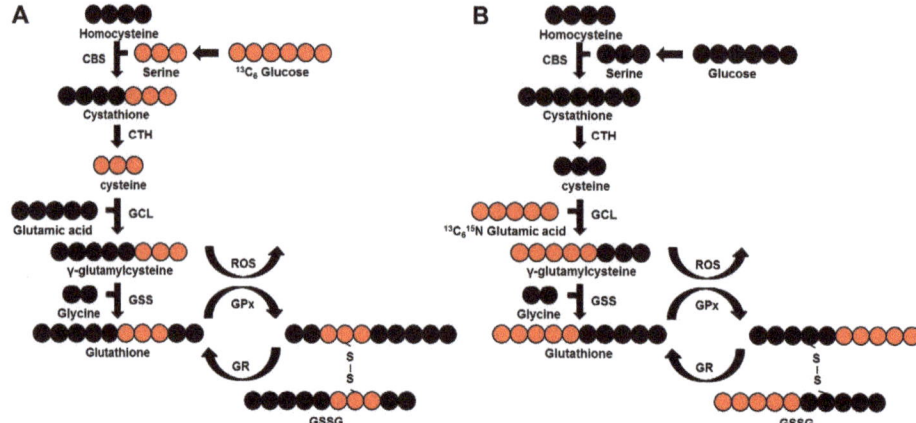

Figure 7. Scheme of the de novo synthesis pathway of glutathione. (**A**) based on $^{13}C_6$ glucose and (**B**) on $^{13}C_5^{15}N$ glutamic acid as tracers. Red circles, $^{13}C_6$; black circles, $^{12}C_6$. CBS, cystathionine b-synthetase; CTH, cystathionase; GCL, glutamate-cysteine ligase; GSS, glutathione synthetase; GPx, glutathione peroxidase; GR, glutathione reductase; GSSG, oxidized GSH. Of note, GSSG can exist in three versions in parallel, as it is made of two GSH molecules: $^{13}C_6$, $^{13}C_3$, and ^{12}C when $^{13}C_6$ glucose is the tracer and $^{13}C_{10}^{15}N_2$, $^{13}C_5^{15}N$, and $^{12}C^{14}N$ when $^{13}C_5^{15}N$ glutamic acid is the tracer.

Only a slight increase was observed for the *de novo* synthesis of GSH and GSSG in Caki-2 cells (1-fold-, 2.8-fold at 24 h) and ACHN cells (2.1-fold-, 2.2-fold at 24 h) compared with HK-2 cells when $^{13}C_6$ glucose was used as the probe (Figure 6G,H). In contrast to this, a significant and dramatic increase of GSH and GSSG de novo synthesis was observed for both, Caki-2 (48.5-fold-, 10.8-fold at 24 h) and ACHN (11-fold-, 12-fold at 24 h) cells, when $^{13}C_5^{15}N$ glutamic acid was used as a probe (Figure 6I,J). Our data demonstrated that GSH de novo synthesis is significantly increased in pRCC cell lines and is based on glutamine consumption, a precursor of glutamate.

2.9. Glutamine Is the Main Nutrient Source in pRCC

In general, glucose and glutamine are the main carbon sources in eukaryotic cells. Tumor cells frequently reduce OXPHOS capacity and are therefore even more dependent on nutrient consumption. Proteome profiling showed that the abundance of proteins involved in proline synthesis, such as CAD protein (CAD, 2-, 5-, 10-fold), aldehyde dehydrogenase family 18 member A1 (ALDH18A1), 1-, 2-, 14-fold; pyrroline-5-carboxylate reductase 1 (PYCR1), nd, nd, 115-fold; and PYCR2, 5-, 7-, 15-fold, Table S2) increase from type I over type II leading to the highest values in metastatic type IIM, indicating a metabolic shift towards proline de novo synthesis originating from glutamine. Based on these results, an isotope tracing experiment was performed in pRCC derived cell lines Caki-2 and ACHN versus HK-2 kidney controls to quantify the consumption of isotopically labeled glutamate for proline de novo synthesis.

Tracing of $^{13}C_5^{15}N$ glutamic acid revealed a significant and (6.3-, 3.9-fold) increase of $^{13}C_5^{15}N$ proline after 12 h in the pRCC derived cell lines Caki-2 and ACHN versus HK-2 (Figure 6K). The high flux in pRCC cell lines correlates well with the abundance of protein in pRCC tissues of enzymes involved in this pathway showing that these tumor cell lines are dependent on glutamine consumption.

3. Discussion

pRCCs are well characterized at the genomic level, with several driver mutations and chromosomal rearrangements having been identified [5]. How these alterations translate to proteome- and metabolome regulation are not well understood, but they determine the fate and progression of tumors. Multi-omics profiling of pRCC was performed, revealing a fundamental reprogramming of the pathways for gluconeogenesis, the respiratory chain, and for glutathione metabolism. These can be regarded as a general hallmark of kidney tumors, as was previously observed in renal oncocytomas [18], chRCCs [28], and in ccRCCs at the transcript level [29]. The anti-correlations that have been identified between genetic and non-genetic profiling argue for focusing on these so far under-studied fields.

Gluconeogenesis, an anabolic and highly endergonic pathway, generates glucose from small carbohydrate precursors, for example from lactate during intense exercise, or over periods of fasting and starvation. This pathway is also regarded as an essential process for tumor cell growth [30], since biosynthetic reactions in cancer cells are highly dependent on glycolytic intermediates [31]. The kidney may be nearly as important as the liver in gluconeogenesis [32] and pRCCs have been shown to moderately accumulated glucose, which further increases the already higher Fuhrman grades [33]. This might be the reason why pRCCs reduce this endergonic pathway, since enough glucose can be imported. Blocking of mTOR activity was shown to augment shuttling of pyruvate into gluconeogenesis, which results in futile cycling of glucose that finally leads to a halt in cancer cell proliferation and ultimately to cell death [34]. Equal amounts of amino acid levels were detected in pRCC and kidney tissues in our study, supporting the idea of a sufficient nutrient supply.

The gluconeogenic gene *FBP1* was previously found to be down-regulated in over 600 ccRCCs and was associated with a poor disease prognosis. Thus, FBP1 has been shown to fulfill two distinct functions, by antagonizing glycolytic flux and thus inhibiting the Warburg effect, and by inhibiting the nuclear function of hypoxia-inducible factor (HIF) in a catalytic-activity-independent manner, leading to reduced expression of HIF targets such as *VEGF*, *LDHA*, and *GLUT1* [29]. This unique dual function of the FBP1 protein explains its ubiquitous loss in ccRCC, distinguishing it from other tumor suppressors that are not consistently mutated in all tumors [29].

Moreover, the inhibition of FBP1 leads to the activation of AMP-activated protein kinase (AMPK). The aldolases (A–C) are required for the formation of a super lysosomal complex containing V-ATPase, ragulator, axin, liver kinase B1 (LKB1), and AMPK in its active form [35]. AMPK activation plays a central role in glucose sensing at the lysosome and acts contrary to other regulatory systems such as the mammalian target of rapamycin (mTOR).

A general shut-down of the entire gluconeogenesis pathway in pRCC was also identified at the proteome level in our study, which has fundamental implications for the metabolic regulation of a cell and organ. Specifically, the two aldolase isoforms A and C, which foster glycolysis were either increased or unchanged, but the aldolase isoform B, necessary for gluconeogenesis was greatly diminished in pRCC (Figure 5C,D). Conversely, an increase of the ALDOB enzyme is frequently found in other tumor species, such as in colon cancer [36], rectal cancer [37], and colorectal adenocarcinoma [38], which was also associated with tumor progression and poor prognosis, and a decrease of the *ALDOB* transcript and ALDOB protein is found in gastric cancer [39] and in chRCC [28], also associated with poor prognosis [39]. This indicates a critical metabolic rewiring of gluconeogenesis in an organ and tumor-specific way.

Also the up-regulation of *ALDOA* has been reported in many cancer types, such as oral squamous cell carcinoma [40], hepatocellular carcinoma [41], and in RCC [42] and of ALDOA in ccRCC [43], osteosarcoma [44], and lung cancer [45]. Specifically, an increase in ALDOA was shown for all RCC types and was associated with metastasis, histological differentiation, and poor prognosis. Furthermore, silencing ALDOA expression in ccRCC cell lines decreased their proliferative, migratory, and invasive abilities, while ALDOA overexpression increased these abilities [42].

In addition, the abundance and enzymatic activities of the P- and V-ATPases were found to be significantly reduced in our pRCC panel. A possible mechanism by which V-ATPases are thought to contribute to cancer cell migration and invasion is to acidify extracellular space to promote the activity of acid-dependent proteases that are involved in invasion [19,46,47]. Besides the classical role of regulating acidity within a cell, recent studies showed that V-ATPases, as part of the V-ATPase-Ragulator complex, serve as a dual sensor for energy/nutrient sufficiency and deficiency and they can initiate the metabolic switch between catalytic and anabolic pathways [48]. It has been further shown and that glycolysis is directly coupled to the V-ATPases by protein-protein interactions [49,50].

The significant reduction of enzymes involved in gluconeogenesis thus has metabolic consequences on multiple layers and is a hallmark of all investigated kidney cancers, such as in pRCC (this study), ccRCC [29], chRCC [28], and renal oncocytomas [18]. By abandoning this endergonic pathway in pRCC the tumor is able to simultaneously reduce other processes involved in the generation of ATP. Indeed, pathways involved in fatty acid metabolism, amino acid metabolism, as well as OXPHOS and the TCA cycle pathways were significantly down-regulated in our pRCC specimen.

Another frequently observed phenomenon in cancer is the diminished oxidative phosphorylation capacity, known already for decades as the "Warburg effect". The abundance of all proteins involved in oxidative phosphorylation and the F_0F_1ATPase, as well as the corresponding enzymatic activities, were significantly reduced in our pRCC panel. This was previously shown for chRCC [28] and only for OXPHOS enzymatic activities and the mtDNA content in ccRCC and pRCC [15]. In contrast, the enhanced expression of lactate dehydrogenase A (LDH-A) and lactic acid was observed in our study and this has been associated with aggressive and metastatic cancers in a variety of tumor types [51–53].

By comparing our proteome- with transcriptome data from TCGA [5], the main differentially regulated pathway was found to be the respiratory chain, which was the most highly decreased pathway on the protein level, but unchanged at the transcript level. A similar discrepancy between transcripts and proteins in the regulation of the respiratory chain was previously observed by us in benign renal oncocytomas [18] and malignant chRCC [28]. Enzymatic activities of the respiratory chain in pRCC and in renal oncocytomas [54] and chRCC [28] matched with protein abundances rather than gene expression. The mechanism for this anti-correlation still remains elusive, but might be directly correlated to the decreased mtDNA level, or also caused by the interference of miRNAs and the stability of transcripts or proteins. This demonstrates the necessity of surveying multiple omics profiles.

The most strikingly increased set of metabolites in pRCC were those involved in glutathione metabolism (GSH, GSSG, cysteine-glutathione disulfide, ophthalmic acid). This is similar to those previously identified in renal oncocytomas [18,55] and chRCC [28,56]. GSH is an important reactive oxygen species (ROS) scavenger [57] and frequently produced by several tumor types to withstand unusual levels of oxidative stress [23]. Therefore increased GSH levels in pRCC may be considered as the main strategy for the tumor to overcome ROS stress originating from a dysregulated respiratory chain.

By probing the metabolic flux for GSH synthesis, a significant increase of the synthesis rate was observed in pRCC derived cell lines over kidney controls when using glutamate as a substrate. This is in agreement with another study, which found that glutamine dependence in ccRCC suppresses oxidative stress [58]. The inhibition of GSH synthesis by a specific glutaminase (GLS) inhibitor and the simultaneous treatment with hydrogen peroxide resulted in a high apoptosis rate in ccRCC [58]. Hence, additional administration of antioxidants during (chemotherapeutic) cancer treatment have been frequently shown to have no or even pro-tumor effects [59,60]. High GSH levels in RCC, which protect the tumor from increased ROS stress, should therefore be therapeutically exploited by reducing the antioxidant levels [61], of GSH, and increasing ROS stress at the same time to a level where healthy cells can still survive, but tumorous cells are forced into apoptosis.

4. Experimental Procedures

4.1. Tissue Dissection and Verification of Papillary RCC

Malignant and non-malignant tissues of 19 nephrectomies performed between 2008 and 2016 at the Department of Urology, Charité—Universitätsmedizin Berlin, were collected in liquid nitrogen immediately after surgery and preserved at −80 °C. The clinical characteristics of the tumors are reported in Table 1. From the collected tissue samples, histologic sections were stained with hematoxylin and eosin. The diagnosis of pRCC and the corresponding matched tumor-free kidney tissue was done according to World Health Organization (WHO) classification criteria. Only cases with a clear diagnosis of pRCC were considered for the study. The study was approved by the institutional Ethics Committee (no. EA1/134/12, Charité – Universitätsmedizin Berlin) and was carried out in accordance with the Declaration of Helsinki. All participants gave informed consent. The ethic commission (Ethikausschuss 1 am Campus Charité Mitte, Berlin, Germany) voted on 14.6.2012 to approve the study with the topic "Nachweis von Biomarkern im Gewebe und in Körperflüssigkeiten für die Diagnose und Prognose bei Patienten mit urologischen Tumoren" (freely translated: Detection of tissue and body fluid biomarkers for diagnosis and prognosis in patients with urological tumors).

4.2. Whole Exome Sequencing (WES)

DNA was isolated from remaining pellets from metabolite extraction using a DNA purification kit following the manufacturer's protocol for tissues (QIAmp DNA Mini Kit, Qiagen, Hilden, Germany). In brief, samples were digested by proteinase K at 56 °C overnight and RNase A treated at 70 °C, before subjecting to exome sequencing.

The library preparation was performed according to Agilent's SureSelect protocol (SureSelectXT Human All Exon V5, protocol version B4 August 2015), (Agilent, Santa Clara, CA, USA) for Illumina paired-end sequencing. In brief, 200 ng of genomic DNA (in 50 µL low Tris-EDTA(TE)) were sheared for 6 × 60 sec on a Covaris™ S2, (Thermo Scientific, Waltham, MA, USA) (duty factor 10%, intensity 5, 200 cycles per burst).

The fragmented DNA (150–200 bp) was purified using AMPure XP beads and subjected to an end-repair reaction. Following another purification step, the DNA was 3'adenylated and furthermore purified. Paired-end adaptors were ligated and the afterward purified library was amplified with 10 amplification cycles. The amplified library was purified, quantified and hybridized to the probe library for exome capture. Captured fragments were purified using streptavidin-coated beads and eluted with 30 µL nuclease-free water. Using Herculase-enzyme, the enriched libraries were amplified and indexed with barcoded primers followed by cleanup and quantification. The resulting libraries were pooled and subjected to Illumina NextSeq4000 (San Diego, CA, USA) paired-end sequencing (six libraries/FC; 2 × 150 bp).

Quantification of the SureSelect captured library: Before sequencing, the samples were re-quantified with two methods. First, the size and concentration was checked on the Agilent 2100 Bioanalyzer and in a second step the enrichment efficiency was estimated by qPCR (Applied Biosystems, Waltham, MA, USA) using a primer set for an enriched exon (forward: ATCCCGGTTG TTCTTCTGTG and reverse: TTCTGGCTCTGCTGTAGGAAG) and a primer set in an intron region as a negative control (forward: AGGTTTGCTGAGGAACCTTGA and reverse: ACCGAAACATCCTGGCTACAG). In general, the cycle threshold (Ct)-values of target and control fragments differed by 6 to 10, thus confirming a very good enrichment of our target regions.

After diluting the captured libraries to 10 nM, Genome Analyzer single-read flow cells were prepared on the supplied Illumina cluster station and 36 bp single-end reads on the Illumina Genome Analyzer IIx platform (Illumina, San Diego, CA, USA) were generated following the manufacturer's protocol. Images from the instrument were processed using the manufacturer's software to generate FASTQ sequence files.

4.3. Analysis of mtDNA Mutations

The FASTQ files were used as input for the MToolBox pipeline [62] in order to extract mitochondrial DNA sequences and quantify each variant allele heteroplasmy and related confidence interval. The same pipeline allows haplogroup prediction of mtDNA sequences, detection of mismatches, insertions and deletions and the functional annotation of the identified variants. The in silico prioritization criteria [63] were used to target the mitochondrial DNA variants of clinical interest. Thus, variants found in the mitochondrial reference sequences The revised Cambridge Reference Sequence (rCRS), the Reconstructed Sapiens Reference Sequence (RSRS) and the macro-haplogroup consensus sequence (MHCS), which occurred in non haplogroup-defining sites with a nucleotide variability lower than the nucleotide variability cutoff (0.0026) and a disease score above the disease score threshold of 0.43 for non-synonymous coding for proteins, 0.35 for tRNA, and 0.60, for rRNA variants were prioritized.

4.4. Sample Preparation for Proteomics

About 10 mg frozen tissue per sample was homogenized under denaturing conditions with a FastPrep instrument (three times for 60 s, 6.5 m × s^{-1}) in a buffer containing 4% sodium dodecyl sulfate (SDS), 0.1 M dithiothreitol (DTT), 0.1 M Tris pH 7.8, followed by sonication for 5 min, boiled at 95 °C for 5 min and precipitated with acetone at −20 °C overnight. Lyophilized proteins were dissolved in 6 M guanidinium chloride, 10 mM tris(2-carboxyethyl)phosphine, 40 mM chloroacetamide, and 100 mM Tris pH 8.5. Samples were boiled for 5 min at 95 °C and sonicated for 15 min in a water sonicator. The lysates were diluted 1:10 with nine times volume of 10% acetonitrile and 25 mM Tris, 8.5 pH, followed by trypsin digestion (1:100) at 37 °C overnight. Subsequent, the peptides were purified with C18 columns. For whole proteome profiling, 90 µg of each sample was fractionated by strong cation exchange (SCX) chromatography. Five µg of each SCX fraction was used for proteome profiling.

4.5. LC-MS Instrument Settings for Shotgun Proteome Profiling and Data Analysis

Liquid chromatography–mass spectrometry (LC-MS/MS) was carried out by nanoflow reverse phase liquid chromatography (Dionex Ultimate 3000, Thermo Scientific) coupled online to a Q-Exactive HF Orbitrap mass spectrometer (Thermo Scientific). Briefly, the LC separation was performed using a PicoFrit analytical column (75 µm ID × 55 cm long, 15 µm Tip ID (New Objectives, Woburn, MA, USA) in-house packed with 3-µm C18 resin (Reprosil-AQ Pur, Dr. Maisch, Ammerbuch-Entringen, Germany). Peptides were eluted using a gradient from 3.8 to 40% solvent B (79.9% acetonitrile, 20% water, 0.1% formic acid) in solvent A (0.1 % formic acid in water) over 120 min at 266 nL per minute flow rate. Nanoelectrospray was generated by applying 3.5 kV. A cycle of one full Fourier transformation scan mass spectrum (300–1750 m/z, resolution of 60,000 at m/z 200, AGC target 1e^6) was followed by 16 data-dependent MS/MS scans (resolution of 30,000, AGC target 5e^5) with a normalized collision energy of 27 eV. In order to avoid repeated sequencing of the same peptides, a dynamic exclusion window of 30 sec was used. In addition, only peptide charge states between two to eight were sequenced.

Raw MS data were processed with MaxQuant software v1.6.0.1 (MPI of Biochemistry, Munich, Germany) [64] and searched against the human proteome database UniProtKB with 70,941 entries, released in 01/2017. Parameters of MaxQuant database searching were: A false discovery rate (FDR) of 0.01 for proteins and peptides, a minimum peptide length of 7 amino acids, a mass tolerance of 4.5 ppm for precursor and 20 ppm for fragment ions were required. A maximum of two missed cleavages was allowed for the tryptic digest. Cysteine carbamidomethylation was set as fixed modification, while N-terminal acetylation and methionine oxidation were set as variable modifications. MaxQuant processed output files can be found in Table S1, showing peptide and protein identification, accession numbers, % sequence coverage of the protein, q-values, and label-free quantification (LFQ) intensities. Contaminants, as well as proteins identified by site modification and proteins derived from the reversed part of the decoy database, were strictly excluded from further analysis. The mass spectrometry proteomics data have been deposited to the ProteomeXchange Consortium via the Pride partner repository [65] with the dataset identifier PXD013523.

4.6. Metabolite Extraction and Profiling by Targeted LC-MS

About 30 mg of 16 pRCC and healthy kidney tissues, shock-frozen in liquid nitrogen, was used for metabolite profiling. Metabolite extraction and tandem LC-MS measurements were done as we have previously reported [18,66]. In brief, methyl-tert-butyl ester (MTBE), methanol, ammonium acetate, and water were used for metabolite extraction. Subsequent separation was performed on an LC instrument (1290 series UHPLC; Agilent, Santa Clara, CA, USA), online coupled to a triple quadrupole hybrid ion trap mass spectrometer QTrap 6500 (Sciex, Foster City, CA, USA), as reported previously [67]. Transition settings for multiple reaction monitoring (MRM) are provided in Table S9.

The mass spectrometry data have been deposited in the publically available repository PeptideAtlas and can be obtained via http://www.peptideatlas.org/PASS/PASS01368.

The metabolite identification was based on three levels: (i) the correct retention time, (ii) up to three MRM's and (iii) a matching MRM ion ratio of tuned pure metabolites as a reference [67]. Relative quantification was performed using MultiQuant software v.2.1.1 (Sciex). The integration setting was a peak splitting factor of 0 and all peaks were reviewed manually. Only the average peak area of the first transition was used for calculations. Normalization was done according to used amounts of tissues and subsequently by internal standards, as indicated in Table S8.

4.7. Cell Culture Conditions for Glutathione and Proline de novo Synthesis

The two pRCC-derived cell lines Caki-2 (ATCC HTB-47, reclassified from ccRCC [68]) and ACHN (ATCC CRL-1611) and the human kidney (HK-2, cortex/proximal tubule, ATCC CRL-2190) cell line were cultivated in Dulbecco's modified Eagle medium (DMEM, Life Technologies, New York, NY, USA) containing 4.5 g/L glucose, supplemented with 10% fetal bovine serum (FBS, Silantes, Munich, Germany) and 1% penicillin–streptomycin–neomycin (Invitrogen, Carlsbad, CA, USA) at 37 °C in a humidified atmosphere of 5% CO_2.

To determine the source for GSH de novo synthesis and potential differences between the pRCC cell lines Caki-2 and ACHN versus HK-2 kidney controls, two isotope tracing experiments were performed. The first experiment employed $^{13}C_6$ labeled glucose, the second $^{13}C_5{}^{15}N$ glutamic acid as probe, a scheme of GSH synthesis is outlined in Figure 7. In addition, proline de novo synthesis was monitored simultaneously within the experimental setting of glutamate as a tracer (Figure 6J).

GSH labeling dynamics were probed by sampling at time points 0, 12, and 24 h, for proline 0 and 12 h were taken in 6-well plate triplicates for all three cell lines. The cells were rinsed twice with PBS and replenished at time point 0 by either a glucose-free DMEM medium with the addition of 5 mM $^{13}C_6$ glucose (Cambridge Isotope Laboratories Inc., Tewksbury, MA, USA), 10% dialyzed FBS and 1% penicillin/streptomycin, or by HBSS solution supplemented with 2 mM $^{13}C_5{}^{15}N$-glutamic acid (Cambridge Isotope Laboratories), 5 mM glucose, 0.4 mM glycine, 10% dialyzed FBS and 1% penicillin/streptomycin. Before metabolite extraction, cells were washed twice by PBS, ice-cold methanol (−80 °C) was added and the cells were scraped from the plate and metabolites were extracted as described for tissues. The MRM method was extended to also include isotope-transitions for metabolites originating from labeled glucose and glutamate (Table S9). As GSSG can be made of either one or two labeled GSH molecules, both versions were measured ($^{13}C_6$ glucose: M+3 and M+6; $^{13}C_5{}^{15}N$-glutamic acid: M+5 and M+10).

4.8. Experimental Design, Statistical Rationale, and Pathway Analyses

Seven pRCC type I, seven pRCC type II, and five pRCC type II metastatic cancer samples were compared with adjacent matched normal kidney tissues. For quantitative proteome profiling, nanoscale liquid chromatography coupled to high-resolution mass spectrometry (nano-LC-MS/MS) was used to quantify the abundance of dysregulated proteins. For quantitative metabolome profiling, a UHPLC coupled to a QTrap instrument (Sciex) was used for the targeted approach (multiple reaction monitoring, MRM) to identify and quantify the abundance of dysregulated metabolites.

For proteome and metabolome data sets, a two-sample *t*-test was performed. Multiple test correction was done by Benjamini-Hochberg with an FDR of 0.05 by using Perseus v1.6.0.2 [69]. Significantly regulated proteins and metabolites were marked by a plus sign in the corresponding Tables S2 and S9. The Pearson correlation was based on "valid values" for each pRCC type in Perseus.

For comprehensive proteome data analyses, gene set enrichment analysis GSEA, v3.0 (Broad institute, San Diego, USA) [70] was applied in order to see, if a priori defined sets of proteins show statistically significant, concordant differences between pRCC and kidney tissues. Only proteins with valid values in at least seven of ten samples in at least one group with replacing missing values from the normal distribution for the other group were used (Table S2). GSEA default settings were applied, except that the minimum size exclusion was set to 5 and KEGG v5.2 was used as a gene set database. The cut-off for significantly regulated pathways was set to a p-value ≤ 0.01 and FDR ≤ 0.10.

For protein-protein interaction (PPI) network analyses, the software tool String v.10.5 (CPR, EMBL, SIB, KU, and UZH) has been used to visualize networks of significantly up- or down-regulated proteins with a confidence level of 0.7 [71]. High blood contamination was identified in the following five samples: pRCC type I kidney 7 and case 5; pRCC type II case 7; pRCC type IIM kidney 3 and case 2; which were then excluded from further proteome and metabolome analysis. These exclusions were based on the individual GSEA pathway and the String PPI network results, where the pathways "coagulation cascade" or "blood particles" were significantly enriched.

5. Conclusions

Key metabolic reprogramming processes, such those for gluconeogenesis, the respiratory chain, and glutathione metabolism are not only the main molecular characteristics for papillary RCC, but rather seem to be a general feature for other kidney tumors as well. Specifically, the reinforcement of glutathione metabolism, reflecting the increased burden of oxidative stress, and abandoning endergonic processes may hold key therapeutic implications as a future treatment option.

Supplementary Materials: The following are available online at http://www.mdpi.com/2072-6694/11/9/1298/s1, Figure S1: Volcano plot of $\log_2$ abundance ratios of (A) pRCC type I, (B) pRCC type II, and (C) pRCC type IIM versus kidney tissues against the $-\log_{10}$ (p-value) of the proteome, Figure S2: Exome-based copy number variation analysis in pRCC, Figure S3: Significantly regulated KEGG pathways between the proteomes of (A) pRCC type II (B) pRCC type IIM versus healthy kidney controls, Figure S4: Protein abundance ratios for all individual complexes of the respiratory chain, shown for (A) pRCC type II and (B) pRCC type IIM, Table S1: MaxQuant output file featuring the proteome profiles of pRCC I, pRCC II, and pRCC IIM with LFQ intensities, Table S2: Significantly regulated proteins between pRCC I, pRCC II, and pRCC IIM and healthy kidneys, Table S3: The percentage of reconstructed genome covered by the assembly, the mean coverage depth, the number of contigs obtained and the best-predicted haplogroup are reported for each sample, Table S4: Identified pathogenic somatic and germline mtDNA mutations, Table S5: Pathway enrichment analysis (GSEA) of proteins between pRCC I, pRCC II, pRCC IIM, and adjacent kidney tissues, Table S6: Significantly regulated transcripts between pRCC and healthy kidneys, Table S7: Pathway enrichment analysis (GSEA) of transcriptome data between pRCC and healthy kidneys, Table S8: Significantly regulated metabolites between pRCC I, pRCC II, and pRCC IIM and healthy kidneys as $\log_2$ peak areas, Table S9: Mass spectrometry settings for targeted metabolite profiling. List of all metabolites with masses, MS conditions, and MRM ion ratios for the targeted LC/MS metabolite approach. The datasets generated during the current study are available as supplementary files and in the following repositories: WES files can be accessed via: https://www.ncbi.nlm.nih.gov/sra; SRA accession number: PRJNA535385; Proteomics data via PRIDE: https://www.ebi.ac.uk/pridePXD013523; Metabolomics data via PeptideAtlas: http://www.peptideatlas.org/PASS/PASS01368.

Author Contributions: Proteome profiling was performed by A.A.A. and V.P., metabolome profiling, data analysis and preparation of figures by A.A.A.; J.F.B. and A.R. recruited pRCC cases, E.K. and S.V. validated histological samples, B.T. performed WES, R.C. and M.A. analyzed WES data; D.M. wrote the manuscript, and conceived and directed the project, A.R. and K.J. reviewed the manuscript.

Acknowledgments: This work is part of the doctoral dissertation of A.A.A. Our work is supported by the Max Planck Society and the Foundation for Urologic Research to A.A.A., A.R., and K.J.

Conflicts of Interest: The authors declare no competing interests.

References

1. Patard, J.J.; Leray, E.; Rioux-Leclercq, N.; Cindolo, L.; Ficarra, V.; Zisman, A.; De La Taille, A.; Tostain, J.; Artibani, W.; Abbou, C.C.; et al. Prognostic value of histologic subtypes in renal cell carcinoma: A multicenter experience. *J. Clin. Oncol.* **2005**, *23*, 2763–2771. [CrossRef]
2. Pai, A.; Brunson, A.; Brown, M.; Pan, C.X.; Lara, P.N., Jr. Evolving epidemiologic trends in nonclear cell renal cell cancer: An analysis of the california cancer registry. *Urology* **2013**, *82*, 840–845. [CrossRef]
3. Delahunt, B.; Eble, J.N. Papillary renal cell carcinoma: A clinicopathologic and immunohistochemical study of 105 tumors. *Mod. Pathol.* **1997**, *10*, 537–544.
4. Klatte, T.; Pantuck, A.J.; Said, J.W.; Seligson, D.B.; Rao, N.P.; LaRochelle, J.C.; Shuch, B.; Zisman, A.; Kabbinavar, F.F.; Belldegrun, A.S. Cytogenetic and molecular tumor profiling for type 1 and type 2 papillary renal cell carcinoma. *Clin. Cancer Res.* **2009**, *15*, 1162–1169. [CrossRef]

5. Cancer Genome Atlas Research, Network; Linehan, W.M.; Spellman, P.T.; Ricketts, C.J.; Creighton, C.J.; Fei, S.S.; Davis, C.; Wheeler, D.A.; Murray, B.A.; Schmidt, L.; et al. Comprehensive molecular characterization of papillary renal-cell carcinoma. *N. Engl. J. Med.* **2016**, *374*, 135–145.
6. Chen, F.; Zhang, Y.; Senbabaoglu, Y.; Ciriello, G.; Yang, L.; Reznik, E.; Shuch, B.; Micevic, G.; De Velasco, G.; Shinbrot, E.; et al. Multilevel genomics-based taxonomy of renal cell carcinoma. *Cell Rep.* **2016**, *14*, 2476–2489. [CrossRef]
7. Kauffman, E.C.; Ricketts, C.J.; Rais-Bahrami, S.; Yang, Y.; Merino, M.J.; Bottaro, D.P.; Srinivasan, R.; Linehan, W.M. Molecular genetics and cellular features of tfe3 and tfeb fusion kidney cancers. *Nat. Rev. Urol.* **2014**, *11*, 465–475. [CrossRef]
8. Shuch, B.; Hahn, A.W.; Agarwal, N. Current treatment landscape of advanced papillary renal cancer. *J. Clin. Oncol.* **2017**, *35*, 2981–2983. [CrossRef]
9. Haake, S.M.; Weyandt, J.D.; Rathmell, W.K. Insights into the genetic basis of the renal cell carcinomas from the cancer genome atlas. *Mol. Cancer Res.* **2016**, *14*, 589–598. [CrossRef]
10. Li, S.; Shuch, B.M.; Gerstein, M.B. Whole-genome analysis of papillary kidney cancer finds significant noncoding alterations. *PLoS Genet.* **2017**, *13*, e1006685. [CrossRef]
11. Ricketts, C.J.; De Cubas, A.A.; Fan, H.; Smith, C.C.; Lang, M.; Reznik, E.; Bowlby, R.; Gibb, E.A.; Akbani, R.; Beroukhim, R.; et al. The cancer genome atlas comprehensive molecular characterization of renal cell carcinoma. *Cell Rep.* **2018**, *23*, 313–326.e5. [CrossRef]
12. Hoadley, K.A.; Yau, C.; Hinoue, T.; Wolf, D.M.; Lazar, A.J.; Drill, E.; Shen, R.; Taylor, A.M.; Cherniack, A.D.; Thorsson, V.; et al. Cell-of-origin patterns dominate the molecular classification of 10,000 tumors from 33 types of cancer. *Cell* **2018**, *173*, 291–304.e6. [CrossRef]
13. Doehn, C.; Grunwald, V.; Steiner, T.; Follmann, M.; Rexer, H.; Krege, S. The diagnosis, treatment, and follow-up of renal cell carcinoma. *Dtsch. Arztebl. Int.* **2016**, *113*, 590–596. [CrossRef]
14. Schaeffeler, E.; Buttner, F.; Reustle, A.; Klumpp, V.; Winter, S.; Rausch, S.; Fisel, P.; Hennenlotter, J.; Kruck, S.; Stenzl, A.; et al. Metabolic and lipidomic reprogramming in renal cell carcinoma subtypes reflects regions of tumor origin. *Eur. Urol. Focus* **2018**. [CrossRef]
15. Meierhofer, D.; Mayr, J.A.; Foetschl, U.; Berger, A.; Fink, K.; Schmeller, N.; Hacker, G.W.; Hauser-Kronberger, C.; Kofler, B.; Sperl, W. Decrease of mitochondrial DNA content and energy metabolism in renal cell carcinoma. *Carcinogenesis* **2004**, *25*, 1005–1010. [CrossRef]
16. Pelletier, J.; Thomas, G.; Volarevic, S. Ribosome biogenesis in cancer: New players and therapeutic avenues. *Nat. Rev. Cancer* **2018**, *18*, 51–63. [CrossRef]
17. Sulima, S.O.; Hofman, I.J.F.; De Keersmaecker, K.; Dinman, J.D. How ribosomes translate cancer. *Cancer Discov.* **2017**, *7*, 1069–1087. [CrossRef]
18. Kurschner, G.; Zhang, Q.; Clima, R.; Xiao, Y.; Busch, J.F.; Kilic, E.; Jung, K.; Berndt, N.; Bulik, S.; Holzhutter, H.G.; et al. Renal oncocytoma characterized by the defective complex i of the respiratory chain boosts the synthesis of the ros scavenger glutathione. *Oncotarget* **2017**, *8*, 105882–105904. [CrossRef]
19. Stransky, L.; Cotter, K.; Forgac, M. The function of v-atpases in cancer. *Physiol. Rev.* **2016**, *96*, 1071–1091. [CrossRef]
20. Penhoet, E.; Rajkumar, T.; Rutter, W.J. Multiple forms of fructose diphosphate aldolase in mammalian tissues. *Proc. Natl. Acad. Sci. USA* **1966**, *56*, 1275–1282. [CrossRef]
21. Saez, D.E.; Slebe, J.C. Subcellular localization of aldolase B. *J. Cell. Biochem.* **2000**, *78*, 62–72. [CrossRef]
22. Droppelmann, C.A.; Saez, D.E.; Asenjo, J.L.; Yanez, A.J.; Garcia-Rocha, M.; Concha, I.I.; Grez, M.; Guinovart, J.J.; Slebe, J.C. A new level of regulation in gluconeogenesis: Metabolic state modulates the intracellular localization of aldolase b and its interaction with liver fructose-1,6-bisphosphatase. *Biochem. J.* **2015**, *472*, 225–237. [CrossRef]
23. Liu, Y.; Hyde, A.S.; Simpson, M.A.; Barycki, J.J. Emerging regulatory paradigms in glutathione metabolism. *Adv. Cancer Res.* **2014**, *122*, 69–101.
24. Soga, T.; Baran, R.; Suematsu, M.; Ueno, Y.; Ikeda, S.; Sakurakawa, T.; Kakazu, Y.; Ishikawa, T.; Robert, M.; Nishioka, T.; et al. Differential metabolomics reveals ophthalmic acid as an oxidative stress biomarker indicating hepatic glutathione consumption. *J. Biol. Chem.* **2006**, *281*, 16768–16776. [CrossRef]
25. Lu, S.C. Glutathione synthesis. *Biochim. Biophys. Acta* **2013**, *1830*, 3143–3153. [CrossRef]

26. Reynaert, N.L.; Ckless, K.; Guala, A.S.; Wouters, E.F.; van der Vliet, A.; Janssen-Heininger, Y.M. In situ detection of s-glutathionylated proteins following glutaredoxin-1 catalyzed cysteine derivatization. *Biochim. Biophys. Acta* **2006**, *1760*, 380–387. [CrossRef]
27. Schilling, S.; Wasternack, C.; Demuth, H.U. Glutaminyl cyclases from animals and plants: A case of functionally convergent protein evolution. *Biol. Chem.* **2008**, *389*, 983–991. [CrossRef]
28. Xiao, Y.; Clima, R.; Busch, J.F.; Rabien, A.; Kilic, E.; Villegas, S.; Türkmen, S.; Timmermann, B.; Attimonelli, M.; Jung, K.; et al. Metabolic reprogramming and elevation of glutathione in chromophobe renal cell carcinomas. *bioRxiv* **2019**, 649046. [CrossRef]
29. Li, B.; Qiu, B.; Lee, D.S.; Walton, Z.E.; Ochocki, J.D.; Mathew, L.K.; Mancuso, A.; Gade, T.P.; Keith, B.; Nissim, I.; et al. Fructose-1,6-bisphosphatase opposes renal carcinoma progression. *Nature* **2014**, *513*, 251–255. [CrossRef]
30. Zhang, P.; Tu, B.; Wang, H.; Cao, Z.; Tang, M.; Zhang, C.; Gu, B.; Li, Z.; Wang, L.; Yang, Y.; et al. Tumor suppressor p53 cooperates with sirt6 to regulate gluconeogenesis by promoting foxo1 nuclear exclusion. *Proc. Natl. Acad. Sci. USA* **2014**, *111*, 10684–10689. [CrossRef]
31. Schulze, A.; Harris, A.L. How cancer metabolism is tuned for proliferation and vulnerable to disruption. *Nature* **2012**, *491*, 364–373. [CrossRef]
32. Gerich, J.E.; Meyer, C.; Woerle, H.J.; Stumvoll, M. Renal gluconeogenesis: Its importance in human glucose homeostasis. *Diabetes Care* **2001**, *24*, 382–391. [CrossRef]
33. Nakajima, R.; Nozaki, S.; Kondo, T.; Nagashima, Y.; Abe, K.; Sakai, S. Evaluation of renal cell carcinoma histological subtype and fuhrman grade using (18)f-fluorodeoxyglucose-positron emission tomography/computed tomography. *Eur. Radiol.* **2017**, *27*, 4866–4873. [CrossRef]
34. Khan, M.W.; Biswas, D.; Ghosh, M.; Mandloi, S.; Chakrabarti, S.; Chakrabarti, P. Mtorc2 controls cancer cell survival by modulating gluconeogenesis. *Cell Death Discov.* **2015**, *1*, 15016. [CrossRef]
35. Zhang, C.S.; Hawley, S.A.; Zong, Y.; Li, M.; Wang, Z.; Gray, A.; Ma, T.; Cui, J.; Feng, J.W.; Zhu, M.; et al. Fructose-1,6-bisphosphate and aldolase mediate glucose sensing by ampk. *Nature* **2017**, *548*, 112–116. [CrossRef]
36. Bu, P.; Chen, K.Y.; Xiang, K.; Johnson, C.; Crown, S.B.; Rakhilin, N.; Ai, Y.; Wang, L.; Xi, R.; Astapova, I.; et al. Aldolase b-mediated fructose metabolism drives metabolic reprogramming of colon cancer liver metastasis. *Cell Metab.* **2018**, *27*, 1249–1262.e4. [CrossRef]
37. Tian, Y.F.; Hsieh, P.L.; Lin, C.Y.; Sun, D.P.; Sheu, M.J.; Yang, C.C.; Lin, L.C.; He, H.L.; Solorzano, J.; Li, C.F.; et al. High expression of aldolase b confers a poor prognosis for rectal cancer patients receiving neoadjuvant chemoradiotherapy. *J. Cancer* **2017**, *8*, 1197–1204. [CrossRef]
38. Li, Q.; Li, Y.; Xu, J.; Wang, S.; Xu, Y.; Li, X.; Cai, S. Aldolase b overexpression is associated with poor prognosis and promotes tumor progression by epithelial-mesenchymal transition in colorectal adenocarcinoma. *Cell. Physiol. Biochem.* **2017**, *42*, 397–406. [CrossRef]
39. He, J.; Jin, Y.; Chen, Y.; Yao, H.B.; Xia, Y.J.; Ma, Y.Y.; Wang, W.; Shao, Q.S. Downregulation of aldob is associated with poor prognosis of patients with gastric cancer. *Onco Targets Ther.* **2016**, *9*, 6099–6109. [CrossRef]
40. Lessa, R.C.; Campos, A.H.; Freitas, C.E.; Silva, F.R.; Kowalski, L.P.; Carvalho, A.L.; Vettore, A.L. Identification of upregulated genes in oral squamous cell carcinomas. *Head Neck* **2013**, *35*, 1475–1481. [CrossRef]
41. Hamaguchi, T.; Iizuka, N.; Tsunedomi, R.; Hamamoto, Y.; Miyamoto, T.; Iida, M.; Tokuhisa, Y.; Sakamoto, K.; Takashima, M.; Tamesa, T.; et al. Glycolysis module activated by hypoxia-inducible factor 1alpha is related to the aggressive phenotype of hepatocellular carcinoma. *Int. J. Oncol.* **2008**, *33*, 725–731.
42. Huang, Z.; Hua, Y.; Tian, Y.; Qin, C.; Qian, J.; Bao, M.; Liu, Y.; Wang, S.; Cao, Q.; Ju, X.; et al. High expression of fructose-bisphosphate aldolase a induces progression of renal cell carcinoma. *Oncol. Rep.* **2018**, *39*, 2996–3006.
43. Na, N.; Li, H.; Xu, C.; Miao, B.; Hong, L.; Huang, Z.; Jiang, Q. High expression of aldolase a predicts poor survival in patients with clear-cell renal cell carcinoma. *Ther. Clin. Risk Manag.* **2017**, *13*, 279–285. [CrossRef]
44. Chen, X.; Yang, T.T.; Zhou, Y.; Wang, W.; Qiu, X.C.; Gao, J.; Li, C.X.; Long, H.; Ma, B.A.; Ma, Q.; et al. Proteomic profiling of osteosarcoma cells identifies aldoa and sult1a3 as negative survival markers of human osteosarcoma. *Mol. Carcinog.* **2014**, *53*, 138–144. [CrossRef]
45. Ojika, T.; Imaizumi, M.; Watanabe, H.; Abe, T.; Kato, K. An immunohistochemical study on three aldolase isozymes in human lung cancer. *Nihon Kyobu Geka Gakkai Zasshi* **1992**, *40*, 382–386.

46. Collins, M.P.; Forgac, M. Regulation of v-atpase assembly in nutrient sensing and function of v-atpases in breast cancer metastasis. *Front. Physiol.* **2018**, *9*, 902. [CrossRef]
47. Cotter, K.; Capecci, J.; Sennoune, S.; Huss, M.; Maier, M.; Martinez-Zaguilan, R.; Forgac, M. Activity of plasma membrane v-atpases is critical for the invasion of mda-mb231 breast cancer cells. *J. Biol. Chem.* **2015**, *290*, 3680–3692. [CrossRef]
48. Zhang, C.S.; Jiang, B.; Li, M.; Zhu, M.; Peng, Y.; Zhang, Y.L.; Wu, Y.Q.; Li, T.Y.; Liang, Y.; Lu, Z.; et al. The lysosomal v-atpase-ragulator complex is a common activator for ampk and mtorc1, acting as a switch between catabolism and anabolism. *Cell Metab.* **2014**, *20*, 526–540. [CrossRef]
49. Lu, M.; Ammar, D.; Ives, H.; Albrecht, F.; Gluck, S.L. Physical interaction between aldolase and vacuolar h+-atpase is essential for the assembly and activity of the proton pump. *J. Biol. Chem.* **2007**, *282*, 24495–24503. [CrossRef]
50. Lu, M.; Sautin, Y.Y.; Holliday, L.S.; Gluck, S.L. The glycolytic enzyme aldolase mediates assembly, expression, and activity of vacuolar h+-atpase. *J. Biol. Chem.* **2004**, *279*, 8732–8739. [CrossRef]
51. Zhao, Y.H.; Zhou, M.; Liu, H.; Ding, Y.; Khong, H.T.; Yu, D.; Fodstad, O.; Tan, M. Upregulation of lactate dehydrogenase a by erbb2 through heat shock factor 1 promotes breast cancer cell glycolysis and growth. *Oncogene* **2009**, *28*, 3689–3701. [CrossRef]
52. Wang, Z.Y.; Loo, T.Y.; Shen, J.G.; Wang, N.; Wang, D.M.; Yang, D.P.; Mo, S.L.; Guan, X.Y.; Chen, J.P. Ldh-a silencing suppresses breast cancer tumorigenicity through induction of oxidative stress mediated mitochondrial pathway apoptosis. *Breast Cancer Res. Treat.* **2012**, *131*, 791–800. [CrossRef]
53. Dong, T.; Liu, Z.; Xuan, Q.; Wang, Z.; Ma, W.; Zhang, Q. Tumor ldh-a expression and serum ldh status are two metabolic predictors for triple negative breast cancer brain metastasis. *Sci.Rep.* **2017**, *7*, 6069. [CrossRef]
54. Mayr, J.A.; Meierhofer, D.; Zimmermann, F.; Feichtinger, R.; Kogler, C.; Ratschek, M.; Schmeller, N.; Sperl, W.; Kofler, B. Loss of complex i due to mitochondrial DNA mutations in renal oncocytoma. *Clin. Cancer Res.* **2008**, *14*, 2270–2275. [CrossRef]
55. Gopal, R.K.; Calvo, S.E.; Shih, A.R.; Chaves, F.L.; McGuone, D.; Mick, E.; Pierce, K.A.; Li, Y.; Garofalo, A.; Van Allen, E.M.; et al. Early loss of mitochondrial complex i and rewiring of glutathione metabolism in renal oncocytoma. *Proc. Natl. Acad. Sci. USA* **2018**, *115*, E6283–E6290. [CrossRef]
56. Priolo, C.; Khabibullin, D.; Reznik, E.; Filippakis, H.; Ogorek, B.; Kavanagh, T.R.; Nijmeh, J.; Herbert, Z.T.; Asara, J.M.; Kwiatkowski, D.J.; et al. Impairment of gamma-glutamyl transferase 1 activity in the metabolic pathogenesis of chromophobe renal cell carcinoma. *Proc. Natl. Acad. Sci. USA* **2018**, *115*, E6274–E6282. [CrossRef]
57. Circu, M.L.; Aw, T.Y. Glutathione and apoptosis. *Free Radic. Res.* **2008**, *42*, 689–706. [CrossRef]
58. Abu Aboud, O.; Habib, S.L.; Trott, J.; Stewart, B.; Liang, S.; Chaudhary, A.J.; Sutcliffe, J.; Weiss, R.H. Glutamine addiction in kidney cancer suppresses oxidative stress and can be exploited for real-time imaging. *Cancer Res.* **2017**, *77*, 6746–6758. [CrossRef]
59. Thyagarajan, A.; Sahu, R.P. Potential contributions of antioxidants to cancer therapy: Immunomodulation and radiosensitization. *Integr. Cancer Ther.* **2018**, *17*, 210–216. [CrossRef]
60. Hsieh, C.L.; Peng, C.C.; Cheng, Y.M.; Lin, L.Y.; Ker, Y.B.; Chang, C.H.; Chen, K.C.; Peng, R.Y. Quercetin and ferulic acid aggravate renal carcinoma in long-term diabetic victims. *J. Agric. Food Chem.* **2010**, *58*, 9273–9280. [CrossRef]
61. Xiao, Y.; Meierhofer, D. Glutathione Metabolism in Renal Cell Carcinoma Progression and Implications for Therapies. *Int. J. Mol. Sci.* **2019**, *20*, 3672. [CrossRef]
62. Calabrese, C.; Simone, D.; Diroma, M.A.; Santorsola, M.; Gutta, C.; Gasparre, G.; Picardi, E.; Pesole, G.; Attimonelli, M. Mtoolbox: A highly automated pipeline for heteroplasmy annotation and prioritization analysis of human mitochondrial variants in high-throughput sequencing. *Bioinformatics* **2014**, *30*, 3115–3117. [CrossRef]
63. Santorsola, M.; Calabrese, C.; Girolimetti, G.; Diroma, M.A.; Gasparre, G.; Attimonelli, M. A multi-parametric workflow for the prioritization of mitochondrial DNA variants of clinical interest. *Hum. Genet.* **2016**, *135*, 121–136. [CrossRef]
64. Cox, J.; Mann, M. Maxquant enables high peptide identification rates, individualized p.P.B.-range mass accuracies and proteome-wide protein quantification. *Nat. Biotechnol.* **2008**, *26*, 1367–1372. [CrossRef]

65. Vizcaino, J.A.; Cote, R.G.; Csordas, A.; Dianes, J.A.; Fabregat, A.; Foster, J.M.; Griss, J.; Alpi, E.; Birim, M.; Contell, J.; et al. The proteomics identifications (pride) database and associated tools: Status in 2013. *Nucleic Acids Res.* **2013**, *41*, D1063–D1069. [CrossRef]
66. Meierhofer, D.; Halbach, M.; Sen, N.E.; Gispert, S.; Auburger, G. Ataxin-2 (atxn2)-knock-out mice show branched chain amino acids and fatty acids pathway alterations. *Mol. Cell. Proteom.* **2016**, *15*, 1728–1739. [CrossRef]
67. Gielisch, I.; Meierhofer, D. Metabolome and proteome profiling of complex i deficiency induced by rotenone. *J. Proteome Res.* **2015**, *14*, 224–235. [CrossRef]
68. Brodaczewska, K.K.; Szczylik, C.; Fiedorowicz, M.; Porta, C.; Czarnecka, A.M. Choosing the right cell line for renal cell cancer research. *Mol. Cancer* **2016**, *15*, 83. [CrossRef]
69. Tyanova, S.; Temu, T.; Sinitcyn, P.; Carlson, A.; Hein, M.Y.; Geiger, T.; Mann, M.; Cox, J. The perseus computational platform for comprehensive analysis of (prote)omics data. *Nat. Methods* **2016**, *13*, 731–740. [CrossRef]
70. Subramanian, A.; Tamayo, P.; Mootha, V.K.; Mukherjee, S.; Ebert, B.L.; Gillette, M.A.; Paulovich, A.; Pomeroy, S.L.; Golub, T.R.; Lander, E.S.; et al. Gene set enrichment analysis: A knowledge-based approach for interpreting genome-wide expression profiles. *Proc. Natl. Acad. Sci. USA* **2005**, *102*, 15545–15550. [CrossRef]
71. Franceschini, A.; Szklarczyk, D.; Frankild, S.; Kuhn, M.; Simonovic, M.; Roth, A.; Lin, J.; Minguez, P.; Bork, P.; von Mering, C.; et al. String v9.1: Protein-protein interaction networks, with increased coverage and integration. *Nucleic Acids Res.* **2013**, *41*, D808–D815. [CrossRef]

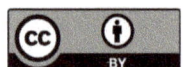

© 2019 by the authors. Licensee MDPI, Basel, Switzerland. This article is an open access article distributed under the terms and conditions of the Creative Commons Attribution (CC BY) license (http://creativecommons.org/licenses/by/4.0/).

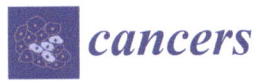

Article

Comprehensive Profiling of Primary and Metastatic ccRCC Reveals a High Homology of the Metastases to a Subregion of the Primary Tumour

Paranita Ferronika [1,2], Joost Hof [1], Gursah Kats-Ugurlu [3], Rolf H. Sijmons [1], Martijn M. Terpstra [1], Kim de Lange [1], Annemarie Leliveld-Kors [4], Helga Westers [1] and Klaas Kok [1,*]

1. Department of Genetics, University of Groningen, University Medical Center Groningen, HPC CB50, 9700 RB Groningen, The Netherlands; p.ferronika@umcg.nl (P.F.); j.hof01@umcg.nl (J.H.); r.h.sijmons@umcg.nl (R.H.S.); m.m.terpstra.cluster@gmail.com (M.M.T.); k.de.lange@umcg.nl (K.d.L.); h.westers@umcg.nl (H.W.)
2. Department of Pathology, Faculty of Medicine, Universitas Gadjah Mada, Public Health, and Nursing, Sekip Utara, 55281 Yogyakarta, Indonesia
3. Department of Pathology and Medical Biology, University of Groningen, University Medical Center Groningen, HPC EA10, 9700 RB Groningen, The Netherlands; g.kats-ugurlu@umcg.nl
4. Department of Urology, University of Groningen, University Medical Center Groningen, HPC CB60, 9700 RB Groningen, The Netherlands; a.m.leliveld@umcg.nl
* Correspondence: k.kok@umcg.nl; Tel.: (+)31-6527224587

Received: 17 May 2019; Accepted: 5 June 2019; Published: 12 June 2019

Abstract: While intratumour genetic heterogeneity of primary clear cell renal cell carcinoma (ccRCC) is well characterized, the genomic profiles of metastatic ccRCCs are seldom studied. We profiled the genomes and transcriptomes of a primary tumour and matched metastases to better understand the evolutionary processes that lead to metastasis. In one ccRCC patient, four regions of the primary tumour, one region of the thrombus in the inferior vena cava, and four lung metastases (including one taken after pegylated (PEG)-interferon therapy) were analysed separately. Each sample was analysed for copy number alterations and somatic mutations by whole exome sequencing. We also evaluated gene expression profiles for this patient and 15 primary tumour and 15 metastasis samples from four additional patients. Copy number profiles of the index patient showed two distinct subgroups: one consisted of three primary tumours with relatively minor copy number changes, the other of a primary tumour, the thrombus, and the lung metastases, all with a similar copy number pattern and tetraploid-like characteristics. Somatic mutation profiles indicated parallel clonal evolution with similar numbers of private mutations in each primary tumour and metastatic sample. Expression profiling of the five patients revealed significantly changed expression levels of 57 genes between primary tumours and metastases, with enrichment in the extracellular matrix cluster. The copy number profiles suggest a punctuated evolution from a subregion of the primary tumour. This process, which differentiated the metastases from the primary tumours, most likely occurred rapidly, possibly even before metastasis formation. The evolutionary patterns we deduced from the genomic alterations were also reflected in the gene expression profiles.

Keywords: intratumour heterogeneity; metastatic ccRCC; copy number alteration; mutation; gene expression

1. Introduction

Kidney cancer is a usually lethal urologic malignancy with an annual mortality rate of 50% and an annual incidence of 337,000 new cases worldwide [1]. About 30% of all kidney cancer patients have metastases at the time of diagnosis, and another 30–40% will develop metastases at a later stage [2].

Clear cell renal cell carcinoma (ccRCC) is the most common type of kidney cancer in adults and metastasizes hematogenously to lungs, bone and liver [3].

Although somatic mutation and RNA expression profiles of primary ccRCC have been extensively described in the Cancer Genome Atlas project [4], the genomic profiles of metastatic ccRCC have not been frequently studied in the context of their primary tumours. In the few reported cases, intra primary tumour and metastasis heterogeneity was identified based on differences in copy number aberrations (CNAs) [5], single nucleotide variants (SNVs) [5,6] and RNA expression patterns [5,7].

Understanding how molecular (genomic) alterations accumulate during tumour evolution is important to gain insight into the development of metastasis and might provide clues to more optimal treatment strategies. As the majority of metastases are thought to establish through hematogenous dissemination [8], studying venous tumour thrombus samples may reveal the mutations of at least some of the cancer cells on their road to distant metastasis [9].

In this study, we extensively analysed samples from a unique ccRCC patient for whom nine samples were available taken from multiple regions of a primary ccRCC tumour, tumour thrombus reaching inferior vena cava, and four pulmonary metastases from different sites in the lung. We analysed the pattern of CNAs, SNVs, and gene expression in these samples to interrogate the process of tumour evolution in this patient. To explore the differences in gene expression among primary ccRCCs and metastases, we then analysed samples from four additional patients.

2. Results

2.1. Copy Number Profiles of Primary and Metastatic ccRCC

Array comparative genomic hybridization (CGH)-based copy number profiles were generated for three primary tumour samples (Pr1, Pr3, and Pr4), the inferior vena cava tumour thrombus (VT), and four lung metastases (M1-M4) of the index patient (Figure 1). All samples had a gain of 5q and a loss of chromosome 3, a small segment of 2q and 10q. In addition to these consistent aberrations, several CNAs were present in either a single sample or a subset of the primary tumour samples. We also observed intermediate copy number states at varying positions in all primary tumour samples, which was indicative of intra-sample heterogeneity in copy number levels. Clear examples of this were a gain of chromosome 2 in Pr1 and loss of 1p and chromosome 4 in Pr3. The most striking copy number differences in the primary tumour samples were observed between Pr1 and Pr3, on the one hand, and Pr4, on the other. Two different samples of primary tumour, Pr1 and Pr3 showed very similar CNA patterns. In contrast, Pr4 showed more extensive CNAs that closely resembled the patterns of the VT and the lung metastases, which shared the loss of 1p, 9 and 13q and the gain of chromosome 7, 12p and 20q as their common feature. The lung metastasis that developed after treatment with pegylated (PEG)-interferon, M4, was distinct from other metastases by several copy number alterations, most prominently the loss of 11q.

A phylogenetic tree based on the CNA data (Figure 2) shows a clear separation, with two primary tumour samples (Pr1 and Pr3) on one branch and the third primary tumour sample (Pr4), VT, and the metastases samples on the other branch. In agreement with the CNA pattern, Pr4 was most closely related to M2, whereas the VT was almost identical to M3. Even though we noticed variations in tumour grade among primary tumours and metastases, we were unable to prove a relationship of regional tumour grade to specific copy number events.

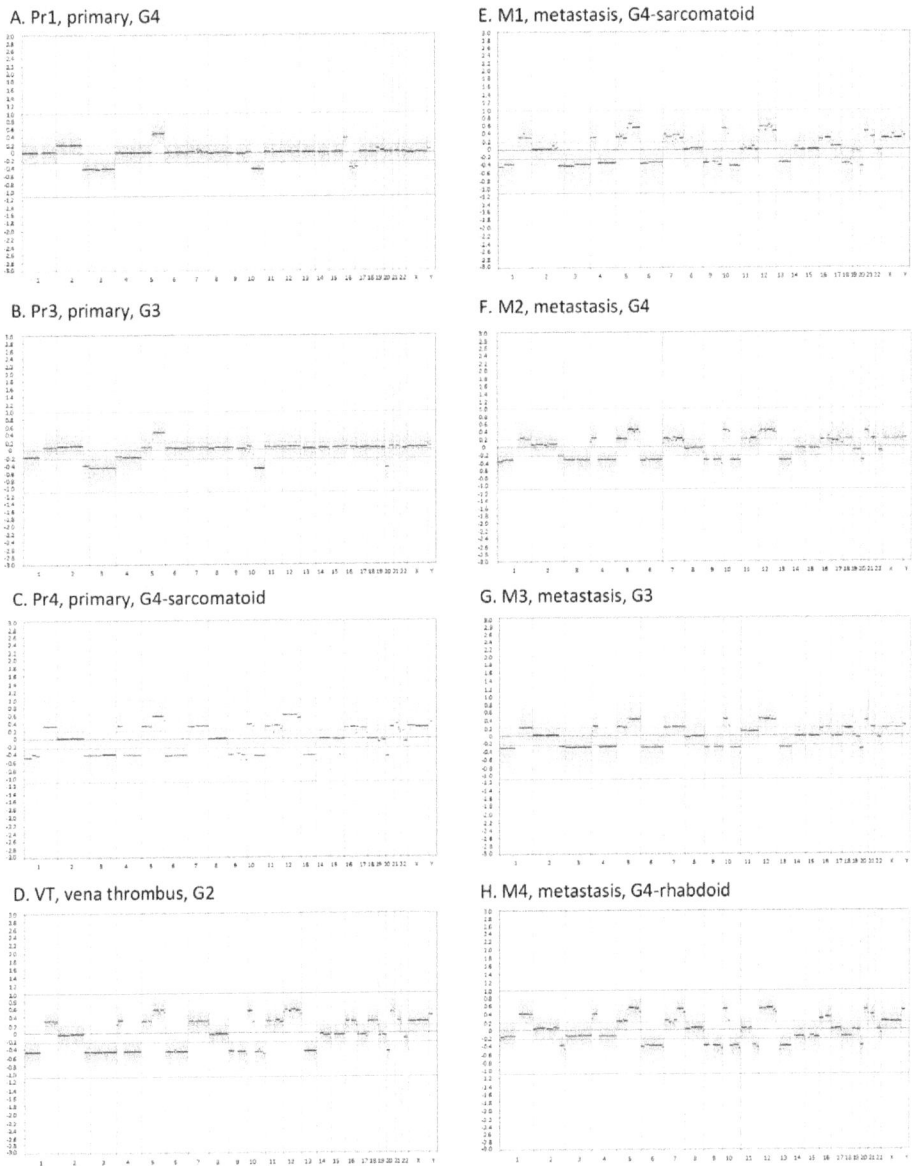

Figure 1. Array comparative genomic hybridization (CGH) plots of eight tumour samples from ccRCC patient 1 (RC1). The x-axes show the genomic position starting from 1pter until Xqter. The y-axes indicate the log2 intensity ratio between tumour and reference. Abbreviations: Pr1, primary tumour 1; Pr3, primary tumour 3; Pr4, primary tumour 4; VT, inferior vena cava tumour thrombus; M1, metastasis 1; M2, metastasis 2; M3, metastasis 3; M4, metastasis 4; G1, tumour grade 1; G2, tumour grade 2; G3, tumour grade 3; G4, tumour grade 4.

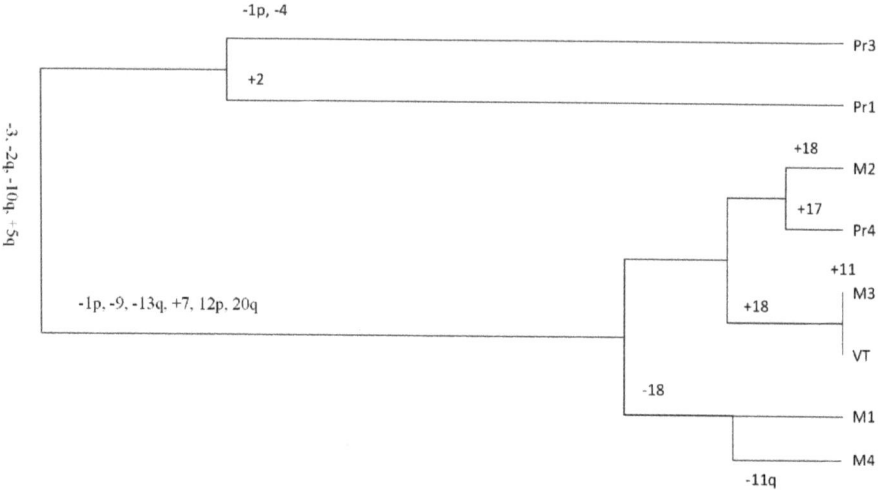

Figure 2. Phylogenetic tree based on copy number alteration (CNA) characteristics from different tumour samples of ccRCC patient 1 (RC1). Abbreviations: Pr1, primary tumour 1; Pr3, primary tumour 3; Pr4, primary tumour 4; VT, inferior vena cava tumour thrombus; M1, metastasis 1; M2, metastasis 2; M3, metastasis 3; M4, metastasis 4.

We generated B-allele frequency (BAF) plots for all samples, including Pr2, for which we had no array CGH data. The BAF plot of Pr2 resembled that of Pr1 and Pr3, indicating a similar CNA pattern (Supplementary Materials Figure S1). We then used the BAF plots to determine absolute chromosomal copy numbers, and thus, the ploidy of the tumour cells. All metastases showed the lowest copy number states for chromosomes 6, 9, and 13 in the array CGH profiles. The BAF data, however, indicated an even number of copies for chromosome 13 in Pr4, VT, and the lung metastases (Supplementary Materials Figure S1 and Table S1). This suggests that the tumour cells of Pr4, VT, and the four lung metastases contained two copies of chromosome 13. The other genomic segments with a similar copy number state in the array CGH plots, including chromosome 3 in all samples except M4, also represented a copy number state of 2. The BAF plots also indicated that all copies of chromosome 3 in Pr4, VT, and the lung metastases originated from the same parental allele. The next level in the CNA plots in Pr4, VT, and the metastases should refer to chromosomal segments for which three copies were present. Indeed, the BAF plots of the germline variants for chromosomes 8, 14, and 15 indicated an odd number of copies in the tumour cells in Pr4, VT, and the lung metastases, consistent with the presence of three copies. Taken together, these data indicated that Pr1–Pr3 had a near diploid genome, while Pr4, VT, and the four lung metastases had a near tetraploid genome.

2.2. Somatic Mutations Identified in Primary and Metastatic ccRCC

Whole exome sequencing (WES) was conducted for all tumour samples of RC1 with matched normal kidney cortex used as control. The mean target coverage for all samples was 57×, with a coverage >10× for 90% of the target region (Supplementary Materials Table S2).

A total of 146 non-synonymous somatic mutations identified in 138 genes were defined as a major clone mutation in at least one tumour sample, adding up to 390 events of major clone mutations in nine tumour samples (Figure 3). In an additional 104 instances, these mutations were classified as minor clone mutations. Targeted sequencing to validate 27 randomly chosen somatic mutations (including both major and minor clone mutations) in nine tumour samples led to a total of 243 validation events, e.g., genomic positions where a mutation should either be present or absent in a specific sample (Supplementary Materials Table S3). Coverage in the targeted sequencing data was sufficient for 207 events. Almost all of the variants, 203 out of 207 (98%), could be validated. The number of major and minor clone mutations that could be validated by targeted sequencing was similar: 127 out of 129 for major clone mutations and seven out of eight for minor clone mutations.

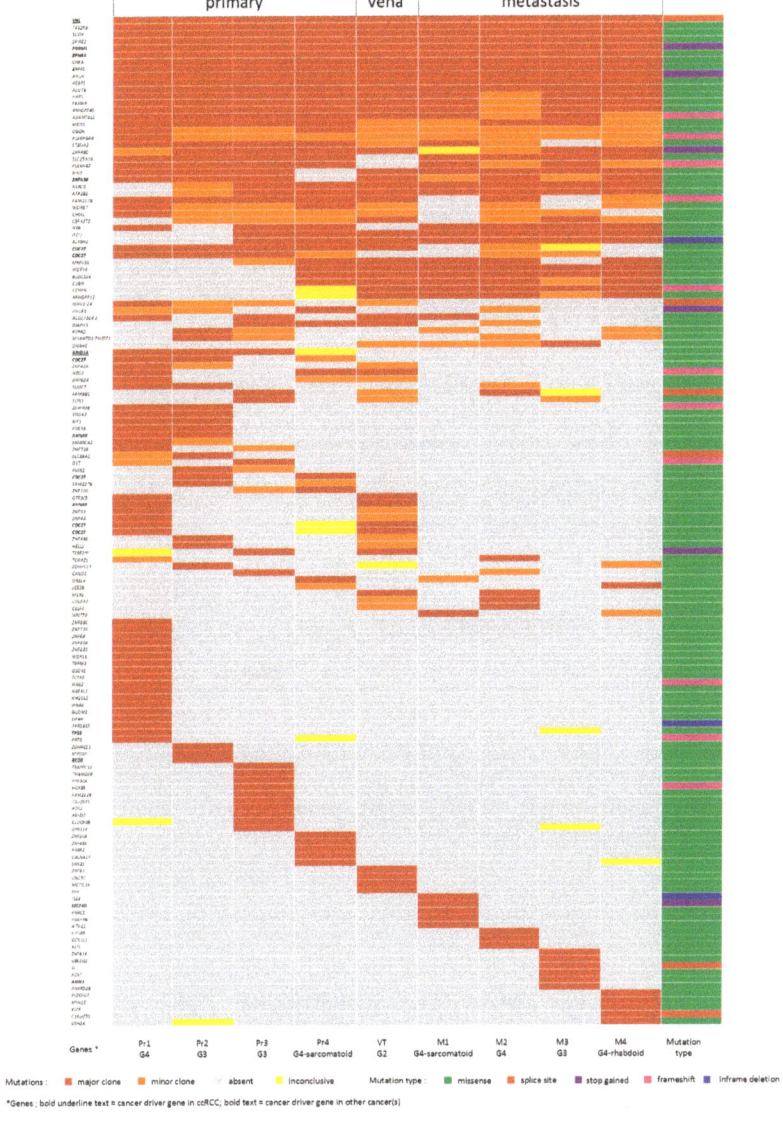

Figure 3. Somatic mutations identified in multiple regions of the primary tumour and metastases detected by whole exome sequencing (WES). The somatic mutations were classified as major or minor clonal as described in the Material and Methods section. Classification of mutations is indicated by the colours in the legend. The somatic mutations encompass 138 genes, including 11 cancer driver genes, as highlighted at the bottom of the figure. Abbreviations: Pr1, primary tumour 1; Pr2, primary tumour 2; Pr3, primary tumour 3; Pr4, primary tumour 4; VT, inferior vena cava tumour thrombus; M1, metastasis 1; M2, metastasis 2; M3, metastasis 3; M4, metastasis 4; G2, tumour grade 2; G3, tumour grade 3; G4, tumour grade 4.

Eighteen of the 146 non-synonymous somatic mutations (12.3%) were shared by all tumour samples. Among these were mutations in two well-known ccRCC cancer driver genes (*VHL* and *PBRM1*) and in *EPHA4*, a lung adenocarcinoma driver gene [10]. Fifty-one mutations (35%) were present in a subset of the primary tumours but not detected in the VT nor in the lung metastases. This included a mutation in a known ccRCC cancer driver gene, *ARID1A*. Twenty mutations were unique for the metastases. We did not observe a clear increase in mutational load consistent with the evolutionary path reflected by CNA patterns depicted in Figure 2. Two primary tumour samples, Pr1 and Pr3 clearly separated in one branch of the phylogenetic tree (Figure 2) and had 18 and 10 unique mutations, respectively. For all other samples, the number of unique mutations fell within the range of 3–6. In Pr4, we identified 10 mutations that were not present in the other primary tumour regions, of which three (in *BLOC1S4*, *WDFY4*, and *CUBN*) were shared with VT and all lung metastases.

2.3. Gene Expression Profiling of Primary and Metastatic ccRCC Samples

We carried out a gene expression analysis to further explore the relationship between the primary tumour and the metastases in the index patient (Supplementary Materials Table S4). Unsupervised hierarchical clustering based on the 500 most variably expressed genes showed a clear distinction between three of the primary tumour samples (Pr1, Pr2, and Pr3) and the remaining samples, including Pr4, VT, and the metastases (Figure 4). The four lung metastases clustered separately from VT and Pr4.

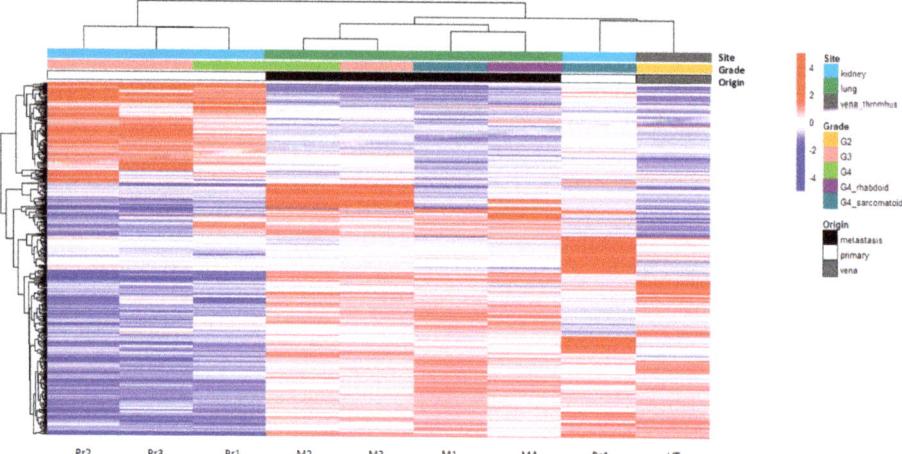

Figure 4. Unsupervised hierarchical clustering of expression profiles generated for ccRCC patient 1 (RC1). Clustering was based on the 500 genes with the highest variance in gene expression across all samples. The respective tumour samples are indicated at the bottom of the graph. For each gene, the mean value across the samples was defined. Expression levels higher than the mean of all samples are indicated in red. Expression levels lower than the mean are indicated in blue. Site of origin and the tumour grade are indicated by the colours at the top of the figure. The overall similarity between tumour samples is depicted by the dendrogram at the top of the figure and is based on the measurement of the Euclidian distance between tumour samples in expressing genes. Abbreviations: Pr1, primary tumour 1; Pr2, primary tumour 2; Pr3, primary tumour 3; Pr4, primary tumour 4; VT, inferior vena cava tumour thrombus; M1, metastasis 1; M2, metastasis 2; M3, metastasis 3; M4, metastasis 4; G2, tumour grade 2; G3, tumour grade 3; G4, tumour grade 4.

To evaluate the performance of gene expression data in visualizing the relationship of primary tumour segments to the metastases of the same patient, we generated gene expression profiles for multiple tumour samples of four additional ccRCC patients (Table 1).

Table 1. Tumour sample characteristics.

Patient	Tumour Origin	Tumour Grade (WHO/ISUP 2012)						Metastatic Site	Method Applied
		G1	G2	G3	G4-epitheloid	G4-sarcomatoid	G4-rhabdoid		
RC1 (pT3bN0M1) Index patient	4 primary samples	-	-	2	1	1	-		WES, Array CGH, RNAseq
	1 vena thrombus	-	1	-	-	-	-	inferior vena cava	
	3 metastasis pre-treatment	-	-	1	1	1	-	lung	
	1 metastasis post-treatment	-	-	-	-	-	1	lung	
RC2 (Pt3N0M1)	4 primary samples	-	3	1	-	-	-		RNAseq
	5 metastasis samples	-	-	3	2	-	-	brain	
RC3 (pT1bN0M1)	4 primary samples	-	-	2	2	-	-		RNAseq
	4 metastasis samples	-	-	-	4	-	-	brain, omentum	
RC4 (pT1N0M1)	4 primary samples	-	2	2	-	-	-		RNAseq
	3 metastasis samples	-	2	-	1	-	-	costae	
RC5 (pT3N0M1)	3 primary samples	-	3	-	-	-	-		RNAseq
	3 metastasis samples	-	1	2	-	-	-	lung	

Abbreviations: pT, pathological tumour size; N, lymph node involvement; M, metastasis; G, tumour grade (World Health Organization/International Society Urological Pathology system, 2012); WES, whole exome sequencing; Array CGH, array comparative genomic hybridization; RNAseq, RNA sequencing.

Unsupervised hierarchical clustering of the most variably expressed genes for each patient indicated that the most distinct separation was between the primary tumour samples and the metastatic samples (Supplementary Materials Figure S2). Within the primary and metastatic samples, the dendrogram branches tended to be further separated based on their regional grades and metastatic sites. In patient RC3, one primary tumour sample clustered together with the metastases, suggesting its role as the tumour region responsible for the metastasis, which was similar to what we observed in our index patient.

2.4. Differentially Expressed Genes in Primary Tumours versus Metastatic Tumours

We next identified genes consistently differentially expressed between primary tumours and metastases of all five patients. As the VT sample of the index patient (RC1) could not be clearly classified as a primary tumour or a metastasis, this sample was not included. The analysis identified 57 genes with an absolute fold change > 3 ($p < 0.01$), 32 of which were upregulated and 25 that were downregulated in metastases versus the primary tumours (Supplementary Materials Table S5). The Database for Annotation, Visualization and Integrated Discovery (DAVID) annotation analysis [11] of these genes showed enrichment for blood micro-particle group ($p < 0.009$) (*CP, FGA, FGB, SERPINA3*, and *ALB*) and extracellular matrix organization ($p < 0.03$) (*ACAN, COL11A1, DCN, FGA, FGB, LAMA2*, and *LOX*). All differentially expressed genes that clustered in the blood micro-particle and extracellular matrix organization groups were upregulated in metastases, except for *ALB* and *ACAN*. Although not indicated as an enriched pathway, seven genes (*COL11A1, DCN, FGA, FOSB, SPOCK1, AQP9*, and *PTGDS*) in this list are related to the epithelial–mesenchymal transition pathway [12–18].

3. Discussion

Application of high-throughput sequencing to multiregional sampled ccRCC has highlighted a marked degree of intratumoural genomic heterogeneity [6,9], but cases with analysis of multiple primary tumour subregions and multiple metastases are still relatively rare. We present a metastatic ccRCC patient for whom multiple samples of the primary tumour, inferior vena cava, and lung metastases were available. Tumour grade heterogeneity is seen both in the primary tumour sections and metastases by haematoxylin and eosin staining. However, we did not observe any significant morphological feature that differentiated metastasis from primary tumour sections. In contrast, through multiregional sampling and extensive genomic analysis, we identified the somatic alterations underlying early and late events in tumour development. We also identified one subclone within the primary tumour that closely matched the profiles of the metastases and is, therefore, likely to be their origin.

When we looked at the pattern of structural alterations to map tumour evolutionary events, we noted two distinct groups. One group, consisting of three primary tumour samples, had a near-diploid genome with few CNAs. The other group, consisting of primary tumour sample Pr4, the vena cava tumour thrombus (VT), and all lung metastases, had a complex, largely similar, copy number profile with tetraploid characteristics. We assumed that conversion of a near diploid tumour cell (Pr1–Pr3) to a near tetraploid state (Pr4) resulted in a tumour–cell lineage with metastatic potential in this patient.

Theoretically, the VT could have acted as a "distribution station" between the primary tumour subclone with metastatic potential and all other metastases, as has been observed by Turajlic et al [9]. Alternatively, and not surprisingly, the primary tumour subclone could have "sent out" multiple cancer cells in parallel, and some of these could have formed the venous thrombus while others metastasized to distant organs, bypassing that thrombus station. Although based on small copy number differences in the metastases group, M2 most closely resembles Pr4, whereas VT and M3 have virtually identical copy number patterns with their only difference being an intra-sample copy number heterogeneity for chr11 in M3. Our data, therefore, suggest that the latter scenario was the most likely one, and Pr4, rather than VT, was the origin of all the metastases we studied. In this scenario, a number of closely related subclones may all have emerged in the region of Pr4 that resulted in the slightly different copy number patterns that we observed in VT and M1–M3. The lung metastasis that developed after treatment of PEG-interferon, M4, featured additional structural alteration in 11q and more copy number levels than the rest of the metastases. However, all the CNAs that characterize the metastases were also present in M4. Thus, M4 seemed derived from the same tumour subclone as the previously developed metastases. The existence of such clones, including very small ones, in different types of cancer matching the distant metastasis profile, was demonstrated by single-cell sequencing experiments including some by our group [19].

Compared to the analysis of the copy number changes, the somatic mutation profiles of the tumours were less informative for reconstructing metastatic origin but did reveal early evolutionary steps. We did not observe a clear difference in the mutation load between Pr1, Pr2, and Pr3, on the one hand, and Pr4, VT, and the lung metastasis, on the other. Only 12% of the somatic mutations were shared between all primary tumour subregions and the metastases. These included mutations in the well-known ccRCC-specific cancer driver genes *VHL* and *PBRM1*, which were, therefore, most likely involved in the initiation of tumour development in this patient. A low number of shared mutations between primary tumours and their metastasis was also reported in a study where single primary tumour samples were compared with a single metastatic sample per patient [20]. We did not see a gradual increase of mutation load. Instead, both the primary tumour sections and metastases we analysed show a more-or-less equal number of unique mutations. The presence of these private mutations might reflect on-going parallel clonal evolution in each of the primary tumour sections and in metastasis regions [21]. It probably reflects independent clonal evolution after the structural variations were established in this patient. The combined data suggest punctuated evolution of structural variations occurred within a short window of time, after which the mutational load of different parts of the primary tumour and all the individual metastasis further increased independently.

We identified several somatic mutations restricted to the different metastatic sites in the lungs, but none of these mutations were shared between all lung metastasis sites. This, again, indicates that metastasis-to-metastasis dissemination of cancer cells, e.g., as seen in prostate cancer [22], did not occur in this patient. Instead, all metastases appeared to have originated individually from the metastasis-resembling region of the primary tumour.

With respect to the mutations that may have facilitated the process of metastasis, we found it interesting that we observed a missense mutation of *ARHGAP12* and a frameshift deletion of *CENPN* in the VT and all lung metastatic samples. Gene *ARHGAP12* encodes a junctional complex protein that affects tumour cell adhesion, scattering, and migration driven by hepatocyte growth factor [23,24]. These processes regulate invasive growth, and when aberrantly expressed in cancer cells, leads to cancer invasion and metastasis [25]. Downregulated *ARHGAP12* has been related to the increased invasive growth of human cancer cell lines from lung epithelial cells, prostate, thyroid, and breast [24]. As it is well known, *CENPN* is important in kinetochore assembly prior to mitosis [26]. Although no literature specifically mentions the involvement of these mutated genes in ccRCC, we speculate that these mutations contributed to metastasis in the index patient. These mutations may already have been present in the primary tumour, but if so, the number of tumour cells in our sample was too small for these mutations to be discovered. Few mutations were only present in area Pr4 of the primary tumour and were shared with VT and all lung metastases, including one missense mutation of *CUBN*. Being expressed in several normal epithelial cell types, including those in the kidney, *CUBN* encodes a receptor for intrinsic factor-vitamin B12 complexes [27]. Low *CUBN* expression has been found by others in venous tumour thrombus and lung metastases, as compared to primary tumours of ccRCC [28]. The same study found low *CUBN* expression was associated with poor overall and cancer-specific survival in ccRCC patients. In our patient's tumours, we did not observe low *CUBN* expression. In fact, none of the genes that showed differential expression between primary tumour and metastases carried a mutation in any of the tumour samples. Conversely, the mutations that occurred in these tumours, apparently did not influence mRNA levels of the mutated genes.

To characterize tumour subclones in primary tumours and metastases based on gene expression, we analysed mRNA profiles of the index patient and four additional ccRCC patients. Through gene expression profiling, we were able to confirm the putative metastatic seeding subclone in the index patient. In the additional patients, we succeeded in one case (RC3). Our inability to identify the putative metastasis-seeding subclone in the other three patients was most likely due to the incomplete sampling and did not exclude the presence of such a subclone in the primary tumour.

Among the 57 differentially expressed genes in the metastatic versus primary tumour samples, six extracellular matrix genes were upregulated, and one was downregulated in the metastases. We also observed upregulation of seven genes related to the epithelial–mesenchymal transition in the metastases, three of which are part of the extracellular matrix pathway as well. Together with intratumoural hypoxia, the extracellular matrix has been suggested to play a crucial role in metastasis development [29] through specific molecular pathways such as the epithelial–mesenchymal transition [30]. Interestingly, upregulation of extracellular matrix genes in the metastases of RCC patients has recently been described [31], which supports our observation.

4. Materials and Methods

4.1. Patient Materials

Formalin-fixed paraffin-embedded (FFPE) tissues were collected from four different regions of the primary tumour, from the venous tumour thrombus and from four metastatic lesions of one ccRCC patient—the index patient (Figure 5). With the exception of one lung metastasis (M4), all tumours were removed prior to PEG-interferon therapy.

For four additional ccRCC patients, multiple regions of a primary ccRCC tumour and metastases were available (Table 1). Haematoxylin and eosin staining was used to grade each tumour sample histomorphologically according to the WHO/ISUP system 2012 [32,33]. The study was performed in accordance with the University Medical Center Groningen Medical Ethical Review board (project number 20190251, approved 4th January 2016) and Dutch ethical guidelines and laws, and complied with the regulations stated in the Declaration of Helsinki. The FFPE tissue section and DNA/RNA isolation are described in the Supplementary Materials Methods.

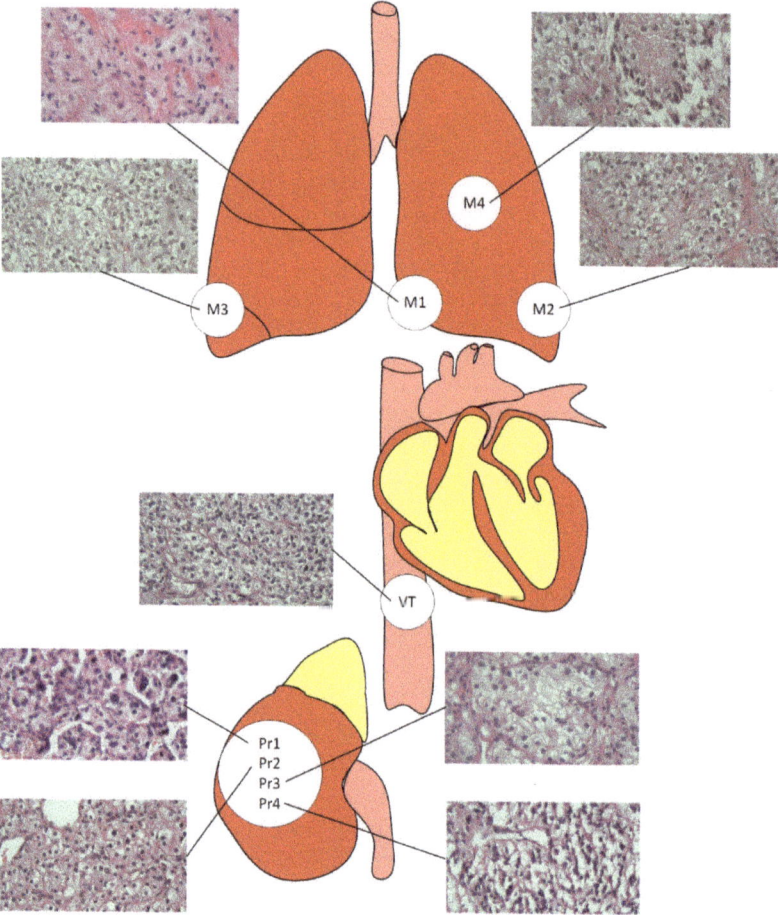

Figure 5. Origin of tumour samples. The primary tumour samples were grade 4 (Pr1), grade 3 (Pr2), grade 4 with sarcomatoid differentiation (Pr4), and grade 3 (Pr3). The venous tumour thrombus of 10 cm length extending to the inferior vena cava was grade 2 (VT). The metastasis in the lingula of the left lung was grade 4 with sarcomatoid differentiation (M1). The metastasis in the dorsal apex, the lower lobe of the left lung, was grade 4 (M2). The metastasis in the lateral basal, the lower lobe of the right lung, had a tumour grade 3 (M3). The metastasis in the upper lobe of the left lung was grade 4 with rhabdoid differentiation and was obtained by lobectomy after PEG-interferon treatment (M4). The haematoxylin and eosin -stained images were made based on 400× magnification.

4.2. CNA Analysis

For all of the index patient's tumour samples, array CGH was carried out using 500 ng genomic DNA from FFPE tumour samples using the Complete Genomic SureTag DNA Enzymatic Labelling Kit protocol and an OligoaCGH/ChIP-on-Chip Hybridization kit (Agilent, Santa Clara, CA, USA), according to the manufacturer's instructions. Normal kidney cortex DNA isolated from FFPE material from the index patient was used as reference. Labelled DNA samples were hybridized on the Agilent Microarray, Custom HD-CGH, 4 × 180 K (Agilent, Santa Clara, CA, USA) following the manufacturer's protocol. After scanning of the arrays, data were analysed with Nexus 7.5 software (BioDiscovery, El Segundo, CA, USA).

4.3. Whole Exome Sequencing

All tumour samples from the index patient were subjected to whole exome sequencing (WES) (Beijing Genomic Institute, China). Exome capturing and subsequent library preparation were conducted using 100 ng of DNA isolated from FFPE material using SureSelect-All exon V2™ (Agilent, Santa Clara, CA, USA). The final library was quantified using an Agilent 2100 Bioanalyzer (Agilent, Santa Clara, CA, USA). Paired-end sequencing with 100 bp reads was performed on the Illumina HiSEQ 4000™ (Illumina, San Diego, CA, USA). Sequencing data were processed using our in-house bioinformatics pipeline (https://github.com/mmterpstra/molgenis-c5-TumorNormal/tree/459417cc9553fae8c3040953970938860dafdfea), as described previously. The GATK HaplotypeCaller (downloaded from https://software.broadinstitute.org/gatk/) was used as variant caller [34]. Variant filtering and somatic mutation identification are described in the Supplementary Materials Methods. All sequencing data are available in the European Nucleotide Archive (ENA) repository (accession number PRJEB32862). To evaluate the CNAs identified by array CGH in more detail, B-allele frequency plots based solely on germline variants were generated for all tumour samples.

4.4. RNA Sequencing

The RNA libraries were prepared for tumour samples from the index patient and four additional patients using the QuantSeq 3' mRNA-Seq library prep kit (Lexogen, Vienna, Austria), according to the protocol for degraded (FFPE) RNA. The enriched libraries were sequenced on the Illumina NextSeq 500 System (Illumina, San Diego, CA, USA). Processing of raw sequence reads and subsequent gene expression analysis are described in the Supplementary Materials Methods.

5. Conclusions

Copy number alteration and somatic mutation profiling from multi-region sampling of the primary tumour and metastases facilitates the identification of somatic alterations that underlie early events in tumour evolution and subsequent events in metastatic development. Gene expression profiling can reveal additional alterations at the transcriptome level. Together, these techniques may help to further identify the genomic profiles in primary renal cell cancer and their metastases, with the ultimate goal of finding patterns that can improve diagnostics and guide clinical management of this severe condition.

Supplementary Materials: The following are available online at http://www.mdpi.com/2072-6694/11/6/812/s1, Figure S1: B-allele frequency (BAF) plots of all tumour samples of patient RC1, Figure S2: Unsupervised hierarchical clustering based on the 500 genes with the highest variance in gene expression across samples from Patient RC2, RC3, RC4, and RC5, Table S1: Minor allele frequency median of normal and all tumour samples of Patient RC1, Table S2: Whole exome sequencing quality report of Patient RC1, Table S3: Validation of somatic mutations by targeted sequencing, Table S4: RNA sequencing quality report of five ccRCC patients, Table S5: Differentially expressed genes primary vs. metastasis groups in five ccRCC patients.

Author Contributions: Conceptualization, P.F., R.H.S., H.W. and K.K.; Data curation, M.M.T. and K.d.L.; Formal analysis, P.F., J.H. and K.K.; Investigation, P.F., J.H. and G.K.-U.; Project administration, R.H.S., H.W. and K.K.; Resources, G.K.-U., K.d.L. and A.L.-K.; Software, M.M.T.; Supervision, R.H.S., H.W. and K.K.; Visualization, P.F.; Writing—original draft, P.F., J.H. and K.K.; Writing—review and editing, G.K.-U., R.H.S., A.L.-K. and H.W.

Funding: This work was supported by a Netherlands Fellowship Program Grant, Netherlands Organization for International Cooperation in Higher Education, NUFFIC (NFP-PhD.13/119 to P.F.).

Acknowledgments: We thank Kate McIntyre for editorial advice.

Conflicts of Interest: None of the authors have conflicts of interest to declare.

References

1. Torre, L.A.; Bray, F.; Siegel, R.L.; Ferlay, J.; Lortet-Tieulent, J.; Jemal, A. Global cancer statistics, 2012. *CA Cancer J. Clin.* **2015**, *65*, 87–108. [CrossRef]
2. Lam, J.S.; Shvarts, O.; Leppert, J.T.; Figlin, R.A.; Belldegrun, A.S. Renal cell carcinoma 2005: New frontiers in staging, prognostication and targeted molecular therapy. *J. Urol.* **2005**, *173*, 1853–1862. [CrossRef]
3. Stewart, G.D.; O'Mahony, F.C.; Powles, T.; Riddick, A.C.; Harrison, D.J.; Faratian, D. What can molecular pathology contribute to the management of renal cell carcinoma? *Nat. Rev. Urol.* **2011**, *8*, 255–265. [CrossRef]
4. Cancer Genome Atlas Research Network. Comprehensive molecular characterization of clear cell renal cell carcinoma. *Nature* **2013**, *499*, 43–49. [CrossRef]
5. Huang, Y.; Gao, S.; Wu, S.; Song, P.; Sun, X.; Hu, X.; Zhang, S.; Yu, Y.; Zhu, J.; Li, C.; et al. Multilayered molecular profiling supported the monoclonal origin of metastatic renal cell carcinoma. *Int. J. Cancer* **2014**, *135*, 78–87. [CrossRef]
6. Gerlinger, M.; Horswell, S.; Larkin, J.; Rowan, A.J.; Salm, M.P.; Varela, I.; Fisher, R.; McGranahan, N.; Matthews, N.; Santos, C.R.; et al. Genomic architecture and evolution of clear cell renal cell carcinomas defined by multiregion sequencing. *Nat. Genet.* **2014**, *46*, 225–233. [CrossRef]
7. Serie, D.J.; Joseph, R.W.; Cheville, J.C.; Ho, T.H.; Parasramka, M.; Hilton, T.; Thompson, R.H.; Leibovich, B.C.; Parker, A.S.; Eckel-Passow, J.E. Clear Cell Type A and B Molecular Subtypes in Metastatic Clear Cell Renal Cell Carcinoma: Tumor Heterogeneity and Aggressiveness. *Eur. Urol.* **2017**, *71*, 979–985. [CrossRef]
8. Chaffer, C.L.; Weinberg, R.A. A perspective on cancer cell metastasis. *Science* **2011**, *331*, 1559–1564. [CrossRef]
9. Turajlic, S.; Xu, H.; Litchfield, K.; Rowan, A.; Chambers, T.; Lopez, J.I.; Nicol, D.; O'Brien, T.; Larkin, J.; Horswell, S.; et al. Tracking Cancer Evolution Reveals Constrained Routes to Metastases: TRACERx Renal. *Cell* **2018**, *173*, 581–594.e12. [CrossRef]
10. Gonzalez-Perez, A.; Perez-Llamas, C.; Deu-Pons, J.; Tamborero, D.; Schroeder, M.P.; Jene-Sanz, A.; Santos, A.; Lopez-Bigas, N. IntOGen-mutations identifies cancer drivers across tumor types. *Nat. Methods* **2013**, *10*, 1081–1082. [CrossRef]
11. Huang da, W.; Sherman, B.T.; Lempicki, R.A. Systematic and integrative analysis of large gene lists using DAVID bioinformatics resources. *Nat. Protoc.* **2009**, *4*, 44–57. [CrossRef] [PubMed]
12. Vazquez-Villa, F.; Garcia-Ocana, M.; Galvan, J.A.; Garcia-Martinez, J.; Garcia-Pravia, C.; Menendez-Rodriguez, P.; Gonzalez-del Rey, C.; Barneo-Serra, L.; de Los Toyos, J.R. COL11A1/(pro)collagen 11A1 expression is a remarkable biomarker of human invasive carcinoma-associated stromal cells and carcinoma progression. *Tumour Biol.* **2015**, *36*, 2213–2222. [CrossRef] [PubMed]
13. Bi, X.; Pohl, N.M.; Qian, Z.; Yang, G.R.; Gou, Y.; Guzman, G.; Kajdacsy-Balla, A.; Iozzo, R.V.; Yang, W. Decorin-mediated inhibition of colorectal cancer growth and migration is associated with E-cadherin in vitro and in mice. *Carcinogenesis* **2012**, *33*, 326–330. [CrossRef] [PubMed]
14. Wang, H.; Meyer, C.A.; Fei, T.; Wang, G.; Zhang, F.; Liu, X.S. A systematic approach identifies FOXA1 as a key factor in the loss of epithelial traits during the epithelial-to-mesenchymal transition in lung cancer. *BMC Genom.* **2013**, *14*, 680. [CrossRef] [PubMed]
15. Pakala, S.B.; Singh, K.; Reddy, S.D.; Ohshiro, K.; Li, D.Q.; Mishra, L.; Kumar, R. TGF-beta1 signaling targets metastasis-associated protein 1, a new effector in epithelial cells. *Oncogene* **2011**, *30*, 2230–2241. [CrossRef] [PubMed]
16. Chen, D.; Zhou, H.; Liu, G.; Zhao, Y.; Cao, G.; Liu, Q. SPOCK1 promotes the invasion and metastasis of gastric cancer through Slug-induced epithelial-mesenchymal transition. *J. Cell. Mol. Med.* **2018**, *22*, 797–807. [CrossRef] [PubMed]
17. Zhang, W.G.; Li, C.F.; Liu, M.; Chen, X.F.; Shuai, K.; Kong, X.; Lv, L.; Mei, Z.C. Aquaporin 9 is down-regulated in hepatocellular carcinoma and its over-expression suppresses hepatoma cell invasion through inhibiting epithelial-to-mesenchymal transition. *Cancer Lett.* **2016**, *378*, 111–119. [CrossRef]
18. Omori, K.; Morikawa, T.; Kunita, A.; Nakamura, T.; Aritake, K.; Urade, Y.; Fukayama, M.; Murata, T. Lipocalin-type prostaglandin D synthase-derived PGD2 attenuates malignant properties of tumor endothelial cells. *J. Pathol.* **2018**, *244*, 84–96. [CrossRef]
19. Ferronika, P.; van den Bos, H.; Taudt, A.; Spierings, D.C.J.; Saber, A.; Hiltermann, T.J.N.; Kok, K.; Porubsky, D.; van der Wekken, A.J.; Timens, W.; et al. Copy number alterations assessed at the single-cell level revealed

mono- and polyclonal seeding patterns of distant metastasis in a small-cell lung cancer patient. *Ann. Oncol.* **2017**, *28*, 1668–1670. [CrossRef]
20. Becerra, M.F.; Reznik, E.; Redzematovic, A.; Tennenbaum, D.M.; Kashan, M.; Ghanaat, M.; Casuscelli, J.; Manley, B.; Jonsson, P.; DiNatale, R.G.; et al. Comparative Genomic Profiling of Matched Primary and Metastatic Tumors in Renal Cell Carcinoma. *Eur. Urol. Focus* **2017**. [CrossRef]
21. Gerlinger, M.; Rowan, A.J.; Horswell, S.; Larkin, J.; Endesfelder, D.; Gronroos, E.; Martinez, P.; Matthews, N.; Stewart, A.; Tarpey, P.; et al. Intratumor heterogeneity and branched evolution revealed by multiregion sequencing. *N. Engl. J. Med.* **2012**, *366*, 883–892. [CrossRef] [PubMed]
22. Gundem, G.; Van Loo, P.; Kremeyer, B.; Alexandrov, L.B.; Tubio, J.M.; Papaemmanuil, E.; Brewer, D.S.; Kallio, H.M.; Hognas, G.; Annala, M.; et al. The evolutionary history of lethal metastatic prostate cancer. *Nature* **2015**, *520*, 353–357. [CrossRef] [PubMed]
23. Matsuda, M.; Kobayashi, Y.; Masuda, S.; Adachi, M.; Watanabe, T.; Yamashita, J.K.; Nishi, E.; Tsukita, S.; Furuse, M. Identification of adherens junction-associated GTPase activating proteins by the fluorescence localization-based expression cloning. *Exp. Cell Res.* **2008**, *314*, 939–949. [CrossRef] [PubMed]
24. Gentile, A.; D'Alessandro, L.; Lazzari, L.; Martinoglio, B.; Bertotti, A.; Mira, A.; Lanzetti, L.; Comoglio, P.M.; Medico, E. Met-driven invasive growth involves transcriptional regulation of Arhgap12. *Oncogene* **2008**, *27*, 5590–5598. [CrossRef] [PubMed]
25. Comoglio, P.M.; Trusolino, L. Invasive growth: From development to metastasis. *J. Clin. Investig.* **2002**, *109*, 857–862. [CrossRef] [PubMed]
26. Fang, J.; Liu, Y.; Wei, Y.; Deng, W.; Yu, Z.; Huang, L.; Teng, Y.; Yao, T.; You, Q.; Ruan, H.; et al. Structural transitions of centromeric chromatin regulate the cell cycle-dependent recruitment of CENP-N. *Genes Dev.* **2015**, *29*, 1058–1073. [CrossRef] [PubMed]
27. Christensen, E.I.; Birn, H. Megalin and cubilin: Multifunctional endocytic receptors. *Nat. Rev. Mol. Cell Biol.* **2002**, *3*, 256–266. [CrossRef]
28. Gremel, G.; Djureinovic, D.; Niinivirta, M.; Laird, A.; Ljungqvist, O.; Johannesson, H.; Bergman, J.; Edqvist, P.H.; Navani, S.; Khan, N.; et al. A systematic search strategy identifies cubilin as independent prognostic marker for renal cell carcinoma. *BMC Cancer* **2017**, *17*, 9. [CrossRef] [PubMed]
29. Gilkes, D.M.; Semenza, G.L.; Wirtz, D. Hypoxia and the extracellular matrix: Drivers of tumour metastasis. *Nat. Rev. Cancer* **2014**, *14*, 430–439. [CrossRef]
30. Jung, H.Y.; Fattet, L.; Yang, J. Molecular pathways: Linking tumor microenvironment to epithelial-mesenchymal transition in metastasis. *Clin. Cancer Res.* **2015**, *21*, 962–968. [CrossRef]
31. Ho, T.H.; Serie, D.J.; Parasramka, M.; Cheville, J.C.; Bot, B.M.; Tan, W.; Wang, L.; Joseph, R.W.; Hilton, T.; Leibovich, B.C.; et al. Differential gene expression profiling of matched primary renal cell carcinoma and metastases reveals upregulation of extracellular matrix genes. *Ann. Oncol.* **2017**, *28*, 604–610. [CrossRef] [PubMed]
32. Dagher, J.; Delahunt, B.; Rioux-Leclercq, N.; Egevad, L.; Srigley, J.R.; Coughlin, G.; Dunglinson, N.; Gianduzzo, T.; Kua, B.; Malone, G.; et al. Clear cell renal cell carcinoma: Validation of World Health Organization/International Society of Urological Pathology grading. *Histopathology* **2017**, *71*, 918–925. [CrossRef] [PubMed]
33. Delahunt, B.; Srigley, J.R.; Egevad, L.; Montironi, R. International Society for Urological Pathology. International Society of Urological Pathology grading and other prognostic factors for renal neoplasia. *Eur. Urol.* **2014**, *66*, 795–798. [CrossRef] [PubMed]
34. McKenna, A.; Hanna, M.; Banks, E.; Sivachenko, A.; Cibulskis, K.; Kernytsky, A.; Garimella, K.; Altshuler, D.; Gabriel, S.; Daly, M.; et al. The Genome Analysis Toolkit: A MapReduce framework for analyzing next-generation DNA sequencing data. *Genome Res.* **2010**, *20*, 1297–1303. [CrossRef] [PubMed]

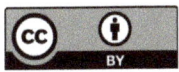

© 2019 by the authors. Licensee MDPI, Basel, Switzerland. This article is an open access article distributed under the terms and conditions of the Creative Commons Attribution (CC BY) license (http://creativecommons.org/licenses/by/4.0/).

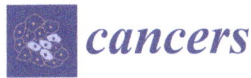

Article

Rising Serum Uric Acid Level Is Negatively Associated with Survival in Renal Cell Carcinoma

Kendrick Yim [1], Ahmet Bindayi [1], Rana McKay [1], Reza Mehrazin [2], Omer A. Raheem [1], Charles Field [1], Aaron Bloch [1], Robert Wake [2], Stephen Ryan [1], Anthony Patterson [2] and Ithaar H. Derweesh [1,*]

1. Department of Urology, University of California at San Diego, La Jolla, CA, 92093, USA; keyim@ucsd.edu (K.Y.); ahmetbindayi@gmail.com (A.B.); rmckay@ucsd.edu (R.M.); oraheem@uw.edu (O.A.R.); c1field@ucsd.edu (C.F.); abloch@ucsd.edu (A.B.); stryan@ucsd.edu (S.R.)
2. Department of Urology, University of Tennessee Health Sciences Center, Memphis, TN 38163, USA; Reza.mehrazin@mountsinai.org (R.M.); rwake@uthsc.edu (R.W.); apatterson@uthsc.edu (A.P.)
* Correspondence: iderweesh@gmail.com; Tel.: +1-858-822-6187; Fax: +1-858-822-6188

Received: 28 February 2019; Accepted: 11 April 2019; Published: 15 April 2019

Abstract: *Aim and Background:* To investigate the association of serum uric acid (SUA) levels along with statin use in Renal Cell Carcinoma (RCC), as statins may be associated with improved outcomes in RCC and SUA elevation is associated with increased risk of chronic kidney disease (CKD). *Methods:* Retrospective study of patients undergoing surgery for RCC with preoperative/postoperative SUA levels between 8/2005–8/2018. Analysis was carried out between patients with increased postoperative SUA vs. patients with decreased/stable postoperative SUA. Kaplan-Meier analysis (KMA) calculated overall survival (OS) and recurrence free survival (RFS). Multivariable analysis (MVA) was performed to identify factors associated with increased SUA levels and all-cause mortality. The prognostic significance of variables for OS and RFS was analyzed by cox regression analysis. *Results:* Decreased/stable SUA levels were noted in 675 (74.6%) and increased SUA levels were noted in 230 (25.4%). A higher proportion of patients with decreased/stable SUA levels took statins (27.9% vs. 18.3%, $p = 0.0039$). KMA demonstrated improved 5- and 10-year OS (89% vs. 47% and 65% vs. 9%, $p < 0.001$) and RFS (94% vs. 45% and 93% vs. 34%, $p < 0.001$), favoring patients with decreased/stable SUA levels. MVA revealed that statin use (Odds ratio (OR) 0.106, $p < 0.001$), dyslipidemia (OR 2.661, $p = 0.004$), stage III and IV disease compared to stage I (OR 1.887, $p = 0.015$ and 10.779, $p < 0.001$, respectively), and postoperative de novo CKD stage III (OR 5.952, $p < 0.001$) were predictors for increased postoperative SUA levels. MVA for all-cause mortality showed that increasing BMI (OR 1.085, $p = 0.002$), increasing ASA score (OR 1.578, $p = 0.014$), increased SUA levels (OR 4.698, $p < 0.001$), stage IV disease compared to stage I (OR 7.702, $p < 0.001$), radical nephrectomy (RN) compared to partial nephrectomy (PN) (OR 1.620, $p = 0.019$), and de novo CKD stage III (OR 7.068, $p < 0.001$) were significant factors. Cox proportional hazard analysis for OS revealed that increasing age (HR 1.017, $p = 0.004$), increasing BMI (Hazard Ratio (HR) 1.099, $p < 0.001$), increasing SUA (HR 4.708, $p < 0.001$), stage III and IV compared to stage I (HR 1.537, $p = 0.013$ and 3.299, $p < 0.001$), RN vs. PN (HR 1.497, $p = 0.029$), and de novo CKD stage III (HR 1.684, $p < 0.001$) were significant factors. Cox proportional hazard analysis for RFS demonstrated that increasing ASA score (HR 1.239, $p < 0.001$, increasing SUA (HR 9.782, $p < 0.001$), and stage II, III, and IV disease compared to stage I (HR 2.497, $p < 0.001$ and 3.195, $p < 0.001$ and 6.911, $p < 0.001$) were significant factors. *Conclusions:* Increasing SUA was associated with poorer outcomes. Decreased SUA levels were associated with statin intake and lower stage disease as well as lack of progression to CKD and anemia. Further investigation is requisite.

Keywords: chronic kidney disease; nephrectomy; overall survival; recurrence free survival; renal cell carcinoma; statins; uric acid

1. Introduction

There is increasing evidence that renal cell carcinoma (RCC) is a metabolically driven disease. Many of the known genes associated with the development of RCC are involved in regulating cellular metabolism within nutrient-deprived tumor microenvironments [1–3]. Moreover, recent studies have identified components of the metabolic syndrome (hypertension, hyperglycemia, hyper-triglyceridemia, and obesity) as independent risk factors for developing RCC [4–6]. These same metabolic derangements are also risk factors for developing chronic kidney disease (CKD) [7,8], with higher morbidity and mortality in CKD patients undergoing extirpative surgery for RCC [9].

Uric acid is the final breakdown product of purine metabolism and is associated with significant health problems. Hyperuricemia, defined as serum uric acid (SUA) elevation, is correlated with development of atherosclerosis, metabolic syndrome, and of CKD after surgery for renal tumors [10,11]. Consequently, SUA elevation may be exploited as a biomarker of disease risk at the intersection of these critical pathophysiologic processes.

A growing body of literature suggests that receiving of statin (HMG-CoA reductase inhibitor) medications may be associated with improved outcomes in RCC through its purported anti-neoplastic activity and renoprotective properties [12,13]. Furthermore, recent reports suggest that SUA may be a marker of response to statin therapy [14]. Different types of statins have various efficacies at reducing SUA levels, and prolonged high-intensity statin therapy has been shown to preserve kidney function and has been associated with decreased SUA levels. [15,16]. In this study, we sought to investigate the relationship between receipt of statin medications, SUA levels, and outcomes in patients with RCC. We hypothesized that increasing uric acid was associated with adverse renal functional and metabolic endpoints which correlated with decreased survival, and that statin therapy was associated with a decreased risk of elevated SUA levels.

2. Results

A total of 905 patients were identified with appropriate SUA data between August 2005 and August 2018. Table 1 lists demographic and clinical disease characteristics.

610 patients underwent radical nephrectomy and 295 underwent partial nephrectomy. Decreased/stable SUA levels were noted in 675 (74.6%) and increased SUA levels were noted in 230 (25.4%). Patients with increased SUA levels were more likely to male ($p = 0.0393$) and obese ($p = 0.0201$). A total of 230 (25%) patients took statins medication. A significantly greater proportion of patients with decreased/stable SUA levels were taking statins (27.9% vs. 18%, $p = 0.004$), had localized RCC (Clinical Stage I/II disease, $p < 0.011$), or underwent nephron sparing surgery ($p < 0.001$).

Table 2 summarizes the renal function and metabolic outcomes in the increased SUA and decreased/stable SUA groups. Patients with increased SUA were more likely to develop de novo eGFR < 60 (38.7% vs. 18.4%, $p < 0.0001$). In addition, patients with increased SUA were more likely to have postoperative proteinuria (30.9% vs. 20.7%, $p = 0.0017$), metabolic acidosis (20.9% vs. 11.7%, $p = 0.0005$), and anemia (47% vs. 25.3%, $p < 0.0001$) when compared to patients with decreased/stable SUA.

Table 1. Demographics and disease characteristics in the decreased/stable uric acid and increased uric acid groups.

Variables	Uric Acid		p
	Decreased/Stable (n = 675)	Increased (n = 230)	
Age, years, mean ± SD	57 + 15.4	58 + 16	0.4734
Gender, n (%)			
Female	253 (37.5)	69 (30.0)	0.0393
Male	421 (62.5)	161 (70.0)	
Race, n (%)			
Caucasian	373 (55.3)	129 (56.1)	0.8273
Other	302 (44.7)	101 (43.9)	
Smoking History, n (%)	423 (62.7)	149 (64.8)	0.7366
BMI, kg/m^2, mean ± SD	27.5 + 4.7	28.5 + 6.0	0.0201
History of DM, n (%)	148 (21.9)	62 (27.0)	0.1186
History of HTN, n (%)	412 (61.0)	150 (65.2)	0.2591
Statin Medications, n (%)	188 (27.9)	42 (18.3)	0.0039
ASA Class, n (%)			
2	264 (42.3)	78 (35.6)	0.0662
3	282 (45.1)	101 (46.1)	
4	79 (12.6)	40 (18.3)	
AJCC Clinical Stage, n (%)			
I	473 (70.1)	127 (55.2)	
II	128 (19.0)	46 (20.0)	<0.001
III	67 (9.9)	41 (17.8)	
IV	7 (1.0)	16 (7.0)	
Pathology, n (%)			
Clear Cell	510 (75.6)	186 (80.9)	0.0986
Other	165 (24.4)	44 (19.1)	
Surgery Type, n (%)			
Radical	432 (64.0)	178 (77.4)	0.0002
Partial	243 (36.0)	52 (22.6)	
Preop SUA	5.45 +2.13	5.59 + 1.243	0.345
Postop SUA	5.173 +1.21	6.42 +1.20	<0.001

BMI, Body mass index; DM, Diabetes mellitus; HTN, hypertension; ASA, American society of Anaesthesiologists' physical status classification; AJCC, American Joint Committee on Cancer.

Table 2. Renal function and metabolic outcomes in the decreased/stable uric acid and increased uric acid groups.

Variable	Uric Acid		p
	Decreased/Stable (n = 675)	Increased (n = 230)	
Preop eGFR < 60	76 (11.3)	45 (19.6)	0.0014
Postop eGFR < 60	203 (30.1)	136 (59.1)	<0.0001
De Novo eGFR < 60	124 (18.4)	89 (38.7)	<0.0001
Preop Proteinuria	72 (10.7)	33 (14.4)	0.1322
Postop Proteinuria	140 (20.7)	71 (30.9)	0.0017
Preop Met Acidosis	22 (3.6)	12 (5.2)	0.1774
Postop Met Acidosis	79 (11.7)	48 (20.9)	0.0005
Preop Osteoporosis	55 (8.2)	27 (11.7)	0.2611
Postop Osteoporosis	110 (16.3)	66 (28.7)	<0.0001
Preop Anemia	106 (15.7)	55 (23.9)	0.0049
Postop Anemia	171 (25.3)	108 (47.0)	<0.0001

In Table 3, UVA and MVA regression analysis were completed for factors associated with increased postoperative SUA. UVA showed that male sex, increasing BMI, statin utilization, dyslipidemia, increasing AJCC stage, RN, and de novo CKD stage III were all significantly associated with increased postoperative SUA. MVA revealed that statin utilization (OR 0.106, 95%CI 0.06–0.19, $p < 0.001$), increasing BMI (OR 1.05, 95% CI 1.01–1.09, $p = 0.009$), dyslipidemia (OR 2.66, 95% CI 1.36–5.2, $p = 0.004$), AJCC stage III and IV disease compared to stage I (OR 1.89, 95% CI 1.13–3.15, $p = 0.015$ and 10.78, 95% CI 4.07–28.52, $p < 0.001$, respectively), and postoperative de novo CKD stage III (OR 5.95, 95% CI 3.95–8.96, $p < 0.001$) were predictors for increased postoperative SUA levels.

In Table 4, UVA and MVA were also completed to identify risk factors for overall mortality. UVA showed that male gender, increasing BMI, increasing American society of Anesthesiologists' physical status classification (ASA score), increased SUA, increasing AJCC stage, de novo CKD stage III, and RN were associated with overall mortality. On MVA, increasing BMI (OR 1.09, 95% CI 1.03–1.14, $p = 0.02$), increasing ASA Score (OR 1.57, 95% CI 1.10–2.27, $p = 0.014$), increased SUA (OR 4.70, 95% CI 2.94–7.50, $p < 0.001$), stage IV compared to stage I disease (OR 7.70, OR 2.87–20.63, $p < 0.001$), RN compared to PN (OR 1.62, 95% CI 1.08–2.42, $p = 0.019$), and de novo CKD stage III (OR 7.07, 95% CI 5.09–9.81, $p < 0.001$) were all significant predictors for all-cause mortality.

Table 5 demonstrates the result of a Cox regression analysis to investigate the association between survival time and a number of predictor variables. In the univariate analysis, increasing age, male sex, increasing BMI, increasing ASA score, increased SUA, stages II, III, and IV compared to stage I, RN compared to PN, and de novo CKD stage III were associated with survival time. On MVA, age (HR 1.02, 95% CI 1.005–1.028, $p = 0.004$), increasing BMI (HR 1.10, 95% CI 1.07–1.13, $p < 0.001$), increased SUA (HR 4.71, 95% CI 3.65–6.08, $p < 0.001$), stage III (HR 1.54, 95% CI 1.10–2.16, $p = 0.013$) and IV (HR 3.29, 95% CI 1.92–5.67, $p < 0.001$) compared stage I disease, RN compared to PN (HR 1.50, 95% CI 1.04–2.15, $p = 0.029$), and de novo CKD stage III (HR 1.68, 95% CI 1.30–2.19, $p < 0.001$) were independent prognostic factors for survival time.

Table 6 shows the result of a Cox regression analysis to investigate the association between time to recurrence and a number of predictor variables. In the univariate analysis, male sex, BMI, ASA score, increased SUA, stage II, III, and IV compared to stage I, RN compared to PN, and de novo CKD stage III were significantly associated with time to recurrence. On MVA, increased SUA (HR 9.78, 95% CI 6.48–14.77, $p < 0.001$), stage II (HR 2.49, 95% CI 1.58–3.94, $p < 0.001$), stage III (HR 3.19, 95% CI 1.99–5.13, $p < 0.001$) and IV (HR 6.91, 95% CI 3.95–12.08, $p < 0.001$) compared stage I disease were independent prognostic factors for recurrence free survival. In Table 7, we observed a positive correlation between clinical stage and increased SUA ($r = 0.188$, $p < 0.001$) and an inverse relationship between survival and increased SUA ($r = -0.317$, $p < 0.001$).

KMA demonstrated improved 5- and 10-year OS (89% vs. 47% and 65% vs. 9%, $p < 0.001$; Figure 1) and RFS (94% vs. 45% and 93% vs. 34%, $p < 0.001$; Figure 2), favoring patients with decreased/stable SUA levels. Estimated rates of OS at 5 years following surgery for the patients with elevated SUA with stage I, II and III disease were 55%, 37%, and 44%, respectively, compared with 91%, 83%, and 91%, respectively, for the patients with decreased/stable SUA ($p < 0.001$; Figure 3). There was no significant OS difference between patients with stage IV disease ($p = 0.437$; Figure 3). Estimated rates of RFS at 5 years following surgery for patients with elevated SUA with stage I, II, and III disease were 66%, 41%, 22% respectively, compared with 98%, 89%, 94%, ($p < 0.001$; Figure 4). There were no significant RFS difference between patients with stage IV disease ($p = 0.276$; Figure 4)

Table 3. Uni and multivariable regression analysis for factors associated with increased postoperative uric acid.

Variable	Univariate Analysis			Multivariate Analysis		
	OR	95% CI (Lower–Upper)	p	OR	95% CI (Lower–Upper)	p
Age (increasing)	1.004	0.994–1.013	0.473			
Sex, male (female ref.)	1.402	1.016–1.935	0.040	1.127	0.790–1.608	0.509
BMI (increasing)	1.039	1.009–1.069	0.009	1.049	1.012–1.088	0.009
ASA Score (increasing)	1.199	0.910–1.579	0.198			
Statin use (positive)	0.579	0.398–0.842	0.004	0.106	0.059–0.193	<0.001
Dyslipidemia (positive)	1.616	1.076–2.426	0.021	2.661	1.361–5.200	0.004
Stage II	1.338	0.906–1.976	0.143	1.123	0.720–1.750	0.610
Stage III	2.279	1.475–3.522	<0.001	1.887	1.131–3.148	0.015
Stage IV	8.513	3.428–21.139	<0.001	10.779	4.074–28.518	<0.001
RN (PN ref.)	1.925	1.361–2.723	<0.001	1.043	0.631–1.456	0.843
De novo CKD stage III	3.364	2.467–4.587	<0.001	5.952	3.954–8.961	<0.001
Preop SUA	1.035	0.963–1.112	0.353			

OR, Odds Ratio.

Table 4. Uni- and multivariate regression analysis of risk factors for all-cause mortality.

Variable	Univariate Analysis			Multivariate Analysis		
	OR	95% CI (Lower–Upper)	p	OR	95% CI (Lower–Upper)	p
Age (increasing)	1.008	0.999–1.017	0.081	0.989	0.970–1.009	0.267
Sex, male (female ref.)	1.459	1.081–1.969	0.014	1.352	0.844–2.166	0.210
BMI (increasing)	1.103	1.072–1.135	<0.001	1.085	1.030–1.142	0.002
ASA Score (increasing)	1.870	1.426–2.450	<0.001	1.578	1.098–2.268	0.014
Increased SUA (dec./stable SUA ref.)	10.068	7.154–14.170	<0.001	4.698	2.943–7.498	<0.001
Stage II	1.628	1.138–2.328	0.008	1.280	0.844–1.940	0.245
Stage III	2.412	1.585–3.669	<0.001	1.543	0.949–2.511	0.080
Stage IV	6.394	2.583–15.831	<0.001	7.702	2.876–20.629	<0.001
RN (PN ref.)	3.040	2.157–4.283	<0.001	1.620	1.084–2.421	0.019
de novo CKD stage III	7.618	5.571–10.418	<0.001	7.068	5.093–9.810	<0.001

Table 5. Cox proportional hazard analysis of prognostic factors for overall survival.

Variable	Univariate Analysis			Multivariate Analysis		
	HR	95% CI (Lower–Upper)	p	HR	95% CI (Lower–Upper)	p
Age (increasing)	1.011	1.004–1.019	0.003	1.017	1.005–1.028	0.004
Sex, male (female ref.)	1.364	1.060–1.756	0.016	1.051	0.803–1.376	0.718
BMI (increasing)	1.095	1.073–1.118	<0.001	1.099	1.070–1.129	<0.001
ASA Score (increasing)	1.731	1.465–2.046	<0.001	1.085	0.843–1.395	0.527
Increased SUA (dec./stable SUA ref.)	6.467	5.088–8.221	<0.001	4.708	3.647–6.078	<0.001
Stage II	1.541	1.152–2.061	0.004	1.336	0.981–1.820	0.066
Stage III	2.025	1.472–2.785	<0.001	1.537	1.095–2.157	0.013
Stage IV	7.119	4.219–12.014	<0.001	3.299	1.919–5.674	<0.001
RN (PN ref.)	2.172	1.600–2.948	<0.001	1.497	1.042–2.150	0.029
de novo CKD stage III	2.534	1.997–3.215	<0.001	1.684	1.297–2.186	<0.001

HR, Hazard Ratio.

Table 6. Cox proportional hazard analysis of prognostic factors for recurrence free survival.

Variable	Univariate Analysis			Multivariate Analysis		
	HR	95% CI (Lower–Upper)	p	HR	95% CI (Lower–Upper)	p
Age (increasing)	1.008	0.997–1.019	0.144	0.983	0.656–1.473	0.933
Sex, male (female ref.)	1.545	1.069–2.233	0.021	1.028	0.993–1.064	0.121
BMI (increasing)	1.037	1.004–1.072	0.030	1.239	0.954–1.609	<0.001
ASA Score (increasing)	1.398	1.101–1.776	0.006	9.782	6.479–14.77	<0.001
Increased SUA (dec./stable SUA ref.)	12.826	8.742–18.818	<0.001	2.497	1.584–3.937	<0.001
Stage II	2.725	1.791–4.147	<0.001	3.195	1.992–5.127	<0.001
Stage III	3.682	2.362–5.741	<0.001	6.911	3.953–12.082	<0.001
Stage IV	16.458	9.857–27.480	<0.001	1.102	0.610–1.990	0.748
RN (PN ref.)	2.146	1.309–3.519	0.002	0.838	0.575–1.221	0.357
de novo CKD stage III	1.634	1.160–2.303	0.005			

Table 7. Pearson correlation coefficient analysis of clinical stage, increased uric acid, and survival.

Variable	Clinical Stage	Increasing SUA	Survival (Months)
Clinical Stage	1		
Increased SUA	0.188 ($p < 0.001$)	1	
Survival (months)	−0.158 ($p < 0.001$)	−0.317 ($p < 0.001$)	1

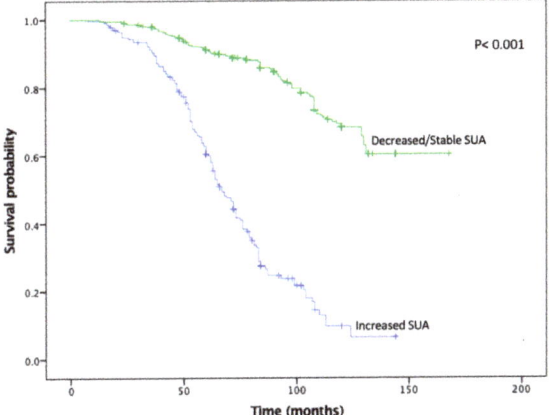

Figure 1. Kaplan-Meier plot for overall survival in the stable/decreased uric acid and increased uric acid groups.

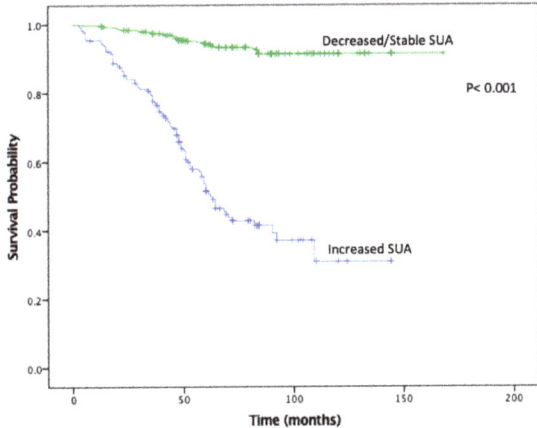

Figure 2. Kaplan-Meier plot for recurrence free survival in the stable/decreased uric acid and increased uric acid groups.

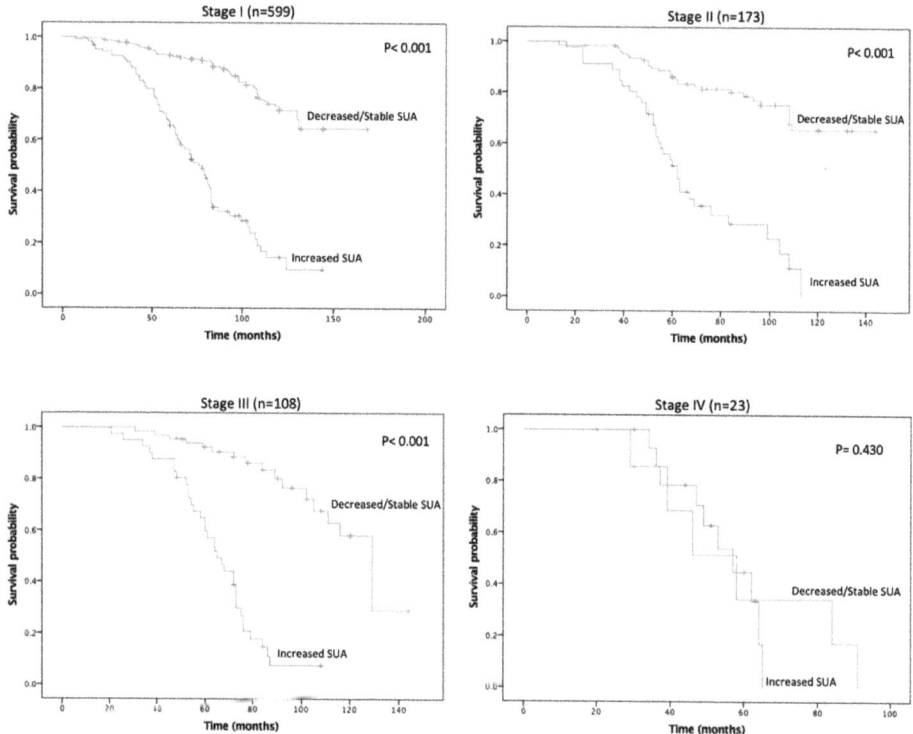

Figure 3. Kaplan-Meier plot for overall survival in the stable/decreased uric acid and increased uric acid groups, separated by disease stage.

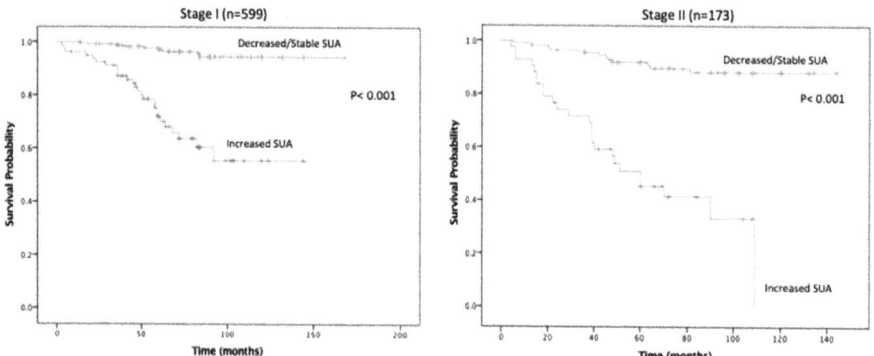

Figure 4. *Cont.*

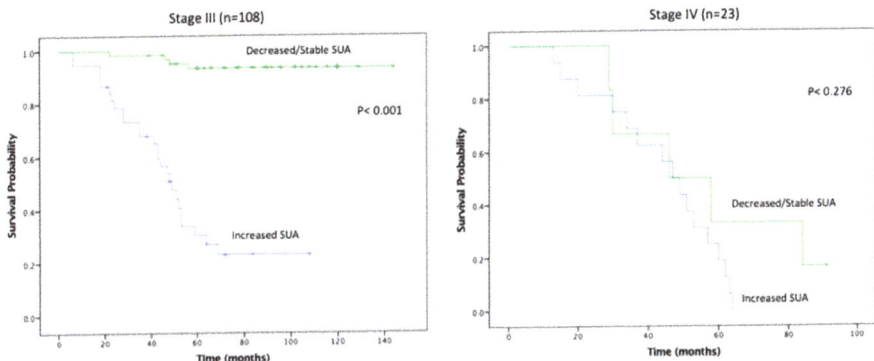

Figure 4. Kaplan-Meier plot for recurrence free survival in the stable/decreased uric acid and increased uric acid groups, separated by disease stage.

3. Discussion

This current study represents the first large and multi-institutional analysis examining changes in preoperative and postoperative SUA as a prognostic marker of survival and renal function. Our findings suggest that changes in SUA levels can predict postoperative renal function, CKD sequelae, and survival in the context of RCC treated with nephrectomy. Patients with increased SUA had increased rates of de novo CKD, proteinuria, metabolic acidosis, osteoporosis, and anemia. In addition, postoperative increase in SUA was predictive of decreased OS and RFS in Stage I-III RCC. Lastly, patients taking statins were associated with decreased SUA and this cohort had significantly longer OS and RFS.

Changes in SUA have been shown to correlate with cancer mortality in a number of non-urologic malignancies through both retrospective and prospective studies. In addition, various preclinical studies have demonstrated that increased intracellular SUA may induce the inflammatory stress response, while elevated extracellular SUA stimulates various transcription factors that promote cellular proliferation, survival, and migration. These cellular changes facilitate the transformation of normally quiescent cells to highly aggressive cancer cells [17]. A retrospective study by Yue et al. analyzed 443 primary breast cancer patients and found that elevated SUA was associated with inferior overall survival (HR 2.13, $p = 0.016$) and was an independent prognostic factor for predicting death [18]. Similarly, a meta-analysis examining 12 prospective studies spanning 632,472 subjects by Yan et al. found that high SUA levels were associated with increased risk of cancer mortality (RR = 1.19, $p = 0.010$), with a larger effect in females (RR= 1.25, $p = 0.004$) in a variety of different cancers [19]. Yuki et al. conducted a retrospective analysis of 89 patients with RCC and noted that an increase of greater than 10% in SUA was predictive for metastases ($p < 0.0001$) [20]. This was the first study to associate increased serum uric acid with oncological endpoints in renal cell carcinoma. We have confirmed these findings by noting that an increase of 10% of more of SUA was independently predictive for RFS (HR 9.782, $p < 0.001$). In addition, our KMA demonstrated improved OS and RFS in patients with decreased/stable SUA levels at both 5 and 10 years. Our subset survival analysis showed improved OS and RFS in the decreased/stable SUA group within stage I-III disease. Expanding upon the work of Yuki et al., we report the first large-scale, multi-institutional study that identifies postoperative SUA as a negative predictor for survival in patients undergoing PN or RN for RCC.

Recent epidemiological studies have demonstrated an independent association between elevated SUA and increased CKD, although the interaction between increased SUA and CKD in the setting of RCC is not well understood [21–23]. Jeon et al. reviewed data from 1534 patients and found that increased baseline SUA was associated with lower preoperative GFR in patients with RCC ($r = -0.313$, $p < 0.001$). In addition, hypertension (OR 1.37, $p = 0.075$) and elevated SUA (OR 1.23, $p = 0.002$) were associated with new onset CKD in patients who underwent PN or RN for RCC [24]. The authors concluded that preoperative SUA might be able to predict CKD after extirpative intervention in patients with RCC. Similarly, in a prospective observational study, Obermayr et al. found that in a cohort of 21,475 patients, those with SUA > 7 mg/dL were nearly twice as likely to develop CKD (OR 1.74, $p < 0.05$), while those with SUA > 9 mg/dL were associated with a tripled risk (OR 3.12, $p < 0.05$) [25]. Instead of looking at SUA as a continuous variable, we stratified postoperative SUA as either increased or decreased/stable in order to better account for the temporal changes in SUA associated with surgical intervention. Our findings are consistent with the findings of these previous reports which demonstrated that patients with postoperative increases in SUA had greater risk for development of de novo CKD. Furthering these findings, we demonstrated that patients with increased SUA had increased frequency of CKD-associated sequelae including: metabolic acidosis, osteoporosis, and anemia. Indeed, our findings and those of Jeon et al. and Overlay et al. suggest that association of rising SUA with CKD and its sequelae may point towards development of surveillance and preventive strategies to identify patients at risk for renal functional degeneration and to attempt to attenuate CKD sequelae by early intervention.

Recent investigations have also focused on identifying interventions that decrease the postoperative drops in eGFR in an effort to reduce complications associated with nephron loss in RN and PN. In a prospective, randomized trial of 54 hyperuricemic patients, Kose et al. found that atorvastatin significantly increased eGFR from 51.1 to 61.8 mL/min/1.73 m^2, while significantly decreasing SUA from 6.38 mg/dL to 5.48 mg/dL in CKD patients [26]. Siu et al. demonstrated that patients treated with 100 to 300 mg of allopurinol had significantly decreased SUA in patients with mild to moderate CKD (9.75 mg/dL to 5.88 mg/dL, $p < 0.001$) and had slower progression of CKD [27]. In addition, statins have been studied for their ability to decrease SUA in addition to other renoprotective effects. A meta-analysis of 88,523 participants by Geng et al. found that statins reduced the decrease in eGFR (SMD 0.14, $p = 0.007$) and decreased proteinuria (SMD -0.19, $p = 0.005$) in patients with early-stage CKD after 3 years of therapy [28]. Although the mechanism of action of statins on SUA has not yet been elucidated, stronger statins such as atorvastatin are more lipophilic thus are more potent at improving endothelial function and increasing glomerular filtration [17]. Additionally, it is thought that statins increase decrease proximal tubular reabsorption of uric acid and this increase urinary uric acid excretion. Our studies approached this question from a different perspective and in a slightly different patient population. We looked at the relationship between statin use and increased or decreased/stable SUA in patients that had undergone extirpative surgery for RCC. Consistent with previous studies, we found that patients taking statins were nearly 10× less likely to have an increased postoperative SUA.

In addition to lowering SUA, improving eGFR and reducing CKD progression, statins may also improve survival in patients with RCC. Recently, Hamilton et al. evaluated the effect of statin medications on RCC progression in a cohort of 2608 patients with localized RCC treated over a 15-year period. Of these patients, 699 (27%) were statin users at surgery. With a median follow-up of 36 months, they noted that statin use attenuated the risk of tumor progression to 23% (hazard ratio 0.77; $p = 0.12$) and augmented the risk reduction in overall survival (hazard ratio 0.71; $p = 0.002$) [29]. In addition, a retrospective study by McKay et al. analyzed 4736 patients treated for metastatic RCC and found that statin use was associated with improved survival (25.6 vs. 18.9 months, $p = 0.025$) [30]. Similarly, in our study, a total of 230/905 (25%) patients received statins and a higher proportion of patients with decreased/stable SUA levels were on statins (28% vs. 18%, $p = 0.004$). Taken together, the findings of McKay et al. and Hamilton et al. suggest a salutory effect of statin agents on RCC outcomes. Furthermore, our findings which demonstrated that decreased/stable SUA correlated with improved OS and RFS, and that receipt of statins was inversely correlated with elevated SUA, suggest utility of SUA as a marker of response and/or efficacy of statin agents in risk reduction for RCC patients.

The present study is limited by its retrospective design, which has inherent potential for selection biases. In addition, because this was not a prospective analysis, we were unable to examine the duration of statin therapy and its potential effects of SUA levels. Nonetheless, our study is strengthened by its multicenter design and validated by our multivariable analysis results. This represents the first attempt to utilize SUA as a biomarker for OS and RFS in RCC. In addition, we were able to confirm that statin therapy is associated with decreased SUA and can predict CKD progression. Ultimately, additional prospective investigation is required to validate these findings, further elucidate the molecular interaction between SUA and RCC and characterize SUA's clinical utility.

4. Materials and Methods

4.1. Study Population

This study was conducted in accordance with the Declaration of Helsinki, and the protocol was approved by the Institutional Review Boards of The University of California (San Diego, CA, USA), and The University of Tennessee Health Science Centre (Memphis, TN, USA). Pre- and postoperative data of 905 patients with RCC who underwent surgery between 2005 and 2018. Patients with no prior preoperative or postoperative SUA levels, history of gout, receipt of allopurinol, or incomplete records were excluded. Six week preoperative and 6 week postoperative SUA levels were recorded. Demographics, clinical characteristics, renal function and oncological outcomes were analyzed and compared.

4.2. Study Design

The primary endpoint was overall survival (OS). Secondary endpoints were recurrence free survival (RFS), development of CKD (estimated GFR [eGFR] < 60 mL/min/1.73 m^2), proteinuria, osteoporosis and anemia. Serum chemistries, including complete metabolic panel and SUA levels, were routinely assessed before surgery as a part of the preoperative evaluation and during postoperative follow up; eGFR was calculated using the modification of diet in renal disease equation [16]. Serum uric acid at both institutions was quantified utilizing a Roche assay (Roche, Basel, Switzerland) and Cobas analyzer (Roche, Basel, Switzerland) that is based on an enzymatic colorimetric method developed by Town et al [31]. Demographics (age, sex, race, body mass index [BMI] and preoperative history of diabetes mellitus, hypertension, smoking and statins medications use), disease characteristics (American Joint Committee on Cancer, TNM classification) [32], and renal functional/metabolic outcomes (development of CKD defined as GFR < 60 mL/min per 1.73 m^2, anemia defined as Hgb < 11.2 gm/dL [F], Hgb < 13.7 gm/dL [M], proteinuria defined as ≥1+ on urinalysis, osteoporosis defined as positive DEXA scan, and metabolic acidosis defined as $HCO3^-$: <23 mEq/L) associated with decreased/stable SUA were recorded.

4.3. Statistical Analysis

We defined 'increased' serum uric acid as an increase of greater than 10%, while all other values were defined as 'decreased/stable'. Our classification was based on the meta-analysis of Ricos et al. who noted an 8.6% range of within-subject biological variability [33]. Furthermore, Yuki et al. found that a threshold of a 10% increase in SUA correlated with adverse oncological outcomes in RCC [20].

Analysis was carried out between two groups: patients with increased postoperative SUA vs. patients with decreased/stable postoperative SUA compared to pre-operative levels. Statistical analysis was conducted to identify factors that were significantly associated with decreased/stable SUA after radical nephrectomy (RN) or partial nephrectomy (PN). Variables were compared between the two groups (decreased/stable SUA vs. increased SUA) using Student's t-test, ANOVA and Fisher's exact/chi-squared tests for continuous and categorical variables, respectively. Kaplan-Meier analysis (KMA) was used to calculate overall survival (OS) and recurrence free survival (RFS) by comparing increased and decreased/stable SUA groups with log-rank test. Univariate logistic regression was performed to identify factors associated with decreased SUA and overall survival. All potential explanatory independent variables identified on univariate analysis were then further examined using multivariate stepwise logistic regression. Independent variables were included in the regression models if ≤0.10 on UVA to allow us to identify the adjusted variables that affected decreased SUA levels. The prognostic significance of variables for OS and RFS was analyzed by cox regression analysis. Pearson correlation coefficient analysis of clinical stage, increasing uric acid, and survival was also conducted. All p values were based on two-sided tests of significance, and $p < 0.05$ was considered to indicate statistical significance. Statistical analysis was performed using SAS version 9.1 (SAS Institute Inc., Cary, NC, USA).

5. Conclusions

This cohort study suggests the utility of SUA as marker for survival in RCC. Increasing SUA levels was associated with worsened outcomes in patients with RCC. Decreased SUA levels were associated with statins intake and lower stage disease as well as lack of CKD and anemia. Future studies are requisite to clarify the etiology of these interactions.

Author Contributions: Conceptualization, I.H.D. and A.P.; Methodology, S.R., K.Y. and A.B. (Ahmet Bindayi); Validation, R.M. (Rana McKay); Formal analysis, K.Y., A.B. (Ahmet Bindayi) and O.A.R.; Investigation, I.H.D., R.M. (Reza Mehrazin), A.P. and R.W.; Data curation, C.F., A.B. (Aaron Bloch), A.P., S.R. and R.W.; Writing—original draft preparation, K.Y., I.H.D., A.B. (Ahmet Bindayi) and O.A.R.; Writing—review and editing, I.H.D., K.Y. and R.M. (Rana McKay); Supervision, I.H.D.; Funding acquisition, I.H.D.

Funding: This research was funded by the Stephen Weissman Kidney Cancer Research Fund.

Conflicts of Interest: The authors declare no conflict of interest.

References

1. Linehan, W.M.; Ricketts, C.J. The Metabolic Basis of Kidney Cancer. *Semin. Cancer Biol.* **2013**, *23*, 46–55. [CrossRef] [PubMed]
2. Wettersten, H.I.; Aboud, O.A.; Lara Jr, P.N.; Weiss, R.H. Metabolic Reprogramming in Clear Cell Renal Cell Carcinoma. *Nat. Rev. Nephrol.* **2017**, *13*, 410–419. [CrossRef] [PubMed]
3. Russo, P. End Stage and Chronic Kidney Disease: Associations with Renal Cancer. *Front. Oncol.* **2012**, *2*, 28. [CrossRef] [PubMed]
4. Van Hemelrijck, M.; Garmo, H.; Hammar, N.; Jungner, I.; Walldius, G.; Lambe, M.; Holmberg, L. The Interplay between Lipid Profiles, Glucose, BMI and Risk of Kidney Cancer in the Swedish AMORIS Study. *Int. J. Cancer* **2012**, *130*, 2118–2128. [CrossRef] [PubMed]
5. Lindblad, P.; Chow, W.H.; Chan, J.; Bergström, A.; Wolk, A.; Gridley, G.; McLaughlin, J.K.; Nyrén, O.; Adami, H.O. The Role of Diabetes Mellitus in the Aetiology of Renal Cell Cancer. *Diabetologia* **1999**, *42*, 107–112. [CrossRef] [PubMed]
6. Chow, W.-H.; Gridley, G.; Fraumeni, J.F.; Järvholm, B. Obesity, Hypertension, and the Risk of Kidney Cancer in Men. *N. Engl. J. Med.* **2000**, *343*, 1305–1311. [CrossRef] [PubMed]
7. Kurella, M.; Lo, J.C.; Chertow, G.M. Metabolic Syndrome and the Risk for Chronic Kidney Disease among Nondiabetic Adults. *J. Am. Soc. Nephrol.* **2005**, *16*, 2134–2140. [CrossRef]
8. Chen, J.; Muntner, P.; Hamm, L.L.; Jones, D.W.; Batuman, V.; Fonseca, V.; Whelton, P.K.; He, J. The Metabolic Syndrome and Chronic Kidney Disease in U.S. Adults. *Ann. Intern. Med.* **2004**, *140*, 167. [CrossRef]
9. Lane, B.R.; Campbell, S.C.; Demirjian, S.; Fergany, A.F. Surgically Induced Chronic Kidney Disease May Be Associated with a Lower Risk of Progression and Mortality than Medical Chronic Kidney Disease. *J. Urol.* **2013**, *189*, 1649–1655. [CrossRef]
10. Huang, W.C.; Levey, A.S.; Serio, A.M.; Snyder, M.; Vickers, A.J.; Raj, G.V.; Scardino, P.T.; Russo, P. Chronic Kidney Disease after Nephrectomy in Patients with Renal Cortical Tumours: A Retrospective Cohort Study. *Lancet Oncol.* **2006**, *7*, 735–740. [CrossRef]
11. Malcolm, J.B.; Bagrodia, A.; Derweesh, I.H.; Mehrazin, R.; DiBlasio, C.J.; Wake, R.W.; Wan, J.Y.; Patterson, A.L. Comparison of Rates and Risk Factors for Developing Chronic Renal Insufficiency, Proteinuria and Metabolic Acidosis after Radical or Partial Nephrectomy. *BJU Int.* **2009**, *104*, 476–481. [CrossRef]
12. Kaffenberger, S.D.; Lin-Tsai, O.; Stratton, K.L.; Morgan, T.M.; Barocas, D.A.; Chang, S.S.; Cookson, M.S.; Herrell, S.D.; Smith, J.A.; Clark, P.E. Statin Use Is Associated with Improved Survival in Patients Undergoing Surgery for Renal Cell Carcinoma. *Urol. Oncol. Semin. Orig. Investig.* **2015**, *33*, 21.e11–21.e17. [CrossRef]

13. Berquist, S.W.; Lee, H.J.; Hamilton, Z.; Bagrodia, A.; Hassan, A.; Beksaç, A.T.; Dufour, C.A.; Wang, S.; Mehrazin, R.; Patterson, A.; et al. Statin Utilization Improves Oncologic and Survival Outcomes in Patients with Dyslipidemia and Surgically Treated Renal Cell Carcinoma. *Minerva Urol. Nefrol.* **2017**. [CrossRef]
14. Athyros, V.G.; Mikhailidis, D.P.; Liberopoulos, E.N.; Kakafika, A.I.; Karagiannis, A.; Papageorgiou, A.A.; Tziomalos, K.; Ganotakis, E.S.; Elisaf, M. Effect of Statin Treatment on Renal Function and Serum Uric Acid Levels and Their Relation to Vascular Events in Patients with Coronary Heart Disease and Metabolic Syndrome: A Subgroup Analysis of the GREek Atorvastatin and Coronary Heart Disease Evaluation (GREACE) Study. *Nephrol. Dial. Transplant.* **2006**, *22*, 118–127. [CrossRef] [PubMed]
15. Strippoli, G.F.M.; Navaneethan, S.D.; Johnson, D.W.; Perkovic, V.; Pellegrini, F.; Nicolucci, A.; Craig, J.C. Effects of Statins in Patients with Chronic Kidney Disease: Meta-Analysis and Meta-Regression of Randomised Controlled Trials. *BMJ* **2008**, *336*, 645–651. [CrossRef]
16. Deedwania, P.C.; Stone, P.H.; Fayyad, R.S.; Laskey, R.E.; Wilson, D.J. Improvement in Renal Function and Reduction in Serum Uric Acid with Intensive Statin Therapy in Older Patients: A Post Hoc Analysis of the SAGE Trial. *Drugs Aging* **2015**, *32*, 1055–1065. [CrossRef]
17. Fini, M.A.; Elias, A.; Johnson, R.J.; Wright, R.M. Contribution of Uric Acid to Cancer Risk, Recurrence, and Mortality. *Clin. Transl. Med.* **2012**, *1*, 16. [CrossRef]
18. Yue, C.F.; Feng, P.N.; Yao, Z.R.; Yu, X.G.; Lin, W.B.; Qian, Y.M.; Guo, Y.M.; Li, L.S.; Liu, M. High Serum Uric Acid Concentration Predicts Poor Survival in Patients with Breast Cancer. *Clin. Chim. Acta* **2017**. [CrossRef]
19. Yan, S.; Zhang, P.; Xu, W.; Liu, Y.; Wang, B.; Jiang, T.; Hua, C.; Wang, X.; Xu, D.; Sun, B. Serum Uric Acid Increases Risk of Cancer Incidence and Mortality: A Systematic Review and Meta-Analysis. *Mediators Inflamm.* **2015**, *2015*, 1–7. [CrossRef]
20. Yuki, H.; Kamai, T.; Murakami, S.; Higashi, S.; Narimatsu, T.; Kambara, T.; Betsunoh, H.; Abe, H.; Arai, K.; Shirataki, H.; et al. Increased Nrf2 Expression by Renal Cell Carcinoma Is Associated with Postoperative Chronic Kidney Disease and an Unfavorable Prognosis. *Oncotarget* **2018**, *9*, 28351–28363. [CrossRef]
21. Tsai, C.-W.; Lin, S.-Y.; Kuo, C.-C.; Huang, C.-C.; Lee, D.; Chen, C. Serum Uric Acid and Progression of Kidney Disease: A Longitudinal Analysis and Mini-Review. *PLoS ONE* **2017**, *12*, e0170393. [CrossRef]
22. Perlstein, T.S.; Gumieniak, O.; Williams, G.H.; Sparrow, D.; Vokonas, P.S.; Gaziano, M.; Weiss, S.T.; Litonjua, A.A. Uric Acid and the Development of Hypertension. *Hypertension* **2006**, *48*, 1031–1036. [CrossRef] [PubMed]
23. Kang, D.-H.; Nakagawa, T.; Feng, L.; Watanabe, S.; Han, L.; Mazzali, M.; Truong, L.; Harris, R.; Johnson, R.J. A Role for Uric Acid in the Progression of Renal Disease. *J. Am. Soc. Nephrol.* **2002**, *13*, 2888–2897. [CrossRef] [PubMed]
24. Jeon, H.G.; Choo, S.H.; Jeong, B.C.; Seo, S.I.; Jeon, S.S.; Choi, H.Y.; Lee, H.M. Uric Acid Levels Correlate with Baseline Renal Function and High Levels Are a Potent Risk Factor for Postoperative Chronic Kidney Disease in Patients with Renal Cell Carcinoma. *J. Urol.* **2013**, *189*, 1249–1254. [CrossRef] [PubMed]
25. Obermayr, R.P.; Temml, C.; Gutjahr, G.; Knechtelsdorfer, M.; Oberbauer, R.; Klauser-Braun, R. Elevated Uric Acid Increases the Risk for Kidney Disease. *J. Am. Soc. Nephrol.* **2008**, *19*, 2407–2413. [CrossRef]
26. Kose, E.; An, T.; Kikkawa, A.; Matsumoto, Y.; Hayashi, H. Effects on Serum Uric Acid by Difference of the Renal Protective Effects with Atorvastatin and Rosuvastatin in Chronic Kidney Disease Patients. *Biol. Pharm. Bull.* **2014**, *37*, 226–231. [CrossRef] [PubMed]
27. Siu, Y.-P.; Leung, K.-T.; Tong, M.K.-H.; Kwan, T.-H. Use of Allopurinol in Slowing the Progression of Renal Disease Through Its Ability to Lower Serum Uric Acid Level. *Am. J. Kidney Dis.* **2006**, *47*, 51–59. [CrossRef] [PubMed]
28. Geng, Q.; Ren, J.; Song, J.; Li, S.; Chen, H. Meta-Analysis of the Effect of Statins on Renal Function. *Am. J. Cardiol.* **2014**, *114*, 562–570. [CrossRef]
29. Hamilton, R.J.; Morilla, D.; Cabrera, F.; Leapman, M.; Chen, L.Y.; Bernstein, M.; Hakimi, A.A.; Reuter, V.E.; Russo, P. The Association between Statin Medication and Progression after Surgery for Localized Renal Cell Carcinoma. *J. Urol.* **2014**, *191*, 914–919. [CrossRef] [PubMed]
30. McKay, R.R.; Lin, X.; Albiges, L.; Fay, A.P.; Kaymakcalan, M.D.; Mickey, S.S.; Ghoroghchian, P.P.; Bhatt, R.S.; Kaffenberger, S.D.; Simantov, R.; et al. Statins and Survival Outcomes in Patients with Metastatic Renal Cell Carcinoma. *Eur. J. Cancer* **2016**, *52*, 155–162. [CrossRef]
31. Town, M.H.; Gehm, S.; Hammer, B.; Ziegenhorn, J. A Sensitive Colorimetric Method for the Enzymatic Determination of Uric Acid. *J. Clin. Chem. Clin. Biochem.* **1985**, *23*, 591.

32. Edge, S.B.; Compton, C.C. The American Joint Committee on Cancer: The 7th Edition of the AJCC Cancer Staging Manual and the Future of TNM. *Ann. Surg. Oncol.* **2010**, *17*, 1471–1474. [CrossRef]
33. Ricos, C.; Alvarez, V.; Cava, F.; Garcia-Lario, J.V.; Hernandez, A.; Jimenez, C.V.; Minchinela, J.; Perich, C.; Simon, M. Desirable Biological Variation Database Specifications. Available online: https://www.westgard.com/biodatabase1.htm (accessed on 3 December 2018).

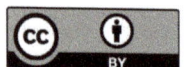

© 2019 by the authors. Licensee MDPI, Basel, Switzerland. This article is an open access article distributed under the terms and conditions of the Creative Commons Attribution (CC BY) license (http://creativecommons.org/licenses/by/4.0/).

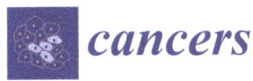

Article

Ghrelin Upregulates Oncogenic Aurora A to Promote Renal Cell Carcinoma Invasion

Tsung-Chieh Lin [1], Yuan-Ming Yeh [1], Wen-Lang Fan [1], Yu-Chan Chang [2], Wei-Ming Lin [3], Tse-Yen Yang [4] and Michael Hsiao [2,5,*]

[1] Genomic Medicine Core Laboratory, Chang Gung Memorial Hospital, Linkou 33305, Taiwan; tclin1980@gmail.com (T.-C.L.); yeh234@gmail.com (Y.-M.Y.); alangfan@gmail.com (W.-L.F.)
[2] Genomics Research Center, Academia Sinica, Taipei 11529, Taiwan; jameskobe0@gmail.com
[3] Department of Diagnostic Radiology, Chang Gung Memorial Hospital, Chiayi Branch, Chang Gung University of Science and Technology, Chiayi 61363, Taiwan; weiming276@gmail.com
[4] Department of Medical Research, China Medical University Hospital, China Medical University, Taichung 40447, Taiwan; hardawayoung@gmail.com
[5] Department of Biochemistry, College of Medicine, Kaohsiung Medical University, Kaohsiung 80708, Taiwan
* Correspondence: mhsiao@gate.sinica.edu.tw; Tel.: +886-2-27871243

Received: 21 January 2019; Accepted: 28 February 2019; Published: 4 March 2019

Abstract: Ghrelin is a peptide hormone, originally identified from the stomach, that functions as an endogenous ligand of the growth hormone secretagogue receptor (GHSR) and promotes growth hormone (GH) release and food intake. Increasing reports point out ghrelin's role in cancer progression. We previously characterized ghrelin's prognostic significance in the clear cell subtype of renal cell carcinoma (ccRCC), and its pro-metastatic ability via Snail-dependent cell migration. However, ghrelin's activity in promoting cell invasion remains obscure. In this study, an Ingenuity Pathway Analysis (IPA)-based investigation of differentially expressed genes in Cancer Cell Line Encyclopedia (CCLE) dataset indicated the potential association of Aurora A with ghrelin in ccRCC metastasis. In addition, a significant correlation between ghrelin and Aurora A expression level in 15 ccRCC cell line was confirmed by variant probes. ccRCC patients with high ghrelin and Aurora A status were clinically associated with poor outcome. We further observed that ghrelin upregulated Aurora A at the protein and RNA levels and that ghrelin-induced ccRCC in vitro invasion and in vivo metastasis occurred in an Aurora A-dependent manner. Furthermore, MMP1, 2, 9 and 10 expressions are associated with poor outcome. In particular, MMP10 is significantly upregulated and required for the ghrelin-Aurora A axis to promote ccRCC invasion. The results of this study indicated a novel signaling mechanism in ccRCC metastasis.

Keywords: ghrelin; aurora A; MMP10; invasion

1. Introduction

Cancer metastasis is one of the leading causes of cancer mortality. Approximately 30% of patients with renal cell carcinoma (RCC) present with metastatic disease [1]. Ghrelin, a peptide hormone, has been reported to promote cancer metastasis and is clinically associated with poor survival in various types of cancers [2]. However, ghrelin's function in RCC remains largely unknown. We previously characterized its impact on cancer biology other than physiological role, and found that ghrelin increased clear cell type RCC (ccRCC) migration [3]. In ccRCC, immunohistochemical analysis of ghrelin indicated that ghrelin expression was increased in cancer tissues compared to normal adjacent tissues. In addition, ghrelin expression in RCC patients was associated with poor outcomes and with lymph node and distant metastasis. Furthermore, we found, for the first time, that ghrelin increased Snail protein levels and its promoter binding activity, leading to the E-cadherin downregulation, subsequently contributing to RCC migration [3]. Importantly, cancer metastasis is a complicated process with the involvement of multiple factors and genetic events which modulate several steps for initiating metastasis including tumor invasion at the primary site [4]. However, the mechanism of ghrelin-mediated RCC invasion has not yet been elucidated.

Aurora A (STK15/BTAK/hARK1/Aurora-2), a member of the serine/threonine Aurora kinase family, plays an important role in ensuring genetic stability in cell division. Aurora A is essential for mitotic spindle formation and accurate chromosome segregation [5]. Overexpression of Aurora A can induce centrosome amplification, aneuploidy and transformation of p53-deficient mammalian cells [6]. Recently, Aurora A was reported to associate with lymph node invasion in patients with breast cancer and renal cell carcinoma [7,8]. In an experimental metastasis model, breast cancer cells with Aurora A overexpression exhibited significant invasion to lung tissue in vivo [7]. Moreover, forced-expression of Aurora A increased the migration of laryngeal squamous cancer cells (LSCC), whereas stable knockdown of Aurora A inhibited cell migration in esophageal squamous cell carcinoma (ESCC) and breast cancer [7,9,10]. In addition, the pro-invasion function of Aurora A is likely to increase matrix metalloproteinase (MMP) expression in cancer cells [11]. These reports indicate a pivotal role and requirement of Aurora A in cancer cell invasion. However, the link between Aurora A and ccRCC metastasis and the signaling mechanism with regard to altered Aurora A function remains obscure.

The results from our clinical study indicate the correlation of the ghrelin-Aurora A axis with ccRCC invasion. To date, the issue of ghrelin-dependent regulation toward Aurora A in ccRCC has not been addressed. In this study, we aimed to investigate whether Aurora A is altered and required for ghrelin-induced ccRCC metastasis.

2. Results

2.1. The Analysis of the Cancer Cell Line Encyclopedia (CCLE) Dataset Via Ingenuity Pathway Analysis (IPA) Indicates that Aurora A Is Potentially Involved in Ghrelin-Mediated ccRCC Metastasis

We first comprehensively examined the impact of high ghrelin expression in ccRCC progression by a genome-wide analysis of differential gene expression in the Cancer Cell Line Encyclopedia (CCLE) [12,13]. 15 ccRCC cell lines were separated into high and low ghrelin groups based on the ranking determined by normalized expression level (GSE36133, Figure 1A). The differentially expressed genes between the two groups were selected (Table S1, threshold: > 1.5 fold change and $p < 0.05$) for further analysis using the IPA.

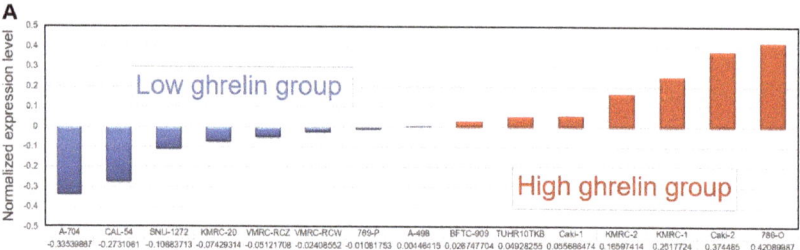

Figure 1. *Cont.*

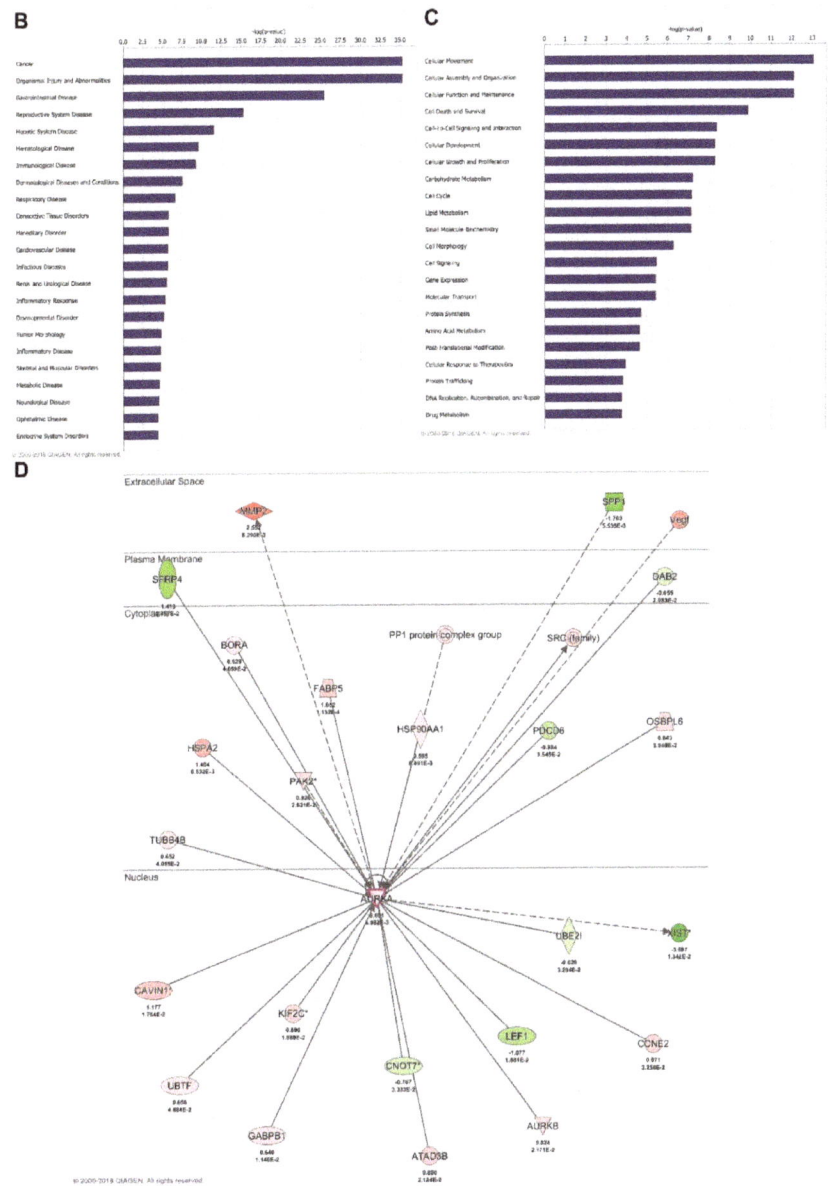

Figure 1. The analysis of Cancer Cell Line Encyclopedia (CCLE) dataset via Ingenuity Pathway Analysis (IPA) points out Aurora A is potentially involved in ghrelin-mediated ccRCC metastasis. (**A**) RCC cell lines and relative ghrelin expressions retrieved from CCLE dataset were listed. (**B**) 15 ccRCC cell lines were separated into high and low ghrelin groups. The differentially expressed genes between two groups were identified (threshold: >1.5 fold change and $p < 0.05$). Canonical pathway analysis was performed to rank the matched (**A**) Diseases and Disorders and (**C**) Molecular and Cellular Function in IPA database. (**D**) Statistical P values and log2 transformed expressions of Aurora A (*AURKA*) and its interactive network were shown. The red and green circles represent upregulation and downregulation, respectively.

Canonical pathway analysis was performed to identify Diseases and Disorders (Figure 1B) and Molecular and Cellular Function (Figure 1C) according to the matched differentially expressed genes in IPA database. The results revealed the association of high ghrelin expression with cancer and cellular movement (ranked top 1, Figure 1B,C). Furthermore, Aurora A was one of upregulated targets identified in high ghrelin group. The oncogenic role of Aurora A has been reported. However, little is known about its function in RCC progression. In addition, Aurora A's interactive network had also been explored based on clinical data that MMP2 and VEGF were also increased in high ghrelin group (Figure 1D), indicating the potential value of studying ghrelin-Aurora A axis in RCC.

2.2. Aurora A Correlates with Poor Outcome in the ccRCC Cohort

To explore the clinical relevance of Aurora A expression in ccRCC patients, a cohort of 562 clear cell-type cases from The Cancer Genome Atlas (TCGA) was analyzed [14]. The Kaplan–Meier plot showed the correlation of high Aurora A expression with poor overall survival ($p = 0.001$, Figure 2A). We confirmed the previously identified ghrelin as a poor prognostic marker in the same cohort (Figure 2B). The combination of ghrelin with Aurora A status showed the prognostic power in predicting poor RCC survival ($p < 0.001$, Figure 2C). A disease-free survival analysis also revealed the association of ghrelin and Aurora A with poor outcome (Figure 2D,E). In addition, univariate and multivariate Cox regression analysis further indicated that high Aurora A level was a significant and independent predictor for high hazard ratios (Table 1). These results show the prognostic value of Aurora A for ccRCC patients.

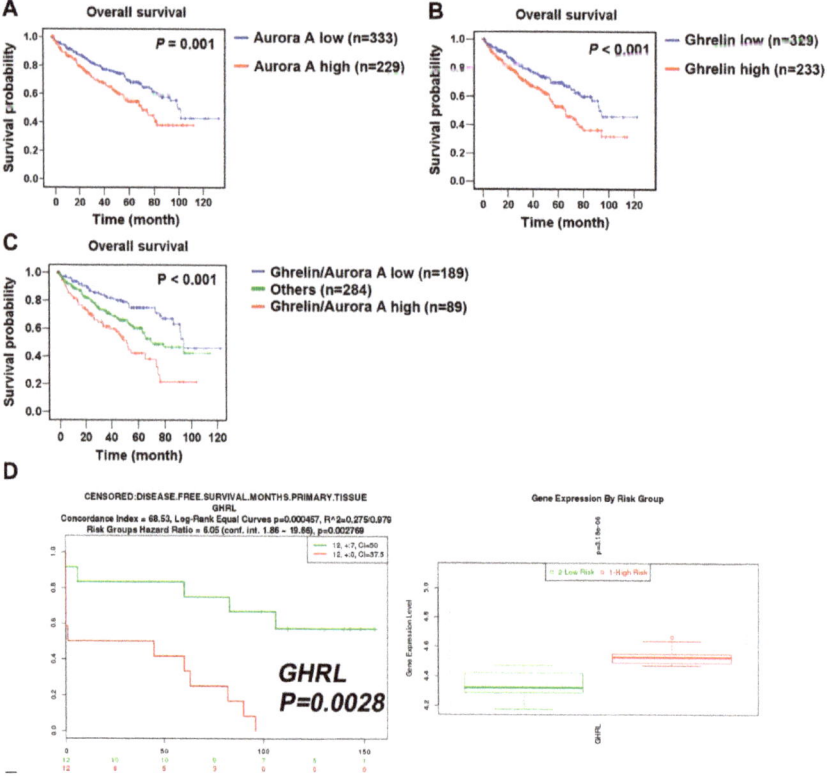

Figure 2. *Cont.*

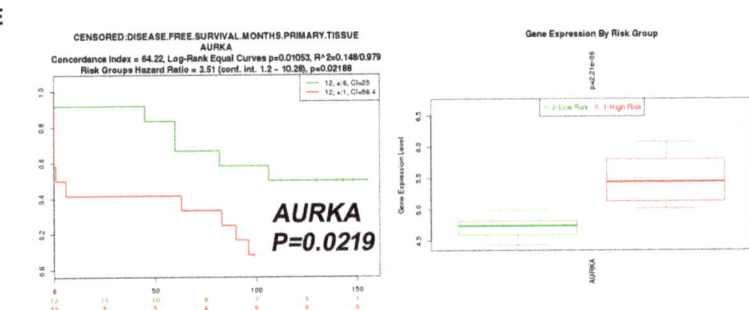

Figure 2. ccRCC patients with high ghrelin and Aurora A expression status correlates with poor outcome. Kaplan–Meier plot of cancer patients divided into high and low expression of Aurora A (**A**) and Ghrelin (**B**) were shown. (**C**) Kaplan–Meier plot of combining Aurora A and Ghrelin expression levels was analyzed. Data of 562 clear cell type RCC cases were retrieved from TCGA (KIRC gene expression (IlluminaHiSeq) dataset). The dataset showed the gene level transcription estimates, as in $log2(x + 1)$ transformed RSEM normalized count. Subgroup was determined according to the ranking in expression level of indicated genes. (**D**) ccRCC patients of high GHRL (**D**) or AURKA (**E**) expression level correlates with poor disease-free survival. Data was analyzed using dataset (Wuttig Wirth Renal Kidney GSE22541), and was retrieved from the SurvExpress database.

Table 1. Cox univariate and multivariate regression analysis of TNM prognostic factors and Aurora A expression for overall survival in 562 renal cell carcinoma patients.

Variable	Comparison	Univariate		Multivariate	
		HR (95% CI)	p	HR (95% CI)	p
T	T1-T2; T3-T4	3.422 (2.488–4.708)	<0.001	2.555 (1.599–4.083)	<0.001
N	N0; N1-N3	2.618 (1.39–4.929)	0.003	1.356 (0.698–2.632)	0.369
M	M0; M1	4.429 (3.208–6.115)	<0.001	2.707 (1.665–4.399)	<0.001
Aurora A	Low; High	1.731 (1.268–2.363)	0.001	1.645 (1.086–2.491)	0.019

Note: Cox proportional hazards regression was used to test independent prognostic contribution of Aurora A after accounting of other potentially important covariates. Abbreviation: HR, hazard ratio; CI: confidence interval.

2.3. Aurora A Expression Is Positively Associated with Ghrelin in ccRCC

We further dissected the expressional correlation between Aurora A and ghrelin. Among ccRCC cell lines in CCLE dataset, the analysis was performed using variant Aurora A probes, and a positive correlation with $\rho = 0.715$ and 0.784 was observed respectively by each Aurora A probe (Figure 3A,B). In addition, endogenous ghrelin and Aurora A protein levels were explored in a panel of seven ccRCC cell lines (Figure 3C). The data further revealed a positive correlation of ghrelin and Aurora A at protein levels in ccRCC cell lines ($\rho = 0.833$).

2.4. Ghrelin Upregulates Aurora A

Ghrelin was stably overexpressed via lentiviral infection in Caki-1 cells. In the results, ghrelin ectopic overexpression elicited Aurora A upregulation at RNA level, respectively in clone 1 and clone 2 (Figure 4A) and ACHN cells (Figure 4B). A similar effect was observed by QPCR method (Figure 4C). In Caki-1 and ACHN cells, the increased Aurora A protein upon ghrelin overexpression was further observed and shown (Figure 4D,E). The data suggest a regulatory impact of ghrelin on Aurora A expression.

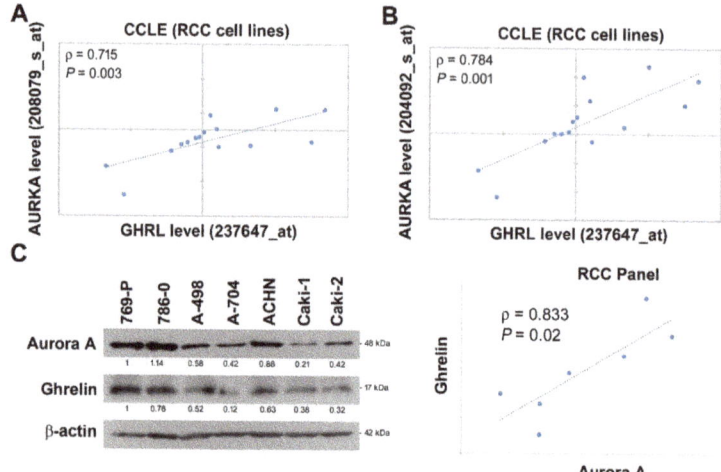

Figure 3. Ghrelin expression correlates with Aurora A in RCC cell lines. (**A**,**B**) Correlations in expression level of ghrelin and Aurora-A in ccRCC cell lines were respectively analyzed using different probes. Raw data was retrieved from CCLE dataset. (**C**) Endogenous Aurora A and ghrelin expression at protein level in ccRCC cell panel was determined by western blot method. Relative protein levels and statistical correlation were analyzed and shown after normalizing with β-actin internal control.

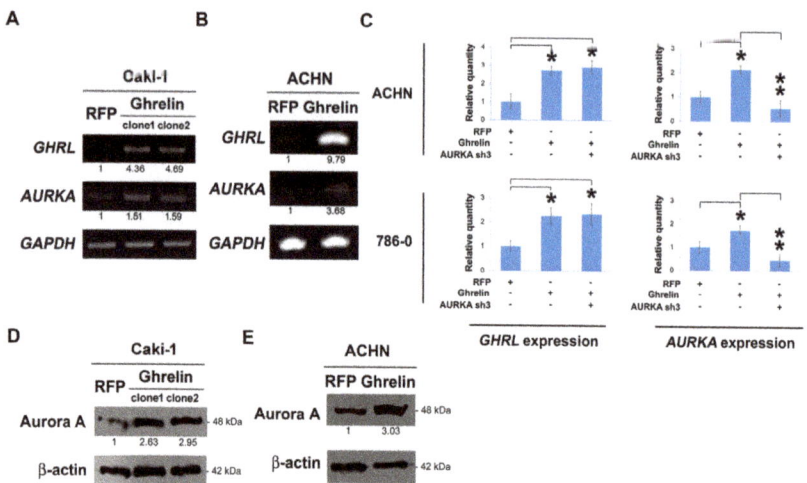

Figure 4. Ghrelin upregulates Aurora A in ccRCC. (**A**) RNA expression levels of indicated molecules were examined upon lentiviral-based ghrelin overexpression in Caki-1 cell clone 1 and clone2. (**B**) Regulation of ghrelin to Aurora A was investigated in ACHN cells using lentiviral-based overexpression method. (**C**) The modulation at RNA level was further examined by QPCR method. (**D**) The regulation of ghrelin overexpression to Aurora A protein was investigated by western blot in Caki-1 (**D**) and in ACHN cells (**E**). Figures were represented from the results of three repeated experiments with similar pattern. * $p < 0.05$, ** $p < 0.01$.

2.5. Aurora A Is Required for Ghrelin-Mediated ccRCC Invasion

Next, we aimed to explore whether ghrelin-induced ccRCC metastasis is dependent on Aurora A. Cell migration ability was first tested in ACHN cells, and the results showed the decrease in migrated cells upon Aurora A silencing in cells overexpressing ghrelin ($p < 0.001$, Figure 5A). Aurora-A was knocked down by 200 nM of specific siRNA in 786-0 cells which was the cell line characterized as having a high Aurora A background (Figure 5B). Aurora A silencing resulted in the reduction of cell invasion compared with the ghrelin treatment (Figure 5C). In in vivo metastasis model, Aurora A expression was stably reduced by shRNA in ACHN (Figure 5D) and 786-0 cells (Figure 5E) after ghrelin overexpression. Cells with Aurora A knockdown revealed the decreased lung metastasis as judged by lung nodules (right, Figure 5D,E). These data indicated the requirement of Aurora A in the ghrelin-mediated in vitro migration, invasion and in vivo metastasis in ccRCC.

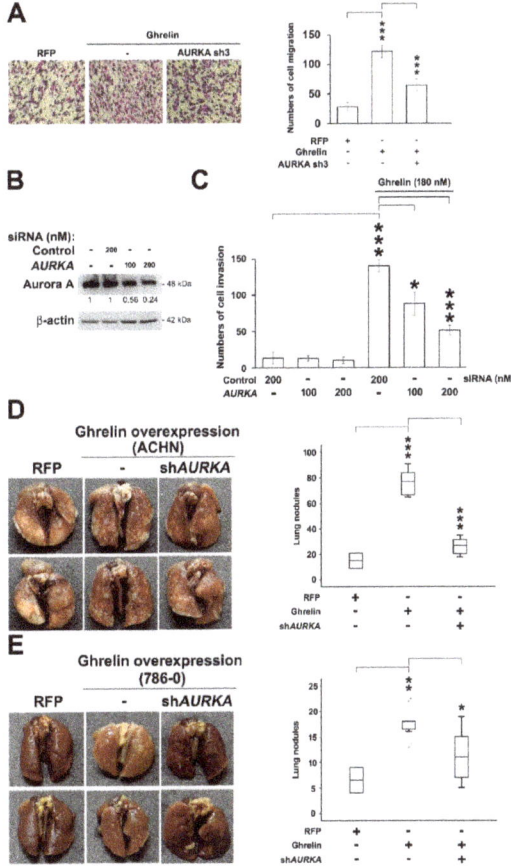

Figure 5. Aurora A is required in ghrelin-mediated RCC metastasis in vitro and in vivo. (**A**) Cell migration assay was performed by transwell devices using stable clones of ACHN cell. Numbers of cell migration in each group were counted after 5h of incubation. (**B**) Knockdown efficacy of Aurora A by specific siRNA in 786-0 cells was examined. Cells were treated with 100 or 200 nM of control siRNA or siRNA specific to Aurora A (**C**) Relative cell invasion ability in 786-0 cells upon Aurora A knockdown was studied. (**D**) RCC metastasis was investigated in ACHN cells (**D**) and in 786-0 cells (**E**) overexpressing ghrelin and combined stable Aurora A silencing. Representative images of lung surface nodule in indicated groups were showed (left). Numbers of lung nodule in each group were quantified 8 weeks after cell injection. $n = 7$ per each group (right). Figures were represented from the results of three repeated experiments with similar pattern. * $p < 0.05$, ** $p < 0.01$, *** $p < 0.001$.

2.6. MMP10 Is the Downstream Effector of the Ghrelin-Aurora A Signaling Axis in ccRCC Invasion

To study the potential regulation of ghrelin toward MMP expression that might be involved in the critical step for initiating cancer cell invasion, the association of MMPs including MMP1, 2, 7, 9, 10, 11 with cancer patient survival was explored to understand the correlation with clinical outcome. The data suggest a potentially pivotal role of indicated MMPs in the RCC invasion. In particular, the prognostic value of MMP10 in RCC was analyzed using The Human Protein Atlas database, which verified the consequences of transcript levels linking to patient survival outcomes [15–19]. The high level of MMP10 in renal cancer patients was found to be associated with poor survival ($p = 0.000284$, Figure 6A). In addition, MMP10 upregulation was reduced after Aurora A silencing in ACHN cells (Figure 6B). The impact of MMP10 alternation was examined in cell invasion test, which showed the decrease in invasive cell numbers upon Aurora A or MMP10 silencing (Figure 6C). The ghrelin receptor, GHS-R1a, was relatively silenced by specific shRNAs (clone sh2 and sh3), and knockdown of GHS-R1a blocked the signaling axis elicited by ghrelin overexpression (Figure 6D). The result indicated the increase in MMP10 level contributed to ccRCC invasion ability, and characterized the importance of the ghrelin-ghrelin receptor-Aurora A-MMP10 signaling pathway in ccRCC metastasis.

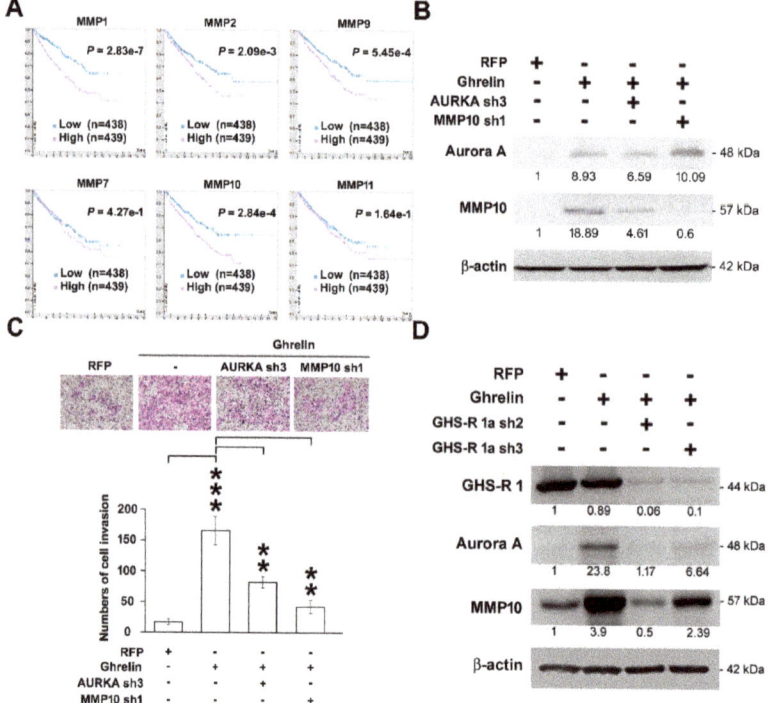

Figure 6. MMP10 is required in the ghrelin-Aurora A signaling axis to promote ccRCC invasion. (**A**) Kaplan–Meier plot showing the association of indicated MMP with RCC (TCGA) patient survival was represented. Data were retrieved from Human Protein Atlas website. (**B**) Representative Aurora A and MMP10 expression pattern in ACHN cells overexpressing ghrelin combined with Aurora A or MMP10 knockdown respectively. (**C**) Alternations in relative ACHN cell invasion ability were shown. Magnification: 100× (**D**) The regulation of ghrelin toward MMP10 expression was further studied in ACHN cells silencing GHS-R1a. Figures were represented from the results of three repeated experiments with similar pattern. ** $p < 0.01$, *** $p < 0.001$.

3. Discussion

Renal cell carcinoma (RCC), also called renal adenocarcinoma, comprises 90–95% of kidney-derived tumors, and is a form of kidney cancer that arises from the cells of the renal tubule [20]. Although RCC is relatively rare compared with other cancers (approximately 2% of malignant tumors), an alarming increase in incidence has been diagnosed and the survival of these patients is poor, with a median survival of less than one year [21]. In addition, about 30% of RCC patients present with metastatic disease, the metastatic RCC (mRCC). The common sites of metastasis include lung, lymph node, bone and brain [1]. In particular, mRCC is generally resistant to chemotherapy. Immunologic therapy with interferon or interleukin-2 (IL-2) has been the most commonly used treatment, despite low a response rate (5–20%) [1]. Hence, it is urgently required to unravel the molecular mechanisms involved in tumorigenesis and metastasis of mRCC for the development of novel target agents. We previously identified a peptide hormone, ghrelin, and investigated the function and mechanism of ghrelin in RCC metastasis [3]. The result of immunohistochemical analysis of ghrelin showed an increase in ghrelin expression in specimens obtained from individuals with disease progression and a progressive ghrelin upregulation in cancer tissues compared to normal adjacent tissues. Furthermore, ghrelin expression is correlated with poor outcome, lymph node and distant metastasis status in RCC patients. Our previous studies indicated that ghrelin could increase Snail protein level and its E-cadherin promoter binding activity via phosphatidylinositol 3-kinase–Akt signaling activation, leading to downregulated E-cadherin expression and subsequently contributing to the development of EMT and RCC migration. The study demonstrated the poor prognostic and pro-metastatic role of ghrelin in RCC. Importantly, cancer metastasis is a complicated process that requires multiple factors to elicit tumor invasion at the primary site. We first observed that MMP10 is increased upon ghrelin treatment in clear cell type of RCC, suggesting a novel function of ghrelin in promoting RCC metastasis.

In this study, we observed Aurora A upregulation by ghrelin, especially at the RNA level, suggesting a potential transcriptional activation of the *AURKA* gene. Recently, increasing reports point out that Aurora A is a target of Wnt/β-catenin signaling pathway, which is involved in multiple myeloma disease progression [22]. In particular, *AURKA* expression is driven by β-catenin transcription in VHL-null ccRCC. However, whether Wnt/β-catenin signaling is activated by ghrelin leading *AURKA* transcriptional activation remains to be explored. An investigation of the synergistic effect of hepatocyte growth factor (HGF) and vascular endothelial growth factor (VEGF) in human endothelial cells revealed the increased expression of human *AURKA* mRNA in cultured cells 24 hours after initial treatment [23]. Furthermore, co-expression of GABPA and GABPB1 proteins significantly increased the promoter (-189-354) activity of human *AURKA* gene [24]. Interestingly, both VEGF and GABPB1 were found to be upregulated in high ghrelin group in the CCLE dataset (Figure 1D), indicating the regulatory mechanism of oncogenic Aurora A upregulation that remains to be studied. In addition, *BORA* is a known Aurora A cofactor required for its kinase activity [25]. The BORA level was also increased in high ghrelin group suggesting a potential role of ghrelin in activating Aurora A in RCC. A report indicated that YY1 could suppress invasion and metastasis by downregulating MMP10 in a MUC4/ErbB2/p38/MEF2C-dependent manner in pancreatic cancer cells, suggesting MEF2C phosphorylation is required for MMP10 expression [26]. Thus far, the link of ghrelin and Aurora kinase A to MEF2C phosphorylation has not yet been studied, and this link might shed light on the molecular mechanism of MMP10 upregulation during RCC metastasis.

Similar function of ghrelin was indicated in gastric cancer invasion of which mechanism was unraveled, that is, via the activation of GHS-R/NFκB signaling pathway [27]. In addition to the modulation of cancer invasion, the ghrelin-ghrelin receptor signaling axis is pivotal in regulating cell motility and cell-cell adhesion, which led to cancer metastasis in many types of cancer [2]. Ghrelin treatment could activate PI3K/GTP-Rac signaling resulting in the actin polymerization in astrocytoma cells [28]. According to the results of a pancreatic adenocarcinoma study, ghrelin promoted cell migration via the activation of GHSR/PI3K/Akt signaling pathway, and the phenotype was inhibited by the addition of ghrelin receptor antagonist [29]. A study in colorectal cancer revealed that the pretreatment of antagonist D(Lys-3)-GHRP-6 inhibited ghrelin-mediated ghrelin receptor function and cell migration ability [30]. Moreover, ghrelin was also observed to induce cell migration by triggering the activation of GHSR/CaMKII/AMPK/NFκB signaling pathway in glioma cells [31]. In our previous study, ghrelin was found to reduce cell-cell contact in cell migration process through Snail-dependent E-cadherin repression. Taken together, the findings demonstrate ghrelin's multi-function in promoting cancer metastasis.

4. Materials and Methods

4.1. Ingenuity Pathway Analysis (IPA)

Differential gene expression signatures of ccRCC cohort divided into high ghrelin and low ghrelin groups were analyzed by Ingenuity® Pathway Analysis (QIAGEN, Hilden, Germany; www.qiagen.com/ingenuity), according to the instructions provided. After comparison of the imported dataset with Ingenuity® Knowledge Base, a list of relevant networks, upstream regulators and algorithmically generated mechanistic networks based on the connectivity was obtained. The Canonical Pathway analysis of IPA was used to rank significant Diseases and Disorders, Molecular and Cellular Functions based on the altered gene signatures.

4.2. Cell Culture

Human renal adenocarcinoma cell lines were all obtained from American Type Culture Collection (Manassas, VA, USA). 786-0 cells were maintained in RPMI 1640 medium supplemented with 10% fetal bovine serum (GIBCO, Grand Island, NY, USA), 10 mM HEPES, 1 mM sodium pyruvate, penicillin (100 unit/mL), and streptomycin (100 µg/mL). 769-P cells were maintained in RPMI 1640 medium supplemented with 10% fetal bovine serum (GIBCO, Grand Island, NY, USA), penicillin (100 unit/mL), and streptomycin (100 µg/mL). ACHN, A-498 and A-704 cells were maintained in MEM medium supplemented with 10% fetal bovine serum, penicillin (100 unit/mL), and streptomycin (100 µg/mL). Caki-1 and Caki-2 cells were maintained in McCoy's 5a medium supplemented with 10% fetal bovine serum, penicillin (100 unit/mL), and streptomycin (100 µg/mL). Cells were incubated in 95% air, 5% CO_2 humidified atmosphere at 37 °C. Ghrelin (n-octanoyl) was obtained from ANASPEC (Fremont, CA, USA). Acylated ghrelin (n-octanoyl) was prepared in ddH_2O.

4.3. Preparation of Ghrelin Expression Plasmid

Ghrelin was cloned from 293T cDNA using TAKARA DNA polymerase (Mountain View, CA, USA) according to the manufacture's instruction. The primer sequences designed were as follows: ACCCAAGCTGGCTAGCATGCCCTCCCCAGGGACCGTC (sense) and TCAAGATCTAGAATTCTCACTTGTCGGCTGGGGCCTC (antisense). The PCR products were gel-purified, digested with NheI/EcoRI, and subcloned into lentiviral expression vector pLAS3W (RNAi Core, Academia Sinica, Taipei, Taiwan). The sequences were confirmed via DNA sequencing by Sequencing Core Facility, SIC, Academia Sinica.

4.4. Animal Study

All animal experiments were conducted in accordance with a protocol approved by the Academia Sinica Institutional Animal Care and Utilization Committee (ethical code: 12-02-319, 18 October 2016). Age-matched male NSG mice (6 to 8 weeks of age) were used. To evaluate metastasis, 1×10^6 cells were resuspended in 0.1 mL of PBS and injected into the lateral tail vein ($n = 7$). Metastatic lung nodules were counted and were further confirmed via HE staining using a dissecting microscope (OLYMPUS, Tokyo, Japan).

4.5. Lentivirus-Based shRNA Production and Infection

The lentiviral shRNA constructs were purchased from Thermo Scientific (Pittsburgh, PA, USA). Lentiviruses were produced via co-transfection of 293T cells with an shRNA-expressing plasmid, an envelope plasmid (pMD.G) and a packaging plasmid (pCMV-dR8.91) using calcium phosphate (Invitrogen, Carlsbad, CA, USA). The 293T cells were incubated for 18 h, followed by replacement of the culture medium. The viral supernatants were harvested and titered at 48 and 72 h post-transfection. The cell monolayers were infected with the indicated lentivirus in the presence of polybrene and were further selected using puromycin (4 µg/mL) for 7 days. The selected stable clones were further cultured in the presence of 2 µg/mL puromycin.

4.6. Western Blot Analysis

The cells were lysed at 4 °C in RIPA buffer containing 50 mM Tris-HCl (pH 7.4), 150 mM NaCl, 1% Triton X-100, 0.25% sodium deoxycholate, 5 mM EDTA (pH 8.0), and 1 mM EGTA supplemented with protease and phosphatase inhibitors. After 20 min of lysis on ice, the cell debris was removed via microcentrifugation, followed by rapid freezing of the supernatants. The protein concentration was determined using the Bradford method. In our experiments, equivalent loads of 25–50 µg of protein were electrophoresed using a SDS-polyacrylamide gel and then electrophoretically transferred from the gel to a PVDF membrane (Millipore, Bedford, MA, USA). After blocking with 5% non-fat milk, the membrane was incubated in specific primary antibodies (Ghrelin: GTX10473, GeneTex, Irvine city, CA, USA, 1:1000; Aurora A: #4718, Cell Signaling, Danvers, MA, USA, 1:1000; MMP10: sc-80197, Santa Cruz, Dallas, TX, USA, 1:1000; β-actin: A5316, Sigma-Aldrich, Louis, MO, USA, 1:5000; GHS-R 1: sc-374515, Santa Cruz, 1:2000) overnight at 4 °C and subsequently incubated in a corresponding horseradish peroxidase-conjugated secondary antibody for 1 h. The membranes were visualized using the ECL-Plus detection kit (PerkinElmer Life Sciences, Boston, MA, USA).

4.7. Invasion and Migration Assay

The in vitro migration and invasion were assessed using Transwell assay (Millipore, Bedford, MA, USA). For invasion assay, transwell was additional pre-coated with 35 µL of 3× diluted matrix matrigel (BD Biosciences Pharmingen, San Diego, CA, USA) for 30 min. Cells of 2×10^5 in serum-free culture medium were added to the upper chamber of the device, and the lower chamber was filled with 10% FBS culture medium. After indicated hours of incubation, upper surface of the filter was carefully removed with a cotton swab. The filter was then fixed, stained and photographed. Cells invasion was quantified by counting the cells in three random fields per filter.

4.8. Semi-Quantitative RT-PCR and Real-Time PCR Amplification Analysis

Total cellular RNA was extracted by TRIzol reagent (Invitrogen, Carlsbad, CA, USA) in accordance with the manufacturer's instructions. One microgram of total RNA was reverse-transcribed using Advantage RT for PCR Kit (Clontech, Mountain View, CA, USA) at 42 °C for 1 h as described in the manufacturer's protocol. PCR conditions for rat leptin were 94 °C for 5 min and 37 cycles at 94 °C for 30 s, 56 °C for 30 s and 72 °C for 60 s, followed by a final extension step at 72 °C for 5 min by Bio-Rad icycler (Bio-Rad, Oxford, UK). For each combination of primers, the kinetics of PCR amplification was studied. The number of cycles corresponding to plateau was determined and PCR was performed at exponential range. PCR products were then electrophoresed through a 1% agarose gel and visualized by ethidium bromide staining in UV irradiation. The mRNA levels were also determined by real-time PCR with ABI StepOnePlus real-time PCR system according to the manufacturer's instructions. GAPDH was used as endogenous control. PCR reaction mixture contained the SYBR PCR master mix, 50 ng cDNA, and primers. Relative gene expression level that the amount of target were normalized to endogenous control gene was calculated using the comparative Ct method formula $E^{-\Delta\Delta Ct}$. The relative primer sequences for semi-qPCR are listed below:

GHRL_F: 5′-GAGCCCTGAAC ACCAGAGAG-3′, GHRL_R: 5′-CCCAGAGGATGTCCTGAAGA-3′ (239 bp); AURKA_F: 5′-TGG AATATGCACCACTTGGA-3′, AURKA_R: 5′-ACTGACCACCCAAAAT CTGC-3′ (208 bp); GAPDH_F: 5′-GCTGAGAACGGGAAGCTTGT-3′, GAPDH_R: 5′-GCCAGGGGTGCTAAGCA GTT-3′ (299 bp). The relative primer sequences for real-time PCR are listed below: GHRL_F: 5′-GGCATCTGACCTCCACTGTT-3′, GHRL_R: 5′-TCTAAACCAGCAACC CCATC-3′ (119 bp); AURKA_F: 5′-TTGGAAGACTTGGGTCCTTG-3′, AURKA_R: 5′-ACGTTTTGGACCTCCAA CTG-3′ (119 bp); GAPDH_F: 5′-GACAGTCAGCCGCATCTTCT-3′, GAPDH_R: 5′-GCGCCCAA TACGACCAAATC-3′ (104 bp).

4.9. Statistical Analysis

Estimates of the survival rates were calculated using the Kaplan-Meier method and were compared using the log-rank test. The association between clinicopathological categorical variables and *AURKA* expression was analyzed using the chi-squared test. Student's *t*-test was used for other statistical analyses. All data are presented as the mean ± S.D. The *p* values at the following levels were considered to be significant: * $p < 0.05$, ** $p < 0.01$, and *** $p < 0.001$. All data was represented based on three repeated experiments with similar pattern.

5. Conclusions

In summary, the analytical results from the CCLE database revealed a significant association between ghrelin and Aurora A expression in ccRCC. In addition, patients with high ghrelin and Aurora A status have poor outcomes. We further observed that ghrelin could upregulate Aurora A at the protein and RNA levels and that Aurora A plays a pivotal role in ghrelin-induced RCC invasion and in vivo metastasis. Among those MMPs identified, MMP10 was associated with poor survival in ccRCC, and the upregulation of MMP10 was induced by the ghrelin-ghrelin receptor-Aurora A signaling axis to promote ccRCC metastasis.

Supplementary Materials: The following are available online at http://www.mdpi.com/2072-6694/11/3/303/s1, Table S1: Supplementary data.

Author Contributions: This study was conceived and designed by T.-C.L., M.H.; Performed the experiments: T.-C.L.; Data analysis: T.-C.L., Y.-M.Y., W.-L.F., Y.-C.C., W.-M.L., M.H., T.-Y.Y.; Manuscript preparation: T.-C.L., M.H. All authors have read and approved the final version of the manuscript.

Funding: This study was funded by Academia Sinica and Ministry of Science and Technology (MOST 106-0210-01-15-02, MOST 107-0210-01-19-01), Taiwan to Michael Hsiao, and by Chang Gung Memorial Hospital, Linkou (CMRPG3G0612) and Ministry of Science and Technology (MOST 106-2314-B-182A-004 -MY2, MOST 107-2314-B-182A-158 -MY3), Taiwan to Tsung-Chieh Lin.

Acknowledgments: The authors thank for the help from Genomic Medicine Core Laboratory, Chang Gung Memorial Hospital, Linkou, Taiwan.

Conflicts of Interest: The authors declare no conflict of interest. The funders had no role in the design of the study; in the collection, analyses, or interpretation of data; in the writing of the manuscript, and in the decision to publish the results.

References

1. Motzer, R.J.; Bander, N.H.; Nanus, D.M. Renal-cell carcinoma. *N. Engl. J. Med.* **1996**, *335*, 865–875. [CrossRef] [PubMed]
2. Lin, T.C.; Hsiao, M. Ghrelin and cancer progression. *Biochim. Biophys. Acta Rev. Cancer* **2017**, *1868*, 51–57. [CrossRef] [PubMed]
3. Lin, T.C.; Liu, Y.P.; Chan, Y.C.; Su, C.Y.; Lin, Y.F.; Hsu, S.L.; Yang, C.S.; Hsiao, M. Ghrelin promotes renal cell carcinoma metastasis via Snail activation and is associated with poor prognosis. *J. Pathol.* **2015**, *237*, 50–61. [CrossRef] [PubMed]
4. Steeg, P.S. Tumor metastasis: Mechanistic insights and clinical challenges. *Nat. Med.* **2006**, *12*, 895–904. [CrossRef] [PubMed]

5. Meraldi, P.; Honda, R.; Nigg, E.A. Aurora kinases link chromosome segregation and cell division to cancer susceptibility. *Curr. Opin. Genet. Dev.* **2004**, *14*, 29–36. [CrossRef] [PubMed]
6. Meraldi, P.; Honda, R.; Nigg, E.A. Aurora-A overexpression reveals tetraploidization as a major route to centrosome amplification in p53−/− cells. *EMBO J.* **2002**, *21*, 483–492. [CrossRef] [PubMed]
7. Wang, L.H.; Xiang, J.; Yan, M.; Zhang, Y.; Zhao, Y.; Yue, C.F.; Xu, J.; Zheng, F.M.; Chen, J.N.; Kang, Z.; et al. The mitotic kinase Aurora-A induces mammary cell migration and breast cancer metastasis by activating the Cofilin-F-actin pathway. *Cancer Res.* **2010**, *70*, 9118–9128. [CrossRef] [PubMed]
8. Mathieu, R.; Patard, J.J.; Stock, N.; Rioux-Leclercq, N.; Guille, F.; Fergelot, P.; Bensalah, K. Study of the expression of Aurora kinases in renal cell carcinoma. *Progres Urol.: J. L'Assoc. Fr. D'Urol. Soc. Fr. D'Urol.* **2010**, *20*, 1200–1205. (in French). [CrossRef] [PubMed]
9. Guan, Z.; Wang, X.R.; Zhu, X.F.; Huang, X.F.; Xu, J.; Wang, L.H.; Wan, X.B.; Long, Z.J.; Liu, J.N.; Feng, G.K.; et al. Aurora-A, a negative prognostic marker, increases migration and decreases radiosensitivity in cancer cells. *Cancer Res.* **2007**, *67*, 10436–10444. [CrossRef] [PubMed]
10. Wang, X.; Dong, L.; Xie, J.; Tong, T.; Zhan, Q. Stable knockdown of Aurora-A by vector-based RNA interference in human esophageal squamous cell carcinoma cell line inhibits tumor cell proliferation, invasion and enhances apoptosis. *Cancer Biol. Ther.* **2009**, *8*, 1852–1859. [CrossRef] [PubMed]
11. Wang, X.; Lu, N.; Niu, B.; Chen, X.; Xie, J.; Cheng, N. Overexpression of Aurora-A enhances invasion and matrix metalloproteinase-2 expression in esophageal squamous cell carcinoma cells. *Mol. Cancer Res.* **2012**, *10*, 588–596. [CrossRef] [PubMed]
12. Barretina, J.; Caponigro, G.; Stransky, N.; Venkatesan, K.; Margolin, A.A.; Kim, S.; Wilson, C.J.; Lehar, J.; Kryukov, G.V.; Sonkin, D.; et al. The Cancer Cell Line Encyclopedia enables predictive modelling of anticancer drug sensitivity. *Nature* **2012**, *483*, 603–607. [CrossRef] [PubMed]
13. Weinstein, J.N. Drug discovery: Cell lines battle cancer. *Nature* **2012**, *483*, 544–545. [CrossRef] [PubMed]
14. Zhu, J.; Sanborn, J.Z.; Benz, S.; Szeto, C.; Hsu, F.; Kuhn, R.M.; Karolchik, D.; Archie, J.; Lenburg, M.E.; Esserman, L.J.; et al. The UCSC Cancer Genomics Browser. *Nat. Methods* **2009**, *6*, 239–240. [CrossRef] [PubMed]
15. Uhlen, M.; Fagerberg, L.; Hallstrom, B.M.; Lindskog, C.; Oksvold, P.; Mardinoglu, A.; Sivertsson, A.; Kampf, C.; Sjostedt, E.; Asplund, A.; et al. Proteomics. Tissue-based map of the human proteome. *Science* **2015**, *347*, 1260419. [CrossRef] [PubMed]
16. Uhlen, M.; Oksvold, P.; Fagerberg, L.; Lundberg, E.; Jonasson, K.; Forsberg, M.; Zwahlen, M.; Kampf, C.; Wester, K.; Hober, S.; et al. Towards a knowledge-based Human Protein Atlas. *Nat. Biotechnol.* **2010**, *28*, 1248–1250. [CrossRef] [PubMed]
17. Thul, P.J.; Akesson, L.; Wiking, M.; Mahdessian, D.; Geladaki, A.; Ait Blal, H.; Alm, T.; Asplund, A.; Bjork, L.; Breckels, L.M.; et al. A subcellular map of the human proteome. *Science* **2017**, *356*. [CrossRef] [PubMed]
18. Uhlen, M.; Zhang, C.; Lee, S.; Sjostedt, E.; Fagerberg, L.; Bidkhori, G.; Benfeitas, R.; Arif, M.; Liu, Z.; Edfors, F.; et al. A pathology atlas of the human cancer transcriptome. *Science* **2017**, *357*. [CrossRef] [PubMed]
19. Uhlen, M.; Bjorling, E.; Agaton, C.; Szigyarto, C.A.; Amini, B.; Andersen, E.; Andersson, A.C.; Angelidou, P.; Asplund, A.; Asplund, C.; et al. A human protein atlas for normal and cancer tissues based on antibody proteomics. *Mol. Cell. Proteom.* **2005**, *4*, 1920–1932. [CrossRef] [PubMed]
20. Pantuck, A.J.; Zisman, A.; Belldegrun, A.S. The changing natural history of renal cell carcinoma. *J. Urol.* **2001**, *166*, 1611–1623. [CrossRef]
21. Campbell, S.C.; Flanigan, R.C.; Clark, J.I. Nephrectomy in metastatic renal cell carcinoma. *Curr. Treat. Option. Oncol.* **2003**, *4*, 363–372. [CrossRef]
22. Dutta-Simmons, J.; Zhang, Y.; Gorgun, G.; Gatt, M.; Mani, M.; Hideshima, T.; Takada, K.; Carlson, N.E.; Carrasco, D.E.; Tai, Y.T.; et al. Aurora kinase A is a target of Wnt/beta-catenin involved in multiple myeloma disease progression. *Blood* **2009**, *114*, 2699–2708. [CrossRef] [PubMed]
23. Gerritsen, M.E.; Tomlinson, J.E.; Zlot, C.; Ziman, M.; Hwang, S. Using gene expression profiling to identify the molecular basis of the synergistic actions of hepatocyte growth factor and vascular endothelial growth factor in human endothelial cells. *Br. J. Pharmacol.* **2003**, *140*, 595–610. [CrossRef] [PubMed]
24. Tanaka, M.; Ueda, A.; Kanamori, H.; Ideguchi, H.; Yang, J.; Kitajima, S.; Ishigatsubo, Y. Cell-cycle-dependent regulation of human aurora A transcription is mediated by periodic repression of E4TF1. *J. Biol. Chem.* **2002**, *277*, 10719–10726. [CrossRef] [PubMed]

25. Macurek, L.; Lindqvist, A.; Lim, D.; Lampson, M.A.; Klompmaker, R.; Freire, R.; Clouin, C.; Taylor, S.S.; Yaffe, M.B.; Medema, R.H. Polo-like kinase-1 is activated by aurora A to promote checkpoint recovery. *Nature* **2008**, *455*, 119–123. [CrossRef] [PubMed]
26. Zhang, J.J.; Zhu, Y.; Xie, K.L.; Peng, Y.P.; Tao, J.Q.; Tang, J.; Li, Z.; Xu, Z.K.; Dai, C.C.; Qian, Z.Y.; et al. Yin Yang-1 suppresses invasion and metastasis of pancreatic ductal adenocarcinoma by downregulating MMP10 in a MUC4/ErbB2/p38/MEF2C-dependent mechanism. *Mol. Cancer* **2014**, *13*, 130. [CrossRef] [PubMed]
27. Tian, C.; Zhang, L.; Hu, D.; Ji, J. Ghrelin induces gastric cancer cell proliferation, migration, and invasion through GHS-R/NF-kappaB signaling pathway. *Mol. Cell. Biochem.* **2013**, *382*, 163–172. [CrossRef] [PubMed]
28. Dixit, V.D.; Weeraratna, A.T.; Yang, H.; Bertak, D.; Cooper-Jenkins, A.; Riggins, G.J.; Eberhart, C.G.; Taub, D.D. Ghrelin and the growth hormone secretagogue receptor constitute a novel autocrine pathway in astrocytoma motility. *J. Biol. Chem.* **2006**, *281*, 16681–16690. [CrossRef] [PubMed]
29. Duxbury, M.S.; Waseem, T.; Ito, H.; Robinson, M.K.; Zinner, M.J.; Ashley, S.W.; Whang, E.E. Ghrelin promotes pancreatic adenocarcinoma cellular proliferation and invasiveness. *Biochem. Biophys. Res. Commun.* **2003**, *309*, 464–468. [CrossRef] [PubMed]
30. Waseem, T.; Javaid Ur, R.; Ahmad, F.; Azam, M.; Qureshi, M.A. Role of ghrelin axis in colorectal cancer: A novel association. *Peptides* **2008**, *29*, 1369–1376. [CrossRef] [PubMed]
31. Chen, J.H.; Huang, S.M.; Chen, C.C.; Tsai, C.F.; Yeh, W.L.; Chou, S.J.; Hsieh, W.T.; Lu, D.Y. Ghrelin induces cell migration through GHS-R, CaMKII, AMPK, and NF-kappaB signaling pathway in glioma cells. *J. Cell. Biochem.* **2011**, *112*, 2931–2941. [CrossRef] [PubMed]

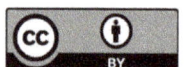

© 2019 by the authors. Licensee MDPI, Basel, Switzerland. This article is an open access article distributed under the terms and conditions of the Creative Commons Attribution (CC BY) license (http://creativecommons.org/licenses/by/4.0/).

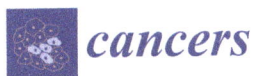

Review

NK Cell-Based Immunotherapy in Renal Cell Carcinoma

Iñigo Terrén [1], Ane Orrantia [1], Idoia Mikelez-Alonso [1,2], Joana Vitallé [1], Olatz Zenarruzabeitia [1] and Francisco Borrego [1,3,*]

[1] Immunopathology Group, Biocruces Bizkaia Health Research Institute, 48903 Barakaldo, Spain; inigo.terrenmartinez@osakidetza.eus (I.T.); ane.orrantiarobles@osakidetza.eus (A.O.); imikelez@cicbiomagune.es (I.M.-A.); joana.vitalleandrade@osakidetza.eus (J.V.); olatz.zenarruzabeitiabelaustegui@osakidetza.eus (O.Z.)
[2] CIC biomaGUNE, 20014 Donostia-San Sebastián, Spain
[3] Ikerbasque, Basque Foundation for Science, 48013 Bilbao, Spain
* Correspondence: francisco.borregorabasco@osakidetza.eus; Tel.: +34-94-600-6000 (ext. 7079)

Received: 4 December 2019; Accepted: 23 January 2020; Published: 29 January 2020

Abstract: Natural killer (NK) cells are cytotoxic lymphocytes that are able to kill tumor cells without prior sensitization. It has been shown that NK cells play a pivotal role in a variety of cancers, highlighting their relevance in tumor immunosurveillance. NK cell infiltration has been reported in renal cell carcinoma (RCC), the most frequent kidney cancer in adults, and their presence has been associated with patients' survival. However, the role of NK cells in this disease is not yet fully understood. In this review, we summarize the biology of NK cells and the mechanisms through which they are able to recognize and kill tumor cells. Furthermore, we discuss the role that NK cells play in renal cell carcinoma, and review current strategies that are being used to boost and exploit their cytotoxic capabilities.

Keywords: NK cells; kidney cancer; renal cell carcinoma; IL-2; cancer immunotherapy; tumor microenvironment

1. Introduction

Natural killer (NK) cells are large granular lymphocytes that were described more than 40 years ago [1,2]. They were initially characterized by their ability to kill cancer cells through, among others, an exocytosis mechanism of cytotoxic granules containing perforin and granzymes. Unlike cytotoxic CD8+ T cells, NK cells can directly induce cell death in the absence of prior sensitization. Over time, it has been described that besides killing tumor cells, they also kill virus-infected cells, and they have important cytotoxic activity against some healthy immune cells, such as activated T cells. In addition to their direct cytotoxic capacity, NK cells also produce cytokines as, for example, interferon gamma (IFNγ) and chemokines, such as the C-C motif chemokine ligand 3 (CCL3) and CCL4, after the ligation of activating receptors that are expressed on their surface and/or following the stimulation with several cytokines [3–10]. While NK cells are better known for their defense against viral infections and for surveillance against tumors, they are also appreciated for their participation in the generation of more efficient T helper type 1 (Th1) immunity, in the modulation of self-reactivity and of immune responses, in which their cytotoxic, as well as cytokine- and chemokine-producing capabilities have an important role [11–13]. Therefore, NK cells are currently considered to have a critical role in the maintenance of homeostasis and in the control of the immune response, promoting inflammation on the one hand, and restricting the adaptive immune response that could lead to excessive inflammation, and even autoimmunity, on the other. Furthermore, although NK cells have long been considered a part of the innate immune system, more recently have been described subpopulations of long-lived NK cells with effector functions characteristic of adaptive immunity [14–18].

2. NK Cell Development, Subsets, and Diversity

NK cells constitute 5–15% of circulating lymphocytes and represent one of the three main human lymphocyte lineages, including T cells and B cells. There are resemblances between NK cells and T cells, mostly with CD8+ T cells [4]. Nevertheless, the developmental pathways of T cells and NK cells, how they detect tumor and infected cells, and the way they get activated are different. T cells develop in the thymus and are specifically activated when their T-cell receptor (TCR) recognizes foreign antigens in the context of major histocompatibility complex (MHC) molecules, called human leukocyte antigens (HLA) in humans [4]. In contrast, NK cells mainly develop outside the thymus, and do not express specific antigen receptors resulting from gene recombination, such as the TCR and B-cell receptor (BCR). NK cells' effector functions are regulated by various types of activating and inhibitory receptors [10,14,19,20].

Currently, NK cells are classified as one of the main members of the family of innate lymphoid cells (ILCs), which are very important effector cells of the innate immune response [21,22]. ILCs respond immediately to infection and cellular damage, and also exert a very relevant influence on the development of the adaptive immune response through cytokine secretion and their cytotoxic activity. ILCs are classified into five subpopulations that could be considered the counterpart of effector T cells. Thus, ILC1 cells would be the counterpart of Th1 lymphocytes, ILC2 of Th2 lymphocytes, and ILC3 of Th17/Th22 lymphocytes. On the other hand, NK cells would be the counterpart of cytotoxic CD8+ T cells. ILCs also include the lymphoid tissue-inducer or LTi cells [21,22]. NK and ILC1 cells have a very similar phenotype, as well as similar effector functions, especially in relation to the pattern of cytokines that they secrete, which is mainly IFNγ. However, they differ in that ILC1 exhibits very little or no cytotoxic activity due to the low or zero levels of perforin and granzymes they express. In addition, they have a different expression pattern of transcription factors. NK cells require and express Eomes and T-bet transcription factors for their development, while ILC1 only express and require T-bet [21,22]. Moreover, with the exception of NK cells, many of which circulate, ILCs are primarily located in tissues.

Human NK cells are classically identified by the absence of TCR/CD3 and the presence of the CD56 molecule. Based on the intensity of CD56 receptor expression, NK cells are basically divided into two subpopulations: CD56^{dim} and CD56^{bright} [3,23,24]. The CD56^{dim} subset expresses low levels of the receptor, constitutes 90–95% of circulating NK cells, and is characterized by increased cytotoxic activity against targets and a lower capacity for cytokine production, such as IFNγ, in response to stimulation with interleukins such as IL-2, IL-12, IL-15, and IL-18. In addition, CD56^{dim} cells express the low affinity receptor for the Fc portion of immunoglobulin G (IgG) or FcγRIII, also called CD16, which is responsible for the antibody-dependent cellular cytotoxicity (ADCC). In contrast, CD56^{bright} cells express high levels of CD56, are the majority in secondary lymphoid tissues (SLT), have a lower cytotoxic capacity, and due to the low or null expression of CD16, also have less ADCC. On the contrary, they secrete higher levels of cytokines in response to the stimulation with interleukins [3,23,24]. In addition to the CD56^{dim} and CD56^{bright} NK cells, two more subsets have been described: CD56^{neg} and unconventional CD56^{dim} (unCD56^{dim}) NK cells, the latter are characterized by the absence of CD16 expression [25]. These two subsets are present at very low frequencies in healthy donors and under homeostatic conditions. However, they are expanded in certain situations. For example, CD56^{neg} NK cells are expanded in human immunodeficiency virus (HIV)-infected patients with high viremia [26,27], and the unCD56^{dim} subset significantly increases in lymphopenic environments of patients after haploidentical hematopoietic stem cell transplantation (haplo-HSCT) [28,29]. Lastly, considering that CD56 is also expressed on ILC1 cells, more precise markers, such as NKp80, are also necessary to unequivocally identify NK cells [23].

Human NK cells develop from CD34+ hematopoietic stem cells (HSC) in the bone marrow [30]. These HSC differentiate first into lymphoid-primed multipotential progenitors (LMPP), which then become a common lymphoid progenitor (CLP). These CLPs further differentiate into NK cell progenitors (NKP) that are classified into three sequential stages of maturation, named NK cell progenitors (stage 1), pre-NK cells (stage 2), and immature NK cells (stage 3). The early stages of NK cell development and differentiation have been characterized in the context of the bone marrow niche, but pre-NK cells can be detected in the circulation, and other data have shown that they are enriched in extramedullary tissues where subpopulations of mature NK cells reside, suggesting that they have developed locally [3,25,31]. It is known that some NKPs are selectively enriched in SLT, such as lymph nodes and tonsils, as well as in the gastrointestinal tract, liver, and uterus [32–37]. The most accepted model of NK cell development occurs in the linear fashion just described above, in which the expression of CD94 marks the commitment to the CD56^{bright} stage (stage 4), that next differentiate into CD56^{dim} NK cells (stages 5 and 6) [25,31]. The differentiation into adaptive (also called memory) CD56^{dim} NK cells could subsequently occur after viral infection, as, for example, the human cytomegalovirus [25]. The CD56^{neg} cells are probably exhausted CD56^{dim} NK cells, although this has not been well-proven yet [25]. Related to the unCD56^{dim} NK cells, it has been suggested that they are an intermediate stage of differentiation between CD56^{bright} and CD56^{dim} NK cells [25]. The support for the linear model comes from analysis of NK cells in SLT and in vitro studies. However, more recent evidence also suggests the existence of a branched model in which different precursor populations can develop independently in distinct subsets of mature NK cells, that is, CD56^{bright}, CD56^{dim}, and adaptive NK cells [38].

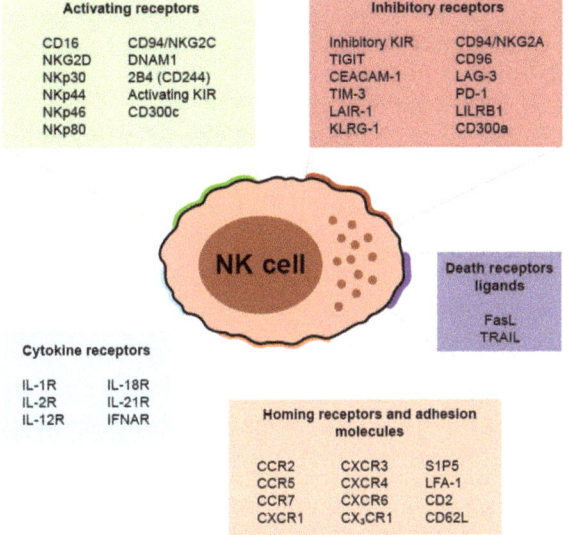

Figure 1. Surface receptor repertoire of human natural killer (NK) cells. DNAM1: DNAX accessory molecule 1. KIR: Killer-cell immunoglobulin-like receptors. TIGIT: T-cell immunoreceptor with Ig and ITIM domains. CEACAM-1: Carcinoembryonic antigen-related cell adhesion molecule 1. TIM-3: T-cell immunoglobulin and mucin-domain containing 3. LAIR-1: Leukocyte-associated immunoglobulin-like receptor 1. KLRG-1: Killer cell lectin-like receptor subfamily G member 1. LAG-3: Lymphocyte activation gene 3. PD-1: Programmed cell death protein 1. LILRB1: Leukocyte immunoglobulin-like receptor subfamily B member 1. FasL: First apoptosis signal ligand. TRAIL: Tumor necrosis factor-related apoptosis-inducing ligand. CCR: C-C chemokine receptor. CXCR: C-X-C chemokine receptor. CX3CR: CX3C chemokine receptor. S1P5: Sphingosine-1-Phosphate receptor 5. LFA-1: Lymphocyte function-associated antigen 1.

NK cells express a wide range of receptors on their surface, some of which are quite cell-specific in their expression [3,14,19,20,23]. Among them, NK cells express activating and inhibitory receptors, death receptor ligands, cytokine receptors, and homing and adhesion molecules (Figure 1). Some of the cell surface receptors are associated with developmental stages. For example, CD94/NKG2A is expressed on all CD56^{bright} NK cells (stage 4) and in a subset of CD56^{dim} NK cells in stage 5, while CD57 is a surface marker of replicative senescence and terminally differentiated CD56^{dim} NK cells in stage 6 [23,25]. Here, it is very important to note that research performed in recent years have established that in each individual and in any tissue, the population of NK cells is much more diverse than previously appreciated in terms of developmental, phenotypic, and functional parameters. In fact, it is clear that the traditional view of the NK cell lineage as a population of cells with very few subsets (i.e., CD56^{bright} and CD56^{dim}), and relatively similar functions, is not entirely accurate. On the contrary, the NK cell lineage is remarkably diverse [23,39]. New technological approaches are helping the scientific community to characterize the NK cell lineage in depth. For example, by simultaneously analyzing 37 parameters on peripheral blood NK cells, an extraordinary degree of diversity was revealed, with there being an estimated 6,000 to 30,000 NK cell subsets within a given individual [40]. Also, single cell transcriptomics studies have revealed tissue-specific gene signatures that allow identification of NK cell populations that differ between tissues [41,42].

3. Cell Surface Receptors and Cytotoxic Mechanisms

NK cells induce cell death primarily through two different mechanisms. The most-studied route is degranulation, through which they release cytotoxic granules containing the pore-forming molecule perforin and death-inducing enzymes, such as granzymes, when activated against the target cell [43–45]. This pathway is triggered by activation signals from cell surface receptors. Other routes by which NK cells can kill target cells are the death receptors' pathways: the tumor necrosis factor (TNF)-related apoptosis-inducing ligand (TRAIL)-TRAIL receptor (TRAILR), and the first apoptosis signal (FAS)-FAS ligand (FASL), also known as the CD95-CD95L pathway. Instead of triggering the release of cytotoxic granules, death receptor pathways induce apoptosis through the activation of caspases within the target cell leading to cytotoxicity regardless of activating receptor-mediated signals that control NK cell degranulation [46–48].

NK cell degranulation and the subsequent killing of the target cell is a very well-regulated process, so that the lytic granules are transported to the interface formed with the target cell and their contents (perforin and granzymes) are secreted in it. To carry this out, it is required for the NK cell to be in contact with the target cell, forming an immunological synapse [49–52]. This is a complex and very dynamic three-dimensional structure with intense activity of biochemical signals between the cells. Numerous molecules that participate in the immunological synapse have been identified, including surface receptors, signaling molecules, cytoskeleton elements, and cellular organelles [49–51]. The formation of a lytic immunological synapse of NK cells involves many stages that occur in a linear manner, in order to guarantee the secretion of perforin and granzymes present in the lytic granules towards the place of contact between the target cell and the NK cell, thus avoiding possible damage to the healthy cells that may be in the vicinity [49,50].

Moreover, NK cells can detect antibody-coated cells through CD16, thereby exerting ADCC and cytokine secretion. CD16 is coupled to the signal transduction polypeptides, also called adaptor proteins, CD3ζ and FcRγ, that contain ITAMs (immunoreceptor tyrosine-based activation motifs) [53,54]. In addition to ADCC, NK cells exert natural (direct) cytotoxicity against target cells in the absence of antibodies. Natural cytotoxicity receptors, or NCRs (NKp46, NKp44, and NKp30) are also potent activating receptors linked to the adaptor proteins CD3ζ, FcRγ, or DAP12 [55]. Other activation receptors include the NKG2D homodimer (which is associated with DAP10), DNAM1, 2B4 (CD244), CD94/NKG2C, CD300c, and so forth [14,56–58]. A characteristic of several NK cell-activating receptors lies in their ability to detect molecules induced under conditions of cellular stress [59,60]. This is the case of the NKG2D receptor, which interacts with several ligands (MICA, MICB, and ULBP1-6), which are not expressed or do so at very low levels in most tissues, but which are overexpressed as a consequence of cellular stress, such as during the DNA damage response [61]. Another example is the B7-H6, an NKp30 receptor ligand, which is not detected in healthy cells but is expressed in certain tumor cells [62].

In the mid-1980s, Kärre and his colleagues pioneered the "missing self" hypothesis, which describes the lack of expression of MHC class I molecules (self) in target cells as the common element that determines their susceptibility to NK cell-mediated lysis [10,63]. Loss of expression of MHC class I molecules can occur when cells are altered by viral infection or malignant transformation, thus being susceptible to NK cell killing. In contrast, healthy cells, by expressing MHC class I molecules, are protected from NK cells' lysis. The recognition of the "missing self" is explained by the expression on the NK cell surface of a variety of specific inhibitory receptors for MHC class I molecules. These receptors include the polygenic and highly polymorphic family of inhibitory KIRs (killer-cell immunoglobulin-like receptors) in humans, Ly49 lectin molecules in mice, and CD94/NKG2A in both species [10,14,19,64,65]. In humans, while the CD94/NKG2A heterodimeric receptor binds to the HLA-E molecule, a non-classical HLA class I molecule, KIRs do bind to the classic HLA-A, -B, and -C molecules [19]. These MHC class I specific inhibitory receptors possess a long intracellular tail with one or more immunoreceptor tyrosine-based inhibitory motifs (ITIMs) that are responsible for the transmission of the inhibitory signal [66,67]. Certain subpopulations of NK cells also express the LILRB1 inhibitor receptor, also known as ILT2 and CD85j, whose ligands are a subgroup of HLA class I molecules [14]. In addition to these MHC class I specific receptors, there are other inhibitory receptors expressed by NK cells, such as TIGIT, LAIR-1, CD300a, and so forth [14,27,68].

The preservation or elimination of target cells with the consequent production of cytokines and chemokines will therefore depend on the result of the integration of activating and inhibitory signals originating from the NK cell surface receptors [20]. NK cells do not lyse healthy cells expressing MHC class I molecules and/or low or null expression of stress-induced molecules and other activating receptor ligands. On the contrary, they selectively kill target cells that have low levels of MHC class I expression and/or are expressing adequate levels of stress-induced molecules, such as NKG2D ligands, and other ligands for activating receptors [57,62] (Figure 2).

In addition to the important role of NK cells in the development of an adequate immune response against tumors and pathogens, it is also essential to maintain tolerance towards the host. This is achieved through a process called education or licensing, which is governed by the interaction of inhibitory receptors (KIR, Ly49, and CD94/NKG2A) with their ligands, the MHC class I molecules, during NK cell development [69–73]. Education could be defined as the process through which a NK cell is programmed to exert its effector functions and is calibrated to be inhibited by its own MHC class I molecules. In general terms, the education of a NK cell by a specific MHC class I molecule is defined by its ability to detect the decrease of that MHC class I molecule in a target cell that can be lysed [69,70,73]. In humans, up to 15 genes on chromosome 19 encode for KIR receptors. *KIR* genes are grouped into haplotypes and expressed in a stochastic manner, so that in a given individual there are various subpopulations of NK cells according to the number of KIR receptors they express [74,75]. Therefore, within a given repertoire, an individual can have educated NK cells, that is, those that during their development have interacted with their own MHC class I molecules, as well as uneducated NK cells, which are those that during their development have not interacted with MHC class I molecules [69,70].

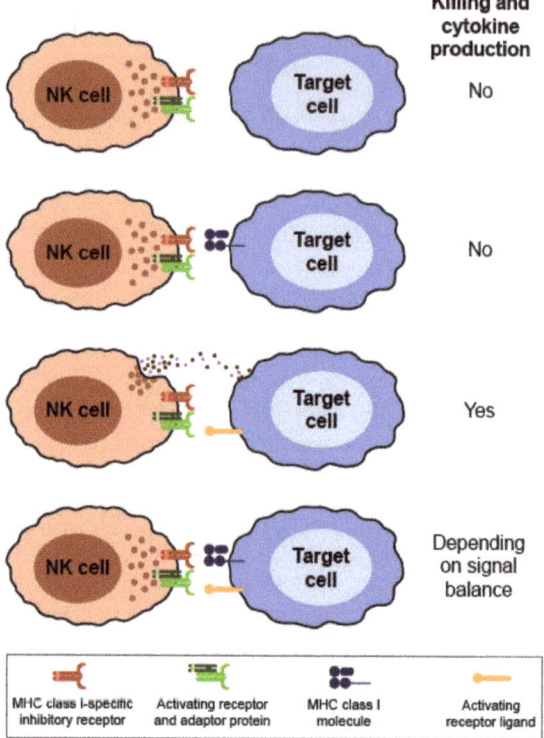

Figure 2. Activating and inhibitory signaling balance determines NK cell killing and cytokine production. Target cells expressing ligands for activating receptors trigger NK activation. When target cells also express ligands for inhibitory receptors, NK cell activation will depend on the signal balance.

4. NK Cells in Cancer Immunotherapy

More than 15 years have passed since the introduction of the pioneering works that established the potential of NK cells to mediate tumor regression. These studies demonstrated that NK cells from a haploidentical donor can prevent relapse after haplo-HSCT and also are able to induce remission after infusion of mature NK cells in patients with acute myeloid leukemia (AML) [76,77].

Several cytokines are currently being used in humans in terms of their ability to stimulate NK cell activity, at least partially, against tumors. Recombinant IL-2 was the first cytokine tested to stimulate the immune response in cancer patients [78–80]. Although early studies established the proof of concept of the therapeutic anti-tumor potential of IL-2, the responses were limited and its toxicity was substantial when used at high doses [81]. Later on, it was shown that a low dose of IL-2 had a lower toxicity profile, and it has been incorporated into an increasing number of assays to induce in vivo expansion and persistence of effector cells, such as NK cells, during adoptive cell therapy [77,82]. However, it should be noted that the use of low doses of IL-2 can also stimulate and expand regulatory T (Treg) cells, which suppress, among others, the proliferation and cytotoxicity of NK cells [83]. New variants of IL-2, such as those that selectively bind to the β-subunit of the IL-2 receptor (IL-2Rβ) expressed on NK cells, rather than the IL-2Rα subunit expressed in Treg cells, could provide better results [79,84,85]. IL-15 selectively stimulates CD8+ T cells and NK cells and prevents undesirable mobilization of Treg cells [86,87]. The first clinical trial with single-chain IL-15 (scIL-15) in cancer patients exhibited high dose-dependent toxicity [88]. Nevertheless, when used after the adoptive infusion of NK cells in patients with AML, scIL-15 promoted the persistence and proliferation of NK cells [80,89]. Importantly, IL-15 superagonists are being developed. An example is ALT-803, a complex consisting of a homodimer of mutated IL-15 linked to a fusion protein formed by the α-chain of IL-15R (IL-15Rα) and the Fc fragment of IgG1 [90,91]. ALT-803 has better pharmacokinetic properties, a longer half-life in lymphoid tissues, and importantly, has greater anti-tumor activity compared to scIL-15 [92]. Other than cytokines, there are several drugs that can directly and/or indirectly increase NK cell function in vivo. For example, lenalidomide indirectly increases the cytotoxicity and proliferation of NK cells through the release of IL-2 and IFNγ from surrounding T cells and the production of cytokines by dendritic cells [80,93].

Immune checkpoint inhibitors provide a blockade of inhibitory receptors [94]. PD-1 (programmed cell death protein 1) is expressed in activated T cells and NK cells [95], and along with its ligand PD-L1, has a central role in tumor recurrence and progression, since signaling through this pathway suppresses lymphocytes, including NK cells [80,95]. In vitro and in vivo experiments have shown that PD-1 and PD-L1 blockades elicit a strong NK cell response that is required for the full effect of the immunotherapy [80,96,97]. PD-1 blockade also increases ADCC mediated by NK cells and improves their traffic to tumors [80,97]. In addition, NK cells are able to express PD-L1, and it has been shown that the anti-PD-L1 monoclonal antibody (mAb) acts on PD-L1+ NK cells against PD-L1- tumor cells [98]. Other checkpoints that are mostly expressed in NK cells include, among others, KIR, CD94/NKG2A, and TIGIT [14,19,64,99,100]. Preclinical studies and clinical trials are currently studying the efficacy of the blockade of these checkpoints [94]. For example, anti-KIR mAbs increase tumor cell lysis mediated by NK cells and enhance ADCC in vitro [101,102]. Also, there are several clinical trials in phase I/II that have been completed or are still recruiting patients with anti-KIR mAbs, alone or in combination with other checkpoint inhibitors [94,103–106]. Related to CD94/NKG2A, it has been demonstrated that blocking its expression by means of a single-chain variable fragment derived from an anti-NKG2A Ab linked to endoplasmic reticulum retention domains overcomes (HLA-E+) tumor resistance to NK cells [107]. Furthermore, it has been demonstrated that the anti-NKG2A mAb monalizumab stimulates anti-tumor immunity by promoting NK cells and CD8+ T cells effector functions [108]. Tumor-associated NK cells also exhibit high expression levels of the checkpoint inhibitory receptor TIGIT, and mAb-mediated blockade of this receptor prevents NK cell exhaustion and elicits potent anti-tumor immunity [109]. Several clinical trials are going on, testing the safety and efficacy of anti-TIGIT mAbs alone or in combination with other mAbs [94].

Antibodies have also been used to direct NK cells to kill tumors. Monoclonal antibodies induce the death of tumor cells through several mechanisms, including growth receptor blockade, complement activation, and ADCC [110]. Also, the impact of polymorphisms on the gene encoding CD16 in response to mAb treatment has demonstrated the importance of NK cells in mediating the anti-tumor responses through ADCC. There is a single nucleotide polymorphism in CD16 that results in an amino acid substitution at position 158 (CD16-F158V), and NK cells with the CD16-158V genotype have a higher affinity for IgG1 and IgG3 than those with the CD16-158F genotype, and perform ADCC more efficiently. This polymorphism reinforces ADCC in vivo, such that, for example, patients with lymphoma that are homozygous for CD16-158V show substantially higher response rates after treatment with rituximab than those with CD16-158F polymorphism [111–113].

BiKEs and TriKEs (bi- and tri-specific killer engagers) are molecules that act through ADCC by cross-linking epitopes in tumor cells with the CD16 receptor in NK cells [7,80,114]. These molecules have advantages over mAbs because they bind to a different epitope of the CD16 molecule, and results in an NK cell with a more potent ADCC [115,116]. In vitro, the CD16xCD33 BiKE is even capable of overcoming the KIR-mediated inhibitory signal, leading to robust cytokine production and the death of myeloid malignant cells [115,116]. In vivo, treatment with the CD16xCD33 BiKE successfully reversed myeloid-derived suppressor cells' (MDSCs) immunosuppression of NK cells and induced killing of CD33+ MDSCs and CD33+ myelodysplastic syndrome (MDS) targets [116]. More recently, it has been shown that NK cells treated with a CD16xCD33xIL-15 TriKE proliferate and became activated to overcome dysfunctional NK cells found in MDS [117]. Moreover, IL-15 treatment alone induces the expression of TIGIT, but not when IL-15 is presented in the context of the TriKE [117]. The design of a trifunctional NK cell engager consisting of mAb fragments targeting the activating receptor NKp46 together with a tumor antigen and an Fc fragment to promote ADCC via CD16 has also been described [118]. The authors showed that this trifunctional NK cell engager exhibited superior killing capacity compared with the available therapeutic mAbs in vitro and in vivo [118].

Another strategy is to make tumor cells more susceptible to NK cell-mediated lysis. In this sense, TRAIL, which is expressed in NK cells, triggers apoptosis in TRAILR-positive tumor cells by initiating excision of caspase 8 [119], and it occurs independently of the signals from inhibitory receptors such as CD94/NKG2A and KIR. Exposing tumor cells to proteasome inhibitors such as bortezomib and carfilzomib, which simultaneously positively regulate the expression of TRAILR, make tumor cells more sensitive to NK cell-mediated lysis [120]. Proteasome inhibitors can also sensitize tumor cells to NK cells through positive regulation of NKG2D ligands on the surface of the tumor cells [121].

Other therapeutic strategies consist in the infusion of NK cells into cancer patients. This allows the possibility of manipulating them before infusion. The adoptive transfer of ex vivo activated allogeneic NK cells in the short term can induce clinical responses in patients with AML and in patients with multiple myeloma [77,122]. Many of these clinical trials involve chemotherapy with fludarabine and cyclophosphamide, with or without irradiation as a preparatory regimen to prevent rejection of infused cells, to provide space for persistence and expansion of infused cells and eradicate suppressor cell populations that inhibit NK cell function. Haploidentical NK cells stimulated for a short period of time with high doses of IL-2 before infusion have been used. In addition, the administration of IL-2 after the transfer of adoptive cells is able to further promote the in vivo expansion of infused NK cells, improving objective response rates [77]. More recently, the efficacy and safety of cytokine-induced memory-like (CIML) NK cells have been explored [123]. These CIML NK cells are generated after their exposure for 16–18 hours to a cocktail of IL-12, IL-15, and IL-18. CIML NK cells have increased effector functions (cytotoxicity and cytokine production) after a resting period and a longer half-life [124–128]. Clinical trials have shown its effectiveness in the treatment of patients with an AML refractory to standard treatments [123]. Other methods of adoptive cell therapy involve the ex vivo expansion of NK cells. In contrast to cytokine stimulation for a short period of time, ex vivo expansion allows the use of multiple infusions of highly activated NK cells [80,129–132]. The development of efficient methods to genetically manipulate NK cells has been seen as a necessity to optimize their persistence in vivo, as well as their location and cytotoxicity against the tumor cells after the adoptive transfer [133–135]. Finally, clinical trials are being conducted in which NK cells expressing CAR (chimeric antigen receptor) are administered to patients, after having proven their efficacy in preclinical models [134–138].

5. NK Cells and Renal Cell Carcinoma

Renal cell carcinoma (RCC) is the most common type of kidney cancer in adults, representing about 85% of diagnoses. This type of cancer develops in the proximal renal tubules, and about 70% of RCCs are made up of clear cells. Other less common kidney cancers include urothelial carcinoma, sarcoma, lymphoma, and the Wilms tumor, where the latter is the most common kidney cancer in children.

Several works have reported the presence of NK cells in RCC [139–143] where they may represent a critical component of the anti-tumor response as shown by the association of the NK cell infiltrate with patients' survival [140,141,144–148]. NK cells also infiltrate RCC lung metastasis, and high NK numbers have been associated with improved survival [145]. Nevertheless, despite the NK cell infiltration, tumors are able to grow, indicating that the tumor microenvironment (TME) negatively affects NK cell functionality. It is well-known that there is an immunosuppressive state in the TME that affects, among others, NK cells [149–152]. Thus, NK cells infiltrated in clear cell RCC have an altered phenotype and poor degranulation activity compared with circulating NK cells and with those from non-tumor kidney cortices [139,141]. The deficient NK cells are characterized by dampened mitogen-activated protein kinase pathway activation that was dependent on high levels of diacylglycerol kinase (DGK)-α.

Restoring NK cell activity was achieved by inhibiting DGK-α and with a brief exposure to IL-2 [141]. Other authors have also shown that NK cells infiltrating clear cell RCC exhibited poor cytotoxic activity against the classical K562 cell target when compared with NK cells from tumor margins and non-tumor tissues. Interestingly, these authors also found that primary tumor cells induced NK cell dysfunction in an exosome-dependent manner [153]. The exosomes were enriched in transforming growth factor (TGF)-β1, which is a well-known mediator that diminishes NK cell-mediated activity in the TME [152–154].

A majority of the RCCs have the von Hippel-Lindau (VHL) gene mutated or functionally inactivated [155]. VHL targets the hypoxia-inducible factor (HIF) family of transcription factors, particularly HIF1α and HIF2α, for ubiquitin-mediated degradation in the proteasome [156–158]. Therefore, inactivation of VHL leads to an increased expression of HIF. Furthermore, HIF2α has been reported to regulate the expression of a unique set of genes and to be involved in the development of RCC [158,159]. In fact, it has been demonstrated that the human 786-0 RCC cell line with mutated VHL was resistant to the NK cells' lysis, while the VHL-corrected cell line was susceptible. The NK cell resistance was due to the HIF2α-induced expression of ITPR1 (inositol triphosphate receptor 1), which inhibited NK cell-mediated lysis through a mechanism that involves the induction of autophagy in the target cell after the interaction with NK cells, resulting in granzyme B degradation and target cell survival [156,160]. Nevertheless, the effect of VHL gene mutations on NK cell effector functions is controversial. In this sense, other authors have described that mutations of the VHL gene confer increased susceptibility to NK cell lysis of RCC cell lines and that overexpression of the wild-type VHL gene decreased it, in a mechanism involving the augmented expression of HLA class I molecules [161]. More recently, Trotta et al. have shown that mutated VHL RCC promotes patients' specific NK cell cytotoxicity. Specifically, they found that IL-2-activated circulating NK cells from RCC patients with mutated VHL exhibited higher degranulation levels and IFNγ production toward a mutated VHL RCC cell line than against a cell line with wild type VHL. Moreover, IL-2-activated NK cells from patients with VHL-mutated RCC displayed higher degranulation levels against autologous RCC cells and a VHL-mutated RCC cell line than against a cell line with wild type VHL [162].

There are several therapeutic approaches to treat renal cancer, including surgery, radiofrequency ablation and cryoablation, radiation therapy, targeted therapy, chemotherapy, and immunotherapy (Table 1). Targeted therapy includes anti-angiogenesis therapy aimed to block the vascular endothelial growth factor (VEGF) by means of antibodies (i.e., bevacizumab) and tyrosine kinase inhibitors (TKI), such as axitinib, sunitinib, sorafenib, and so forth. Targeted therapies also include the mTOR inhibitors, everolimus and temsirolimus. Within immunotherapies in renal cancer, some of the current approved treatments include IL-2, IFNα, and immune checkpoint inhibitors (e.g., nivolumab, ipilimumab, pembrolizumab). It is important to note that there are several approved combination therapies. For example, the FDA has approved the combination of TKI axitinib and the checkpoint inhibitor pembrolizumab for the treatment of advanced RCC.

Table 1. Selected clinical trials on Renal Cell Carcinoma and NK cells (ClinicalTrials.gov).

NCT number	Treatment	NK cell-related analysis	Title of the clinical trial
NCT02843607	Cryosurgery + NK cell infusion	Not specified	Combination of Cryosurgery and NK Immunotherapy for Advanced Kidney Cancer
NCT00328861	Chemotherapy + IL-2 (Aldesleukin) + NK cell infusion	Not specified	Natural Killer Cells Plus IL-2 Following Chemotherapy to Treat Advanced Melanoma or Kidney Cancer
NCT03319459	Group 1: activated NK cell infusion (FATE-NK100) Group 2: activated NK cell infusion (FATE-NK100) + anti-HER-2 (Trastuzumab) Group 3: activated NK cell infusion (FATE-NK100) + anti-EGFR (Cetuximab)	% NK cells	FATE-NK100 as Monotherapy and in Combination With Monoclonal Antibody in Subjects With Advanced Solid Tumors
NCT03841110	Group 1: Lympho-conditioning chemotherapy + iPSC-derived NK cell infusion (FT500) Group 2: Lympho-conditioning chemotherapy + iPSC-derived NK cell infusion (FT500) + anti-PD-1 (Nivolumab or Pembrolizumab) or anti-PD-L1 (Atezolizumab)	iPSC-derived NK cell persistence	FT500 as Monotherapy and in Combination With Immune Checkpoint Inhibitors in Subjects With Advanced Solid Tumors
NCT04106167	iPSC-derived NK cell infusion (FT500)	Not specified	Long-term, Non-interventional, Observational Study Following Treatment With Fate Therapeutics FT500 Cellular Immunotherapy
NCT01727076	IL-15	NK cell effector functions % NK cells	Recombinant Interleukin-15 in Treating Patients With Advanced Melanoma, Kidney Cancer, Non-small Cell Lung Cancer, or Squamous Cell Head and Neck Cancer
NCT01274273	IL-2 (Aldesleukin) + IFNα + anti-VEGF (Bevacizumab)	NK cell assessment	Study of Interleukin-2, Interferon-alpha and Bevacizumab in Metastatic Kidney Cancer
NCT01550367	Autophagy blocking therapy (HC) + IL-2 (Aldesleukin)	% NK cells	Study of Hydroxychloroquine and Aldesleukin in Renal Cell Carcinoma Patients (RCC)
NCT03891485	anti-PD-1 (Nivolumab)	NK cell effector functions	Nivolumab in mRCC Patients: Treg Function, T-cell Access and NK Interactions to Predict and Improve Efficacy
NCT03628859	Group 1: anti-PD-1 (Nivolumab) Group 2: TKI (Axitinib or Cabozantinib) Group 3: mTOR inhibitor (Everolimus)	NK cell effector functions NK cell phenotype	BIOREN (Predictive BIOmarkers in Metastatic RENal Cancer)
NCT01144169	Autophagy blocking therapy (HC) + Surgery	NK cell effector functions NK cell phenotype % NK cells	Study of Hydroxychloroquine Before Surgery in Patients With Primary Renal Cell Carcinoma

Abbreviations: TKI: tyrosine kinase inhibitor; HC: Hydroxychloroquine; iPSC: induced pluripotent stem cell.

Both TKI and mTOR inhibitors exert antiangiogenic and immunomodulatory functions [163]. In addition to their action on tumor cells, these inhibitors may also inhibit signaling pathways in immune effector cells, such as NK cells. For example, resting and IL-2 activated NK cells exhibited less degranulation and cytokine production when exposed to pharmacological doses of sorafenib, but not sunitinib, in a mechanism involving impaired PI3K and ERK phosphorylation [164]. Other studies have also shown that sunitinib does not impair NK cell function in patients with RCC [165]. On the other hand, sunitinib has been found to induce the expression of MICA, MICB, and ULBP1-3, all of them ligands of the activating NKG2D receptor, on nasopharyngeal cancer cell lines that lead to an increase in their susceptibility to NK cell-mediated cytoxicity [166]. Axitinib is another TKI, which in addition to its direct proapoptotic effect on renal carcinoma cells, is able to increase NKG2D ligands through the DNA damage response (DDR) and, therefore, increasing NK cell recognition and degranulation against a RCC cell line in a reactive oxygen species (ROS)-dependent manner [167]. The combination of sunitinib and immunotherapy has been tested in mouse preclinical models. Specifically, in a mouse model of metastatic RCC, a synergistic anti-tumor response with the combined treatment of sunitinib and an agonistic mAb against the glucocorticoid-induced TNFR related protein (GITR) was shown [168]. Among others, this combined treatment induced a very significant increase in the infiltration and activation of CD8+ T cells and NK cells in liver metastasis [168]. Moreover, cell depletion experiments demonstrated that CD8+ T cells, macrophages, and NK cells infiltrating the metastatic liver contributed to the anti-tumor effect of this combination therapy [168].

In search of prognostic markers that could be associated with the evolution of metastatic RCC patients, levels of Eomes mRNA in peripheral blood were studied before the treatment with sorafenib [169]. Multivariate analysis, including clinical features, identified Eomes mRNA expression levels as a good prognostic marker for progression-free survival and overall survival in these patients treated with sorafenib [169]. Moreover, at protein levels, Eomes was highly expressed on circulating NK cells [169], suggesting that NK cells may play a role in the tumor response in RCC patients treated with sorafenib. On the other hand, in patients with metastatic RCC, the systemic effect of the mTOR inhibitor everolimus was shown to induce immunological alterations in circulating immune cells, including NK cells [170]. Specifically, a significant decrease in the frequency of the $CD56^{bright}$ NK cell subset and the conventional DCs was found, along with an increase in Treg cells and monocyte MDSCs. These data suggest that everolimus may favor immunosuppression and, therefore, that it should be carefully considered in the treatment of these patients [170].

Targeting immune checkpoints, such as PD-1 and CTLA-4, is a success story in the fight against cancer. For example, cancer immunotherapies targeting the PD-1/PD-L1 axis has shown remarkable efficacy in the treatment of many cancers [171–176], including RCC [175–179]. Nevertheless, not all patients respond to the therapy, and the identification of treatment response biomarkers is a real need. More importantly, information about blood markers, rather than tumor markers, that are associated with the response to checkpoint inhibition is very scarce. Recently, the changes in blood immune cell subsets and soluble mediators after anti-PD-1 therapy were studied [180]. The authors found that in blood samples from non-small cell lung cancer and RCC patients before treatment, an increased frequency of central memory CD4+ T cells and leukocyte count was associated with a response, while an increased percentage of PD-L1+ NK cells and naïve CD4+ T cells was associated with a lack of response [180]. Considering that it has been proposed that anti-PD-L1 antibodies activate PD-L1+ NK cells to control tumor growth [98] and that the mutated VHL gene induces PD-L1 expression in RCC cells [181], treating patients that have a high frequency of PD-L1+ NK cells with anti-PD-L1 rather than anti-PD-1 antibodies should be considered. Combination therapy of checkpoint inhibitors with other drugs is another reality in the current arsenal for treating RCC patients, and more combination therapies are being tested in preclinical models. For example, the combination of checkpoint inhibitor (CTLA-4) and oncolytic virotherapy has been found to be very complex, and many factors, including viral strains, are critical for the synergistic effects [182]. Once the best condition for the combined administration of anti-CTLA4 antibodies and the oncolytic virus was identified in a mouse model of RCC, it was shown that the synergistic effects of the combined therapy required the participation of CD8+ T cells, NK cells, and IFNγ for the anti-tumor response [182]. Interestingly, HLA-E expression has been reported in RCC tumors [183,184]. However, whether the use of anti-NKG2A Abs could benefit RCC patients remains unexplored.

Tumor-associated antigens are also a focus for the implementation of new therapeutic strategies. Carbonic anhydrase IX (CAIX) is one of the best-characterized antigens associated to RCC [185,186]. Results have shown that human anti-CAIX mAbs induce NK cell-mediated ADCC against RCC cells.

Furthermore, engineered anti-CAIX mAbs to enhance the binding affinity to Fc gamma receptors (i.e., CD16) enhanced their ADCC effector function [187]. In an in vivo orthotopic RCC mouse model using human peripheral blood mononuclear cells, it was shown that the anti-CAIX mAbs induced human responses, including NK cell tumor infiltration [187]. Other mAbs are being tested in preclinical models of RCC. In this context, CCR4 is highly expressed in human RCC biopsies and, in a mouse model of RCC, anti-CCR4 mAb was shown to exhibit anti-tumor activity. Interestingly, this anti-CCR4 mAb induced a modification of the immune cell infiltrate in the TME, leading, among others, to an increase in NK cell numbers [188]. More specifically, anti-CCR4 mAb, among other effects, increased the numbers of infiltrating NK cells [188], suggesting that these may participate in tumor elimination following anti-CCR4 mAb administration. Also, it has been shown that SIRPα is highly expressed in human RCC cells, and anti-SIRPα mAbs decreased tumor formation in syngeneic mice [189]. Interestingly, the anti-tumor effect of anti-SIRPα mAbs required not only macrophages, but also NK cells and CD8+ T cells [189].

IL-2 was the first cytokine to be molecularly cloned. The high-affinity IL-2 receptor (IL-2R) is composed of three chains (α, β, and γ), and it is highly expressed in Treg cells, while the intermediate-affinity IL-2R is only composed of the β and γ chains, and is expressed in the majority of T and NK cells [190–192]. Soon after the discovery that this cytokine stimulates T and NK cell proliferation and the generation of effector T cells, clinical trials were carried out to evaluate its ability to stimulate anti-tumor responses in patients with renal cancer, melanoma, and other tumors [78,79,85,190]. In fact, high doses of IL-2 were approved by the FDA in 1992 to treat patients with metastatic RCC [78,193]. Evaluating data from a cohort of patients treated with high doses of IL-2, it was found that when the higher-affinity genotypes for FCGR2A, FCGR3A, and FCGR2C were considered together, they were associated with increased tumor shrinkage and prolonged survival [194]. FCGR3A encodes for CD16 expressed on NK cells. On the other hand, in the same cohort of patients, an association of the KIR/KIR-ligand genotype with patient outcomes was not found [195]. IL-2 has also been administered to RCC patients in combination with IFNα, which has been proven to enhance NK cell cytotoxicity and expansion [196,197]. However, several studies have also pointed out that insufficient activation of RCC tumor-infiltrating NK cells contributed to the failure of IL-2 treatment alone or in combination with other agents, such as IFNα [147,198,199].

IL-15 is another cytokine that signals through the IL-2Rβγ, and it is being tested in clinical trials for cancer immunotherapy, including patients with metastatic RCC. A clinical trial has demonstrated acute lymphocyte dynamics with a redistribution of NK cells and CD8+ T cells, followed by hyperproliferation and increased numbers of NK cells (and T cells) after 2–3 days of the infusion. Cell numbers returned to baseline levels around 6 weeks after IL-15 infusion [88]. Another trial using subcutaneous IL-15 administration induced a profound expansion of NK cells, especially the CD56^{bright} subset. In this trial, objective responses were not observed, although some patients had disease stabilization [200] (NCT01727076). Finally, a trial with ALT-803, a complex containing two molecules of mutated IL-15 and two molecules of the IL-15Rα "sushi" domain fused to human IgG1 Fc, also demonstrated expansion and activation of NK cells [201].

Adoptive cell therapy has also been used for the treatment of metastatic RCC. Infusion of activated NK cells in combination with IL-2 [81,202,203], and the adoptive transfer of allogeneic NK cells [77] and NK cell lines, such as NK-92 [204], have been tested [142,205]. Infusions of NK cells have also been combined with other therapeutic procedures. For example, combining allogeneic NK cell therapy with percutaneous cryoablation had a synergistic effect, improving the quality of life of the patients, and also exhibited clinical efficacy [206] (NCT02843607). Also, genetically modified NK cells are being studied for their potential use in the clinic [142]. Given that there are higher concentrations of CXCR2 ligands in tumors compared with the plasma of RCC patients, the properties of NK cells engineered to express CXCR2 were tested [207]. CXCR2 expressing NK cells were able to migrate along a chemokine gradient of RCC tumor supernatants, and this enhanced trafficking resulted in an increased killing of target cells [207]. CAR-engineered NK cells are also being tested in preclinical models. Some examples include the ability of NK-92 cells expressing an ErbB2 (Her2)-specific CAR to reduce lung metastasis in a RCC model [208], how the combination of cabozantinib and NK-92 cells expressing an EGFR-specific CAR exhibit synergistic therapeutic efficacy against the human RCC xenograft model [209], and how bortezomib improves adoptive CAIX-specific CAR-modified NK-92 cell therapy in mouse models of RCC as well [210].

6. Conclusions

As summarized in this review, NK cells present several features that make them suitable for fighting against malignant pathologies, and RCC is not an exception. Multiple strategies have been developed to enhance anti-tumor activities of NK cells, and some of them are currently being tested in clinical trials with RCC patients. Therefore, based on current knowledge, we consider that NK cell-based immunotherapies represent a promising tool in the treatment of renal cancers.

Author Contributions: All authors have made a substantial, direct and intellectual contribution to the work, and approved it for publication. All authors have read and agreed to the published version of the manuscript.

Funding: Supported by the following grants: AECC-Spanish Association Against Cancer (PROYE16074BORR) and Health Department, Basque Government (2018222038). Iñigo Terrén is recipient of a fellowship from the Jesús de Gangoiti Barrera Foundation (FJGB18/002) and a predoctoral contract funded by the Department of Education, Basque Government (PRE_2019_2_0109). Joana Vitallé is recipient of a predoctoral contract funded by the Department of Education, Basque Government (PRE_2018_2_0211). Olatz Zenarruzabeitia is recipient of a postdoctoral contract funded by "Instituto de Salud Carlos III-Contratos Sara Borrell 2017 (CD17/00128)" and the European Social Fund (ESF)-The ESF invests in your future. Francisco Borrego is an Ikerbasque Research Professor, Ikerbasque, Basque Foundation for Science.

Conflicts of Interest: The authors declare that the research was conducted in the absence of any commercial or financial relationships that could be construed as a potential conflict of interest.

References

1. Herberman, R.B.; Nunn, M.E.; Holden, H.T.; Lavrin, D.H. Natural cytotoxic reactivity of mouse lymphoid cells against syngeneic and allogeneic tumors. II. Characterization of effector cells. *Int. J. Cancer* **1975**, *16*, 230–239. [CrossRef]
2. Kiessling, R.; Klein, E.; Pross, H.; Wigzell, H. „Natural" killer cells in the mouse. II. Cytotoxic cells with specificity for mouse Moloney leukemia cells. Characteristics of the killer cell. *Eur. J. Immunol.* **1975**, *5*, 117–121. [CrossRef]
3. Caligiuri, M.A. Human natural killer cells. *Blood* **2008**, *112*, 461–469. [CrossRef]
4. Sun, J.C.; Lanier, L.L. NK cell development, homeostasis and function: parallels with CD8+ T cells. *Nat. Rev. Immunol.* **2011**, *11*, 645–657. [CrossRef] [PubMed]
5. Morvan, M.G.; Lanier, L.L. NK cells and cancer: you can teach innate cells new tricks. *Nat. Rev. Cancer* **2016**, *16*, 7–19. [CrossRef] [PubMed]
6. Cerwenka, A.; Lanier, L.L. Natural killer cell memory in infection, inflammation and cancer. *Nat. Rev. Immunol.* **2016**, *16*, 112–123. [CrossRef] [PubMed]
7. Chiossone, L.; Dumas, P.-Y.; Vienne, M.; Vivier, E. Natural killer cells and other innate lymphoid cells in cancer. *Nat. Rev. Immunol.* **2018**, *18*, 671–688. [CrossRef]
8. Ali, A.; Gyurova, I.E.; Waggoner, S.N. Mutually assured destruction: the cold war between viruses and natural killer cells. *Curr. Opin. Virol.* **2019**, *34*, 130–139. [CrossRef]
9. Welsh, R.M.; Waggoner, S.N. NK cells controlling virus-specific T cells: Rheostats for acute vs. persistent infections. *Virology* **2013**, *435*, 37–45. [CrossRef]
10. Vitale, M.; Cantoni, C.; Della Chiesa, M.; Ferlazzo, G.; Carlomagno, S.; Pende, D.; Falco, M.; Pessino, A.; Muccio, L.; De Maria, A.; et al. An Historical Overview: The Discovery of How NK Cells Can Kill Enemies, Recruit Defense Troops, and More. *Front. Immunol.* **2019**, *10*, 1415. [CrossRef]
11. Martín-Fontecha, A.; Thomsen, L.L.; Brett, S.; Gerard, C.; Lipp, M.; Lanzavecchia, A.; Sallusto, F. Induced recruitment of NK cells to lymph nodes provides IFN-γ for TH1 priming. *Nat. Immunol.* **2004**, *5*, 1260–1265. [CrossRef]

12. Van Kaer, L.; Postoak, J.L.; Wang, C.; Yang, G.; Wu, L. Innate, innate-like and adaptive lymphocytes in the pathogenesis of MS and EAE. *Cell. Mol. Immunol.* **2019**, *16*, 531–539. [CrossRef]
13. Zitti, B.; Bryceson, Y.T. Natural killer cells in inflammation and autoimmunity. *Cytokine Growth Factor Rev.* **2018**, *42*, 37–46. [CrossRef]
14. Vivier, E.; Raulet, D.H.; Moretta, A.; Caligiuri, M.A.; Zitvogel, L.; Lanier, L.L.; Yokoyama, W.M.; Ugolini, S. Innate or Adaptive Immunity? The Example of Natural Killer Cells. *Science (80-.).* **2011**, *331*, 44–49. [CrossRef] [PubMed]
15. O'Sullivan, T.E.; Sun, J.C.; Lanier, L.L. Natural Killer Cell Memory. *Immunity* **2015**, *43*, 634–645. [CrossRef]
16. Min-Oo, G.; Kamimura, Y.; Hendricks, D.W.; Nabekura, T.; Lanier, L.L. Natural killer cells: walking three paths down memory lane. *Trends Immunol.* **2013**, *34*, 251–258. [CrossRef]
17. Muntasell, A.; Vilches, C.; Angulo, A.; López-Botet, M. Adaptive reconfiguration of the human NK-cell compartment in response to cytomegalovirus: A different perspective of the host-pathogen interaction. *Eur. J. Immunol.* **2013**, *43*, 1133–1141. [CrossRef]
18. Holmes, T.D.; Bryceson, Y.T. Natural killer cell memory in context. *Semin. Immunol.* **2016**, *28*, 368–376. [CrossRef]
19. Borrego, F.; Kabat, J.; Kim, D.-K.; Lieto, L.; Maasho, K.; Peña, J.; Solana, R.; Coligan, J.E. Structure and function of major histocompatibility complex (MHC) class I specific receptors expressed on human natural killer (NK) cells. *Mol. Immunol.* **2002**, *38*, 637–660. [CrossRef]
20. Long, E.O.; Sik Kim, H.; Liu, D.; Peterson, M.E.; Rajagopalan, S. Controlling Natural Killer Cell Responses: Integration of Signals for Activation and Inhibition. *Annu. Rev. Immunol.* **2013**, *31*, 227–258. [CrossRef]
21. Vivier, E.; Artis, D.; Colonna, M.; Diefenbach, A.; Di Santo, J.P.; Eberl, G.; Koyasu, S.; Locksley, R.M.; McKenzie, A.N.J.; Mebius, R.E.; et al. Innate Lymphoid Cells: 10 Years On. *Cell* **2018**, *174*, 1054–1066. [CrossRef] [PubMed]
22. Colonna, M. Innate Lymphoid Cells: Diversity, Plasticity, and Unique Functions in Immunity. *Immunity* **2018**, *48*, 1104–1117. [CrossRef] [PubMed]
23. Freud, A.G.; Mundy-Bosse, B.L.; Yu, J.; Caligiuri, M.A. The Broad Spectrum of Human Natural Killer Cell Diversity. *Immunity* **2017**, *47*, 820–833. [CrossRef] [PubMed]
24. Cooper, M.A.; Fehniger, T.A.; Caligiuri, M.A. The biology of human natural killer-cell subsets. *Trends Immunol.* **2001**, *22*, 633–640. [CrossRef]
25. Di Vito, C.; Mikulak, J.; Mavilio, D. On the Way to Become a Natural Killer Cell. *Front. Immunol.* **2019**, *10*, 1812. [CrossRef] [PubMed]
26. Mavilio, D.; Lombardo, G.; Benjamin, J.; Kim, D.; Follman, D.; Marcenaro, E.; O'Shea, M.A.; Kinter, A.; Kovacs, C.; Moretta, A.; et al. Characterization of CD56-/CD16+ natural killer (NK) cells: A highly dysfunctional NK subset expanded in HIV-infected viremic individuals. *Proc. Natl. Acad. Sci.* **2005**, *102*, 2886–2891. [CrossRef]
27. Vitallé, J.; Terrén, I.; Orrantia, A.; Pérez-Garay, R.; Vidal, F.; Iribarren, J.A.; Rodríguez, C.; Lirola, A.M.L.; Bernal, E.; Zenarruzabeitia, O.; et al. CD300a inhibits CD16-mediated NK cell effector functions in HIV-1-infected patients. *Cell. Mol. Immunol.* **2019**, *16*, 940–942. [CrossRef]
28. Roberto, A.; Di Vito, C.; Zaghi, E.; Mazza, E.M.C.; Capucetti, A.; Calvi, M.; Tentorio, P.; Zanon, V.; Sarina, B.; Mariotti, J.; et al. The early expansion of anergic NKG2A^{pos}/CD56^{dim}/CD16^{neg} natural killer represents a therapeutic target in haploidentical hematopoietic stem cell transplantation. *Haematologica* **2018**, *103*, 1390–1402. [CrossRef]
29. Vulpis, E.; Stabile, H.; Soriani, A.; Fionda, C.; Petrucci, M.; Mariggio', E.; Ricciardi, M.; Cippitelli, M.; Gismondi, A.; Santoni, A.; et al. Key Role of the CD56lowCD16low Natural Killer Cell Subset in the Recognition and Killing of Multiple Myeloma Cells. *Cancers (Basel).* **2018**, *10*, 473. [CrossRef]
30. Freud, A.G.; Caligiuri, M.A. Human natural killer cell development. *Immunol. Rev.* **2006**, *214*, 56–72. [CrossRef]
31. Freud, A.G.; Yokohama, A.; Becknell, B.; Lee, M.T.; Mao, H.C.; Ferketich, A.K.; Caligiuri, M.A. Evidence for discrete stages of human natural killer cell differentiation in vivo. *J. Exp. Med.* **2006**, *203*, 1033–1043. [CrossRef] [PubMed]
32. Hughes, T.; Becknell, B.; Freud, A.G.; McClory, S.; Briercheck, E.; Yu, J.; Mao, C.; Giovenzana, C.; Nuovo, G.; Wei, L.; et al. Interleukin-1β Selectively Expands and Sustains Interleukin-22+ Immature Human Natural Killer Cells in Secondary Lymphoid Tissue. *Immunity* **2010**, *32*, 803–814. [CrossRef] [PubMed]

33. Chinen, H.; Matsuoka, K.; Sato, T.; Kamada, N.; Okamoto, S.; Hisamatsu, T.; Kobayashi, T.; Hasegawa, H.; Sugita, A.; Kinjo, F.; et al. Lamina propria c-kit+ immune precursors reside in human adult intestine and differentiate into natural killer cells. *Gastroenterology* **2007**, *133*, 559–573. [CrossRef] [PubMed]
34. Moroso, V.; Famili, F.; Papazian, N.; Cupedo, T.; van der Laan, L.J.W.; Kazemier, G.; Metselaar, H.J.; Kwekkeboom, J. NK cells can generate from precursors in the adult human liver. *Eur. J. Immunol.* **2011**, *41*, 3340–3350. [CrossRef] [PubMed]
35. Vacca, P.; Vitale, C.; Montaldo, E.; Conte, R.; Cantoni, C.; Fulcheri, E.; Darretta, V.; Moretta, L.; Mingari, M.C. CD34+ hematopoietic precursors are present in human decidua and differentiate into natural killer cells upon interaction with stromal cells. *Proc. Natl. Acad. Sci.* **2011**, *108*, 2402–2407. [CrossRef]
36. Freud, A.G.; Yu, J.; Caligiuri, M.A. Human natural killer cell development in secondary lymphoid tissues. *Semin. Immunol.* **2014**, *26*, 132–137. [CrossRef]
37. Yu, J.; Freud, A.G.; Caligiuri, M.A. Location and cellular stages of natural killer cell development. *Trends Immunol.* **2013**, *34*, 573–582. [CrossRef]
38. Cichocki, F.; Grzywacz, B.; Miller, J.S. Human NK Cell Development: One Road or Many? *Front. Immunol.* **2019**, *10*, 2078. [CrossRef]
39. Wilk, A.J.; Blish, C.A. Diversification of human NK cells: Lessons from deep profiling. *J. Leukoc. Biol.* **2018**, *103*, 629–641. [CrossRef]
40. Horowitz, A.; Strauss-Albee, D.M.; Leipold, M.; Kubo, J.; Nemat-Gorgani, N.; Dogan, O.C.; Dekker, C.L.; Mackey, S.; Maecker, H.; Swan, G.E.; et al. Genetic and Environmental Determinants of Human NK Cell Diversity Revealed by Mass Cytometry. *Sci. Transl. Med.* **2013**, *5*, 208ra145. [CrossRef]
41. Crinier, A.; Milpied, P.; Escalière, B.; Piperoglou, C.; Galluso, J.; Balsamo, A.; Spinelli, L.; Cervera-Marzal, I.; Ebbo, M.; Girard-Madoux, M.; et al. High-Dimensional Single-Cell Analysis Identifies Organ-Specific Signatures and Conserved NK Cell Subsets in Humans and Mice. *Immunity* **2018**, *49*, 971–986.e5. [CrossRef] [PubMed]
42. Yang, C.; Siebert, J.R.; Burns, R.; Gerbec, Z.J.; Bonacci, B.; Rymaszewski, A.; Rau, M.; Riese, M.J.; Rao, S.; Carlson, K.-S.; et al. Heterogeneity of human bone marrow and blood natural killer cells defined by single-cell transcriptome. *Nat. Commun.* **2019**, *10*, 3931. [CrossRef] [PubMed]
43. Smyth, M.J.; Thia, K.Y.T.; Street, S.E.A.; MacGregor, D.; Godfrey, D.I.; Trapani, J.A. Perforin-Mediated Cytotoxicity Is Critical for Surveillance of Spontaneous Lymphoma. *J. Exp. Med.* **2000**, *192*, 755–760. [CrossRef] [PubMed]
44. Voskoboinik, I.; Whisstock, J.C.; Trapani, J.A. Perforin and granzymes: function, dysfunction and human pathology. *Nat. Rev. Immunol.* **2015**, *15*, 388–400. [CrossRef] [PubMed]
45. Krzewski, K.; Coligan, J.E. Human NK cell lytic granules and regulation of their exocytosis. *Front. Immunol.* **2012**, *3*, 335. [CrossRef]
46. Screpanti, V.; Wallin, R.P.A.; Grandien, A.; Ljunggren, H.-G. Impact of FASL-induced apoptosis in the elimination of tumor cells by NK cells. *Mol. Immunol.* **2005**, *42*, 495–499. [CrossRef]
47. Cretney, E.; Takeda, K.; Yagita, H.; Glaccum, M.; Peschon, J.J.; Smyth, M.J. Increased Susceptibility to Tumor Initiation and Metastasis in TNF-Related Apoptosis-Inducing Ligand-Deficient Mice. *J. Immunol.* **2002**, *168*, 1356–1361. [CrossRef]
48. Finnberg, N.; Klein-Szanto, A.J.P.; El-Deiry, W.S. TRAIL-R deficiency in mice promotes susceptibility to chronic inflammation and tumorigenesis. *J. Clin. Invest.* **2008**, *118*, 111–123. [CrossRef]
49. Orange, J.S. Formation and function of the lytic NK-cell immunological synapse. *Nat. Rev. Immunol.* **2008**, *8*, 713–725. [CrossRef]
50. Mace, E.M.; Dongre, P.; Hsu, H.-T.; Sinha, P.; James, A.M.; Mann, S.S.; Forbes, L.R.; Watkin, L.B.; Orange, J.S. Cell biological steps and checkpoints in accessing NK cell cytotoxicity. *Immunol. Cell Biol.* **2014**, *92*, 245–255. [CrossRef]
51. Dustin, M.L.; Long, E.O. Cytotoxic immunological synapses. *Immunol. Rev.* **2010**, *235*, 24–34. [CrossRef] [PubMed]
52. Lagrue, K.; Carisey, A.; Oszmiana, A.; Kennedy, P.R.; Williamson, D.J.; Cartwright, A.; Barthen, C.; Davis, D.M. The central role of the cytoskeleton in mechanisms and functions of the NK cell immune synapse. *Immunol. Rev.* **2013**, *256*, 203–221. [CrossRef] [PubMed]
53. Lanier, L.L.; Yu, G.; Phillips, J.H. Co-association of CD3ζ with a receptor (CD16) for IgG Fc on human natural killer cells. *Nature* **1989**, *342*, 803–805. [CrossRef] [PubMed]

54. Blázquez-Moreno, A.; Park, S.; Im, W.; Call, M.J.; Call, M.E.; Reyburn, H.T. Transmembrane features governing Fc receptor CD16A assembly with CD16A signaling adaptor molecules. *Proc. Natl. Acad. Sci. USA* **2017**, *114*, E5645–E5654. [CrossRef] [PubMed]
55. Kruse, P.H.; Matta, J.; Ugolini, S.; Vivier, E. Natural cytotoxicity receptors and their ligands. *Immunol. Cell Biol.* **2014**, *92*, 221–229. [CrossRef]
56. Martinet, L.; Smyth, M.J. Balancing natural killer cell activation through paired receptors. *Nat. Rev. Immunol.* **2015**, *15*, 243–254. [CrossRef]
57. Lanier, L.L. NKG2D Receptor and Its Ligands in Host Defense. *Cancer Immunol. Res.* **2015**, *3*, 575–582. [CrossRef]
58. Dimitrova, M.; Zenarruzabeitia, O.; Borrego, F.; Simhadri, V.R. CD300c is uniquely expressed on CD56bright Natural Killer Cells and differs from CD300a upon ligand recognition. *Sci. Rep.* **2016**, *6*, 23942. [CrossRef]
59. Raulet, D.H.; Gasser, S.; Gowen, B.G.; Deng, W.; Jung, H. Regulation of Ligands for the NKG2D Activating Receptor. *Annu. Rev. Immunol.* **2013**, *31*, 413–441. [CrossRef]
60. Lam, A.R.; Le Bert, N.; Ho, S.S.W.; Shen, Y.J.; Tang, M.L.F.; Xiong, G.M.; Croxford, J.L.; Koo, C.X.; Ishii, K.J.; Akira, S.; et al. RAE1 Ligands for the NKG2D Receptor Are Regulated by STING-Dependent DNA Sensor Pathways in Lymphoma. *Cancer Res.* **2014**, *74*, 2193–2203. [CrossRef]
61. Cerboni, C.; Fionda, C.; Soriani, A.; Zingoni, A.; Doria, M.; Cippitelli, M.; Santoni, A. The DNA Damage Response: A Common Pathway in the Regulation of NKG2D and DNAM-1 Ligand Expression in Normal, Infected, and Cancer Cells. *Front. Immunol.* **2014**, *4*, 508. [CrossRef] [PubMed]
62. Brandt, C.S.; Baratin, M.; Yi, E.C.; Kennedy, J.; Gao, Z.; Fox, B.; Haldeman, B.; Ostrander, C.D.; Kaifu, T.; Chabannon, C.; et al. The B7 family member B7-H6 is a tumor cell ligand for the activating natural killer cell receptor NKp30 in humans. *J. Exp. Med.* **2009**, *206*, 1495–1503. [CrossRef] [PubMed]
63. Ljunggren, H.G.; Kärre, K. In search of the "missing self": MHC molecules and NK cell recognition. *Immunol. Today* **1990**, *11*, 237–244. [CrossRef]
64. Long, E.O.; Barber, D.F.; Burshtyn, D.N.; Faure, M.; Peterson, M.; Rajagopalan, S.; Renard, V.; Sandusky, M.; Stebbins, C.C.; Wagtmann, N.; et al. Inhibition of natural killer cell activation signals by killer cell immunoglobulin-like receptors (CD158). *Immunol. Rev.* **2001**, *181*, 223–233. [CrossRef]
65. Borrego, F.; Ulbrecht, M.; Weiss, E.H.; Coligan, J.E.; Brooks, A.G. Recognition of Human Histocompatibility Leukocyte Antigen (HLA)-E Complexed with HLA Class I Signal Sequence–derived Peptides by CD94/NKG2 Confers Protection from Natural Killer Cell–mediated Lysis. *J. Exp. Med.* **1998**, *187*, 813–818. [CrossRef]
66. Kabat, J.; Borrego, F.; Brooks, A.; Coligan, J.E. Role That Each NKG2A Immunoreceptor Tyrosine-Based Inhibitory Motif Plays in Mediating the Human CD94/NKG2A Inhibitory Signal. *J. Immunol.* **2002**, *169*, 1948–1958. [CrossRef]
67. Burshtyn, D.N.; Lam, A.S.; Weston, M.; Gupta, N.; Warmerdam, P.A.; Long, E.O. Conserved residues amino-terminal of cytoplasmic tyrosines contribute to the SHP-1-mediated inhibitory function of killer cell Ig-like receptors. *J. Immunol.* **1999**, *162*, 897–902.
68. Lankry, D.; Rovis, T.L.; Jonjic, S.; Mandelboim, O. The interaction between CD300a and phosphatidylserine inhibits tumor cell killing by NK cells. *Eur. J. Immunol.* **2013**, *43*, 2151–2161. [CrossRef]
69. Kim, S.; Poursine-Laurent, J.; Truscott, S.M.; Lybarger, L.; Song, Y.-J.; Yang, L.; French, A.R.; Sunwoo, J.B.; Lemieux, S.; Hansen, T.H.; et al. Licensing of natural killer cells by host major histocompatibility complex class I molecules. *Nature* **2005**, *436*, 709–713. [CrossRef]
70. Anfossi, N.; André, P.; Guia, S.; Falk, C.S.; Roetynck, S.; Stewart, C.A.; Breso, V.; Frassati, C.; Reviron, D.; Middleton, D.; et al. Human NK Cell Education by Inhibitory Receptors for MHC Class I. *Immunity* **2006**, *25*, 331–342. [CrossRef]
71. Elliott, J.M.; Yokoyama, W.M. Unifying concepts of MHC-dependent natural killer cell education. *Trends Immunol.* **2011**, *32*, 364–372. [CrossRef] [PubMed]
72. Boudreau, J.E.; Hsu, K.C. Natural Killer Cell Education and the Response to Infection and Cancer Therapy: Stay Tuned. *Trends Immunol.* **2018**, *39*, 222–239. [CrossRef] [PubMed]
73. Boudreau, J.E.; Hsu, K.C. Natural killer cell education in human health and disease. *Curr. Opin. Immunol.* **2018**, *50*, 102–111. [CrossRef] [PubMed]
74. Hsu, K.C.; Chida, S.; Geraghty, D.E.; Dupont, B. The killer cell immunoglobulin-like receptor (KIR) genomic region: gene-order, haplotypes and allelic polymorphism. *Immunol. Rev.* **2002**, *190*, 40–52. [CrossRef] [PubMed]

75. Valiante, N.M.; Uhrberg, M.; Shilling, H.G.; Lienert-Weidenbach, K.; Arnett, K.L.; D'Andrea, A.; Phillips, J.H.; Lanier, L.L.; Parham, P. Functionally and structurally distinct NK cell receptor repertoires in the peripheral blood of two human donors. *Immunity* **1997**, *7*, 739–751. [CrossRef]
76. Ruggeri, L.; Capanni, M.; Urbani, E.; Perruccio, K.; Shlomchik, W.D.; Tosti, A.; Posati, S.; Rogaia, D.; Frassoni, F.; Aversa, F.; et al. Effectiveness of Donor Natural Killer Cell Alloreactivity in Mismatched Hematopoietic Transplants. *Science (80-.)*. **2002**, *295*, 2097–2100. [CrossRef]
77. Miller, J.S.; Soignier, Y.; Panoskaltsis-Mortari, A.; McNearney, S.A.; Yun, G.H.; Fautsch, S.K.; McKenna, D.; Le, C.; Defor, T.E.; Burns, L.J.; et al. Successful adoptive transfer and in vivo expansion of human haploidentical NK cells in patients with cancer. *Blood* **2005**, *105*, 3051–3057. [CrossRef]
78. Rosenberg, S.A. IL-2: The First Effective Immunotherapy for Human Cancer. *J. Immunol.* **2014**, *192*, 5451–5458. [CrossRef]
79. Sim, G.C.; Radvanyi, L. The IL-2 cytokine family in cancer immunotherapy. *Cytokine Growth Factor Rev.* **2014**, *25*, 377–390. [CrossRef]
80. Childs, R.W.; Carlsten, M. Therapeutic approaches to enhance natural killer cell cytotoxicity against cancer: the force awakens. *Nat. Rev. Drug Discov.* **2015**, *14*, 487–498. [CrossRef]
81. Rosenberg, S.A.; Lotze, M.T.; Muul, L.M.; Leitman, S.; Chang, A.E.; Ettinghausen, S.E.; Matory, Y.L.; Skibber, J.M.; Shiloni, E.; Vetto, J.T.; et al. Observations on the Systemic Administration of Autologous Lymphokine-Activated Killer Cells and Recombinant Interleukin-2 to Patients with Metastatic Cancer. *N. Engl. J. Med.* **1985**, *313*, 1485–1492. [CrossRef] [PubMed]
82. Curti, A.; Ruggeri, L.; D'Addio, A.; Bontadini, A.; Dan, E.; Motta, M.R.; Trabanelli, S.; Giudice, V.; Urbani, E.; Martinelli, G.; et al. Successful transfer of alloreactive haploidentical KIR ligand-mismatched natural killer cells after infusion in elderly high risk acute myeloid leukemia patients. *Blood* **2011**, *118*, 3273–3279. [CrossRef] [PubMed]
83. Ito, S.; Bollard, C.M.; Carlsten, M.; Melenhorst, J.J.; Biancotto, A.; Wang, E.; Chen, J.; Kotliarov, Y.; Cheung, F.; Xie, Z.; et al. Ultra-low Dose Interleukin-2 Promotes Immune-modulating Function of Regulatory T Cells and Natural Killer Cells in Healthy Volunteers. *Mol. Ther.* **2014**, *22*, 1388–1395. [CrossRef] [PubMed]
84. Levin, A.M.; Bates, D.L.; Ring, A.M.; Krieg, C.; Lin, J.T.; Su, L.; Moraga, I.; Raeber, M.E.; Bowman, G.R.; Novick, P.; et al. Exploiting a natural conformational switch to engineer an interleukin-2 "superkine". *Nature* **2012**, *484*, 529–533. [CrossRef]
85. Abbas, A.K.; Trotta, E.; R Simeonov, D.; Marson, A.; Bluestone, J.A. Revisiting IL-2: Biology and therapeutic prospects. *Sci. Immunol.* **2018**, *3*, eaat1482. [CrossRef]
86. Becknell, B.; Caligiuri, M.A. Interleukin-2, Interleukin-15, and Their Roles in Human Natural Killer Cells. In *Advances in Immunology*; Academic Press: Cambridge, MA, USA, 2005; Volume 86, pp. 209–239.
87. Leclercq, G.; Debacker, V.; de Smedt, M.; Plum, J. Differential effects of interleukin-15 and interleukin-2 on differentiation of bipotential T/natural killer progenitor cells. *J. Exp. Med.* **1996**, *184*, 325–336. [CrossRef]
88. Conlon, K.C.; Lugli, E.; Welles, H.C.; Rosenberg, S.A.; Fojo, A.T.; Morris, J.C.; Fleisher, T.A.; Dubois, S.P.; Perera, L.P.; Stewart, D.M.; et al. Redistribution, hyperproliferation, activation of natural killer cells and CD8 T cells, and cytokine production during first-in-human clinical trial of recombinant human interleukin-15 in patients with cancer. *J. Clin. Oncol.* **2015**, *33*, 74–82. [CrossRef]
89. Miller, J.S. Therapeutic applications: natural killer cells in the clinic. *Hematology* **2013**, *2013*, 247–253. [CrossRef]
90. Rosario, M.; Liu, B.; Kong, L.; Collins, L.I.; Schneider, S.E.; Chen, X.; Han, K.; Jeng, E.K.; Rhode, P.R.; Leong, J.W.; et al. The IL-15-Based ALT-803 Complex Enhances FcγRIIIa-Triggered NK Cell Responses and In Vivo Clearance of B Cell Lymphomas. *Clin. Cancer Res.* **2016**, *22*, 596–608. [CrossRef]
91. Xu, W.; Jones, M.; Liu, B.; Zhu, X.; Johnson, C.B.; Edwards, A.C.; Kong, L.; Jeng, E.K.; Han, K.; Marcus, W.D.; et al. Efficacy and Mechanism-of-Action of a Novel Superagonist Interleukin-15: Interleukin-15 Receptor Su/Fc Fusion Complex in Syngeneic Murine Models of Multiple Myeloma. *Cancer Res.* **2013**, *73*, 3075–3086. [CrossRef] [PubMed]
92. Han, K.; Zhu, X.; Liu, B.; Jeng, E.; Kong, L.; Yovandich, J.L.; Vyas, V.V.; Marcus, W.D.; Chavaillaz, P.-A.; Romero, C.A.; et al. IL-15:IL-15 receptor alpha superagonist complex: High-level co-expression in recombinant mammalian cells, purification and characterization. *Cytokine* **2011**, *56*, 804–810. [CrossRef] [PubMed]

93. Reddy, N.; Hernandez-Ilizaliturri, F.J.; Deeb, G.; Roth, M.; Vaughn, M.; Knight, J.; Wallace, P.; Czuczman, M.S. Immunomodulatory drugs stimulate natural killer-cell function, alter cytokine production by dendritic cells, and inhibit angiogenesis enhancing the anti-tumour activity of rituximab in vivo. *Br. J. Haematol.* **2008**, *140*, 36–45. [CrossRef] [PubMed]
94. Sun, H.; Sun, C. The Rise of NK Cell Checkpoints as Promising Therapeutic Targets in Cancer Immunotherapy. *Front. Immunol.* **2019**, *10*, 2354. [CrossRef]
95. Keir, M.E.; Butte, M.J.; Freeman, G.J.; Sharpe, A.H. PD-1 and Its Ligands in Tolerance and Immunity. *Annu. Rev. Immunol.* **2008**, *26*, 677–704. [CrossRef]
96. Hsu, J.; Hodgins, J.J.; Marathe, M.; Nicolai, C.J.; Bourgeois-Daigneault, M.-C.; Trevino, T.N.; Azimi, C.S.; Scheer, A.K.; Randolph, H.E.; Thompson, T.W.; et al. Contribution of NK cells to immunotherapy mediated by PD-1/PD-L1 blockade. *J. Clin. Invest.* **2018**, *128*, 4654–4668. [CrossRef]
97. Benson, D.M.; Bakan, C.E.; Mishra, A.; Hofmeister, C.C.; Efebera, Y.; Becknell, B.; Baiocchi, R.A.; Zhang, J.; Yu, J.; Smith, M.K.; et al. The PD-1/PD-L1 axis modulates the natural killer cell versus multiple myeloma effect: a therapeutic target for CT-011, a novel monoclonal anti–PD-1 antibody. *Blood* **2010**, *116*, 2286–2294. [CrossRef]
98. Dong, W.; Wu, X.; Ma, S.; Wang, Y.; Nalin, A.P.; Zhu, Z.; Zhang, J.; Benson, D.M.; He, K.; Caligiuri, M.A.; et al. The Mechanism of Anti–PD-L1 Antibody Efficacy against PD-L1–Negative Tumors Identifies NK Cells Expressing PD-L1 as a Cytolytic Effector. *Cancer Discov.* **2019**, *9*, 1422–1437. [CrossRef]
99. Stanietsky, N.; Simic, H.; Arapovic, J.; Toporik, A.; Levy, O.; Novik, A.; Levine, Z.; Beiman, M.; Dassa, L.; Achdout, H.; et al. The interaction of TIGIT with PVR and PVRL2 inhibits human NK cell cytotoxicity. *Proc. Natl. Acad. Sci.* **2009**, *106*, 17858–17863. [CrossRef]
100. Sanchez-Correa, B.; Valhondo, I.; Hassouneh, F.; Lopez-Sejas, N.; Pera, A.; Bergua, J.M.; Arcos, M.J.; Bañas, H.; Casas-Avilés, I.; Durán, E.; et al. DNAM-1 and the TIGIT/PVRIG/TACTILE Axis: Novel Immune Checkpoints for Natural Killer Cell-Based Cancer Immunotherapy. *Cancers (Basel).* **2019**, *11*, 877. [CrossRef]
101. Benson, D.M.; Bakan, C.E.; Zhang, S.; Collins, S.M.; Liang, J.; Srivastava, S.; Hofmeister, C.C.; Efebera, Y.; Andre, P.; Romagne, F.; et al. IPH2101, a novel anti-inhibitory KIR antibody, and lenalidomide combine to enhance the natural killer cell versus multiple myeloma effect. *Blood* **2011**, *118*, 6387–6391. [CrossRef] [PubMed]
102. Romagné, F.; André, P.; Spee, P.; Zahn, S.; Anfossi, N.; Gauthier, L.; Capanni, M.; Ruggeri, L.; Benson, D.M.; Blaser, B.W.; et al. Preclinical characterization of 1-7F9, a novel human anti–KIR receptor therapeutic antibody that augments natural killer–mediated killing of tumor cells. *Blood* **2009**, *114*, 2667–2677. [CrossRef] [PubMed]
103. Carlsten, M.; Korde, N.; Kotecha, R.; Reger, R.; Bor, S.; Kazandjian, D.; Landgren, O.; Childs, R.W. Checkpoint Inhibition of KIR2D with the Monoclonal Antibody IPH2101 Induces Contraction and Hyporesponsiveness of NK Cells in Patients with Myeloma. *Clin. Cancer Res.* **2016**, *22*, 5211–5222. [CrossRef] [PubMed]
104. Vey, N.; Bourhis, J.-H.; Boissel, N.; Bordessoule, D.; Prebet, T.; Charbonnier, A.; Etienne, A.; Andre, P.; Romagne, F.; Benson, D.; et al. A phase 1 trial of the anti-inhibitory KIR mAb IPH2101 for AML in complete remission. *Blood* **2012**, *120*, 4317–4323. [CrossRef]
105. Vey, N.; Karlin, L.; Sadot-Lebouvier, S.; Broussais, F.; Berton-Rigaud, D.; Rey, J.; Charbonnier, A.; Marie, D.; André, P.; Paturel, C.; et al. A phase 1 study of lirilumab (antibody against killer immunoglobulin-like receptor antibody KIR2D; IPH2102) in patients with solid tumors and hematologic malignancies. *Oncotarget* **2018**, *9*, 17675–17688. [CrossRef]
106. Bagot, M.; Porcu, P.; Marie-Cardine, A.; Battistella, M.; William, B.M.; Vermeer, M.; Whittaker, S.; Rotolo, F.; Ram-Wolff, C.; Khodadoust, M.S.; et al. IPH4102, a first-in-class anti-KIR3DL2 monoclonal antibody, in patients with relapsed or refractory cutaneous T-cell lymphoma: an international, first-in-human, open-label, phase 1 trial. *Lancet Oncol.* **2019**, *20*, 1160–1170. [CrossRef]
107. Kamiya, T.; Seow, S.V.; Wong, D.; Robinson, M.; Campana, D. Blocking expression of inhibitory receptor NKG2A overcomes tumor resistance to NK cells. *J. Clin. Invest.* **2019**, *129*, 2094–2106. [CrossRef]
108. André, P.; Denis, C.; Soulas, C.; Bourbon-Caillet, C.; Lopez, J.; Arnoux, T.; Bléry, M.; Bonnafous, C.; Gauthier, L.; Morel, A.; et al. Anti-NKG2A mAb Is a Checkpoint Inhibitor that Promotes Anti-tumor Immunity by Unleashing Both T and NK Cells. *Cell* **2018**, *175*, 1731–1743.e13. [CrossRef]

109. Zhang, Q.; Bi, J.; Zheng, X.; Chen, Y.; Wang, H.; Wu, W.; Wang, Z.; Wu, Q.; Peng, H.; Wei, H.; et al. Blockade of the checkpoint receptor TIGIT prevents NK cell exhaustion and elicits potent anti-tumor immunity. *Nat. Immunol.* **2018**, *19*, 723–732. [CrossRef]
110. Jiang, X.-R.; Song, A.; Bergelson, S.; Arroll, T.; Parekh, B.; May, K.; Chung, S.; Strouse, R.; Mire-Sluis, A.; Schenerman, M. Advances in the assessment and control of the effector functions of therapeutic antibodies. *Nat. Rev. Drug Discov.* **2011**, *10*, 101–111. [CrossRef]
111. Cartron, G.; Dacheux, L.; Salles, G.; Solal-Celigny, P.; Bardos, P.; Colombat, P.; Watier, H. Therapeutic activity of humanized anti-CD20 monoclonal antibody and polymorphism in IgG Fc receptor FcgammaRIIIa gene. *Blood* **2002**, *99*, 754–758. [CrossRef] [PubMed]
112. Weng, W.-K.; Levy, R. Two Immunoglobulin G Fragment C Receptor Polymorphisms Independently Predict Response to Rituximab in Patients With Follicular Lymphoma. *J. Clin. Oncol.* **2003**, *21*, 3940–3947. [CrossRef]
113. Pander, J.; Gelderblom, H.; Antonini, N.F.; Tol, J.; van Krieken, J.H.J.M.; van der Straaten, T.; Punt, C.J.A.; Guchelaar, H.-J. Correlation of FCGR3A and EGFR germline polymorphisms with the efficacy of cetuximab in KRAS wild-type metastatic colorectal cancer. *Eur. J. Cancer* **2010**, *46*, 1829–1834. [CrossRef] [PubMed]
114. Gleason, M.K.; Verneris, M.R.; Todhunter, D.A.; Zhang, B.; McCullar, V.; Zhou, S.X.; Panoskaltsis-Mortari, A.; Weiner, L.M.; Vallera, D.A.; Miller, J.S. Bispecific and Trispecific Killer Cell Engagers Directly Activate Human NK Cells through CD16 Signaling and Induce Cytotoxicity and Cytokine Production. *Mol. Cancer Ther.* **2012**, *11*, 2674–2684. [CrossRef] [PubMed]
115. Wiernik, A.; Foley, B.; Zhang, B.; Verneris, M.R.; Warlick, E.; Gleason, M.K.; Ross, J.A.; Luo, X.; Weisdorf, D.J.; Walcheck, B.; et al. Targeting Natural Killer Cells to Acute Myeloid Leukemia In Vitro with a CD16 x 33 Bispecific Killer Cell Engager and ADAM17 Inhibition. *Clin. Cancer Res.* **2013**, *19*, 3844–3855. [CrossRef]
116. Gleason, M.K.; Ross, J.A.; Warlick, E.D.; Lund, T.C.; Verneris, M.R.; Wiernik, A.; Spellman, S.; Haagenson, M.D.; Lenvik, A.J.; Litzow, M.R.; et al. CD16xCD33 bispecific killer cell engager (BiKE) activates NK cells against primary MDS and MDSC CD33+ targets. *Blood* **2014**, *123*, 3016–3026. [CrossRef]
117. Sarhan, D.; Brandt, L.; Felices, M.; Guldevall, K.; Lenvik, T.; Hinderlie, P.; Curtsinger, J.; Warlick, E.; Spellman, S.R.; Blazar, B.R.; et al. 161533 TriKE stimulates NK-cell function to overcome myeloid-derived suppressor cells in MDS. *Blood Adv.* **2018**, *2*, 1459–1469. [CrossRef]
118. Gauthier, L.; Morel, A.; Anceriz, N.; Rossi, B.; Blanchard-Alvarez, A.; Grondin, G.; Trichard, S.; Cesari, C.; Sapet, M.; Bosco, F.; et al. Multifunctional Natural Killer Cell Engagers Targeting NKp46 Trigger Protective Tumor Immunity. *Cell* **2019**, *177*, 1701–1713.e16. [CrossRef]
119. Thorburn, A. Death receptor-induced cell killing. *Cell. Signal.* **2004**, *16*, 139–144. [CrossRef]
120. Lundqvist, A.; Yokoyama, H.; Smith, A.; Berg, M.; Childs, R. Bortezomib treatment and regulatory T-cell depletion enhance the antitumor effects of adoptively infused NK cells. *Blood* **2009**, *113*, 6120–6127. [CrossRef]
121. Vales-Gomez, M.; Chisholm, S.E.; Cassady-Cain, R.L.; Roda-Navarro, P.; Reyburn, H.T. Selective Induction of Expression of a Ligand for the NKG2D Receptor by Proteasome Inhibitors. *Cancer Res.* **2008**, *68*, 1546–1554. [CrossRef]
122. Shi, J.; Tricot, G.; Szmania, S.; Rosen, N.; Garg, T.K.; Malaviarachchi, P.A.; Moreno, A.; Dupont, B.; Hsu, K.C.; Baxter-Lowe, L.A.; et al. Infusion of haplo-identical killer immunoglobulin-like receptor ligand mismatched NK cells for relapsed myeloma in the setting of autologous stem cell transplantation. *Br. J. Haematol.* **2008**, *143*, 641–653. [CrossRef] [PubMed]
123. Romee, R.; Rosario, M.; Berrien-Elliott, M.M.; Wagner, J.A.; Jewell, B.A.; Schappe, T.; Leong, J.W.; Abdel-Latif, S.; Schneider, S.E.; Willey, S.; et al. Cytokine-induced memory-like natural killer cells exhibit enhanced responses against myeloid leukemia. *Sci. Transl. Med.* **2016**, *8*, 357ra123. [CrossRef] [PubMed]
124. Cooper, M.A.; Elliott, J.M.; Keyel, P.A.; Yang, L.; Carrero, J.A.; Yokoyama, W.M. Cytokine-induced memory-like natural killer cells. *Proc. Natl. Acad. Sci.* **2009**, *106*, 1915–1919. [CrossRef]
125. Romee, R.; Schneider, S.E.; Leong, J.W.; Chase, J.M.; Keppel, C.R.; Sullivan, R.P.; Cooper, M.A.; Fehniger, T.A. Cytokine activation induces human memory-like NK cells. *Blood* **2012**, *120*, 4751–4760. [CrossRef] [PubMed]
126. Simhadri, V.R.; Mariano, J.L.; Zenarruzabeitia, O.; Seroogy, C.M.; Holland, S.M.; Kuehn, H.S.; Rosenzweig, S.D.; Borrego, F. Intact IL-12 signaling is necessary for the generation of human natural killer cells with enhanced effector function after restimulation. *J. Allergy Clin. Immunol.* **2014**, *134*, 1190–1193.e1. [CrossRef]

127. Simhadri, V.R.; Dimitrova, M.; Mariano, J.L.; Zenarruzabeitia, O.; Zhong, W.; Ozawa, T.; Muraguchi, A.; Kishi, H.; Eichelberger, M.C.; Borrego, F. A Human Anti-M2 Antibody Mediates Antibody-Dependent Cell-Mediated Cytotoxicity (ADCC) and Cytokine Secretion by Resting and Cytokine-Preactivated Natural Killer (NK) Cells. *PLoS One* **2015**, *10*, e0124677. [CrossRef]
128. Terrén, I.; Mikelez, I.; Odriozola, I.; Gredilla, A.; González, J.; Orrantia, A.; Vitallé, J.; Zenarruzabeitia, O.; Borrego, F. Implication of Interleukin-12/15/18 and Ruxolitinib in the Phenotype, Proliferation, and Polyfunctionality of Human Cytokine-Preactivated Natural Killer Cells. *Front. Immunol.* **2018**, *9*, 737. [CrossRef]
129. Mehta, R.S.; Rezvani, K.; Olson, A.; Oran, B.; Hosing, C.; Shah, N.; Parmar, S.; Armitage, S.; Shpall, E.J. Novel Techniques for Ex Vivo Expansion of Cord Blood: Clinical Trials. *Front. Med.* **2015**, *2*, 89. [CrossRef]
130. Garg, T.K.; Szmania, S.M.; Khan, J.A.; Hoering, A.; Malbrough, P.A.; Moreno-Bost, A.; Greenway, A.D.; Lingo, J.D.; Li, X.; Yaccoby, S.; et al. Highly activated and expanded natural killer cells for multiple myeloma immunotherapy. *Haematologica* **2012**, *97*, 1348–1356. [CrossRef]
131. Lapteva, N.; Durett, A.G.; Sun, J.; Rollins, L.A.; Huye, L.L.; Fang, J.; Dandekar, V.; Mei, Z.; Jackson, K.; Vera, J.; et al. Large-scale ex vivo expansion and characterization of natural killer cells for clinical applications. *Cytotherapy* **2012**, *14*, 1131–1143. [CrossRef] [PubMed]
132. Lapteva, N.; Parihar, R.; Rollins, L.A.; Gee, A.P.; Rooney, C.M. Large-Scale Culture and Genetic Modification of Human Natural Killer Cells for Cellular Therapy. In *Natural Killer Cells*; Humana Press: New York, NY, USA, 2016; Volume 1441, pp. 195–202.
133. Carlsten, M.; Childs, R.W. Genetic Manipulation of NK Cells for Cancer Immunotherapy: Techniques and Clinical Implications. *Front. Immunol.* **2015**, *6*, 266. [CrossRef] [PubMed]
134. Daher, M.; Rezvani, K. Next generation natural killer cells for cancer immunotherapy: the promise of genetic engineering. *Curr. Opin. Immunol.* **2018**, *51*, 146–153. [CrossRef]
135. Rezvani, K. Adoptive cell therapy using engineered natural killer cells. *Bone Marrow Transplant.* **2019**, *54*, 785–788. [CrossRef]
136. Mehta, R.S.; Rezvani, K. Chimeric Antigen Receptor Expressing Natural Killer Cells for the Immunotherapy of Cancer. *Front. Immunol.* **2018**, *9*, 283. [CrossRef]
137. Quintarelli, C.; Sivori, S.; Caruso, S.; Carlomagno, S.; Falco, M.; Boffa, I.; Orlando, D.; Guercio, M.; Abbaszadeh, Z.; Sinibaldi, M.; et al. Efficacy of third-party chimeric antigen receptor modified peripheral blood natural killer cells for adoptive cell therapy of B-cell precursor acute lymphoblastic leukemia. *Leukemia* **2019**. [CrossRef]
138. Zhang, C.; Oberoi, P.; Oelsner, S.; Waldmann, A.; Lindner, A.; Tonn, T.; Wels, W.S. Chimeric Antigen Receptor-Engineered NK-92 Cells: An Off-the-Shelf Cellular Therapeutic for Targeted Elimination of Cancer Cells and Induction of Protective Antitumor Immunity. *Front. Immunol.* **2017**, *8*, 533. [CrossRef]
139. Schleypen, J.S.; von Geldern, M.; Weiß, E.H.; Kotzias, N.; Rohrmann, K.; Schendel, D.J.; Falk, C.S.; Pohla, H. Renal cell carcinoma-infiltrating natural killer cells express differential repertoires of activating and inhibitory receptors and are inhibited by specific HLA class I allotypes. *Int. J. Cancer* **2003**, *106*, 905–912. [CrossRef]
140. Schleypen, J.S. Cytotoxic Markers and Frequency Predict Functional Capacity of Natural Killer Cells Infiltrating Renal Cell Carcinoma. *Clin. Cancer Res.* **2006**, *12*, 718–725. [CrossRef]
141. Prinz, P.U.; Mendler, A.N.; Brech, D.; Masouris, I.; Oberneder, R.; Noessner, E. NK-cell dysfunction in human renal carcinoma reveals diacylglycerol kinase as key regulator and target for therapeutic intervention. *Int. J. Cancer* **2014**, *135*, 1832–1841. [CrossRef] [PubMed]
142. Murphy, K.A.; James, B.R.; Guan, Y.; Torry, D.S.; Wilber, A.; Griffith, T.S. Exploiting natural anti-tumor immunity for metastatic renal cell carcinoma. *Hum. Vaccin. Immunother.* **2015**, *11*, 1612–1620. [CrossRef] [PubMed]
143. Chevrier, S.; Levine, J.H.; Zanotelli, V.R.T.; Silina, K.; Schulz, D.; Bacac, M.; Ries, C.H.; Ailles, L.; Jewett, M.A.S.; Moch, H.; et al. An Immune Atlas of Clear Cell Renal Cell Carcinoma. *Cell* **2017**, *169*, 736–749.e18. [CrossRef] [PubMed]
144. Eckl, J.; Buchner, A.; Prinz, P.U.; Riesenberg, R.; Siegert, S.I.; Kammerer, R.; Nelson, P.J.; Noessner, E. Transcript signature predicts tissue NK cell content and defines renal cell carcinoma subgroups independent of TNM staging. *J. Mol. Med.* **2012**, *90*, 55–66. [CrossRef] [PubMed]

145. Remark, R.; Alifano, M.; Cremer, I.; Lupo, A.; Dieu-Nosjean, M.-C.; Riquet, M.; Crozet, L.; Ouakrim, H.; Goc, J.; Cazes, A.; et al. Characteristics and Clinical Impacts of the Immune Environments in Colorectal and Renal Cell Carcinoma Lung Metastases: Influence of Tumor Origin. *Clin. Cancer Res.* **2013**, *19*, 4079–4091. [CrossRef] [PubMed]
146. Cózar, J.M.; Canton, J.; Tallada, M.; Concha, A.; Cabrera, T.; Garrido, F.; Ruiz-Cabello Osuna, F. Analysis of NK cells and chemokine receptors in tumor infiltrating CD4 T lymphocytes in human renal carcinomas. *Cancer Immunol. Immunother.* **2005**, *54*, 858–866. [CrossRef]
147. Donskov, F.; von der Maase, H. Impact of Immune Parameters on Long-Term Survival in Metastatic Renal Cell Carcinoma. *J. Clin. Oncol.* **2006**, *24*, 1997–2005. [CrossRef]
148. Kowalczyk, D.; Skorupski, W.; Kwias, Z.; Nowak, J. Flow cytometric analysis of tumour-infiltrating lymphocytes in patients with renal cell carcinoma. *BJU Int.* **1997**, *80*, 543–547. [CrossRef]
149. Terrén, I.; Orrantia, A.; Vitallé, J.; Zenarruzabeitia, O.; Borrego, F. NK Cell Metabolism and Tumor Microenvironment. *Front. Immunol.* **2019**, *10*, 2278. [CrossRef]
150. Vitale, M.; Cantoni, C.; Pietra, G.; Mingari, M.C.; Moretta, L. Effect of tumor cells and tumor microenvironment on NK-cell function. *Eur. J. Immunol.* **2014**, *44*, 1582–1592. [CrossRef]
151. Stojanovic, A.; Correia, M.P.; Cerwenka, A. Shaping of NK cell responses by the tumor microenvironment. *Cancer Microenviron.* **2013**, *6*, 135–146. [CrossRef] [PubMed]
152. Zenarruzabeitia, O.; Vitallé, J.; Astigarraga, I.; Borrego, F. Natural Killer Cells to the Attack: Combination Therapy against Neuroblastoma. *Clin. Cancer Res.* **2017**, *23*, 615–617. [CrossRef] [PubMed]
153. Xia, Y.; Zhang, Q.; Zhen, Q.; Zhao, Y.; Liu, N.; Li, T.; Hao, Y.; Zhang, Y.; Luo, C.; Wu, X. Negative regulation of tumor-infiltrating NK cell in clear cell renal cell carcinoma patients through the exosomal pathway. *Oncotarget* **2017**, *8*, 37783–37795. [CrossRef] [PubMed]
154. Tran, H.C.; Wan, Z.; Sheard, M.A.; Sun, J.; Jackson, J.R.; Malvar, J.; Xu, Y.; Wang, L.; Sposto, R.; Kim, E.S.; et al. TGFβR1 Blockade with Galunisertib (LY2157299) Enhances Anti-Neuroblastoma Activity of the Anti-GD2 Antibody Dinutuximab (ch14.18) with Natural Killer Cells. *Clin. Cancer Res.* **2017**, *23*, 804–813. [CrossRef]
155. Kaelin, W.G. The von Hippel-Lindau Tumor Suppressor Protein and Clear Cell Renal Carcinoma. *Clin. Cancer Res.* **2007**, *13*, 680s–684s. [CrossRef] [PubMed]
156. Messai, Y.; Noman, M.Z.; Hasmim, M.; Escudier, B.; Chouaib, S. HIF-2α/ITPR1 axis: A new saboteur of NK-mediated lysis. *Oncoimmunology* **2015**, *4*, e985951. [CrossRef] [PubMed]
157. Iliopoulos, O.; Kibel, A.; Gray, S.; Kaelin, W.G. Tumour suppression by the human von Hippel-Lindau gene product. *Nat. Med.* **1995**, *1*, 822–826. [CrossRef]
158. Kaelin Jr, W.G. The von Hippel–Lindau tumour suppressor protein: O2 sensing and cancer. *Nat. Rev. Cancer* **2008**, *8*, 865–873. [CrossRef]
159. Kondo, K.; Kim, W.Y.; Lechpammer, M.; Kaelin, W.G. Inhibition of HIF2alpha is sufficient to suppress pVHL-defective tumor growth. *PLoS Biol.* **2003**, *1*, E83. [CrossRef]
160. Messai, Y.; Noman, M.Z.; Hasmim, M.; Janji, B.; Tittarelli, A.; Boutet, M.; Baud, V.; Viry, E.; Billot, K.; Nanbakhsh, A.; et al. ITPR1 Protects Renal Cancer Cells against Natural Killer Cells by Inducing Autophagy. *Cancer Res.* **2014**, *74*, 6820–6832. [CrossRef]
161. Perier, A.; Fregni, G.; Wittnebel, S.; Gad, S.; Allard, M.; Gervois, N.; Escudier, B.; Azzarone, B.; Caignard, A. Mutations of the von Hippel–Lindau gene confer increased susceptibility to natural killer cells of clear-cell renal cell carcinoma. *Oncogene* **2011**, *30*, 2622–2632. [CrossRef] [PubMed]
162. Trotta, A.M.; Santagata, S.; Zanotta, S.; D'Alterio, C.; Napolitano, M.; Rea, G.; Camerlingo, R.; Esposito, F.; Lamantia, E.; Anniciello, A.; et al. Mutated Von Hippel-Lindau-renal cell carcinoma (RCC) promotes patients specific natural killer (NK) cytotoxicity. *J. Exp. Clin. Cancer Res.* **2018**, *37*, 297. [CrossRef] [PubMed]
163. Santoni, M.; Berardi, R.; Amantini, C.; Burattini, L.; Santini, D.; Santoni, G.; Cascinu, S. Role of natural and adaptive immunity in renal cell carcinoma response to VEGFR-TKIs and mTOR inhibitor. *Int. J. Cancer* **2014**, *134*, 2772–2777. [CrossRef] [PubMed]
164. Krusch, M.; Salih, J.; Schlicke, M.; Baessler, T.; Kampa, K.M.; Mayer, F.; Salih, H.R. The Kinase Inhibitors Sunitinib and Sorafenib Differentially Affect NK Cell Antitumor Reactivity In Vitro. *J. Immunol.* **2009**, *183*, 8286–8294. [CrossRef] [PubMed]
165. Moeckel, J.; Staiger, N.; Mackensen, A.; Meidenbauer, N.; Ullrich, E. Sunitinib does not impair natural killer cell function in patients with renal cell carcinoma. *Oncol. Lett.* **2017**, *14*, 1089–1096. [CrossRef] [PubMed]

166. Huang, Y.; Wang, Y.; Li, Y.; Guo, K.; He, Y. Role of sorafenib and sunitinib in the induction of expressions of NKG2D ligands in nasopharyngeal carcinoma with high expression of ABCG2. *J. Cancer Res. Clin. Oncol.* **2011**, *137*, 829–837. [CrossRef] [PubMed]

167. Morelli, M.B.; Amantini, C.; Santoni, M.; Soriani, A.; Nabissi, M.; Cardinali, C.; Santoni, A.; Santoni, G. Axitinib induces DNA damage response leading to senescence, mitotic catastrophe, and increased NK cell recognition in human renal carcinoma cells. *Oncotarget* **2015**, *6*, 36245–36259. [CrossRef]

168. Yu, N.; Fu, S.; Xu, Z.; Liu, Y.; Hao, J.; Zhang, A.; Wang, B. Synergistic antitumor responses by combined GITR activation and sunitinib in metastatic renal cell carcinoma. *Int. J. cancer* **2016**, *138*, 451–462. [CrossRef]

169. Dielmann, A.; Letsch, A.; Nonnenmacher, A.; Miller, K.; Keilholz, U.; Busse, A. Favorable prognostic influence of T-box transcription factor Eomesodermin in metastatic renal cell cancer patients. *Cancer Immunol. Immunother.* **2016**, *65*, 181–192. [CrossRef]

170. Huijts, C.M.; Santegoets, S.J.; de Jong, T.D.; Verheul, H.M.; de Gruijl, T.D.; van der Vliet, H.J. Immunological effects of everolimus in patients with metastatic renal cell cancer. *Int. J. Immunopathol. Pharmacol.* **2017**, *30*, 341–352. [CrossRef]

171. Brahmer, J.; Reckamp, K.L.; Baas, P.; Crinò, L.; Eberhardt, W.E.E.; Poddubskaya, E.; Antonia, S.; Pluzanski, A.; Vokes, E.E.; Holgado, E.; et al. Nivolumab versus Docetaxel in Advanced Squamous-Cell Non–Small-Cell Lung Cancer. *N. Engl. J. Med.* **2015**, *373*, 123–135. [CrossRef] [PubMed]

172. Ferris, R.L.; Blumenschein, G.; Fayette, J.; Guigay, J.; Colevas, A.D.; Licitra, L.; Harrington, K.; Kasper, S.; Vokes, E.E.; Even, C.; et al. Nivolumab for Recurrent Squamous-Cell Carcinoma of the Head and Neck. *N. Engl. J. Med.* **2016**, *375*, 1856–1867. [CrossRef] [PubMed]

173. Hodi, F.S.; Chesney, J.; Pavlick, A.C.; Robert, C.; Grossmann, K.F.; McDermott, D.F.; Linette, G.P.; Meyer, N.; Giguere, J.K.; Agarwala, S.S.; et al. Combined nivolumab and ipilimumab versus ipilimumab alone in patients with advanced melanoma: 2-year overall survival outcomes in a multicentre, randomised, controlled, phase 2 trial. *Lancet Oncol.* **2016**, *17*, 1558–1568. [CrossRef]

174. Robert, C.; Long, G.V.; Brady, B.; Dutriaux, C.; Maio, M.; Mortier, L.; Hassel, J.C.; Rutkowski, P.; McNeil, C.; Kalinka-Warzocha, E.; et al. Nivolumab in Previously Untreated Melanoma without *BRAF* Mutation. *N. Engl. J. Med.* **2015**, *372*, 320–330. [CrossRef]

175. Motzer, R.J.; Escudier, B.; McDermott, D.F.; George, S.; Hammers, H.J.; Srinivas, S.; Tykodi, S.S.; Sosman, J.A.; Procopio, G.; Plimack, E.R.; et al. Nivolumab versus Everolimus in Advanced Renal-Cell Carcinoma. *N. Engl. J. Med.* **2015**, *373*, 1803–1813. [CrossRef]

176. Motzer, R.J.; Tannir, N.M.; McDermott, D.F.; Arén Frontera, O.; Melichar, B.; Choueiri, T.K.; Plimack, E.R.; Barthélémy, P.; Porta, C.; George, S.; et al. Nivolumab plus Ipilimumab versus Sunitinib in Advanced Renal-Cell Carcinoma. *N. Engl. J. Med.* **2018**, *378*, 1277–1290. [CrossRef]

177. Brahmer, J.R.; Tykodi, S.S.; Chow, L.Q.M.; Hwu, W.-J.; Topalian, S.L.; Hwu, P.; Drake, C.G.; Camacho, L.H.; Kauh, J.; Odunsi, K.; et al. Safety and Activity of Anti–PD-L1 Antibody in Patients with Advanced Cancer. *N. Engl. J. Med.* **2012**, *366*, 2455–2465. [CrossRef]

178. Motzer, R.J.; Rini, B.I.; McDermott, D.F.; Redman, B.G.; Kuzel, T.M.; Harrison, M.R.; Vaishampayan, U.N.; Drabkin, H.A.; George, S.; Logan, T.F.; et al. Nivolumab for Metastatic Renal Cell Carcinoma: Results of a Randomized Phase II Trial. *J. Clin. Oncol.* **2015**, *33*, 1430–1437. [CrossRef]

179. McDermott, D.F.; Sosman, J.A.; Sznol, M.; Massard, C.; Gordon, M.S.; Hamid, O.; Powderly, J.D.; Infante, J.R.; Fassò, M.; Wang, Y.V.; et al. Atezolizumab, an Anti-Programmed Death-Ligand 1 Antibody, in Metastatic Renal Cell Carcinoma: Long-Term Safety, Clinical Activity, and Immune Correlates From a Phase Ia Study. *J. Clin. Oncol.* **2016**, *34*, 833–842. [CrossRef]

180. Juliá, E.P.; Mandó, P.; Rizzo, M.M.; Cueto, G.R.; Tsou, F.; Luca, R.; Pupareli, C.; Bravo, A.I.; Astorino, W.; Mordoh, J.; et al. Peripheral changes in immune cell populations and soluble mediators after anti-PD-1 therapy in non-small cell lung cancer and renal cell carcinoma patients. *Cancer Immunol. Immunother.* **2019**, *68*, 1585–1596. [CrossRef]

181. Messai, Y.; Gad, S.; Noman, M.Z.; Le Teuff, G.; Couve, S.; Janji, B.; Kammerer, S.F.; Rioux-Leclerc, N.; Hasmim, M.; Ferlicot, S.; et al. Renal Cell Carcinoma Programmed Death-ligand 1, a New Direct Target of Hypoxia-inducible Factor-2 Alpha, is Regulated by von Hippel–Lindau Gene Mutation Status. *Eur. Urol.* **2016**, *70*, 623–632. [CrossRef] [PubMed]

182. Rojas, J.J.; Sampath, P.; Hou, W.; Thorne, S.H. Defining Effective Combinations of Immune Checkpoint Blockade and Oncolytic Virotherapy. *Clin. Cancer Res.* **2015**, *21*, 5543–5551. [CrossRef] [PubMed]

183. Seliger, B.; Jasinski-Bergner, S.; Quandt, D.; Stoehr, C.; Bukur, J.; Wach, S.; Legal, W.; Taubert, H.; Wullich, B.; Hartmann, A. HLA-E expression and its clinical relevance in human renal cell carcinoma. *Oncotarget* **2016**, *7*, 67360–67372. [CrossRef] [PubMed]
184. Kren, L.; Valkovsky, I.; Dolezel, J.; Capak, I.; Pacik, D.; Poprach, A.; Lakomy, R.; Redova, M.; Fabian, P.; Krenova, Z.; et al. HLA-G and HLA-E specific mRNAs connote opposite prognostic significance in renal cell carcinoma. *Diagn. Pathol.* **2012**, *7*, 58. [CrossRef]
185. Genega, E.M.; Ghebremichael, M.; Najarian, R.; Fu, Y.; Wang, Y.; Argani, P.; Grisanzio, C.; Signoretti, S. Carbonic Anhydrase IX Expression in Renal Neoplasms. *Am. J. Clin. Pathol.* **2010**, *134*, 873–879. [CrossRef]
186. Tostain, J.; Li, G.; Gentil-Perret, A.; Gigante, M. Carbonic anhydrase 9 in clear cell renal cell carcinoma: A marker for diagnosis, prognosis and treatment. *Eur. J. Cancer* **2010**, *46*, 3141–3148. [CrossRef]
187. Chang, D.-K.; Moniz, R.J.; Xu, Z.; Sun, J.; Signoretti, S.; Zhu, Q.; Marasco, W.A. Human anti-CAIX antibodies mediate immune cell inhibition of renal cell carcinoma in vitro and in a humanized mouse model in vivo. *Mol. Cancer* **2015**, *14*, 119. [CrossRef]
188. Berlato, C.; Khan, M.N.; Schioppa, T.; Thompson, R.; Maniati, E.; Montfort, A.; Jangani, M.; Canosa, M.; Kulbe, H.; Hagemann, U.B.; et al. A CCR4 antagonist reverses the tumor-promoting microenvironment of renal cancer. *J. Clin. Invest.* **2017**, *127*, 801–813. [CrossRef]
189. Yanagita, T.; Murata, Y.; Tanaka, D.; Motegi, S.; Arai, E.; Daniwijaya, E.W.; Hazama, D.; Washio, K.; Saito, Y.; Kotani, T.; et al. Anti-SIRPα antibodies as a potential new tool for cancer immunotherapy. *JCI Insight* **2017**, *2*, e89140. [CrossRef]
190. Wrangle, J.M.; Patterson, A.; Johnson, C.B.; Neitzke, D.J.; Mehrotra, S.; Denlinger, C.E.; Paulos, C.M.; Li, Z.; Cole, D.J.; Rubinstein, M.P. IL-2 and Beyond in Cancer Immunotherapy. *J. Interferon Cytokine Res.* **2018**, *38*, 45–68. [CrossRef]
191. Kovanen, P.E.; Leonard, W.J. Cytokines and immunodeficiency diseases: critical roles of the gamma(c)-dependent cytokines interleukins 2, 4, 7, 9, 15, and 21, and their signaling pathways. *Immunol. Rev.* **2004**, *202*, 67–83. [CrossRef] [PubMed]
192. Fehniger, T.A.; Cooper, M.A.; Caligiuri, M.A. Interleukin-2 and interleukin-15: immunotherapy for cancer. *Cytokine Growth Factor Rev.* **2002**, *13*, 169–183. [CrossRef]
193. Bhatia, S.; Tykodi, S.S.; Thompson, J.A. Treatment of metastatic melanoma: an overview. *Oncology (Williston Park)*. **2009**, *23*, 488–496. [PubMed]
194. Erbe, A.K.; Wang, W.; Goldberg, J.; Gallenberger, M.; Kim, K.; Carmichael, L.; Hess, D.; Mendonca, E.A.; Song, Y.; Hank, J.A.; et al. FCGR Polymorphisms Influence Response to IL2 in Metastatic Renal Cell Carcinoma. *Clin. Cancer Res.* **2017**, *23*, 2159–2168. [CrossRef]
195. Wang, W.; Erbe, A.K.; Gallenberger, M.; Kim, K.; Carmichael, L.; Hess, D.; Mendonca, E.A.; Song, Y.; Hank, J.A.; Cheng, S.-C.; et al. Killer immunoglobulin-like receptor (KIR) and KIR–ligand genotype do not correlate with clinical outcome of renal cell carcinoma patients receiving high-dose IL2. *Cancer Immunol. Immunother.* **2016**, *65*, 1523–1532. [CrossRef]
196. Pavone, L.; Andrulli, S.; Santi, R.; Majori, M.; Buzio, C. Long-term treatment with low doses of interleukin-2 and interferon-alpha: immunological effects in advanced renal cell cancer. *Cancer Immunol. Immunother.* **2001**, *50*, 82–86. [CrossRef]
197. Pavone, L.; Fanti, G.; Bongiovanni, C.; Goldoni, M.; Alberici, F.; Bonomini, S.; Cristinelli, L.; Buzio, C. Natural killer cell cytotoxicity is enhanced by very low doses of rIL-2 and rIFN-alpha in patients with renal cell carcinoma. *Med. Oncol.* **2009**, *26*, 38–44. [CrossRef]
198. Donskov, F.; Bennedsgaard, K.M.; von der Maase, H.; Marcussen, N.; Fisker, R.; Jensen, J.J.; Naredi, P.; Hokland, M. Intratumoural and peripheral blood lymphocyte subsets in patients with metastatic renal cell carcinoma undergoing interleukin-2 based immunotherapy: association to objective response and survival. *Br. J. Cancer* **2002**, *87*, 194–201. [CrossRef]
199. Toliou, T.; Stravoravdi, P.; Polyzonis, M.; Vakalikos, J. Natural killer cell activation after interferon administration in patients with metastatic renal cell carcinoma: an ultrastructural and immunohistochemical study. *Eur. Urol.* **1996**, *29*, 252–256.
200. Miller, J.S.; Morishima, C.; McNeel, D.G.; Patel, M.R.; Kohrt, H.E.K.; Thompson, J.A.; Sondel, P.M.; Wakelee, H.A.; Disis, M.L.; Kaiser, J.C.; et al. A First-in-Human Phase I Study of Subcutaneous Outpatient Recombinant Human IL15 (rhIL15) in Adults with Advanced Solid Tumors. *Clin. Cancer Res.* **2018**, *24*, 1525–1535. [CrossRef]

201. Margolin, K.; Morishima, C.; Velcheti, V.; Miller, J.S.; Lee, S.M.; Silk, A.W.; Holtan, S.G.; Lacroix, A.M.; Fling, S.P.; Kaiser, J.C.; et al. Phase I Trial of ALT-803, A Novel Recombinant IL15 Complex, in Patients with Advanced Solid Tumors. *Clin. Cancer Res.* **2018**, *24*, 5552–5561. [CrossRef] [PubMed]
202. Law, T.M.; Motzer, R.J.; Mazumdar, M.; Sell, K.W.; Walther, P.J.; O'Connell, M.; Khan, A.; Vlamis, V.; Vogelzang, N.J.; Bajorin, D.F. Phase III randomized trial of interleukin-2 with or without lymphokine-activated killer cells in the treatment of patients with advanced renal cell carcinoma. *Cancer* **1995**, *76*, 824–832. [CrossRef]
203. Rosenberg, S.A.; Yang, J.C.; Topalian, S.L.; Schwartzentruber, D.J.; Weber, J.S.; Parkinson, D.R.; Seipp, C.A.; Einhorn, J.H.; White, D.E. Treatment of 283 consecutive patients with metastatic melanoma or renal cell cancer using high-dose bolus interleukin 2. *JAMA* **1994**, *271*, 907–913. [CrossRef] [PubMed]
204. Tam, Y.K.; Martinson, J.A.; Doligosa, K.; Klingemann, H.-G. Ex vivo expansion of the highly cytotoxic human natural killer-92 cell-line under current good manufacturing practice conditions for clinical adoptive cellular immunotherapy. *Cytotherapy* **2003**, *5*, 259–272.
205. Wong, Y.N.S.; Joshi, K.; Pule, M.; Peggs, K.S.; Swanton, C.; Quezada, S.A.; Linch, M. Evolving adoptive cellular therapies in urological malignancies. *Lancet. Oncol.* **2017**, *18*, e341–e353. [CrossRef]
206. Lin, M.; Xu, K.; Liang, S.; Wang, X.; Liang, Y.; Zhang, M.; Chen, J.; Niu, L. Prospective study of percutaneous cryoablation combined with allogenic NK cell immunotherapy for advanced renal cell cancer. *Immunol. Lett.* **2017**, *184*, 98–104. [CrossRef]
207. Kremer, V.; Ligtenberg, M.A.; Zendehdel, R.; Seitz, C.; Duivenvoorden, A.; Wennerberg, E.; Colón, E.; Scherman-Plogell, A.-H.; Lundqvist, A. Genetic engineering of human NK cells to express CXCR2 improves migration to renal cell carcinoma. *J. Immunother. Cancer* **2017**, *5*, 73. [CrossRef]
208. Schönfeld, K.; Sahm, C.; Zhang, C.; Naundorf, S.; Brendel, C.; Odendahl, M.; Nowakowska, P.; Bönig, H.; Köhl, U.; Kloess, S.; et al. Selective Inhibition of Tumor Growth by Clonal NK Cells Expressing an ErbB2/HER2-Specific Chimeric Antigen Receptor. *Mol. Ther.* **2015**, *23*, 330–338. [CrossRef]
209. Zhang, Q.; Tian, K.; Xu, J.; Zhang, H.; Li, L.; Fu, Q.; Chai, D.; Li, H.; Zheng, J. Synergistic Effects of Cabozantinib and EGFR-Specific CAR-NK-92 Cells in Renal Cell Carcinoma. *J. Immunol. Res.* **2017**, *2017*, 1–14. [CrossRef]
210. Zhang, Q.; Xu, J.; Ding, J.; Liu, H.; Li, H.; Li, H.; Lu, M.; Miao, Y.; Wang, Z.; Fu, Q.; et al. Bortezomib improves adoptive carbonic anhydrase IX-specific chimeric antigen receptor-modified NK92 cell therapy in mouse models of human renal cell carcinoma. *Oncol. Rep.* **2018**, *40*, 3714–3724. [CrossRef]

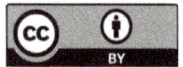

© 2020 by the authors. Licensee MDPI, Basel, Switzerland. This article is an open access article distributed under the terms and conditions of the Creative Commons Attribution (CC BY) license (http://creativecommons.org/licenses/by/4.0/).

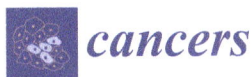 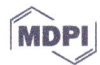

Review

ESC, ALK, HOT and LOT: Three Letter Acronyms of Emerging Renal Entities Knocking on the Door of the WHO Classification

Farshid Siadat and Kiril Trpkov *

Department of Pathology and Laboratory Medicine, University of Calgary and Alberta Precision Laboratories, Rockyview General Hospital, 7007 14 Street, Calgary, AB T2V 1P9, Canada; Farshid.Siadat@albertaprecisionlabs.ca
* Correspondence: kiril.trpkov@albertaprecisionlabs.ca

Received: 4 December 2019; Accepted: 6 January 2020; Published: 9 January 2020

Abstract: Kidney neoplasms are among the most heterogeneous and diverse tumors. Continuous advancement of this field is reflected in the emergence of new tumour entities and an increased recognition of the expanding morphologic, immunohistochemical, molecular, epidemiologic and clinical spectrum of renal tumors. Most recent advances after the 2016 World Health Organization (WHO) classification of renal cell tumors have provided new evidence on some emerging entities, such as anaplastic lymphoma kinase rearrangement-associated RCC (ALK-RCC), which has already been included in the WHO 2016 classification as a provisional entity. Additionally, several previously unrecognized entities, not currently included in the WHO classification, have also been introduced, such as eosinophilic solid and cystic renal cell carcinoma (ESC RCC), low-grade oncocytic renal tumor (LOT) and high-grade oncocytic renal tumor (HOT) of kidney. Although pathologists play a crucial role in the recognition and classification of these new tumor entities and are at the forefront of the efforts to characterize them, the awareness and the acceptance of these entities among clinicians will ultimately translate into more nuanced management and improved prognostication for individual patients. In this review, we summarise the current knowledge and the novel data on these emerging renal entities, with an aim to promote their increased diagnostic recognition and better characterization, and to facilitate further studies that will hopefully lead to their formal recognition and consideration in the future classifications of kidney tumors.

Keywords: kidney; emerging entity; new entity; oncocytic renal tumor; unclassified renal cell carcinoma; unclassified renal tumor; anaplastic lymphoma kinase rearrangement; ALK; ESC; HOT; LOT

---

1. Eosinophilic Solid and Cystic Renal Cell Carcinoma (ESC RCC)

Eosinophilic solid and cystic renal cell carcinoma (ESC RCC) has been recently characterized as an emerging renal entity that exhibits a set of well-defined clinical, pathological, immunohistochemical and molecular features [1–3]. Because it was described very recently, it is not yet included in the 2016 WHO classification of genitourinary tumors [4]. These types of tumors have likely been previously designated as "unclassified renal cell carcinoma" or "unclassified renal neoplasm (or renal cell carcinoma) with oncocytic or eosinophilic morphology". Great majority of ESC RCC are sporadic and are found in non-syndromic setting, although a subset of identical tumors have been documented in patients with a tuberous sclerosis complex (TSC) [5,6]. The great majority of ESC RCC are small, solitary tumors of low stage that are found in female patients, and generally exhibit indolent behaviour, although rare cases have been documented with metastatic disease [1,2,7–10]. The most salient features of ESC RCC and the other emerging entities included in this review are summarized in Table 1.

Table 1. Summary of the features of emerging renal tumors eosinophilic solid and cystic renal cell carcinoma (ESC RCC), anaplastic lymphoma kinase rearrangement-associated RCC (ALK-RCC), low-grade oncocytic renal tumor (LOT) and high-grade oncocytic renal tumor (HOT).

Emerging Renal Tumor	Clinical Features	Morphology	Immunohistochemistry	Molecular Features	Prognosis
Eosinophilic solid and cystic RCC (ESC RCC)	Mostly females and solitary tumors, ~10% in TSC patients	Solid and cystic growth, often scattered histiocytes and lymphocytes, voluminous eosinophilic cells, cytoplasmic coarse granularity (stippling)	CK20+ either focal or diffuse (note: 10%–15% CK20-), CK7-, CD117-	Somatic bi-allelic loss or mutation of *TSC1* and *TSC2*	Typically good, but rare cases documented with adverse prognosis
Anaplastic lymphoma kinase rearrangement-associated RCC (ALK-RCC)	Adults (younger middle age or older); children or adolescent with the sickle cell trait	Variable and admixed morphologies in adults, often mucinous background present; renal medullary carcinoma-like morphology in children	ALK1+, remaining IHC nonspecific; rare cases in children TFE3+ (but without translocation by FISH)	*ALK* rearrangement with various fusion partners: *VCL*, *TPM3*, *EML4*, *STRN*, *HOOK1*, *CLIP1* and *KIF5 B*	~1/3 adverse prognosis (metastatic disease at presentation)
High-grade oncocytic tumor (HOT)	Wide age range, female/male = 4/1; can occur rarely in TSC patients; typically smaller tumors	Solid growth, oncocytic/eosinophilic cells, prominent cytoplasmic vacuoles round to oval nuclei, often very large nucleoli	Cathepsin K+, CD10+, CD117+, CK7- (only rare scattered cells +)	Limited data: non-overlapping mutations in either *TSC1*, or *TSC2*, or *MTOR* genes; by aCGH loss of 19 p or chr. 1	Indolent tumors (limited follow-up)
Low-grade oncocytic tumor (LOT)	Older patients, solitary and non-syndromic tumors, small size	Solid growth with sharp transition to edematous areas with loose cell arrangement; low-grade oncocytic cells, round to oval nuclei and frequent perinuclear halos	CD117- (rarely very weak+), CK7+	Limited data: by aCGH deletions at 19p13.3, 1 p36.33 and 19q13; also disomic status in some	Indolent tumors (limited follow up)

1.1. Clinical Features

ESC RCC are typically sporadic tumors, not associated with TSC; however, about 10% or less of these tumors with virtually identical features have been documented in TSC patients [1–3,5]. ESC RCC are typically solitary, unifocal tumors of small size and low stage (mostly pT1, rarely pT2 or pT3) [1–3,11]. Occasional multifocal and bilateral cases have also been reported [2,8,12]. The patients are overwhelmingly females, and only rare cases have been reported in males. In an unselected patient cohort, the median age was 55 years, with a broad patient age range (32–79 years) [1,2]. However, a recent study of previously 'unclassified' eosinophilic renal tumors in younger patients (defined as age 35 years or younger), found 10 ESC RCC, which represented 30% of this cohort, with a median age of 27 years [12]. The true incidence of this tumor is currently unknown.

Although the great majority of ESC RCC exhibit indolent behavior, four cases have so far been reported with metastases, which justifies the "RCC" designation for this entity and reiterates the need for an ongoing clinical surveillance for these patients [1,2,7–9]. Additional studies are needed to fully determine the biologic behavior of ESC RCC, because to date, there are only few well-documented series with sufficient follow-up [1,2,10].

1.2. Pathological Features

1.2.1. Gross Features

The proposed name of this tumor entails the designations "solid and cystic" which succinctly conveys the main gross features [1–5]. ESC RCC are well-delineated tumors, showing mixed macrocystic and solid patterns (Figure 1A) [1,2]. The cysts are often multifocal and vary in size from few millimeters to few centimeters; the presence of macrocysts is one of the key gross features. Rare cases demonstrated almost exclusively solid growth with only rare identifiable microscopic cysts [1,2]. The tumor cut surface is yellow/gray/tan. Most of the reported tumors were smaller than 5 cm (median: 3.1 cm, mean

4.2 cm), but the reported tumor size was variable, from 1.2 to as 13.5 cm in greatest dimension, based on the largest series by Trpkov et al. [1,2].

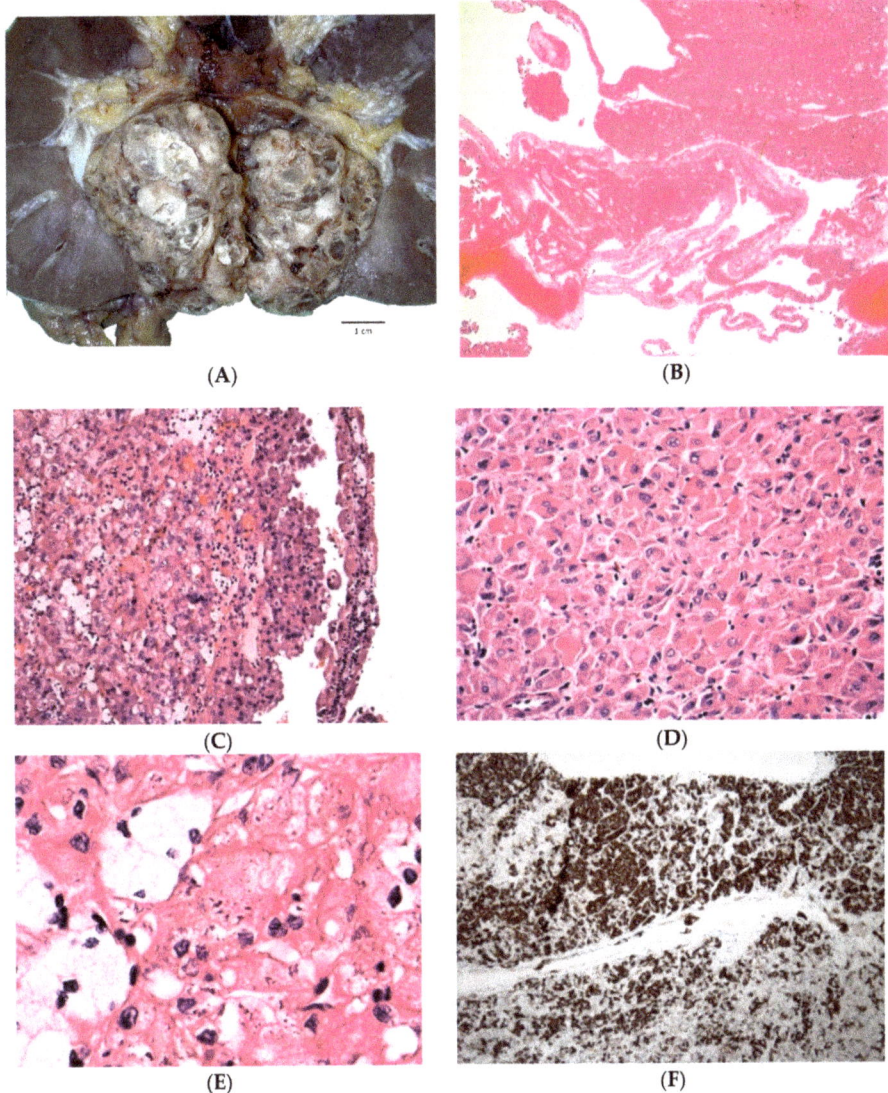

Figure 1. Eosinophilic solid and cystic renal cell carcinoma (ESC RCC) show grossly mixed macrocystic and solid appearances (**A**). Solid and cystic areas can also be appreciated at low power (**B**). The solid areas demonstrate diffuse and compact growth with adjacent cyst trabeculae showing hobnailing (**C**). Eosinophilic cells exhibit voluminous cytoplasm with readily recognizable coarse cytoplasmic granules ('stippling'); aggregates of foamy histiocytes and lymphocytes are often found (**D**,**E**). CK20 is positive in the majority of ESC RCC (**F**).

1.2.2. Microscopic Features

ESC RCC are circumscribed tumors, but without a well-formed capsule at the periphery.

The epithelial lining of the cysts has a hobnail arrangement and the cyst trabeculae (i.e., the solid parts between the cysts) can vary in thickness (Figure 1B,C) [1,2]. The solid tumor areas have identical appearances as seen in the trabeculae between the cysts, showing diffuse, compact acinar or compact nested growth (Figure 1D). Scattered aggregates of foamy histiocytes and lymphocytes are often found (Figure 1C,E). The cells typically show eosinophilic, voluminous cytoplasm, with readily identifiable coarse, basophilic to purple, cytoplasmic granules ('stippling'), which represents a very helpful morphologic feature; these granules correspond to aggregates of rough endoplasmic reticulum, observed on electron microscopy (Figure 1E) [1]. The nuclei are round to oval with focally prominent nucleoli, equivalent to WHO/ISUP grade 2 or 3 (Figure 1D,E). Focal nuclear irregularities can also be seen.

Other less common or less specific features can also be present, including focal papillary growth, focal "clear cell" areas, as well as focal insular or tubular growth and clusters of multinucleated cells [1,2]. Cell size variations or architectural pattern variations can also be observed within individual cases. Intracytoplasmic vacuolization, either microvesicular or macrovesicular, is also common and psammoma bodies can be found in about half of the cases [1,2].

1.2.3. Immunohistochemical and Molecular Features

Immunohistochemistry (IHC) for CK20 is positive in great majority of ESC RCC (Figure 1F), either as diffuse or focal reactivity, and it is usually paired with a negative or only focally positive CK7 (in about a quarter of cases) [1,2]. Of note, negative CK20 can also be observed in about 10%–15% of otherwise typical cases, together with either negative or focally positive CK7 [1–3]. To our knowledge, none of the reported ESC RCC cases so far demonstrated a CK20 negative/CK7 positive immunophenotype, which may be helpful in differentiating ESC RCC from other eosinophilic renal tumors. Other positive stains also include PAX8, AE1/AE3, CK8/18 and vimentin; rare cases can be negative or only focally positive for cytokeratin AE1/AE3 [1,2]. Cathepsin K is also reactive in great majority of ESC RCC, either as diffuse or focal positivity (personal unpublished observations), in line with some of the reported observations of cathepsin K reactivity in ESC RCC [10,12]. Negative stains include CD117, CA9, HMB45 and melan A [1,2].

The molecular characterization of ESC RCC by next generation sequencing (NGS) revealed recurrent and mutually exclusive somatic bi-allelic loss or mutations in of TSC gene family, including *TSC2* and *TSC1* in 85% (6/7) of evaluated cases [13]. Parilla et al. characterized two cases of sporadic ESC RCC in patients without clinical features of tuberous sclerosis, which demonstrated pathogenic somatic TSC2 gene mutations [9]. These mutations were without other alterations in any other genes associated with RCC, suggesting that sporadic ESC RCC may be characterized by somatic tuberous sclerosis gene mutations (TSC2) [9]. Palsgrove and al have also confirmed a consistent presence of either TSC1 or TSC2 gene mutations in pediatric ESC RCC (8/9 cases) and adult ESC RCC (6/6 cases). These included a metastatic ESC RCC which had a complete response to mTOR targeted therapy [10]. Molecular karyotype profiling of ESC RCC has also shown common and recurring genomic changes, including copy number (CN) gains at 16p13-16q23, 7p21-7q36, 13q14, and 19p12 and CN losses at Xp11.21 and 22q11 [2]. Loss of heterozygosity (LOH) alterations were identified at 16p11.2-11.1, Xq11-13, Xq13-21, 11p11, 9q21-22, and 9q33 [2]. Many of the genes and gene sets in the affected regions are involved in the regulation of *MTOR* signaling pathway and indicate that ESC RCC genomic alterations are different from those found in the currently recognized renal neoplasms [2,9,10]. Although these molecular alterations are neither pathognomonic nor specific for ESC RCC, taken together with the morphologic and immunohistochemical features seen in ESC RCC, signify a relatively compact and distinct morpho-molecular entity.

1.3. Differential Diagnosis

The wide spectrum of the renal tumours with eosinophilic cells should all be considered in the differential diagnosis of ESC RCC, which includes primarily renal oncocytoma and the eosinophilic variant of chromophobe renal cell carcinoma (Chr RCC), as well as some less common entities, such as succinate dehydrogenase (SDH)-deficient RCC, MiTF translocation RCC (particularly TFEB), and epithelioid angiomyolipoma (AML), as shown in Table 2. However, the morphologic features of ESC RCC observed on H&E and its immunohistochemical profile are generally sufficient for the diagnosis.

Table 2. Key distinguishing features of the emerging renal tumors vs. other eosinophilic/oncocytic renal tumors.

Diagnosis	Key Distinguishing Features	Immunohistochemistry
Eosinophilic, solid and cystic RCC (ESC RCC)	Great majority females, solid and cystic growth, cytoplasmic stippling, lacks perinuclear halos	CK20+ (diffuse or focal; rarely CK20-), CK7-, CD117-
Anaplastic lymphoma kinase rearrangement-associated RCC (ALK RCC)	Variable and mixed morphology in adults, often mucinous background. Renal medullary carcinoma-like morphology in children	ALK1+, rare TFE3+ (FISH-)
High-grade oncocytic tumor (HOT)	Solid growth, voluminous oncocytic cells with high grade nuclei, large cytoplasmic vacuoles	CD117+, CK7- (only scattered cells CK7+), Cathepsin K+, CD10+
Low-grade oncocytic tumor(LOT)	Solid growth with gradual transition to trabecular areas; sharply delineated edematous stromal areas with loose and irregular cell arrangement	CD117-, CK7+ (diffuse)
Oncocytoma	Solid growth at the periphery, can show tubulocystic growth, central 'archipelaginous' areas, cells lack perinuclear halos	CD117+, CK7- (usually only scattered cells CK7+)
Chromophobe RCC, eosinophilic	Solid growth, loose stromal areas absent, cells with more prominent membranes, irregular ('raisinoid') nuclei, perinuclear halos	CD117+, CK7+
Clear cell RCC, eosinophilic	At least focal clear cell areas, delicate vasculature in the background	CA9+, CD117-
Papillary RCC, oncocytic/solid	Papillary growth (at least focally)	AMACR+, CK7+, CD10+
Epithelioid angiomyolipoma	Epithelioid cells, may be pleomorphic, lacks perinuclear halos	PAX8-, Cathepsin K+, HMB45+, AE1/AE3-
SDH-deficient RCC	Low-grade oncocytic cells with at least focal flocculent (fluffy) cytoplasm and inclusions; lacks perinuclear halos	CD117-, SDHB-, AE1/AE3- (often)

2. ALK Rearrangement-Associated RCC (ALK-RCC)

ALK rearrangement-associated RCC (ALK-RCC) is another novel renal entity that has already been included in the 2016 WHO classification as an "emerging/provisional" entity [3,4]. It encompasses renal carcinomas demonstrating translocation that result in a fusion of the ALK gene with various gene partners. ALK is located at 2p23 and it is a member of the receptor tyrosine kinase family and the insulin receptor superfamily [14]. Chromosomal rearrangements resulting in ALK fusion with several partner genes lead to aberrant ALK activation through the formation of oncogenic chimeric proteins. However, rearrangement of ALK is not restricted only to ALK-RCC, but has also been previously documented in other non-renal tumors, such as non-small-cell lung adenocarcinoma, anaplastic thyroid carcinoma, anaplastic large-cell lymphoma, and others [15]. Since the first report in 2011, less than 30 cases of ALK-RCC have been reported [16–32]. These tumors demonstrate considerable morphologic diversity, but their underlying commonality includes the ALK rearrangement that can be documented either by IHC or by molecular studies, such as fluorescence in situ hybridisation (FISH).

2.1. Clinical Features

ALK RCC are solitary tumors, typically not associated with any clinical syndromes. They are documented in patients with diverse racial background, including African American, Caucasian and Asian patients. However, a large study of 1019 kidney tumors in adult Polish patient cohort failed to identify a single ALK-RCC by using three different clones of anti-ALK antibodies for immunohistochemical evaluation [33].

ALK-RCC occurs slightly more often in male patients (M:F = 1.5:1) and has been documented in patients of wide age range, with clustering in children and adolescents (range, 3–19 years), younger and middle aged adults (range, 30–49 years), and in patients older than 50 years (range, 52–85 years). Some pediatric cases demonstrating *VCL–ALK* and *TPM3–ALK* fusions have been documented in African American patients with the sickle-cell trait [19,27,28].

Although the clinical behavior and the histopathologic characteristics of this tumor have not been fully established, they may exhibit adverse prognosis, including metastatic disease and death, which has been documented in about 30% of the cases, clearly substantiating their malignant potential [16,24,32]. The interest in this tumor has also been fortified by the availability of targeted therapies, such as ALK inhibitors alectinib and crizotinib in tumors demonstrating ALK rearrangement. A recent report described three patients with "metastatic ALK-rearranged papillary RCC" with documented ALK fusion (all with *EML4-ALK*), who were treated with alectinib, and all patients showed a demonstrable short term clinical and radiographic response [32]. Based on the provided data in the report, these three case likely represent types of tumors within the spectrum of the reported ALK-RCC [32].

2.2. Pathological Features

2.2.1. Gross Features

ALK-RCC are solitary, solid or solid–cystic tumors that show white-grey to yellow and variegated cut surface and range in size from 3 to 7 cm (Figure 2A). Most of the reported pediatric cases with *VCL-ALK* fusion were located in the medulla or the renal pelvis, while the remaining cases were mostly located in the renal cortex. Grossly identifiable necrosis and hemorrhage were also noted in some cases.

2.2.2. Microscopic Features

Pediatric cases demonstrating *VCL–ALK* and *TPM3–ALK* fusions exhibited morphologic similarities to adult renal medullary carcinoma and collecting duct carcinoma, such as diffuse solid or reticular/syncytial/tubular growth, with a background of prominent and delicate vascular network, often admixed with significant lymphoplasmacytic inflammatory infiltrate and stromal desmoplasia [19–21,27,28]. The neoplastic cells in these pediatric cases were typically discohesive and showed variable cytomorphologies, including polygonal, spindle, cuboidal and low columnar. They also exhibited voluminous eosinophilic cytoplasm with common intracytoplasmic lumina; the nuclei were round to oval with focally prominent nucleoli.

The remaining types of ALK-RCC showed variable and complex morphologies, typically demonstrating multiple growth patterns in a single case, including solid, tubular or tubulo-cystic, papillary (or pseudopapillary), cribriform, trabecular, and signet-ring individual cell growth (Figure 2B–E). An extensive mucinous background, as well as intracytoplasmic mucin have been frequently found in these cases and may be a helpful clue for the diagnosis [16,18,23]. The cells had eosinophilic cytoplasm and showed variable morphologies, including rhabdoid, vacuolated, pleomorphic giant cell and small cell (metanephric adenoma-like) morphology. Occasional psammoma bodies were also present and coagulative necrosis and mitoses have also been found in these cases [16,24].

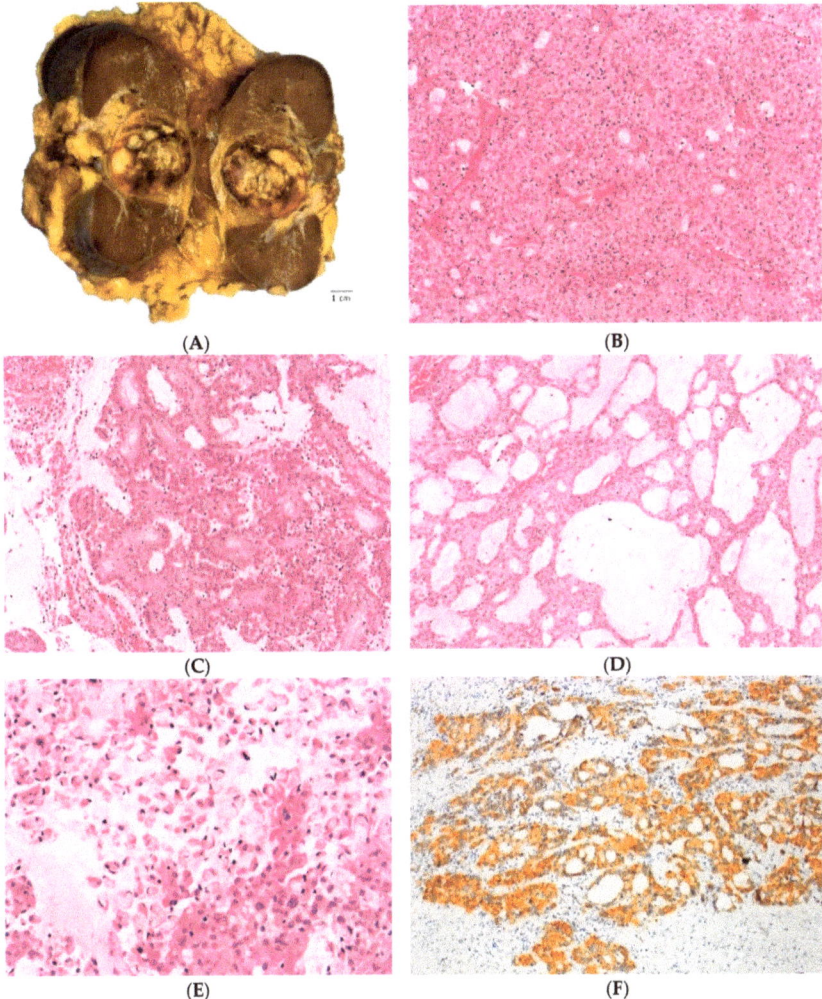

Figure 2. ALK rearrangement-associated RCC (ALK-RCC) shows a variegated gross appearance (**A**). On microscopy, multiple growth patterns can be seen in a single tumor, including solid (**B**), papillary (**C**), tubular and tubulocystic (**D**). Intracytoplasmic vacuoles and individual signet ring cells can also be found (**E**) often with a mucinous background (**D,E**). There is ALK1 protein expression on immunohistochemistry (**F**).

2.2.3. Immunohistochemistry, Electron Microscopy and Molecular Features

Patients with ALK-RCC demonstrate diffuse cytoplasmic and membranous ALK protein expression by IHC, which can aid in screening suspicious cases (Figure 2F). However, for a definitive diagnosis, an ALK-rearrangement by FISH is necessary, typically showing an ALK split signal in the majority of tumor cells. ALK-RCCs are usually reactive for CK7, 34βE12, AMACR and vimentin; INI-1 expression is retained and Ki67 proliferation index is relatively low [19]. Melanocytic markers such as melan A, S100, HMB45, and cathepsin K are negative [16]. Immunoreactivity for TFE3, but without genuine TFE3-rearrangement by FISH, has been reported in some pediatric cases [19–21,25] and in one adult patient with ALK-RCC showing *TPM3-ALK* fusion [18].

Electron microscopy of ALK-RCC demonstrated the presence of microvilli, tight desmosomes, numerous lipofuscin-like structures, and a well-developed cytoskeleton in the cytoplasm [21,25,27].

Genetic studies have identified, so far, several ALK fusion gene partners, but in some cases none of these partners were found, which indicates the possibility that some additional gene partners have yet to be discovered. Until recently, *VCL-ALK* has been documented only in pediatric patients of African American descent with the sickle-cell trait [19,21,27,28]. However, a recent report identified *VCL-ALK* fusion in a 57 year-old Chinese woman, without any evidence of the sickle cell trait [31]. Four other ALK fusion gene partners have been also identified, both in pediatric and adult patients: *TPM3-ALK*, *EML4-ALK*, striatin *(STRN)-ALK*, and *HOOK1-ALK* [16–18,20–23]. Most recently, in a multi-institutional study of 12 novel ALK-RCC, we identified three new, previously unreported ALK gene partners: *CLIP1*, *KIF5B* and *KIAA1217* (data presented in part at the United States Canadian Academy of Pathology Annual Meeting 2019) [34].

2.3. Differential Diagnosis

The differential diagnosis of ALK-RCC is quite broad, primarily due to the presence of variable and diverse morphologies that can be observed in ALK-RCC, which may mimic other renal entities, such as renal medullary carcinoma (in children and adolescents), collective duct carcinoma, papillary RCC, MiTF RCC (TFE3 and TFEB), mucinous tubular and spindle cell carcinoma, and thyroid-like follicular RCC. However, ALK-RCC usually shows multiple, admixed growth patterns, often set in a mucinous background, generally demonstrates lesser degree of cytologic atypia, lack significant stromal desmoplasia and are non-infiltrative. ALK positive IHC or ALK rearrangements demonstrated by FISH are crucial in establishing the diagnosis. A notable pitfall in misdiagnosing ALK RCC as Xp11.2 translocation RCC may be due to its positivity for TFE3 by IHC in some cases; however, TFE3 rearrangement by FISH is lacking in these cases [19,20,25,27,28].

3. High-Grade Oncocytic Tumor (HOT) of Kidney

High-grade oncocytic tumor (HOT) is an entity with unique and readily recognizable morphology, composed predominantly of oncocytic cells with high-grade nuclei, prominent intracytoplasmic vacuoles, and demonstrates a relatively consistent IHC profile. HOT of kidney has recently been proposed [35] to represent a previously unrecognized and potentially new renal entity that is currently not listed in the 2016 WHO classification [4]. The first published study on this tumor in 2018 by He et al. described a multi-institutional series of 14 tumors, designated as "HOT" of kidney [35]. Soon thereafter, Chen et al. reported a single-institutional series of seven morphologically identical tumors that they designated "sporadic renal cell carcinomas with eosinophilic and vacuolated cytoplasm" [36]. Most recently, an example of an identical type of tumor was reported by Trpkov et al. in a patient with a Tuberous Sclerosis Complex (TSC) [37], in contrast to the sporadic cases included in the initial two series [35,36]. The tumors designated as "HOT" and "sporadic renal cell carcinomas with eosinophilic and vacuolated cytoplasm", in our view, represent the same entity. In this review, we will use the designation "HOT" for this novel tumor, which we proposed initially as a provisional name for this entity [35]. The term "sporadic renal cell carcinomas with eosinophilic and vacuolated cytoplasm" used by Chen et al. despite being somewhat long, inaccurately stipulates that this tumor is a "carcinoma" prima-facie, without providing either evidence or justification for this terminology [36]. Importantly, the case reported in a TSC patient also argues against the use of the descriptor "sporadic" for these tumors [37].

HOT of kidney emerged from the spectrum of oncocytic (or eosinophilic) tumours that include renal oncocytoma, chromophobe renal cell carcinoma (Chr RCC), as well as previously reported tumors with "hybrid" morphology of oncocytoma-Chr RCC, either as sporadic "hybrid-oncocytic" tumors, or tumors found in a syndromic setting, such as Birt–Hogg–Dubé (BHD) syndrome, renal oncocytosis and TSC [5,38–42]. Indeed, it is not uncommon to encounter oncocytic tumors with mixed and unusual morphologies either in a syndromic or sporadic setting that are not easy to classify because they do not fit into any of the currently recognized renal tumor categories [38].

3.1. Clinical Features

All patients included in the He et al. and Chen et al. studies presented with non-syndromic, solitary tumors. HOT was found more often in females (M:F = 1:2.5), with median age of 50 and 55 years respectively, within a broad age range (range, 25 to 73 years) [35,36]. During the documented follow-up, all tumors demonstrated an indolent behavior, and although the follow-up was relatively limited in both series, some cases had a follow-up of more than 10 years. The prevalence of this type of tumor is currently unknown.

Of note, the one renal HOT reported in a TSC patient, was found in a 48 year old female with a known TSC, who had bilateral renal masses on routine ultrasound screening [37]. The tumor measured 1.3 cm and represented a solid, tan-brown neoplasm. Multiple small adjacent AML tumorlets were also found, as well as a small renal cell carcinoma with angioleiomyomatous (or smooth muscle) stroma, a type of renal neoplasm documented in a setting of TSC [5].

3.2. Pathological Features

3.2.1. Gross Features

All sporadic tumors were typically solid (except one case that showed focal gross cysts), small size and low-stage (pT1) [36,37]. The mean tumor size was 3.4 cm (range, 1.5 to 7 cm) [35,36]. The cut surface demonstrated tan/mahogany-brown color, often mimicking the color of the adjacent kidney parenchyma, as often seen in renal oncocytoma, without a gross evidence of necrosis or hemorrhage (Figure 3A).

3.2.2. Microscopic Features

At low power, HOT is a well-circumscribed, but non-encapsulated tumor that demonstrates solid to nested growth with focal tubulocystic features (Figure 3B). Prominent intratumoral vessels of medium to large caliber and rare entrapped renal tubules can be found at the periphery [35]. The nested growth is more typically found in a loose stroma. The cells show voluminous eosinophilic cytoplasm and frequent large intracytoplasmic vacuoles, which can be quite prominent and easily recognizable at low to mid-power (Figure 3B–D) [35]. The nuclei are round to oval with conspicuously enlarged nucleoli that focally mimic viral inclusions and invoke a "high-grade" appearance, which at first impression can be worrisome [35]. Perinuclear halos and nuclear irregularities are typically not found.

3.2.3. Immunohistochemical Features, Electron Microscopy and Molecular Findings

HOT shows frequent reactivity for CD117 with CK7 only focally positive in scattered cells, an immunoprofile mimicking the one typically found in renal oncocytoma (oncocytoma-like immunoprofile) [35,36]. Cathepsin K is, however, invariably positive, either as diffuse or focal (Figure 3E) and CD10 was positive in great majority of reported cases [35]. All cases reported by He et al. were also reactive for PAX8, AE1/AE3, CK18, antimitochondrial antigen, and SDHB, and were negative for vimentin, TFE3, HMB45, and melan-A [35]. None of the evaluated cases showed *TFEB* and *TFE3* gene rearrangements [35].

We have also studied two HOT cases by electron microscopy and both cases demonstrated an 'oncocytoma-like' appearances with numerous intracytoplasmic mitochondria (Figure 3F).

Using NGS, Chen et al. found somatic inactivating mutations of *TSC2* or activating mutations of *MTOR* with a loss of chromosome 1 in the evaluated cases, consistent with a hyperactive *MTOR* complex [36]. None of their evaluated patients had a documented TSC [36]. Using array comparative genomic hybridization (aCGH), He et al. found frequent losses of chromosome 1, chromosome 19, and a loss of heterozygosity on 16p11.2-11.1 and 7q31.31 [35]. Of note, some similarities in these molecular findings in HOT, such as losses of *TSC2* and *TSC1* and activation of the *MTOR* pathway have also been found in ESC RCC, another emerging renal entity, covered in this review, that nevertheless shows quite different morphology from HOT [1,2,5,9,10,13].

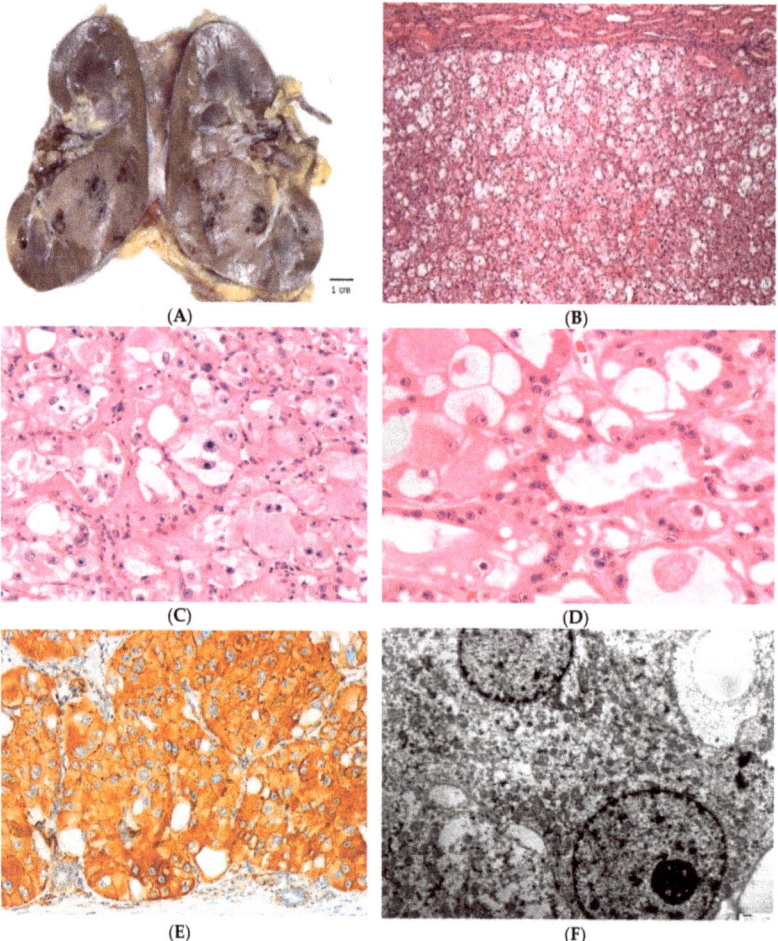

Figure 3. High-grade Oncocytic Tumor (HOT) of kidney often mimics the color of the adjacent renal parenchyma (**A**). It demonstrates solid growth of mostly eosinophilic cells, admixed with 'clear' cells with intracytoplasmic vacuoles (**B**). The eosinophilic cells have voluminous cytoplasm with large intracytoplasmic vacuoles; the nuclei show prominent to often very large nucleoli (**C,D**). Cathepsin K is positive on immunohistochemistry (**E**). On electron microscopy, numerous intracytoplasmic mitochondria are present (**F**).

3.3. Differential Diagnosis

The main differential diagnosis for HOT includes renal oncocytoma, Chr RCC and the broad category of "hybrid" oncocytic tumors, seen in the sporadic or syndromic setting.

Although various morphologic patterns and atypical features of renal oncocytoma have been well documented [43], the typical "high-grade" morphology, as seen in HOT, is essentially beyond the permissible morphology for renal oncocytoma, despite the IHC similarities that include the positive CD117, accompanied by CK7 reactivity restricted to rare scattered cells.

Although conspicuous "plant like" growth that is seen in classic Chr RCC can superficially mimic the vacuolated morphology of HOT, Chr RCC lacks marked cytoplasmic vacuoles; importantly, the "high-grade" nuclear features seen in HOT are not part of the Chr RCC morphologic spectrum. Chr RCC also typically exhibits irregular ("raisinoid") nuclei with perinuclear halos, which are not seen in HOT. On IHC, CK7 is typically diffusely positive in Chr RCC, but CK7 is only reactive in rare cells in HOT. Importantly, cathepsin K and CD10 reactivity seen in HOT are typically absent both in renal oncocytoma and Chr RCC.

The main differential diagnosis for the HOT are the so-called "hybrid tumors" that can be seen either in either a syndromic or sporadic setting [5,38–42]. These "hybrid tumors" are, however, typically multifocal, when encountered in patients with BHD syndrome, renal oncocytosis and TSC. We have also encountered solitary "HOT-like" cases on morphology, that demonstrated *FLCN* mutation (either as a new mutation or in a patient with previously unrecognized BHD), which can be conclusively distinguished from HOT only by molecular analysis (unpublished data).

Other, less common renal tumors that can potentially mimic HOT include MiTF RCC (TFEB and TFE3), oncocytic papillary RCC, SDH-deficient RCC, and ESC RCC and their key distinguishing features are summarized in Table 2.

4. Low-Grade Oncocytic Tumor (LOT) of Kidney

Low-grade oncocytic tumor (LOT) has been recently proposed as a distinct renal entity, emerging from the spectrum of oncocytic renal tumors that are difficult to classify [44]. In the only published study to date, consisting of 28 cases collected from four large institutional renal tumor archives, LOT showed fairy consistent morphologic features and immunoprofile characterized by lack of CD117 reactivity and diffuse positivity for CK7 [44]. Although LOT demonstrates an overlapping morphology with renal oncocytoma and eosinophilic Chr RCC, it does not fit completely into either of these entities. Some of these tumors were, and likely still are, labeled using designations such as "eosinophilic Chr RCC", "oncocytic renal tumor, NOS", "unclassified/low-grade oncocytic tumor", "hybrid or hybrid oncocytoma-chromophobe tumor" or "borderline/uncertain/low malignant potential" tumors [38].

To our knowledge, this emerging entity is morphologically similar to the four cases labelled 'eosinophilic Chr RCC' that were included in the study by Davis et al., that lacked any copy number alterations; however, no IHC profile was provided for these cases [45]. Another recent study by Ohashi et al. also showed a complete absence of any chromosomal losses in 10/24 (41.7%) of cases designated as "eosinophilic Chr RCC" in a large Japanese-Swiss combined cohort of Chr RCC, whereas only 6/69 (8%) of the "classic Chr RCC" showed absence of any chromosomal loss [46]. The authors pointed out correctly that no stringent diagnostic criteria exist to classify eosinophilic Chr RCC, based on the current 2016 WHO classification, which stipulates that eosinophilic Chr RCC should be "almost purely composed of eosinophilic cells" [47]. Although no overall survival differences were found between the "classic Chr RCC" and the "eosinophilic Chr RCC" cases, their study did not provide more granular outcome data, for example on disease-specific survival or disease-specific progression in these subgroups [46].

LOT is typically a single, small tumor that shows low stage and, based on the available data, it exhibits an indolent clinical behavior [44]. The awareness of the constellation of the clinical, morphologic and immunophenotypic features of this tumor that we provisionally named "LOT" will hopefully increase its recognition and will prompt re-evaluation of similar oncocytic tumors that were diagnosed using various terms.

4.1. Clinical Features

LOT is typically a single and sporadic tumor, found in a non-syndromic setting and in older patients (median age 66 years). There is a female predilection (M:F = 1:1.8) [44]. During the follow-up, these tumors behaved indolently, with no evidence of disease progression, although this is based on a single study with a relatively limited follow-up (mean 31.8 months) [44].

4.2. Pathological Features

4.2.1. Gross Features

LOT is typically a tan/yellow-brown, solid tumor; some examples showed macrocysts (Figure 4A). Multiple tumors or bilateral kidney involvement have not been documented so far. Median tumor size was 3 cm (range 1.1–13 cm) and the great majority (88%) of tumors were stage pT1a (68%) or pT1b (20%) [44].

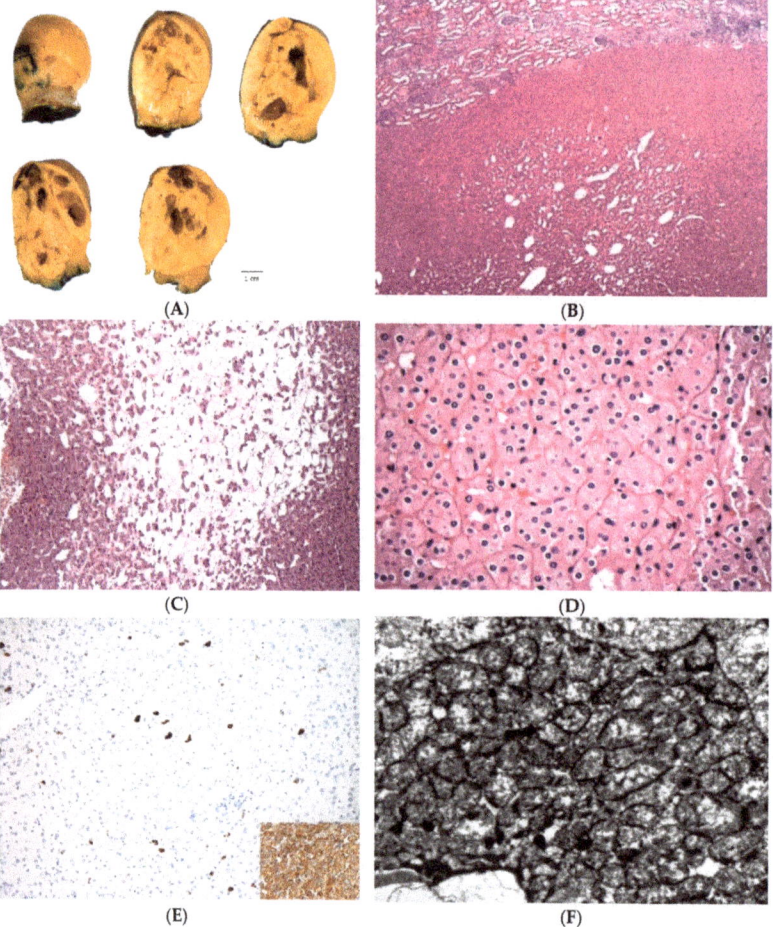

Figure 4. Low-grade oncocytic tumor (LOT) of kidney grossly shows tan to yellow cut surface (**A**). LOT is a non-encapsulated tumor showing mostly solid growth; focal tubular-tubuloreticular patterns can be present more centrally (**B**). There are frequent, sharply delineated edematous areas containing single cells and irregularly cell cords (**C**). The eosinophilic cells show 'low-grade', round to oval nuclei, often with delicate perinuclear clearing (**D**). On immunostains, CD117 is typically negative and there is diffuse reactivity for CK7 (insert) (**E**). Electron microscopy shows densely packed intracytoplasmic mitochondria (**F**).

4.2.2. Microscopic Features

LOT of kidney is a non-encapsulated neoplasm that exhibits solid, compact nested or focal tubular and tubuloreticular growth, particularly to the more central parts (Figure 4B) [44]. Sharply delineated lose stromal, edematous areas are frequently found, containing cells that show irregular, loose reticular, cord-like and individual cell growth, often resembling disorganized tissue culture (Figure 4C) [44]. Focal lymphocytic clusters or more delicate and irregular intercellular lymphocytic clusters can be often seen in the more solid tumor areas. The cells show homogeneous oncocytic cytoplasm, round to oval nuclei that typically lack significant irregularities and "raisinoid" shapes. The nuclei may focally show delicate perinuclear halos or clearings (Figure 4D). No atypical or potentially worrisome morphologic features were noted, such as significant cell atypia, pleomorphism, mitotic activity or coagulative necrosis.

4.2.3. Immunohistochemical Features, Electron Microscopy, Molecular Features

LOT of kidney is invariably CD117-negative and diffusely CK7-positive, which is a typical and constant immunopattern (Figure 4E) [44]. Of note, rare cases may show only focal and weak CD117 reactivity. LOT is also positive for AE1/AE3, PAX8, E-cadherin, BerEP4 and MOC31; fumarate hydratase is retained [44]. LOT is negative for CA9, CK20, CK5/6, p63, CD15, HMB45, melan-A, and vimentin [44]. CD10 and AMACR are mostly negative or only focally positive. Muller–Mowry colloidal iron staining was either negative or only luminal positive.

On electron microscopy, LOT demonstrates abundant, closely packed intracytoplasmic mitochondria, similar to oncocytoma, which supports the descriptor "oncocytic" for this entity (Figure 4F).

Only limited molecular data are available so far that show no consistent chromosomal losses or gains of multiple chromosomes; in some cases a disomic chromosomal status was found [44]. Evaluated cases showed frequent deletions at 19p13.3, 1p36.33 and 19q13.11 [44].

4.3. Differential Diagnosis

The main differential diagnosis for LOT includes renal oncocytoma and Chr RCC. The similarities with oncocytoma include: an absence of capsule, mostly diffuse solid growth, cells with uniform oncocytic cytoplasm and typically round to oval nuclei. In contrast to oncocytoma, LOT has areas of edematous stroma that are sharply delineated from the solid areas. These hypocellular areas show disorganized "tissue culture-like" cell arrangement and contain cells forming irregular cords and single cells. These areas are somewhat different from the typical "archipelaginous" areas that are often found in the more central parts of the renal oncocytoma. The cell of renal oncocytoma, in contrast to LOT, also lack perinuclear halos, and are usually diffusely reactive for CD117, whereas CK7 stains only scattered cells.

LOT exhibits as well some similarities with the eosinophilic variant of Chr RCC that include: absence of a peripheral capsule, presence of diffuse and solid growth, cells with perinuclear clearings (halos), and diffuse CK7 reactivity. In contrast to LOT, eosinophilic Chr RCC typically lacks the focal edematous and hypocellular areas; the cells exhibit more prominent membranes, and the nuclei demonstrate more irregular shapes and perinuclear halos. CD117 is also diffusely positive in great majority of Chr RCC, including the eosinophilic Chr RCC.

An extended differential diagnosis that includes other renal tumors with oncocytic or eosinophilic features include several additional entities, which are usually easily distinguished from the core group of renal "oncocytic" tumors, that include oncocytoma, eosinophilic Chr RCC and the broader group of "borderline/hybrid" oncocytic tumors. A summary of the features that are helpful in distinguishing LOT from the other kidney tumors with oncocytic/eosinophilic cytoplasm is shown in Table 2.

5. Conclusions

In this review we summarized the current knowledge and available data on four emerging, provisional renal entities, that include ALK-RCC, which is already included in the WHO 2016 classification as an 'emerging/provisional' entity, as well as three previously unrecognized entities that are not currently included in the WHO classification, eosinophilic solid and cystic renal cell carcinoma (ESC RCC), low-grade oncocytic renal tumor (LOT) and high-grade oncocytic renal tumor (HOT) of kidney. Importantly, the recognition of these novel entities rests primarily on their distinct morphologic features with the aid of IHC. We hope that this review will promote an awareness of these emerging renal tumor entities and additional studies for their further evaluation and characterization.

Funding: This research received no external funding.

Conflicts of Interest: The authors declare no conflict of interest.

References

1. Trpkov, K.; Hes, O.; Bonert, M.; Lopez, J.I.; Bonsib, S.M.; Nesi, G.; Comperat, E.; Sibony, M.; Berney, D.M.; Martinek, P.; et al. Eosinophilic, solid, and cystic renal cell carcinoma: Clinicopathologic study of 16 unique, sporadic neoplasms occurring in women. *Am. J. Surg. Pathol.* **2016**, *40*, 60–71. [CrossRef] [PubMed]
2. Trpkov, K.; Abou-Ouf, H.; Hes, O.; Lopez, J.I.; Nesi, G.; Comperat, E.; Sibony, M.; Osunkoya, A.O.; Zhou, M.; Gokden, N.; et al. Eosinophilic solid and cystic renal cell carcinoma (ESC RCC): Further morphologic and molecular characterization of ESC RCC as a distinct entity. *Am. J. Surg. Pathol.* **2017**, *41*, 1299–1308. [CrossRef] [PubMed]
3. Trpkov, K.; Hes, O. New and emerging renal entities: A perspective post-WHO 2016 classification. *Histopathology* **2019**, *74*, 31–59. [CrossRef] [PubMed]
4. Moch, H.; Humphrey, P.A.; Ulbright, T.M.; Reuter, V.E. *WHO Classification of Tumours of the Urinary System and Male Genital Organs*, 4th ed.; International Agency for Research on Cancer: Lyon, France, 2016.
5. Guo, J.; Tretiakova, M.S.; Troxell, M.L.; Osunkoya, A.O.; Fadare, O.; Sangoi, A.R.; Shen, S.S.; Lopez-Beltran, A.; Mehra, R.; Heider, A.; et al. Tuberous sclerosis-associated renal cell carcinoma: A clinicopathologic study of 57 separate carcinomas in 18 patients. *Am. J. Surg. Pathol.* **2014**, *38*, 1457–1467. [CrossRef] [PubMed]
6. Park, J.H.; Lee, C.; Chang, M.S.; Kim, K.; Choi, S.; Lee, H.; Lee, H.S.; Moon, K.C. Molecular characterization and putative pathogenic pathways of tuberous sclerosis complex-associated renal cell carcinoma. *Transl. Oncol.* **2018**, *11*, 962–970. [CrossRef] [PubMed]
7. McKenney, J.K.; Przybycin, C.; Trpkov, K.; Magi-Galluzzi, C. Eosinophilic solid and cystic (ESC) renal cell carcinomas have metastatic potential. *Histopathology* **2018**, *42*. [CrossRef]
8. Tretiakova, M.S. Eosinophilic solid and cystic renal cell carcinoma mimicking epithelioid angiomyolipoma: Series of 4 primary tumors and 2 metastases. *Hum. Pathol.* **2018**, *80*, 65–75. [CrossRef]
9. Parilla, M.; Kadri, S.; Patil, S.A.; Ritterhouse, L.; Segal, J.; Henriksen, K.J.; Antic, T. Are sporadic eosinophilic solid and cystic renal cell carcinomas characterized by somatic tuberous sclerosis gene mutations? *Am. J. Surg. Pathol.* **2018**, *42*, 911–917. [CrossRef]
10. Palsgrove, D.N.; Li, Y.; Pratilas, C.A.; Lin, M.T.; Pallavajjalla, A.; Gocke, C.; De Marzo, A.M.; Matoso, A.; Netto, G.J.; Epstein, J.I.; et al. Eosinophilic solid and cystic (ESC) renal cell carcinomas harbor tsc mutations: Molecular analysis supports an expanding clinicopathologic spectrum. *Am. J. Surg. Pathol.* **2018**, *42*, 1166–1181. [CrossRef]
11. Fenelon, S.S.; Santos, J.; Faraj, S.F.; Mattedi, R.L.; Trpkov, K.; Nahas, W.C.; Garcia, M.R.T.; Viana, P.C.C. Eosinophilic solid and cystic renal cell carcinoma: Imaging features of a novel neoplasm. *Urology* **2018**, *114*, e9–e10. [CrossRef]
12. Li, Y.; Reuter, V.E.; Matoso, A.; Netto, G.J.; Epstein, J.I.; Argani, P. Re-evaluation of 33 'unclassified' eosinophilic renal cell carcinomas in young patients. *Histopathology* **2018**, *72*, 588–600. [CrossRef] [PubMed]
13. Mehra, R.; Vats, P.; Cao, X.; Su, F.; Lee, N.D.; Lonigro, R.; Premkumar, K.; Trpkov, K.; McKenney, J.K.; Dhanasekaran, S.M.; et al. Somatic Bi-allelic loss of TSC Genes in eosinophilic solid and cystic renal cell carcinoma. *Eur. Urol.* **2018**, *74*, 483–486. [CrossRef] [PubMed]

14. Pulford, K.; Lamant, L.; Morris, S.; Butler, L.; Wood, K.M.; Stroud, D.; Delsol, G.; Mason, D. Detection of anaplastic lymphoma kinase (ALK) and nucleolar protein nucleophosmin (NPM)-ALK proteins in normal and neoplastic cells with the monoclonal antibody ALK1. *Blood* **1997**, *89*, 1394–1404. [CrossRef] [PubMed]
15. Mano, H. ALKoma: A cancer subtype with a shared target. *Cancer Discov.* **2012**, *2*, 495–502. [CrossRef]
16. Kusano, H.; Togashi, Y.; Akiba, J.; Moriya, F.; Baba, K.; Matsuzaki, N.; Yuba, Y.; Shiraishi, Y.; Kanamaru, H.; Kuroda, N.; et al. Two cases of renal cell carcinoma harboring a novel STRN-ALK fusion gene. *Am. J. Surg. Pathol.* **2016**, *40*, 761–769. [CrossRef]
17. Bodokh, Y.; Ambrosetti, D.; Kubiniek, V.; Tibi, B.; Durand, M.; Amiel, J.; Pertuit, M.; Barlier, A.; Pedeutour, F. ALK-TPM3 rearrangement in adult renal cell carcinoma: Report of a new case showing loss of chromosome 3 and literature review. *Cancer Genet.* **2018**, *221*, 31–37. [CrossRef]
18. Yu, W.; Wang, Y.; Jiang, Y.; Zhang, W.; Li, Y. Genetic analysis and clinicopathological features of ALK-rearranged renal cell carcinoma in a large series of resected Chinese renal cell carcinoma patients and literature review. *Histopathology* **2017**, *71*, 53–62. [CrossRef]
19. Smith, N.E.; Deyrup, A.T.; Marino-Enriquez, A.; Fletcher, J.A.; Bridge, J.A.; Illei, P.B.; Netto, G.J.; Argani, P. VCL-ALK renal cell carcinoma in children with sickle-cell trait: The eighth sickle-cell nephropathy? *Am. J. Surg. Pathol.* **2014**, *38*, 858–863. [CrossRef]
20. Thorner, P.S.; Shago, M.; Marrano, P.; Shaikh, F.; Somers, G.R. TFE3-positive renal cell carcinomas are not always Xp11 translocation carcinomas: Report of a case with a TPM3-ALK translocation. *Pathol. Res. Pract.* **2016**, *212*, 937–942. [CrossRef]
21. Cajaiba, M.M.; Jennings, L.J.; Rohan, S.M.; Perez-Atayde, A.R.; Marino-Enriquez, A.; Fletcher, J.A.; Geller, J.I.; Leuer, K.M.; Bridge, J.A.; Perlman, E.J. ALK-rearranged renal cell carcinomas in children. *Genes Chromosomes Cancer* **2016**, *55*, 442–451. [CrossRef]
22. Cajaiba, M.M.; Jennings, L.J.; George, D.; Perlman, E.J. Expanding the spectrum of ALK-rearranged renal cell carcinomas in children: Identification of a novel HOOK1-ALK fusion transcript. *Genes Chromosomes Cancer* **2016**, *55*, 814–817. [CrossRef] [PubMed]
23. Sugawara, E.; Togashi, Y.; Kuroda, N.; Sakata, S.; Hatano, S.; Asaka, R.; Yuasa, T.; Yonese, J.; Kitagawa, M.; Mano, H.; et al. Identification of anaplastic lymphoma kinase fusions in renal cancer: Large-scale immunohistochemical screening by the intercalated antibody-enhanced polymer method. *Cancer* **2012**, *118*, 4427–4436. [CrossRef] [PubMed]
24. Sukov, W.R.; Hodge, J.C.; Lohse, C.M.; Akre, M.K.; Leibovich, B.C.; Thompson, R.H.; Cheville, J.C. ALK alterations in adult renal cell carcinoma: Frequency, clinicopathologic features and outcome in a large series of consecutively treated patients. *Mod. Pathol.* **2012**, *25*, 1516–1525. [CrossRef] [PubMed]
25. Oyama, Y.; Nishida, H.; Kusaba, T.; Kadowaki, H.; Arakane, M.; Daa, T.; Watanabe, D.; Akita, Y.; Sato, F.; Mimata, H.; et al. A case of anaplastic lymphoma kinase-positive renal cell carcinoma coincident with Hodgkin lymphoma. *Pathol. Int.* **2017**, *67*, 626–631. [CrossRef] [PubMed]
26. Jeanneau, M.; Gregoire, V.; Desplechain, C.; Escande, F.; Tica, D.P.; Aubert, S.; Leroy, X. ALK rearrangements-associated renal cell carcinoma (RCC) with unique pathological features in an adult. *Pathol. Res. Pract.* **2016**, *212*, 1064–1066. [CrossRef] [PubMed]
27. Marino-Enriquez, A.; Ou, W.B.; Weldon, C.B.; Fletcher, J.A.; Perez-Atayde, A.R. ALK rearrangement in sickle cell trait-associated renal medullary carcinoma. *Genes Chromosomes Cancer* **2011**, *50*, 146–153. [CrossRef]
28. Debelenko, L.V.; Raimondi, S.C.; Daw, N.; Shivakumar, B.R.; Huang, D.; Nelson, M.; Bridge, J.A. Renal cell carcinoma with novel VCL-ALK fusion: New representative of ALK-associated tumor spectrum. *Mod. Pathol.* **2011**, *24*, 430–442. [CrossRef]
29. Lee, C.; Park, J.W.; Suh, J.H.; Nam, K.H.; Moon, K.C. ALK-positive renal cell carcinoma in a large series of consecutively resected korean renal cell carcinoma patients. *Korean J. Pathol.* **2013**, *47*, 452–457. [CrossRef]
30. Yang, J.; Dong, L.; Du, H.; Li, X.B.; Liang, Y.X.; Liu, G.R. ALK-TPM3 rearrangement in adult renal cell carcinoma: A case report and literature review. *Diagn. Pathol.* **2019**, *14*, 112. [CrossRef]
31. Wang, X.T.; Fang, R.; Ye, S.B.; Zhang, R.S.; Li, R.; Wang, X.; Ji, R.H.; Lu, Z.F.; Ma, H.H.; Zhou, X.J.; et al. Targeted next-generation sequencing revealed distinct clinicopathologic and molecular features of VCL-ALK RCC: A unique case from an older patient without clinical evidence of sickle cell trait. *Pathol. Res. Pract.* **2019**, *215*, 152651. [CrossRef]

32. Pal, S.K.; Bergerot, P.; Dizman, N.; Bergerot, C.; Adashek, J.; Madison, R.; Chung, J.H.; Ali, S.M.; Jones, J.O.; Salgia, R. Responses to alectinib in ALK-rearranged papillary renal cell carcinoma. *Eur. Urol.* **2018**, *74*, 124–128. [CrossRef] [PubMed]
33. Gorczynski, A.; Czapiewski, P.; Korwat, A.; Budynko, L.; Prelowska, M.; Okon, K.; Biernat, W. ALK-rearranged renal cell carcinomas in Polish population. *Pathol. Res. Pract.* **2019**, *215*, 152669. [CrossRef] [PubMed]
34. Kuroda, N.; Liu, Y.; Tretiakova, M.; Ulamec, M.; Takeuchi, K.; Przybycin, C.; Maggi-Galuzzi, C.; Agaimy, A.; Yilmaz, A.; Trpkov, K.; et al. Clinicopathological study of seven cases of ALK-postitive renal tumor identification of new fusion partners including CLIP1 and KIF5B genes. *Mod. Pathol.* **2019**, *32*, 885.
35. He, H.; Trpkov, K.; Martinek, P.; Isikci, O.T.; Maggi-Galuzzi, C.; Alaghehbandan, R.; Gill, A.J.; Tretiakova, M.; Lopez, J.I.; Williamson, S.R.; et al. "High-grade oncocytic renal tumor": Morphologic, immunohistochemical, and molecular genetic study of 14 cases. *Virchows Arch.* **2018**, *473*, 725–738. [CrossRef] [PubMed]
36. Chen, Y.; Mirsadraei, L.; Jayakumaran, G.; Al-Ahmadie, H.; Fine, S.; Gopalan, A.; Sirintrapun, S.J.; Tickoo, S.; Reuter, V. Somatic mutations of TSC2 or MTOR characterize a morphologically distinct subset of sporadic renal cell carcinoma with eosinophilic and vacuolated cytoplasm. *Am. J. Surg. Pathol.* **2019**, *43*, 121–131. [CrossRef] [PubMed]
37. Trpkov, K.; Bonert, M.; Gao, Y.; Kapoor, A.; He, H.; Yilmaz, A.; Gill, A.J.; Williamson, S.R.; Comperat, E.; Tretiakova, M.; et al. High-grade oncocytic tumour (HOT) of kidney in a patient with tuberous sclerosis complex. *Histopathology* **2019**, *75*, 440–442. [CrossRef]
38. Williamson, S.R.; Gadde, R.; Trpkov, K.; Hirsch, M.S.; Srigley, J.R.; Reuter, V.E.; Cheng, L.; Kunju, L.P.; Barod, R.; Rogers, C.G.; et al. Diagnostic criteria for oncocytic renal neoplasms: A survey of urologic pathologists. *Hum. Pathol.* **2017**, *63*, 149–156. [CrossRef]
39. Petersson, F.; Gatalica, Z.; Grossmann, P.; Perez Montiel, M.D.; Alvarado Cabrero, I.; Bulimbasic, S.; Swatek, A.; Straka, L.; Tichy, T.; Hora, M.; et al. Sporadic hybrid oncocytic/chromophobe tumor of the kidney: A clinicopathologic, histomorphologic, immunohistochemical, ultrastructural, and molecular cytogenetic study of 14 cases. *Virchows Arch.* **2010**, *456*, 355–365. [CrossRef]
40. Delongchamps, N.B.; Galmiche, L.; Fiss, D.; Rouach, Y.; Vogt, B.; Timsit, M.O.; Vlelllefond, A.; Mejean, A. Hybrid tumour 'oncocytoma-chromophobe renal cell carcinoma' of the kidney: A report of seven sporadic cases. *BJUI Int.* **2009**, *103*, 1381–1384. [CrossRef]
41. Mai, K.T.; Dhamanaskar, P.; Belanger, E.; Stinson, W.A. Hybrid chromophobe renal cell neoplasm. *Pathol. Res. Pract.* **2005**, *201*, 385–389. [CrossRef]
42. Hes, O.; Petersson, F.; Kuroda, N.; Hora, M.; Michal, M. Renal hybrid oncocytic/chromophobe tumors–A review. *Histol. Histopathol.* **2013**, *28*, 1257–1264. [PubMed]
43. Trpkov, K.; Yilmaz, A.; Uzer, D.; Dishongh, K.M.; Quick, C.M.; Bismar, T.A.; Gokden, N. Renal oncocytoma revisited: A clinicopathological study of 109 cases with emphasis on problematic diagnostic features. *Histopathology* **2010**, *57*, 893–906. [CrossRef] [PubMed]
44. Trpkov, K.; Williamson, S.R.; Gao, Y.; Martinek, P.; Cheng, L.; Sangoi, A.R.; Yilmaz, A.; Wang, C.; San Miguel Fraile, P.; Perez Montiel, D.M.; et al. Low-grade oncocytic tumor of kidney (CD117 negative, cytokeratin 7 positive): A distinct entity? *Histopathology* **2019**, *75*, 174–184. [CrossRef]
45. Davis, C.F.; Ricketts, C.J.; Wang, M.; Yang, L.; Cherniack, A.D.; Shen, H.; Buhay, C.; Kang, H.; Kim, S.C.; Fahey, C.C.; et al. The somatic genomic landscape of chromophobe renal cell carcinoma. *Cancer Cell* **2014**, *26*, 319–330. [CrossRef]
46. Ohashi, R.; Schraml, P.; Angori, S.; Batavia, A.; Rupp, N.; Ohe, C.; Otsuki, Y.; Kawasaki, T.; Kobayashi, H.; Kobayashi, K.; et al. Classic chromophobe renal cell carcinoma incur a larger number of chromosomal losses than seen in the eosinophilic subtype. *Cancers* **2019**, *11*, 1492. [CrossRef] [PubMed]
47. Paner, G.; Amin, M.; Moch, H.; Storke, L.S. Chromophobe renal cell carcinoma. In *WHO Classification of Tumours of the Urinary System and Male Genital Organs*; Moch, H., Ulbright, T.M., Reuter, V.E., Eds.; International Agency for Research on Cancer: Lyon, France, 2016; pp. 27–28.

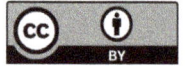

© 2020 by the authors. Licensee MDPI, Basel, Switzerland. This article is an open access article distributed under the terms and conditions of the Creative Commons Attribution (CC BY) license (http://creativecommons.org/licenses/by/4.0/).

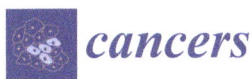

Review

The Future of Immunotherapy-Based Combination Therapy in Metastatic Renal Cell Carcinoma

Rohan Garje [1,*], Josiah An [1], Austin Greco [2], Raju Kumar Vaddepally [3] and Yousef Zakharia [1]

1. Holden Comprehensive Cancer Center, University of Iowa, Iowa City, IA 52242, USA; josiah-an@uiowa.edu (J.A.); yousef-zakharia@uiowa.edu (Y.Z.)
2. Department of Internal Medicine, University of Iowa, Iowa City, IA 52242, USA; austin-greco@uiowa.edu
3. Yuma Regional Medical Center, Yuma, AZ 85364, USA; rkvaddepally@gmail.com
* Correspondence: rohan-garje@uiowa.edu; Tel.: +1-319-356-7831

Received: 8 December 2019; Accepted: 6 January 2020; Published: 7 January 2020

Abstract: In the past two decades, there has been a significant improvement in the understanding of the molecular pathogenesis of Renal Cell Carcinoma (RCC). These insights in the biological pathways have resulted in the development of multiple agents targeting vascular endothelial growth factor (VEGF), as well as inhibitors of the mammalian target of the rapamycin (mTOR) pathway. Most recently, checkpoint inhibitors were shown to have excellent clinical efficacy. Although the patients are living longer, durable complete responses are rarely seen. Historically, high dose interleukin 2 (IL2) therapy has produced durable complete responses in 5% to 8% highly selected patients—albeit with significant toxicity. A durable complete response is a surrogate for a long-term response in the modern era of targeted therapy and checkpoint immunotherapy. Numerous clinical trials are currently exploring the combination of immunotherapy with various targeted therapeutic agents to develop therapies with a higher complete response rate with acceptable toxicity. in this study, we provide a comprehensive review of multiple reported and ongoing clinical trials evaluating the combination of PD-1/PD-L1 inhibitors with either ipilimumab (a cytotoxic T-lymphocyte-associated protein 4, CTLA-4 inhibitor) or with anti-VEGF targeted therapy.

Keywords: renal cell carcinoma; checkpoint inhibitors; VEGF inhibitors; mTOR inhibitors

1. Introduction

Kidney cancer is the second most common malignancy arising from the urinary system. In 2019, about 73,820 new cases and 14,770 deaths were estimated to occur in the United States [1]. According to the SEER (Surveillance, Epidemiology, and End Results) program, about 16% patients with RCC present with distant metastatic disease and have a 5-year survival rate of 11.6%. Clear cell is the most common histological subtype of renal cell carcinoma (ccRCC) and accounts for about 75% of the cases. The remaining 25% non-clear cell subtypes include papillary, chromophobe, medullary, collecting duct, sarcomatoid, and unclassified types. Advanced, unresectable, or relapsed RCC is treated with palliative systemic therapy.

In the past two decades, there has been significant progress in the understanding of the molecular pathogenesis of ccRCC. These insights in the biological pathways have resulted in the development of multiple agents targeting vascular endothelial growth factors (VEGF) such as sunitinib, pazopanib, cabozantinib, axitinib, and lenvatinib, as well as inhibitors of the mammalian target of rapamycin pathway (mTOR) such as temsirolimus and everolimus. These agents have improved the objective response rates (ORR) and overall survival (OS); however, they are short-lived. The ability of the tumor cells to evade the host immune surveillance by PD-1-PD-L1 interaction, lead to the development of checkpoint inhibitors that target either PD-1 or PD-L1, and restore immune competence. Nivolumab, a fully human IgG4 programmed death 1 (PD-1) checkpoint inhibitor selectively blocks the interaction between PD-1 (expressed on activated T cells) and PD ligands (expressed on immune cells and tumor cells). In a Phase III trial of patients previously treated with one or two VEGF inhibitors, nivolumab, when compared to everolimus, showed significantly longer overall survival along with fewer adverse events [2]. Despite the addition of several agents to the therapeutic armamentarium of ccRCC, durable complete responses are rarely seen. Historically, high dose interleukin 2 (IL2) has achieved durable complete responses, but only in 5% to 8% of highly selected patients, and at the cost of significant toxicities [3,4]. Patients who withstand this toxic therapy and achieve complete response can essentially be cured. This points to the fact that achieving a complete response is a surrogate for long term response in the modern era of targeted therapy and checkpoint immunotherapy. Newer treatment strategies that aim to achieve complete response similar to IL-2, albeit with less toxicity, is a plausible therapeutic avenue. One such approach is to explore the synergy of checkpoint inhibitors with various targeted therapeutic agents, which, if successful, is a step closer to achieve potential cure.

2. The Rationale to Combine Immunotherapy with Angiogenesis Inhibitors

Vascular endothelial growth factors (VEGF) play a crucial role in tumor angiogenesis by binding to VEGF receptors. In addition to a proangiogenic effect, they also exert immunosuppression in the tumor microenvironment by not only inducing the accumulation of myeloid-derived suppressor cells and regulatory T cells but also by impeding the migration of T lymphocytes towards the tumor microenvironment. VEFG inhibition can restore antitumor immunity by normalizing the vasculature and endothelial cell activation [5]. Additionally, PD-1 blockage also promotes cytotoxic T-cell infiltration into the tumor and significantly enhances antitumor immunity. The synergy of both VEGF inhibition and PD-1 blockade was successfully demonstrated in murine cancer models [6]. The clinical evidence and correlative biomarkers of synergism were initially reported in a Phase II clinical trial, where atezolizumab, a PD-L1 inhibitor, in combination with bevacizumab, was compared to sunitinib in patients with treatment naïve metastatic ccRCC. This study evaluated molecular biomarkers predicting response by utilizing the genes signatures associated angiogenesis ($Angio^{High}$ or $Angio^{low}$), anti-tumor immune response (T_{eff}^{High} or T_{eff}^{Low}), and myeloid inflammation ($Myeloid^{High}$ or $Myeloid^{Low}$) [7–10]. In tumors with high angiogenesis, these were no progression-free survival (PFS) differences with either sunitinib monotherapy or the combination of atezolizumab and bevacizumab. On the contrary, in the $Angio^{low}$ subgroup, the combination therapy had better PFS when compared to sunitinib. Additionally, the high T_{eff} gene signature expression, a maker of a high preexisting anti-tumor immune response, was associated with improved PFS with atezolizumab + bevacizumab when compared to sunitinib monotherapy. A higher level of PD-L1 expression by immunohistochemistry was also predictive of a better response to the combination therapy. However, tumor mutation and neoantigen burden did not correlate with PFS [9,10]. Finally, higher expression of myeloid inflammation gene signatures (associated with impaired antitumor T cell response), did not show any difference between the combination therapy versus sunitinib [9,10]. This study—with its correlative biomarkers—shows evidence of the potential synergy of immune checkpoint inhibitors and VEGF inhibitors.

Numerous of these combinational studies are ongoing, and some have been recently published. In this review, we summarize the clinical trials evaluating the combination of PD1/PDL1 inhibitors with either ipilimumab (a cytotoxic T-lymphocyte-associated protein 4, CTLA-4 inhibitor) or angiogenesis inhibitors.

3. Nivolumab in Combination with Ipilimumab versus Sunitinib Monotherapy

In Checkmate 214, a Phase III randomized open-label multicenter trial, nivolumab (3 mg/kg) + ipilimumab (1 mg/kg) was compared with sunitinib monotherapy (50 mg daily for 4 weeks on and 2 weeks off every cycle) in patients with treatment naïve metastatic ccRCC [11] (summarized in Table 1). Of the 1096 enrolled patients, 550 received nivolumab + ipilimumab, and 546 received sunitinib; 425 and 422, respectively, had intermediate or poor-risk disease as per the International Metastatic Renal-Cell Carcinoma Database Consortium (IMDC) prognostic model [12]. At a median follow-up of 25.2 months, the 18-month overall survival of the intermediate and poor-risk patients was 75% with nivolumab +

ipilimumab and 60% with sunitinib. The median OS was not reached with the combination therapy vs. 26.0 months with sunitinib (hazard ratio for death, 0.63; $p < 0.001$). Progression-free survival (PFS) and overall response rates (ORR) also favored the checkpoint inhibitors when compared to sunitinib and were 11.6 months vs. 8.4 months and 42% vs. 27% ($p < 0.001$), respectively. The complete response (CR) rate was 9% in the combination immunotherapy arm. However, the PFS and ORR were better with sunitinib monotherapy in patients with IMDC favorable risk cancer. Additionally, PDL-L1 status was not predictive of response to the combination therapy. Treatment-related grade 3 or 4 adverse events (AE) occurred in 250 (46%) and 335 (63%) patients in nivolumab + ipilimumab and sunitinib groups, respectively. The most common grade 3 or 4 AEs in the combination group were elevated lipase levels, fatigue, and diarrhea. While in the sunitinib group, the most common grade 3 or 4 AEs were hypertension, fatigue, palmar-plantar erythrodysesthesia, and elevated lipase levels. About 35% of patients in the combination immunotherapy group required high-dose steroids for the management of immune-mediated adverse events. There were eight treatment-related deaths in the combination group and four in the sunitinib group. Based on the study results, the US Food and Drug Administration (FDA) approved the combination immunotherapy for intermediate and poor-risk patients in the first-line setting for metastatic ccRCC and also received a category 1 recommendation by the National Comprehensive Cancer Network (NCCN). Additionally, Grunwald and colleagues studied the depth of response as an indicator for long term survival among the 1096 patients in Checkmate 214 with previously untreated ccRCC [13]. They found that patients who received nivolumab + ipilimumab had similar OS between >50–≤75% and >75% tumor reduction. Receiver operating characteristic analysis was utilized to show that >50% depth of reduction indicated the most OS benefit in nivolumab + ipilimumab. This study showed that nivolumab + ipilimumab treatment resulted in prolonged OS in comparison to sunitinib, and depth of response may reflect the possibility of long-term survival for ccRCC patients who receive nivolumab + ipilimumab [13].

Table 1. Immunotherapy based combination trials in treatment-naive mRCC with results.

Study	N	Compounds	Median OS, mo (95% CI)	Median PFS, mo (95% CI)	CRR	ORR (95% CI)	Grade 3 and 4 TRAEs	Treatment-Related Deaths	Treatment Discontinuation Rate	IRAE Needing ≥40 mg Total Daily Dose of Prednisone or Equivalent
Checkmate 214 [11]	1096	Intermediate and poor risk: Nivolumab + ipilimumab vs. sunitinib	NR vs. 26.0 HR = 0.63; $p < 0.001$.	11.6 vs. 8.4 (HR = 0.82; $p = 0.0331$.	9% vs. 1%	42% vs. 27%	46% vs. 63%	1.5% vs. 0.74%	22% vs. 12%	35%
KEYNOTE-426 [14]	861	Pembrolizumab + axitinib vs. sunitinib	NR, HR 0.53; $p < 0.0001$ 12-mo OS: 90% vs. 78%	15.1 vs. 11.1 HR 0.69; 0.57-0.84; $p = 0.0001$)	5.8% vs. 1.9%	59.3% vs. 35.7%; $p < 0.00001$	62.9% vs. 58.1%	0.9% vs. 1.6%	both drugs: 30.5%, sunitinib: 13.9%	N/a
JAVELIN Renal 101 [15]	886	Avelumab plus axitinib vs. sunitinib	NR: 12-mo: 86% vs. 83% (HR 0.78; 0.55 to 1.08; $p = 0.14$)	13.8 vs 8.4 (HR 0.69; 0.56 to 0.84; $p < 0.0001$)	3.4% vs 1.8%	51.4% vs. 25.7 %	71.2% vs. 71.5%	0.7% vs. 0.2%	7.6 vs.13.4	11.1%
IMmotion151 [16]	915; PDL1+: 362	Atezolizumab + bevacizumab vs. sunitinib	NR, 24-mo: 63% vs. 60% (HR 0.93; 0.76 to 1.14; $p = 0.4751$)	ITT: 11.2 vs. 8.4 (HR 0.83; 0.70-0.97; $p = 0.0219$) PDL1+: 11.2 vs. 7.7	ITT: 5% vs. 2%; PD-L1+: 9% vs. 4%	ITT: 37% vs. 33% PD-L1+: 43% vs. 35%	40% vs. 54%	1.1% vs. 0.22%	5% vs. 8%	9%

OS, overall survival; CI, confidence interval; PFS, progression-free survival; ORR, objective response rate; CRR, complete response rate; NR, not reached; N/a, not available; HR, hazard ratio; mo, months; TRAEs, treatment-related adverse events; IRAE, immune-related adverse events.

4. Pembrolizumab in Combination with Axitinib in Metastatic ccRCC

In Phase III, randomized KEYNOTE-426 clinical trial of the efficacy of checkpoint PD-1 inhibitor, pembrolizumab (200 mg IV every 3 weeks) in combination with axitinib (5 mg orally twice daily) was compared to sunitinib monotherapy in previously untreated patients with metastatic ccRCC [14]. In this study, 861 patients were randomized to receive treatment in one of these two groups until disease progression or intolerable toxicities. The median PFS was both clinically and statistically significant with the pembrolizumab—axitinib group when compared to sunitinib (15.1 months vs. 11.1 months, HR 0.69; $p < 0.001$) irrespective of IMDC risk groups and PDL1 status. The median OS was not reached, but the risk of death was 47% lower with combination therapy when compared to sunitinib. This OS benefit was also evidenced in all subgroups irrespective of age, metastatic sites, and IMDC risk groups. The ORRs were better with the combination therapy when compared to sunitinib and were 59.3% vs. 35.7%, respectively. The most common grade 3 and 4 treatment-related adverse events in both groups were diarrhea and hypertension. The incidence of hepatic toxicity was higher in the pembrolizumab-axitinib group; however, there were no deaths related to hepatotoxicity. Based on the significant efficacy and acceptable toxicity profile, this combination therapy was approved by the FDA for treatment naïve metastatic ccRCC, irrespective of PDL1 status or IMDC risk stratification. Brian Rini and colleagues presented a subgroup analysis of KEYNOTE-426 during the American Society of Clinical Oncology (ASCO) annual meeting in June 2019, examining intermediate and poor-risk groups in addition to the sarcomatoid group [17]. Analysis of 592 patients with intermediate and poor-risk mCCRCC patients showed 1 year OS, median PFS, ORR, and complete response rate at 87.3%, 12.6 months, 55.8%, and 4.8% in the pembrolizumab + axitinib group compared to the sunitinib group at 71.3%, 8.2 months, 29.5%, and 0.7%. In addition, 105 patients with sarcomatoid features were examined and results showed improved 12 months OS, PFS, ORR, and complete response rate at 83.4%, median PFS not reached, 58.8%, 11.8% in pembrolizumab + axitinib group while sunitinib group showed 79.5%, 8.4 months, 31.5%, and 0% [17]. This study confirmed the benefit of pembrolizumab + axitinib intermediate and poor IMDC risk groups and in tumors with sarcomatoid features.

5. Avelumab in Combination with Axitinib in Metastatic ccRCC

TK Choueiri and colleagues evaluated the combination of avelumab, a PD-L1 antibody with axitinib in a Phase 1b clinical trial, where it was not only shown to be safe, but also had 58% objective response rate in patients with metastatic ccRCC [18]. These encouraging results lead to Phase III, randomized clinical trial (JAVELIN Renal 101), which evaluated the efficacy of avelumab (10 mg/kg IV every 2 weeks) along with axitinib (5 mg twice a day) and compared to sunitinib in the first-line setting for metastatic ccRCC. Of the 886 patients, 442 were randomly assigned to the combination group, and 444 were assigned to receive sunitinib; 560 (63.2%) patients had PD-L1 positive tumor defined as ≥1% of immune cells staining positive within the tumor area with Ventana PD-L1 (SP263) assay [15]. The median PFS was significantly longer with the combination therapy when compared to sunitinib and was 13.8 vs. 8.4 months in the overall population and 13.8 vs. 7.2 months in PD-L1 positive patients, respectively. Additionally, irrespective of PD-L1 status, the objective response rates and complete response rates were almost doubled with combination therapy as compared to sunitinib and were 51.4% vs. 25.7% and 3.4% vs. 1.8%, respectively [15]. On subgroup analysis of PDL1 positive patients, irrespective of IMDC prognostic risk group the combination therapy was better than sunitinib in terms of median PFS and objective response rates. Interestingly, patients did better for those who underwent nephrectomy in the combination group, but no difference was noted if patients did not undergo nephrectomy. However, only a small fraction of patients do not undergo nephrectomy in this subgroup. In terms of safety, grade 3 or higher adverse events were seen in 71.2% and 71.5% in the combination therapy and sunitinib groups, respectively. About 166 patients (38.2%) who received avelumab and axitinib had immune-mediated adverse events, and about 11% required high dose glucocorticoids. The data was premature for overall survival analysis and a further follow up is needed [15]. Another subgroup analysis of the JAVELIN Renal 101 trial presented at the European Society for Medical

Oncology (ESMO) annual meeting held in September 2019 included 117 patients with advanced ccRCC who did not undergo upfront cytoreductive nephrectomy and had renal lesions [19]. In this study, Albiges and colleagues found that 34.5% of the patients that received avelumab and axitinib had ≥30% shrinkage in renal lesions in comparison to 9.6% who received sunitinib, indicating future areas of research in neoadjuvant therapy with immunotherapy and tyrosine kinase inhibitor [19].

6. Atezolizumab in Combination with Bevacizumab versus Sunitinib Monotherapy in Metastatic ccRCC

In a Phase II randomized study (IMmotion150) reported by McDermott et al., atezolizumab monotherapy or in combination with bevacizumab was compared with sunitinib in 305 patients with treatment naïve metastatic renal cell carcinoma. In the intention to treat population, the median PFS was 11.7 months vs. 6.1 months vs. 8.4 months (HR = 1.00; 95% CI = 0.69–1.45) with atezolizumab plus bevacizumab ($n = 101$), atezolizumab alone ($n = 103$) and sunitinib ($n = 101$), respectively, and was not statistically significantly. In PD-L1 positive patients (defined as ≥1% PD-L1 expression on IC by IHC), the atezolizumab plus bevacizumab arm had a PFS of 14.7 months as opposed to 7.8 months with sunitinib. Treatment-related grade 3 or 4 adverse events were seen in 40% vs. 17% vs. 57% in atezolizumab plus bevacizumab, atezolizumab, alone, and sunitinib arms, respectively. In the atezolizumab plus bevacizumab group, proteinuria was the most common adverse event leading to treatment discontinuation. While in the atezolizumab monotherapy group, it was nephritis, pancreatitis, and demyelination. In the sunitinib group, there was increased blood creatinine and palmar-plantar erythrodysesthesia syndrome. Of note, there were two treatment-related AEs leading to death in the sunitinib group secondary to sudden death and intestinal hemorrhage, and one in the atezolizumab plus bevacizumab group secondary to intracranial hemorrhage [9].

The above findings were further supported in the interim results of IMmotion151, a randomized Phase III trial comparing atezolizumab plus bevacizumab combined therapy vs. Sunitinib in treatment naïve patients with metastatic renal cell carcinoma [20]. OS was immature at the time of interim analysis and results for this were not reported. PFS in intention-to-treat patients was greater in the atezolizumab plus bevacizumab group at 11.2 months as compared to 8.4 months in the sunitinib group. Of note, this PFS benefit was shown across analyzed subgroups including MSKCC risk, liver metastases, and sarcomatoid histology. Also, in patients who had disease with positive PD-LI status (characterized as >/=1%) PFS for atezolizumab plus bevacizumab group was longer than in the sunitinib group at 11.2 months and 7.7 months, respectively. Grade 3 and 4 AEs occurred in 40% of the atezolizumab plus bevacizumab group and 54% of the sunitinib group. Discontinuation of therapy secondary to all grade AEs occurred in 12% and 8% for the two groups, respectively. Subgroup analysis of IMmotion151 examined 142 patients with sarcomatoid histology and found that median PFS, median OS, ORR, and complete response rate were 8.3 months, median OS not reached, 49%, and 10% in atezolizumab + bevacizumab group compared to sunitinib group with 5.3 months, 15 months, 14%, and 3%. MD Anderson Symptom Inventory (MDASI) scale analysis indicated median time to deterioration was 11.3 months in atezolizumab + bevacizumab group compared to 4.9 months in sunitinib group. In addition, biomarker analysis with angiogenesis signature subset and T-effector gene expression subset were higher in sarcomatoid histology when compared to non-sarcomatoid tumors, while PD-L1 positive tumors were seen in greater proportion in sarcomatoid histology at 63% compared to 39%. This study showed that biomarker analysis was consistent with the improved survival seen in atezolizumab + bevacizumab group compared to sunitinib group in tumors with sarcomatoid histology [17]. Table 1 provides a summary of all the studies with results.

In addition to the above Phase III trials, there are multiple other combination therapies with preliminary Phase I results and ongoing Phase III studies.

7. Nivolumab in Combination with Tivozanib in mRCC

In an open-labeled non-randomized Phase Ib/II study, tivozanib was studied in combination with nivolumab in patients with metastatic renal cell carcinoma and previously treated with one oral TKI [21]. Tivozanib is a highly selective VEGF receptor tyrosine kinase inhibitor with minimal off-target action and presumably lower AE profile. In the dose-escalation phase, six patients were enrolled, and no dose-limiting toxicities (DLTs) were observed. The maximum tolerated dose (MTD) was found to be full dose tivozanib, 1.5 mg/day, in combination with nivolumab. In the Phase II cohort, an additional 22 patients were enrolled, and grade 3 and 4 AEs were seen in 60% of patients, with hypertension being the most common. The objective response rate was 56%, with one patient achieving complete response [22]. Median PFS was 18.5 months for patients who were previously untreated and did not reach PFS for patients who were previously treated at the time of analysis [23]. ORR was 56% and results were premature for OS analysis.

8. Nivolumab in Combination with Sunitinib or Pazopanib in mRCC

CheckMate 016 study was a Phase I trial dose-escalation and expansion study, which evaluated the safety and efficacy of nivolumab, in combination with either sunitinib or pazopanib in patients with metastatic renal cell carcinoma [24].

Twenty patients were enrolled in the nivolumab plus pazopanib group. However, 4 DLTs were seen with this combination, including elevated liver enzymes ($n = 3$) and fatigue ($n = 1$). Also, 70% (14/20) patients experienced grade 3 and 4 treatment-related AEs. This study arm was subsequently closed due to significant toxicities. The objective response rate was 45%, and all were partial responses. The median PFS and OS were 7.2 months and 27.9 months, respectively.

In the nivolumab plus sunitinib cohort, 33 patients were enrolled. There were no DLTs. In this cohort as well, grade 3 and 4 treatment-related AEs were seen in 82% (27/33) patients, and the most common were hypertension, hepatotoxicity, diarrhea, and fatigue. The objective response rate was 54.5%, with two complete responses and 16 partial responses. The median PFS was 12.7 months, and median OS was not reached. Though there were signals for antitumor efficacy, due to significant toxicities, this combination was also not considered for further evaluation [24].

9. Pembrolizumab in Combination with Bevacizumab in mRCC

In the Big Ten Cancer Research Consortium sponsored Phase Ib/II clinical trial, the safety and antitumor activity of pembrolizumab in combination with bevacizumab was evaluated in 61 patients with metastatic ccRCC, who at received at least one prior systemic therapy [25]. No dose-limiting toxicities had been reported. The 200 mg fixed dose of pembrolizumab and 15 mg/kg dose of bevacizumab, both given every three weeks, was determined to be safe and recommended for a multicenter Phase 2 study. The overall response rate was 60.9% with median time on treatment of 298 days and median PFS was found to be 17.0 months. The most common grade 3 or 4 AEs were hypertension, proteinuria, and adrenal insufficiency. One death was reported due to heart failure [25].

10. Pembrolizumab in Combination with Lenvatinib in mRCC

Lenvatinib is an oral multi kinase inhibitor that targets VEGFR1–3, FGFR1–4, PDGFRα, and the oncogenes *RET* and *KIT* [26]. A Phase Ib/II multicenter open-label study of lenvatinib plus pembrolizumab in patients with clear cell metastatic RCC was performed to assess the safety and antitumor activity [27]. Patients with measurable metastatic RCC with or without prior systemic therapy with ECOG status ≤1 were enrolled. Lenvatinib 20 mg daily plus pembrolizumab 200 mg intravenously every three weeks was deemed as the maximum tolerated dose and recommended for Phase 2 evaluation. Of the 33 patients enrolled, the objective response rate was 52% with disease control rate of 94% [28]. Median follow up time for PFS was 4.2 months. Median PFS was not reached, but the PFS rate at 3, 6, and 9 months were 93.1%, 73.8%, and 64.6%, respectively. Response duration of ≥6 months was seen in 80.8% of patients. The most common therapy-related adverse events were fatigue, followed by dysphonia, diarrhea, stomatitis, hypertension, dry mouth, nausea, proteinuria, and hand-foot syndrome. Treatment was discontinued in 9% of patients due to adverse events [28].

11. Pembrolizumab and Pazopanib in Patients with Advanced or mRCC

Preliminary safety and antitumor effects of the Phase I part of the KEYNOTE-018 study were presented at the ASCO annual meeting 2017 [29]. Twenty patients were enrolled in two cohorts to study safety in pembrolizumab and pazopanib combination therapy and determine the maximum tolerated dose. Cohort A evaluated pembrolizumab 2 mg/kg every three weeks and pazopanib 800 mg daily. Cohort B evaluated pembrolizumab at the same dose and pazopanib at 600 mg daily. Seven out of 20 patients experienced DLTs primarily in the form of hepatotoxicity. Subsequently, 15 patients were added to Cohort C, where pazopanib was started with nine weeks run-in, followed by combination therapy to limit toxicities. In the initial five patients enrolled, three had DLTs that included pneumonitis, bowel perforation and grade 4 lipase levels. Due to significant DLTs and grade 3 and 4 adverse events, the combination of pazopanib and pembrolizumab has overall limited tolerability and was not suitable for evaluation in a larger cohort [29].

12. Cabozantinib in Combination with Atezolizumab in Advance Renal Cell Carcinoma

COSMIC-021 clinical trial is a Phase Ib, multicenter trial that evaluated the safety and efficacy of the combination of cabozantinib (VEGFR/MET/AXL inhibitor) at 40 mg or 60 mg daily dose along with atezolizumab 1200 mg every three weeks in seven genitourinary cohorts, including a cohort of advanced RCC. There were no DLTs but the 40 mg cabozantinib dose was chosen for the expansion cohort. Of the 10 evaluable patients, the ORR was 50% with 1 CR, 4 PR. The most common grade 3 AEs were hypertension, diarrhea and hypophosphatemia [30].

Several other studies investigating other combinations of antiangiogenic agents and immunotherapies in mRCC are ongoing. Ongoing trials include VEGF/PD-1 blockade combination, including lenvatinib with everolimus and pembrolizumab, and nivolumab with cabozantinib as first-line treatment in patients with mRCC are summarized in Table 2 with their current accrual status.

Table 2. Select ongoing VEGF/PD-1 blockade combination studies in mRCC.

National Clinical Trial ID Number (Study)	Treatment	Phase	Clinical Trial Status	Treatment Line	Patients	Primary Outcome Measures
Lenvatinib						
NCT02811861 (CLEAR)	Lenvatinib with everolimus or pembrolizumab compared to SOC sunitinib	III, randomized 1:1:1, open label	active, not-recruiting	First-line treatment of subjects with advanced renal cell carcinoma	1069	PFS by independent review
Cabozantinib						
NCT03141177 (CheckMate 9ER)	Nivolumab + Cabozantinib vs. Sunitinib	Phase III, randomized, open-label study	active, not recruiting	First line, metastatic RCC	638	PFS per blinded independent central review (BICR)
NCT03937219 (COSMIC-313)	Cabozantinib + nivolumab + ipilimumab vs. Nivolumab + ipilimumab	III, randomized, 1:1, double-blind	recruiting	First line, intermediate- or poor-risk metastatic RCC	676	PFS by blinded independent radiology committee (BIRC)
NCT03793166 (PDIGREE study)	Nivolumab and Ipilimumab followed by Nivolumab vs. Cabozantinib with Nivolumab	III, randomized, open label	recruiting	First line	1046	OS
NCT03149822	Pembrolizumab plus Cabozantinib	I/II, open label, single arm	recruiting	First or second line	55	ORR (CR + PR)
NCT03200587	Avelumab and Cabozantinib	Ib, open label	recruiting	First line	20	DLTs, AEs, RP2D

OS, overall survival; PFS, progression-free survival; ORR, objective response rate; CR, complete response; PR partial response; DLT, dose limiting toxicity; AE, adverse event; RP2D, recommended Phase 2 dose.

13. Discussion

The therapeutic landscape of renal cell carcinoma has rapidly advanced in the past decade. The combination strategies of checkpoint inhibitors along with ipilimumab or antiangiogenic agents have demonstrated good synergy. Most notably, for the IMDC intermediate and poor-risk patients, the dual checkpoint inhibitor combination of nivolumab with ipilimumab and the combination of pembrolizumab with axitinib have shown improved response and overall survival leading to FDA approval in the first-line setting. Similarly, for the IMDC favorable-risk, the combination of pembrolizumab with axitinib or single-agent VEGF inhibitors such as sunitinib and pazopanib are preferred first-line options [31]. The combination of avelumab and axitinib is also an alternative option in the first-line setting based on improved response rate and PFS, but there was no OS benefit at the time of data cut off [15]. Figure 1 illustrates the first-line treatment approach for mRCC. The benefit of the combination therapy was seen in a reasonable number of patients irrespective of any specific biomarkers, such as PD-L1 positivity. Also, the complete response rates were higher from the combination strategies, whether this translates to long term survival or potentially a cure is unknown. Long-term follow-up data from these studies are needed.

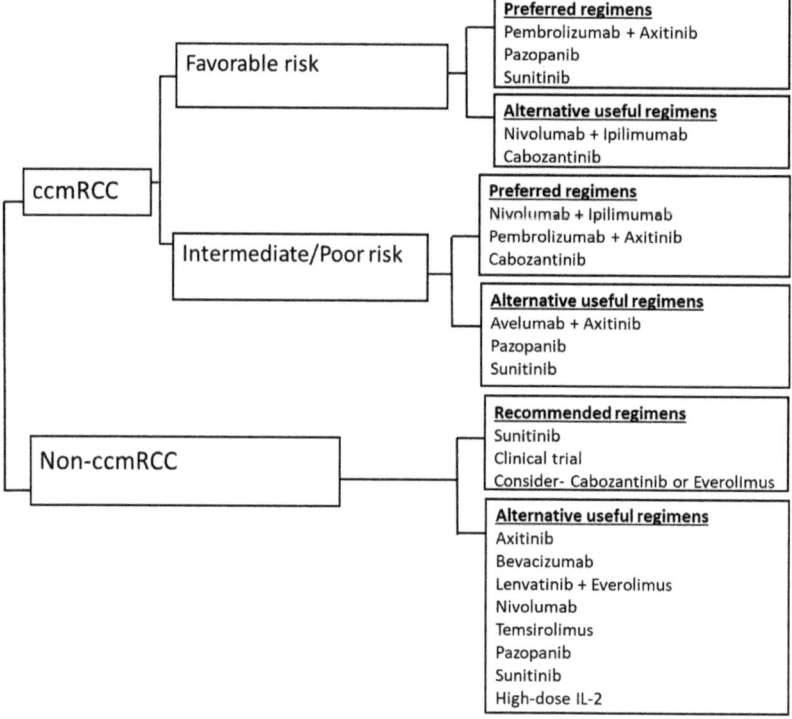

Figure 1. Overview of treatment strategy for treatment naïve metastatic RCC, based on IMDC risk-stratification. ccmRCC, clear cell metastatic renal cell carcinoma; non-ccmRCC, non-clear cell metastatic renal cell carcinoma; risk stratification based on International Metastatic Renal Cell Carcinoma Database Consortium (IMDC) criteria. The International Metastatic RCC Database Consortium (IMDC) prognostic model integrates six adverse factors: Karnofsky performance status (KPS) <80 percent, time from diagnosis to treatment < 1-year, hemoglobin concentration < lower limit of normal, serum calcium > upper limit of normal, neutrophil count > upper limit of normal, platelet count > upper limit of normal. (Favorable risk: no risk factors, intermediate risk: 1 or 2 risk factors, poor risk: 3 or more risk factors).

It is imperative to understand that not all patients benefit from combination therapy, and some have a higher incidence of serious toxicities. Biomarkers and genomic studies that can predict the efficacy of either monotherapy or combination therapy should be explored to individualize the treatment. A few combinations appeared to be beneficial in limited cases with specific histology and immunologic biomarkers and may be considered in particular situations, as seen in atezolizumab and bevacizumab in comparison to sunitinib monotherapy, where PFS was more significant in sarcomatoid variant mRCC and PD-L1 expressing tumors [10]. Not all combination therapies are safe. The combination of pazopanib with either nivolumab or pembrolizumab was associated with significant hepatoxicity and not deemed safe for further study. Even the combination of axitinib and pembrolizumab had high grade 3 and 4 elevations of hepatic enzymes. The exact mechanism of such toxicity is unknown. Caution should be maintained before initiating such combination therapies in patients with liver dysfunction at baseline.

Combination therapy can be associated with severe side effects, with a significant overlap in the toxicity profile of the drugs. For example, diarrhea and hepatoxicity are common side effects that can be associated with either axitinib or checkpoint inhibitors. The management varies based on the etiology and also the severity, i.e., treatment discontinuation/dose reduction and use of loperamide for diarrhea in case of axitinib and timely initiation of high dose corticosteroids for autoimmune colitis and hepatitis secondary to checkpoint inhibitors. Checkpoint inhibitor and antiangiogenic combination therapy requires intense monitoring on treatment that entails frequent office visits, physician and nurse assessments, investment of health-care resources, and higher financial burden on the patient. A multidisciplinary approach and an in-depth knowledge of complications are crucial before embarking on the combination therapy.

14. Conclusions

In summary, the combination of checkpoint inhibitors and anti-angiogenic agents is a valuable addition in the therapeutic armamentarium for mRCC. The choice of combination therapy or monotherapy should be individualized after a thorough discussion between the physician and patients based on cost, efficacy, and toxicity profile.

Funding: This research received no external funding.

Acknowledgments: The authors from University of Iowa are supported by National Institutes of Health grant P30 CA086862.

Conflicts of Interest: R.G., J.A., A.G., R.V. declare no conflict of interest. Y.Z. Advisory Board: Amgen, Roche Diagnostics, Novartis, Jansen, Eisai, Exelixis, Castle Bioscience, Array, Bayer, Pfizer, Clovis, EMD Serono. Grant/research support from: Institution clinical trial support from NewLink Genetics, Pfizer, Exelixis, Eisai. DSMC: Jansen.

References

1. Siegel, R.L.; Miller, K.D.; Jemal, A. Cancer statistics, 2019. *CA A Cancer J. Clin.* **2019**, *69*, 7–34. [CrossRef]
2. Motzer, R.J.; Escudier, B.; McDermott, D.F.; George, S.; Hammers, H.J.; Srinivas, S.; Tykodi, S.S.; Sosman, J.A.; Procopio, G.; Plimack, E.R.; et al. Nivolumab versus Everolimus in Advanced Renal-Cell Carcinoma. *N. Engl. J. Med.* **2015**, *373*, 1803–1813. [CrossRef]
3. Belldegrun, A.S.; Klatte, T.; Shuch, B.; LaRochelle, J.C.; Miller, D.C.; Said, J.W.; Riggs, S.B.; Zomorodian, N.; Kabbinavar, F.F.; Dekernion, J.B.; et al. Cancer-specific survival outcomes among patients treated during the cytokine era of kidney cancer (1989–2005): A benchmark for emerging targeted cancer therapies. *Cancer* **2008**, *113*, 2457–2463. [CrossRef]
4. Fyfe, G.; Fisher, R.I.; Rosenberg, S.A.; Sznol, M.; Parkinson, D.R.; Louie, A.C. Results of treatment of 255 patients with metastatic renal cell carcinoma who received high-dose recombinant interleukin-2 therapy. *J. Clin. Oncol.* **1995**, *13*, 688–696. [CrossRef]
5. Voron, T.; Marcheteau, E.; Pernot, S.; Colussi, O.; Tartour, E.; Taieb, J.; Terme, M. Control of the immune response by pro-angiogenic factors. *Front. Oncol.* **2014**, *4*, 70. [CrossRef]

6. Yasuda, S.; Sho, M.; Yamato, I.; Yoshiji, H.; Wakatsuki, K.; Nishiwada, S.; Yagita, H.; Nakajima, Y. Simultaneous blockade of programmed death 1 and vascular endothelial growth factor receptor 2 (VEGFR2) induces synergistic anti-tumour effect in vivo. *Clin. Exp. Immunol.* **2013**, *172*, 500–506. [CrossRef]
7. Brauer, M.J.; Zhuang, G.; Schmidt, M.; Yao, J.; Wu, X.; Kaminker, J.S.; Jurinka, S.S.; Kolumam, G.; Chung, A.S.; Jubb, A.; et al. Identification and Analysis of In Vivo VEGF Downstream Markers Link VEGF Pathway Activity with Efficacy of Anti-VEGF Therapies. *Clin. Cancer Res.* **2013**, *19*, 3681–3692. [CrossRef]
8. Powles, T.; Nickles, D.; Van Allen, E.; Chappey, C.; Zou, W.; Kowanetz, M.; Kadel, E.; Denker, M.; Boyd, Z.; Vogelzang, N.; et al. Immune biomarkers associated with clinical benefit from atezolizumab (MPDL3280a; anti-PD-L1) in advanced urothelial bladder cancer (UBC). *J. Immunother. Cancer* **2015**, *3*, P83. [CrossRef]
9. McDermott, D.F.; Huseni, M.A.; Atkins, M.B.; Motzer, R.J.; Rini, B.I.; Escudier, B.; Fong, L.; Joseph, R.W.; Pal, S.K.; Reeves, J.A.; et al. Clinical activity and molecular correlates of response to atezolizumab alone or in combination with bevacizumab versus sunitinib in renal cell carcinoma. *Nat. Med.* **2018**, *24*, 749–757. [CrossRef]
10. Wallin, J.J.; Bendell, J.C.; Funke, R.; Sznol, M.; Korski, K.; Jones, S.; Hernandez, G.; Mier, J.; He, X.; Hodi, F.S.; et al. Atezolizumab in combination with bevacizumab enhances antigen-specific T-cell migration in metastatic renal cell carcinoma. *Nat. Commun.* **2016**, *7*, 12624. [CrossRef]
11. Motzer, R.J.; Tannir, N.M.; McDermott, D.F.; Arén Frontera, O.; Melichar, B.; Choueiri, T.K.; Plimack, E.R.; Barthélémy, P.; Porta, C.; George, S.; et al. Nivolumab plus Ipilimumab versus Sunitinib in Advanced Renal-Cell Carcinoma. *N. Engl. J. Med.* **2018**, *378*, 1277–1290. [CrossRef]
12. Ko, J.J.; Xie, W.; Kroeger, N.; Lee, J.L.; Rini, B.I.; Knox, J.J.; Bjarnason, G.A.; Srinivas, S.; Pal, S.K.; Yuasa, T.; et al. The International Metastatic Renal Cell Carcinoma Database Consortium model as a prognostic tool in patients with metastatic renal cell carcinoma previously treated with first-line targeted therapy: A population-based study. *Lancet Oncol.* **2015**, *16*, 293–300. [CrossRef]
13. Grünwald, V.; Choueiri, T.K.; Rini, B.I.; Powles, T.; George, S.; Grimm, M.-O.; McHenry, M.B.; Maurer, M.; Motzer, R.J.; Hammers, H.J.; et al. 950PAssociation between depth of response and overall survival: Exploratory analysis in patients with previously untreated advanced renal cell carcinoma (aRCC) in CheckMate 214. *Ann. Oncol.* **2019**, *30*, mdz249-046. [CrossRef]
14. Rini, B.I.; Plimack, E.R.; Stus, V.; Gafanov, R.; Hawkins, R.; Nosov, D.; Pouliot, F.; Alekseev, B.; Soulieres, D.; Melichar, B.; et al. Pembrolizumab plus Axitinib versus Sunitinib for Advanced Renal-Cell Carcinoma. *N. Engl. J. Med.* **2019**, *380*, 1116–1127. [CrossRef]
15. Motzer, R.J.; Penkov, K.; Haanen, J.; Rini, B.; Albiges, L.; Campbell, M.T.; Venugopal, B.; Kollmannsberger, C.; Negrier, S.; Uemura, M.; et al. Avelumab plus Axitinib versus Sunitinib for Advanced Renal-Cell Carcinoma. *N. Engl. J. Med.* **2019**, *380*, 1103–1115. [CrossRef]
16. Rini, B.I.; Powles, T.; Atkins, M.B.; Escudier, B.; McDermott, D.F.; Suarez, C.; Bracarda, S.; Stadler, W.M.; Donskov, F.; Lee, J.L.; et al. Atezolizumab plus bevacizumab versus sunitinib in patients with previously untreated metastatic renal cell carcinoma (IMmotion151): A multicentre, open-label, phase 3, randomised controlled trial. *Lancet* **2019**, *393*, 2404–2415. [CrossRef]
17. Rini, B.I.; Plimack, E.R.; Stus, V.; Gafanov, R.; Hawkins, R.; Nosov, D.; Pouliot, F.; Soulieres, D.; Melichar, B.; Vynnychenko, I.; et al. Pembrolizumab (pembro) plus axitinib (axi) versus sunitinib as first-line therapy for metastatic renal cell carcinoma (mRCC): Outcomes in the combined IMDC intermediate/poor risk and sarcomatoid subgroups of the phase 3 KEYNOTE-426 study. *J. Clin. Oncol.* **2019**, *37*, 4500. [CrossRef]
18. Choueiri, T.K.; Larkin, J.; Oya, M.; Thistlethwaite, F.; Martignoni, M.; Nathan, P.; Powles, T.; McDermott, D.; Robbins, P.B.; Chism, D.D.; et al. Preliminary results for avelumab plus axitinib as first-line therapy in patients with advanced clear-cell renal-cell carcinoma (JAVELIN Renal 100): An open-label, dose-finding and dose-expansion, phase 1b trial. *Lancet Oncol.* **2018**, *19*, 451–460. [CrossRef]
19. Albiges, L.; Rini, B.I.; Haanen, J.B.A.G.; Motzer, R.J.; Kollmannsberger, C.K.; Negrier, S.; Nole, F.; Bedke, J.; Bilen, M.A.; Nathan, P.; et al. 908PDPrimary renal tumour shrinkage in patients (pts) who did not undergo upfront cytoreductive nephrectomy (uCN): Subgroup analysis from the phase III JAVELIN Renal 101 trial of first-line avelumab + axitinib (A + Ax) vs sunitinib (S) for advanced renal cell carcinoma (aRCC). *Ann. Oncol.* **2019**, *30*, mdz249-007. [CrossRef]
20. Motzer, R.J.; Powles, T.; Atkins, M.B.; Escudier, B.; McDermott, D.F.; Suarez, C.; Bracarda, S.; Stadler, W.M.; Donskov, F.; Lee, J.-L.; et al. IMmotion151: A Randomized Phase III Study of Atezolizumab Plus Bevacizumab vs Sunitinib in Untreated Metastatic Renal Cell Carcinoma (mRCC). *J. Clin. Oncol.* **2018**, *36*, 578. [CrossRef]

21. Escudier, B.; Barthelemy, P.; Ravaud, A.; Negrier, S.; Needle, M.N.; Albiges, L. Tivozanib combined with nivolumab: Phase Ib/II study in metastatic renal cell carcinoma (mRCC). *J. Clin. Oncol.* **2018**, *36*, 618. [CrossRef]
22. Barthelemy, P.; Escudier, B.; Ravaud, A.; Negrier, S.; Needle, M.N.; Albiges, L. 878PTiNivo—Tivozanib combined with nivolumab: Safety and efficacy in patients with metastatic renal cell carcinoma (mRCC). *Ann. Oncol.* **2018**, *29*, mdy283-087. [CrossRef]
23. Barthelemy, P.; Escudier, B.; Negrier, S.; Ravaud, A.; Needle, M.N.; Albiges, L. 947PTiNivo: Tivozanib combined with nivolumab results in prolonged progression free survival in patients with metastatic renal cell carcinoma (mRCC): Final results. *Ann. Oncol.* **2019**, *30*, mdz249-043. [CrossRef]
24. Amin, A.; Plimack, E.R.; Ernstoff, M.S.; Lewis, L.D.; Bauer, T.M.; McDermott, D.F.; Carducci, M.; Kollmannsberger, C.; Rini, B.I.; Heng, D.Y.C.; et al. Safety and efficacy of nivolumab in combination with sunitinib or pazopanib in advanced or metastatic renal cell carcinoma: The CheckMate 016 study. *J. Immunother. Cancer* **2018**, *6*, 109. [CrossRef]
25. Dudek, A.Z.; Sica, R.A.; Sidani, A.; Jha, G.G.; Xie, H.; Alva, A.S.; Stein, M.N.; Singer, E.A. Phase Ib study of pembrolizumab in combination with bevacizumab for the treatment of metastatic renal cell carcinoma: Big Ten Cancer Research Consortium BTCRC-GU14-003. *J. Clin. Oncol.* **2016**, *34*, 559. [CrossRef]
26. Matsui, J.; Yamamoto, Y.; Funahashi, Y.; Tsuruoka, A.; Watanabe, T.; Wakabayashi, T.; Uenaka, T.; Asada, M. E7080, a novel inhibitor that targets multiple kinases, has potent antitumor activities against stem cell factor producing human small cell lung cancer H146, based on angiogenesis inhibition. *Int. J. Cancer* **2008**, *122*, 664–671. [CrossRef]
27. Lee, C.-H.; Makker, V.; Rasco, D.W.; Taylor, M.H.; Stepan, D.E.; Shumaker, R.C.; Schmidt, E.V.; Guo, M.; Dutcus, C.E.; Motzer, R.J. Lenvatinib + pembrolizumab in patients with renal cell carcinoma: Updated results. *J. Clin. Oncol.* **2018**, *36*, 4560. [CrossRef]
28. Lee, C.-H.; Shah, A.Y.; Makker, V.; Taylor, M.H.; Shaffer, D.; Hsieh, J.J.; Cohn, A.L.; DiSimone, C.; Marin, A.P.; Rasco, D.W.; et al. 1187PDPhase II study of lenvatinib plus pembrolizumab for disease progression after PD-1/PD-L1 immune checkpoint inhibitor in metastatic clear cell renal cell carcinoma (mccRCC): Results of an interim analysis. *Ann. Oncol.* **2019**, *30*, mdz253-013. [CrossRef]
29. Chowdhury, S.; McDermott, D.F.; Voss, M.H.; Hawkins, R.E.; Aimone, P.; Voi, M.; Isabelle, N.; Wu, Y.; Infante, J.R. A phase I/II study to assess the safety and efficacy of pazopanib (PAZ) and pembrolizumab (PEM) in patients (pts) with advanced renal cell carcinoma (aRCC). *J. Clin. Oncol.* **2017**, *35*, 4506. [CrossRef]
30. Agarwal, N.; Vaishampayan, U.; Green, M.; di Nucci, F.; Chang, P.-Y.; Scheffold, C.; Pal, S. 872PPhase Ib study (COSMIC-021) of cabozantinib in combination with atezolizumab: Results of the dose escalation stage in patients (pts) with treatment-naïve advanced renal cell carcinoma (RCC). *Ann. Oncol.* **2018**, *29*, mdy283-081. [CrossRef]
31. Kidney Cancer NCCN Clinical Practice Guidelines in Oncology. Available online: https://www.nccn.org/professionals/physician_gls/pdf/kidney.pdf (accessed on 15 December 2019).

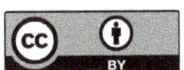

© 2020 by the authors. Licensee MDPI, Basel, Switzerland. This article is an open access article distributed under the terms and conditions of the Creative Commons Attribution (CC BY) license (http://creativecommons.org/licenses/by/4.0/).

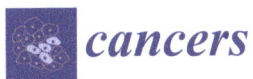

Review

Sarcomatoid Dedifferentiation in Renal Cell Carcinoma: From Novel Molecular Insights to New Clinical Opportunities

Véronique Debien [1,2,†], Jonathan Thouvenin [1,2,†], Véronique Lindner [3], Philippe Barthélémy [2], Hervé Lang [4], Ronan Flippot [5,‡] and Gabriel G. Malouf [1,2,*,‡]

1. Department of Oncology, Institut de Cancérologie de Strasbourg, Hôpitaux Universitaires de Strasbourg, Université de Strasbourg, 67200 Strasbourg, France; veronique.debien@chru-strasbourg.fr (V.D.); jonathan.thouvenin@chru-strasbourg.fr (J.T.)
2. Department of Cancer and Functional Genomics, Institute of Genetics and Molecular and Cellular Biology, CNRS/INSERM/UNISTRA, 67400 Illkirch, France; p.barthelemy@icans.eu
3. Department of Pathology, Centre Hospitalier Universitaire Régional de Strasbourg, 67200 Strasbourg, France; veronique.lindner@chru-strasbourg.fr
4. Department of Urology, Centre Hospitalier Universitaire Régional de Strasbourg, 67000 Strasbourg, France; herve.lang@chru-strasbourg.fr
5. Department of Cancer Medicine, Gustave Roussy, 94800 Villejuif, France; ronan.flippot@gustaveroussy.fr
* Correspondence: g.malouf@icans.eu or gabriel.malouf@chru-strasbourg.fr; Tel.: +33-368-767-217
† These authors contributed equally to this paper.
‡ These authors contributed equally to this paper.

Received: 29 October 2019; Accepted: 20 December 2019; Published: 31 December 2019

Abstract: Sarcomatoid features in renal cell carcinoma (RCC) have long been associated with dismal prognosis and poor response to therapy, while biological mechanisms underpinning sarcomatoid dedifferentiation remained obscure. Several efforts have been conducted to break down the molecular profile of sarcomatoid RCC and investigate different targeted therapeutic approaches. Mutations enriched for in sarcomatoid RCC involve, notably, *TP53*, *BAP1*, cell cycle, and chromatin-remodeling genes. The immunological landscape of these tumors is also gradually being uncovered, showing frequent expression of programmed cell death ligand-1 (PD-L1) and high levels of tumor-infiltrating lymphocytes. These features may be major determinants for the activity of immune checkpoint inhibitors in this population, which has been confirmed by retrospective studies and subgroup analyses of large randomized phase 3 trials. Combinations based on PD-1/PD-L1 inhibition have demonstrated response rates and complete responses in >50% and >10% of patients in the first-line metastatic setting, respectively, with median overall survival exceeding two years. This remarkable improvement in outcomes effectively establishes immune checkpoint inhibitor combinations as a new standard of care in patients with sarcomatoid RCC. New research fields, including epigenetic regulations and tumor–microenvironment interactions, may further sharpen understanding of sarcomatoid RCC and advance therapeutic developments.

Keywords: renal cell carcinoma; sarcomatoid; immunotherapy

1. Introduction

Renal cell carcinoma (RCC) is the third most frequent urologic malignancy, affecting more than 400,000 patients each year [1]. Approximately half of these patients will present with metastatic disease, either at diagnosis or after initial treatment of localized disease. While five-year overall survival (OS) rates do not exceed 15% in the Western world [2], vascular endothelial growth receptor

(VEGFR)-directed therapies and immune checkpoint inhibitor combinations have progressively improved the prognosis of these tumors.

The landscape of RCC remains largely heterogeneous. Most RCCs (75%) consist of clear-cell subtypes, while the remaining 25% consist of different tumor subtypes grouped under the umbrella term of non-clear-cell RCC [3]. Non-clear-cell RCCs are usually more aggressive diseases than clear-cell RCCs [4] and include papillary, chromophobe, collecting duct, translocation, and medullary carcinomas. Sarcomatoid dedifferentiation is a histological feature that can be found in approximately 10% of tumors in any RCC subtype and confers aggressive behavior characterized by swift progression and dismal outcomes [5,6]; however, molecular and immunologic determinants of sarcomatoid dedifferentiation remain unclear. As survival commonly remains <12 months in patients with sarcomatoid RCC (sRCC) treated in the era of targeted molecular therapies [5], it is essential to improve our understanding of the natural history of sRCC and evaluate new therapeutic avenues in this aggressive disease.

The clinical and translational research field of sRCC is hopefully growing fast. Clinical trials of immune checkpoint inhibitors have demonstrated encouraging activity results, while an increasing number of studies have continued to provide new insights into sRCC biology. As the landscape of sRCC is being redefined, this review aims to explore the most recent advances in molecular and immune characterization of sRCC and discuss how new therapeutic developments can transform the standard of care in this population.

2. Pathological Implications of Sarcomatoid Renal Cell Carcinoma

sRCC is a pathological entity defined by the presence of spindle-shaped cells in a varying proportion of the tumor area, which can account for a sarcoma-like aspect [7]. Indeed, sarcomatoid cells in RCCs have been reported to be engaged in epithelial–mesenchymal transition (EMT) [8,9], expressing mesenchymal markers including N-cadherin and vimentin, while expression of the epithelial marker e-cadherin is lost. Sarcomatoid cells also harbor increased Snail levels, a transcription factor enabling the expression of genes involved in EMT [10]. As such, the main differential diagnoses of sRCC with extensive sarcomatoid dedifferentiation are retroperitoneal leiomyosarcoma or liposarcoma. Immunohistochemistry assays may refine diagnosis, with expression of epithelial markers as keratin, cytokeratin 7, or epithelial membrane antigen (EMA) with expression of PAX8, CD10, and CAIX accounting for a renal origin [11,12]. Most often, however, sarcomatoid areas of sRCC coexist with their parent histology to make for an easier diagnosis. Rarely, some RCCs might harbor low-grade spindle cell proliferation, an entity that is distinct from sRCC and less aggressive [13].

Among aggressive subsets of RCCs, the International Society of Urologist Pathologists (ISUP) classification distinguishes sRCC and rhabdoid RCC[1,7]. Any of these features can be present in RCC regardless of the histological subtype, and they may coexist. The presence of sarcomatoid or rhabdoid features in any proportion would classify any clear-cell or papillary RCC as an ISUP grade 4 tumor [14]. Some sRCCs with extensive sarcomatoid dedifferentiation encompassing the whole tumor without clear evidence of any parent histology may be considered as unclassified RCCs [15]. The occurrence of sarcomatoid dedifferentiation may vary according to the parent histology. Sarcomatoid features have thus been reported in 9% of chromophobe RCCs, 5% of clear-cell RCCs, and 2% of papillary RCCs in a large retrospective study [16].

The aggressiveness of sRCC is highlighted by the high frequency of distant metastases at diagnosis, reported in approximately two-thirds of patients with sRCC of any histology compared to approximately 30% of patients without sarcomatoid features [17,18]. The proportion of sarcomatoid features also plays a role in the definition of prognosis, as a higher percentage has been shown to be associated with higher risk of relapse in a localized setting, and worse overall survival [17,19]. While the quantification of sarcomatoid features is an important prognostic indicator, accurate evaluation might be compromised by the extent of tumor heterogeneity. It has been shown that biopsies are up to two-fold less likely to identify sarcomatoid features compared to the analysis of nephrectomy specimens [20], while some tumors may harbor sarcomatoid features exclusively in distant metastases [19], which may lead to an underestimation of the prevalence of sRCC in kidney cancer patients. It is yet unknown whether sarcomatoid dedifferentiation can also occur as a late event upon disease progression, an element that could have prognostic and therapeutic implications for late-stage disease.

3. Molecular Landscape of Sarcomatoid Renal Cell Carcinoma

Multiple studies have aimed to unravel the molecular picture of sRCC and events leading to sarcomatoid dedifferentiation, an important effort considering the low incidence of these tumors and the heterogeneity of parent histologies. The theory of a common cell of origin for the epithelial and sarcomatoid components in sRCC has been confirmed by several studies. As demonstrated in sRCC of clear-cell type, sarcomatoid and epithelial components share most copy number alterations, X chromosome inactivation patterns, and single nucleotide variants [21–23]. Notably, clear-cell sRCC harbor a lower frequency of 3p loss, locus of the *VHL* gene, but also of chromatin remodeling genes *BAP1* and *PBRM1* [22,24]. More surprisingly, clear-cell sRCC are also devoid of 9p and 14q alterations usually associated with poor prognosis and high grade in clear-cell RCC [22].

Likewise, the transcriptomic profile of clear-cell sRCC harbors differences compared to that of nonsarcomatoid clear-cell RCC, with activation of pathways involved in aggressiveness and epithelial mesenchymal transition. It has been shown that clear-cell sRCCs harbor higher expression of VEGF and TGFβ1 pathways, while the TP53 pathway is repressed [22,24]. Clear-cell sRCC expression profile is also enriched in genes involved in the poor prognostic signature ccB [25] compared to non sarcomatoid clear-cell RCC, consistent with their clinical aggressiveness [22]. A few studies have pinpointed differences between the transcriptional profiles of sarcomatoid and epithelial components in a single tumor [22–24]. These have shown that several genes involved in EMT may have increased expression in the sarcomatoid component of clear-cell sRCC, which could account for the mesenchymal phenotype of these cells [22]. Additional insights from an independent cohort showed that sarcomatoid components might harbor increased Aurora kinase-1 expression, suggested to drive malignancy by increasing mammalian target of rapamycin (mTOR) activation [26].

More differences may be found in exploring the genomic alterations of sRCC, which reveals several potential drivers of sarcomatoid dedifferentiation (Figure 1). A study of 26 sRCCs using tumor microdissection from mixed parent histologies by targeted sequencing showed that sRCC harbored frequent mutations in *TP53*, *VHL*, *CDKN2A*, and *NF2* in 42%, 35%, 27%, and 19% of tumors, respectively [27]. *TP53* mutations were not associated with a specific histological subtype and were significantly enriched compared to non sarcomatoid RCC cohorts as those were found in only 2% of clear-cell RCC from the Cancer Genome Atlas (TCGA) dataset [28]. Likewise, *NF2* mutations only involved 1% of clear-cell RCC from the TCGA. Additional studies have depicted the mutational landscape of sRCC with focus on specific histologies. Whole-exome sequencing of sRCC from clear-cell origin confirmed the high prevalence of *TP53* alterations in two independent cohorts [23,24]. Additional recurrent mutations in sRCC from clear-cell origin include Hippo regulators *FAT1/2/3* and chromatin remodeling gene *ARID1A* [23] as well as tumor suppressor *PTEN* and TGFβ regulator *RELN* [24]. Comparison of sarcomatoid and epithelial components of clear-cell sRCC hint at a higher mutational burden in the sarcomatoid component and a higher frequency of *TP53*, *BAP1*, and *ARID1A* mutations [23]. Mutations in those three genes have been described as mutually exclusive, suggesting potential driver events [23]. *TP53* alterations have also been described in sRCC from papillary origin, along with alterations of Hippo member *NF2*, while mutations in *RELN* are reported to be enriched in sRCC regardless of the parent histology [24].

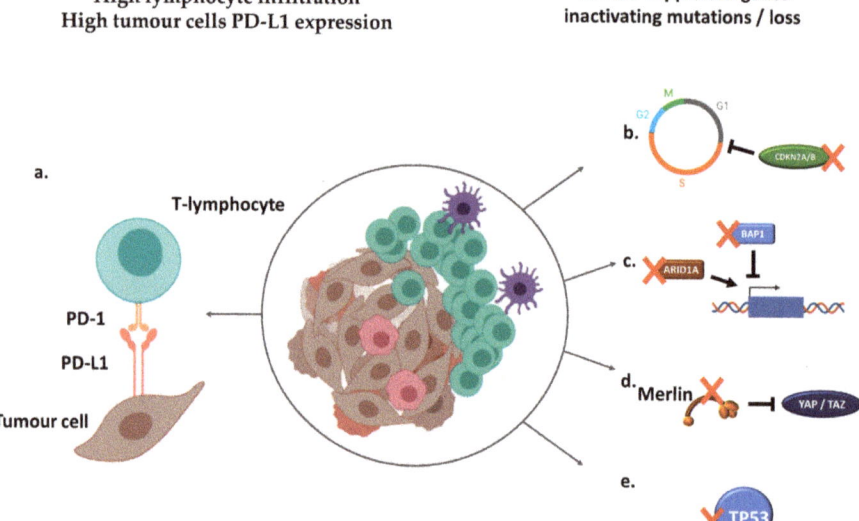

Figure 1. Immunologic and genomic hallmarks of sarcomatoid dedifferentiation in renal cell carcinoma (RCC). (**a**) Sarcomatoid renal cell carcinomas (sRCCs) are associated with higher programmed cell death ligand-1 (PD-L1) expression on tumor cells and higher lymphocyte infiltration. (**b**) Recurrent alterations of cell cycle inhibitors *CDKN2A/B* promote cell proliferation and epithelial/mesenchymal transition. (**c**) Loss of chromatin-remodeling genes *BAP1* and *ARID1A* induce genome-wide expression deregulation. (**d**) Loss of Merlin, encoded by the *NF2* gene, promotes Hippo pathway activation, leading to growth and aggressiveness. (**e**) Loss of tumor suppressor gene *TP53* favors survival and proliferation.

While these studies do not provide a unique explanation for the emergence of sarcomatoid features, recurrent mutations might participate in driving this aggressive phenotype, along with other deregulations of cellular processes. Likewise, an updated analysis of the TCGA dataset identified a subset of metabolically divergent chromophobe RCC, characterized by low expression of genes involved in the Krebs cycle, the electron transport chain, repression of the AMPK, and overexpression of genes involved in the ribose synthesis [29]. This signature was associated with poor outcomes and, strikingly, four of the six patients (67%) with metabolically deficient chromophobe RCC had a disease that presented with sarcomatoid dedifferentiation. Other particular phenotypes may include hypermutated tumors, which was found in 2 of 21 (10%) clear-cell sRCC in a single institution cohort [23]; this phenotype had not been encountered in the larger, non-sRCC TCGA dataset. This hypermutated phenotype was due to somatic *MSH2* and *POLE* mutations, which could have favored the emergence of the sarcomatoid phenotype in these tumors.

A better understanding of sarcomatoid transformation may also be achieved by studying aggressive unclassified RCC (uRCC), which may include tumors with an exclusive sarcomatoid or rhabdoid component [15]. A molecular study of 62 uRCC identified a *NF2*-deficient subgroup encompassing 26% of tumors and characterized by worse outcomes [30]. This subgroup of tumors also displayed more frequent *SETD2* alterations and 3p loss. As such, alterations of the Hippo pathway may be an important event for tumor aggressiveness and progression regardless of pathological features of RCC, which may have translational and therapeutic relevance for targeted approaches [31].

Several aspects of sRCC as a disease remain unknown. The relationship between molecular heterogeneity and response to therapy is yet to be defined, while the natural history of the disease may also be heavily influenced by the tumor microenvironment. In the era of immune checkpoint inhibitors, immune infiltration and exploration of immune markers will be key factors for the management of sRCC.

4. The Immune Microenvironment of Sarcomatoid Renal Cell Carcinoma

The biology of sRCC may account for a particular immune context when compared to non-sRCC (Figure 1). The expression of the immune checkpoint programmed cell death ligand-1 (PD-L1), promoting immune tolerance and targeted by several immune checkpoint inhibitors, is increased on the surface of sRCC cells compared to non-sRCC ones (Figure 2) regardless of parent histology and non-sRCC tumor grade [32,33]. Interestingly, there is a clear difference in PD-L1 expression between the different components of sRCC. While sarcomatoid components of sRCC display the highest PD-L1 expression, levels of PD-L1 expression on epithelial components of sRCC are similar to those of non-sRCC [32]. As such, PD-L1 expression levels are associated with the extent of sarcomatoid dedifferentiation [33]. Data from prospective clinical trials have confirmed the high levels of PD-L1 expression on sRCC of clear-cell type, with ≥50% of patients displaying PD-L1 expression ≥1% on tumor cells [34] or immune-infiltrating cells [35,36].

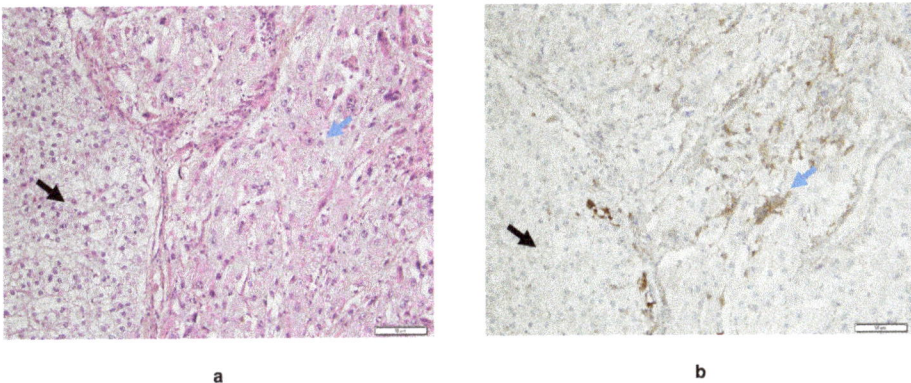

Figure 2. (a) Interface between areas of classical clear-cell carcinoma (black arrow) and its sarcomatoid component (blue arrow), Hematoxylin Eosin staining. (b) A higher density of tumor-infiltrating mononuclear inflammatory cells expressing PD-L1 is observed in the sRCC area compared to the clear-cell RCC one (monoclonal mouse antibody clone 22C3, hematoxylin counter staining). In this case, there is no PD-L1 expression on tumor cells.

sRCC also present with a higher density of tumor-infiltrating lymphocytes (TILs) compared to non-sRCC regardless of histology (Figure 2), and most of these lymphocytes have been reported to express PD-1 [33]. Up to 40% of sarcomatoid components of 118 sRCC from any histology were reported to harbor both PD-L1 expression and TIL infiltration in a single center study, compared to 8% of epithelial components of sRCC and 1% of control clear-cell RCCs [32]. This pattern has been suggested to be associated with immune resistance and may confer sensitivity to immune checkpoint inhibitors. This is corroborated by the high concomitant expression of PD-L1 in tumor cells and PD-1 in TIL, which was reported in up to 50% of sRCC of any subtype compared to less than 5% of non-sRCC in another retrospective cohort, suggesting that the PD-1/PD-L1 axis is active in sRCC [33].

Molecular studies provide additional basis for the immunogenic potential of sRCC. Study of gene expression signatures in the IMmotion151 phase 3 trial of atezolizumab plus bevacizumab versus sunitinib reported that clear-cell sRCC had a higher T-effector signature (54% versus 40%), a lower angiogenesis signature (34% versus 65%), and a higher expression of PD-L1 (63% versus 39%) compared to nonsarcomatoid clear-cell RCC [37]. Along with concordant clinical outcomes showing potent activity of atezolizumab plus bevacizumab in this population (Table 1), these data corroborate the immunogenicity of these tumors and the potential for immune-directed approaches.

Table 1. Activity of immune checkpoint inhibitors in clear-cell sRCC from subgroup analyses of phase 3 trials.

Trials	Population	Agents	N	ORR	CRR	Median PFS	Median OS
Keynote-426	Intent-to-treat	pembrolizumab + axitinib vs. sunitinib	51 vs. 54	59% vs. 32%	13% vs. 2%	8.4 months vs. NR	NR vs. NR
CheckMate-214	IMDC poor or intermediate risk	nivolumab + ipilimumab vs. sunitinib	60 vs. 52	57% vs. 19%	18% vs. 0%	8.4 months vs. 4.9 months	31.2 months vs. 13.6 months
IMmotion151	Intent-to-treat	atezolizumab + bevacizumab vs. sunitinib	68 vs. 74	49% vs. 14%	10% vs. 3%	8.3 months vs. 5.3 months	21.7 months vs. 15.4 months
JAVELIN Renal 101	Intent-to-treat	avelumab + axitinib vs. sunitinib	47 vs. 61	47% vs. 21%	4% vs. 0%	7.0 months vs. 4.0 months	NA

Abbreviations: ORR: objective response rate, CRR: complete response rate, PFS: progression-free survival, OS: overall survival, NR: not reached, NA: not available, CPS: combined positive score.

Tumor mutational burden is another hallmark that has been suggested to predict outcomes to immunotherapy in solid tumors through the formation of immunogenic neoantigens that would elicit antitumor immune response [38]. Data on sRCC remain equivocal. In a large retrospective study based on targeted sequencing of 79 sarcomatoid or rhabdoid RCC from any parent histology, mutational burden was not significantly different from nonsarcomatoid and nonrhabdoid tumors [39]. While a higher rate of somatic mutations has been described in unselected sRCC from another small dataset, these did not significantly affect relevant cancer-related genes [24]. Some data suggest that TP53 alterations may be associated with higher mutational load, but the clinical relevance is yet unclear [27].

Overall, there is consistent data demonstrating that sRCC may constitute a more immunogenic subtype of cancer than non-sRCC regardless of histology, which provide an interesting basis for the study of immune checkpoint inhibitors in these populations. Additional exploration of the immune microenvironment [40], specific mutation profiles including small insertions and deletions [41], and expression of other immune checkpoints [42] should be pursued to improve our understanding of sRCC immunity.

5. Improving Therapeutic Strategies through Immune Checkpoint Inhibition

Therapeutic management of sRCC shares similarities with that of non-sRCC. In a context of nonresectable or metastatic disease, patients have so far been treated with systemic therapies based on VEGFR-targeted agents. Data from patients treated with sunitinib and sorafenib, however, show very limited efficacy, with objective response rates (ORR) below 20% and median progression-free survival (PFS) and OS below 6 and 12 months, respectively [43]. Additional chemotherapy-based strategies have been used, assuming that antimitotic agents would be effective against this highly proliferative disease. In phase 2 trials, combination of gemcitabine with doxorubicin [44] as well as gemcitabine plus capecitabine and bevacizumab [45] demonstrated some activity regardless of the histological subtype of sRCC, with ORR between 16% and 20%, PFS of 3.5 to 5.5 months, and OS of 8.8 to 12 months. More recently, the combination of gemcitabine and sunitinib showed mild antitumor activity in unselected sRCC with an ORR of 26% and PFS and OS of 5 and 10 months, respectively. Subgroup analyses showed an improved response rate in tumors with more than 10% of sarcomatoid features and improved survival in patients with poor-risk disease [46].

These poor outcomes may be improved by immune checkpoint inhibitors, which has become the standard of care in patients with clear-cell RCC in monotherapy or combination. Notably, nivolumab plus ipilimumab [47] and pembrolizumab plus axitinib [48] have both demonstrated improved OS in intermediate/poor risk patients and all comers, respectively, while atezolizumab plus bevacizumab [37] and avelumab plus axitinib [47] demonstrated PFS improvement compared to sunitinib in the first-line metastatic setting. First subgroup analyses, including patients with sarcomatoid tumors, are being reported with promising efficacy results (Table 1).

The Keynote-426 trial assessing the pembrolizumab plus axitinib combination and the JAVELIN Renal 101 trial of avelumab plus axitinib both demonstrated improved outcomes in patients with clear-cell sRCC compared with sunitinib [36,49]. The ORR with those combinations were strikingly high at 59% and 47%, with complete responses (CR) in 12% and 4% of patients, respectively. These data translated into increased PFS compared to sunitinib with hazard ratios (HR) of 0.54 (95% confidence interval (CI) 0.29–1.00) and 0.57 (95% CI 0.32–1.00) for OS, respectively. Similarly, interesting results were reported with the IMmotion151 trial, which evaluated the combination of atezolizumab plus bevacizumab in the same population. An ORR of 49%, including a complete response rate of 10%, and a HR for PFS of 0.52 (95% CI 0.34–0.79) and 0.64 (95% CI 0.41–1.01) in sRCC were reported [35].

The combination of two immune checkpoint inhibitors may also provide impressive results in sRCC patients, as demonstrated by the CheckMate-214 study of nivolumab plus ipilimumab. In patients with intermediate or poor-risk clear-cell sRCC, PFS and OS were improved in the experimental arm, with HR of 0.61 (95% CI 0.38–0.97) and 0.55 (95% CI 0.33–0.90), respectively, compared to sunitinib. Importantly, the ORR achieved by the combination of nivolumab plus ipilimumab was as high as 57%, with an impressive proportion (18%) of patients achieving complete response (Table 1). These results are encouraging as complete response to immunotherapy has been recently suggested to be a potential surrogate marker for very long-term survival [50].

Additional data stems from phase 2 trials spanning across uncommon histologies. In a phase 2 trial of atezolizumab plus bevacizumab, patients with clear-cell RCC and sarcomatoid dedifferentiation >20% had an ORR of 50% [34]. Data from the cohort B of the Keynote-427 study evaluating pembrolizumab monotherapy showed an ORR of 42% in patients with sRCC of non-clear-cell subtypes [51].

Prospective clinical trial data thus show convincing efficacy of immune checkpoint inhibitors in sRCC patients and is in line with translational work suggesting that sRCC may be immune-reactive tumors. The use of immunotherapy combinations should be considered as standard of care in these populations, while biomarker analyses are awaited to better inform patient selection.

6. Perspectives

The study of sRCC has become a dynamic field, sparking hope for sustained improvement in outcomes in this aggressive subset of tumors. It is now established that sRCC are immunologically "hot" tumors that demonstrate excellent responses to immune checkpoint inhibitors and prolonged survival with combination-based strategies. Current efforts to unravel the molecular landscape of these tumors might help develop targeted strategies to overcome resistance to current therapies.

Many questions about sRCC biology have yet to be answered to get to this point. The mechanisms underlying sarcomatoid dedifferentiation are still mostly unknown. Despite evidence of recurrent genomic alterations, those are not specific to sRCC and may not be enough to drive this aggressive phenotype. In addition, the relevance of these alterations for targeted therapies has yet to be investigated in dedicated clinical trials. More answers could lie in epigenetics and regulatory processes that trigger transcriptional programs involved in sarcomatoid transformation. Such processes may be impacted by the cellular context, including alterations of cellular metabolism [29] as well as interactions between tumor cells and their surrounding microenvironment [52]. The noncoding genome also needs to be explored in the future. In particular, alterations affecting regulatory RNAs may impact cell machinery and disrupt gene expression toward epithelial–mesenchymal transition [53]. The impact of parent histologies on such cellular processes also needs to be determined as the diversity of RCC subtypes may account for wide genetic and epigenetic variations.

The encouraging results of immune checkpoint inhibitor combinations in a disease known to be refractory to past standard of care therapies brings new optimism in the field. Biomarkers of response to therapy remain to be found, similar to non-sRCC, where PD-L1 expression [54], tumor mutational burden [38], or gene expression profiles [55] have yet to prove their clinical utility to accurately stratify patients. Additional combinations using modified proinflammatory cytokines [56] or novel checkpoint inhibitors [57] have the potential to further improve the efficacy of PD-1/PD-L1-based regimens. Approaches based on multimodal therapy, such as combining stereotactic radiation therapy to bolster immunity, could be interesting to explore in these inflamed tumors [58]. Opportunities for targeted therapies should also be evaluated: cell cycle inhibitors could be interesting in tumors with alterations of cell cycle proteins [59]; approaches targeting chromatin remodeling complexes in tumors already deficient in one or multiple chromatin-remodeling genes, such as *ARID1A*, could promote synthetic lethality, as demonstrated in other solid tumors [60]; *NF2*-deficient tumors could be targeted in preclinical models by YAP/TAZ depletion associated with MEK inhibition [31]. The progress made in the metastatic setting may also translate into localized disease. Multiple trials are ongoing for evaluating immune checkpoint inhibition perioperatively, including nivolumab (NCT03055013) and pembrolizumab (NCT03142334), which could be beneficial to these tumors at high risk of recurrence.

7. Conclusions

Clinical and translational research efforts have transformed the understanding of sRCC: from a hard-to-treat disease with limited biological understanding, it is becoming part of a burgeoning research field with major advances in outcomes and new paths to innovative therapeutic developments. Evaluation of novel treatment strategies and potential biomarkers of response to therapy are needed to improve patient selection and the prognosis of this aggressive disease.

Funding: This research received no external funding.

Conflicts of Interest: The authors declare no conflict of interest related to this work.

References

1. Bray, F.; Ferlay, J.; Soerjomataram, I.; Siegel, R.L.; Torre, L.A.; Jemal, A. Global cancer statistics 2018: GLOBOCAN estimates of incidence and mortality worldwide for 36 cancers in 185 countries. *CA Cancer J. Clin.* **2018**, *68*, 394–424. [CrossRef] [PubMed]
2. Kyriakopoulos, C.E.; Chittoria, N.; Choueiri, T.K.; Kroeger, N.; Lee, J.-L.; Srinivas, S.; Knox, J.J.; Bjarnason, G.A.; Ernst, S.D.; Wood, L.A.; et al. Outcome of patients with metastatic sarcomatoid renal cell carcinoma: Results from the International Metastatic Renal Cell Carcinoma Database Consortium. *Clin. Genitourin. Cancer* **2015**, *13*, e79–e85. [CrossRef] [PubMed]
3. Albiges, L.; Flippot, R.; Rioux-Leclercq, N.; Choueiri, T.K. Non-Clear Cell Renal Cell Carcinomas: From Shadow to Light. *J. Clin. Oncol.* **2018**, *36*, 3624–3631. [CrossRef] [PubMed]
4. Kroeger, N.; Xie, W.; Lee, J.-L.; Bjarnason, G.A.; Knox, J.J.; Mackenzie, M.J.; Wood, L.; Srinivas, S.; Vaishamayan, U.N.; Rha, S.-Y.; et al. Metastatic non-clear cell renal cell carcinoma treated with targeted therapy agents: Characterization of survival outcome and application of the International mRCC Database Consortium criteria. *Cancer* **2013**, *119*, 2999–3006. [CrossRef] [PubMed]
5. Molina, A.M.; Tickoo, S.K.; Ishill, N.; Trinos, M.J.; Schwartz, L.H.; Patil, S.; Feldman, D.R.; Reuter, V.E.; Russo, P.; Motzer, R.J. Sarcomatoid-variant Renal Cell Carcinoma Treatment Outcome and Survival in Advanced Disease. *Am. J. Clin. Oncol.* **2011**, *34*, 454–459. [CrossRef] [PubMed]
6. Zhang, L.; Wu, B.; Zha, Z.; Zhao, H.; Feng, Y. The prognostic value and clinicopathological features of sarcomatoid differentiation in patients with renal cell carcinoma: A systematic review and meta-analysis. *Cancer Manag. Res.* **2018**, *10*, 1687–1703. [CrossRef]
7. Moch, H.; Cubilla, A.L.; Humphrey, P.A.; Reuter, V.E.; Ulbright, T.M. The 2016 WHO Classification of Tumours of the Urinary System and Male Genital Organs—Part A: Renal, Penile, and Testicular Tumours. *Eur. Urol.* **2016**, *70*, 93–105. [CrossRef]
8. He, H.; Magi-Galluzzi, C. Epithelial-to-mesenchymal transition in renal neoplasms. *Adv. Anat. Pathol.* **2014**, *21*, 174–180. [CrossRef]

9. Boström, A.-K.; Möller, C.; Nilsson, E.; Elfving, P.; Axelson, H.; Johansson, M.E. Sarcomatoid conversion of clear cell renal cell carcinoma in relation to epithelial-to-mesenchymal transition. *Hum. Pathol.* **2012**, *43*, 708–719. [CrossRef]
10. Conant, J.L.; Peng, Z.; Evans, M.F.; Naud, S.; Cooper, K. Sarcomatoid renal cell carcinoma is an example of epithelial–mesenchymal transition. *J. Clin. Pathol.* **2011**, *64*, 1088–1092. [CrossRef]
11. Yu, W.; Wang, Y.; Jiang, Y.; Zhang, W.; Li, Y. Distinct immunophenotypes and prognostic factors in renal cell carcinoma with sarcomatoid differentiation: A systematic study of 19 immunohistochemical markers in 42 cases. *BMC Cancer* **2017**, *17*, 293. [CrossRef] [PubMed]
12. Reuter, V.E.; Argani, P.; Zhou, M.; Delahunt, B. Members of the ISUP Immunohistochemistry in Diagnostic Urologic Pathology Group Best practices recommendations in the application of immunohistochemistry in the kidney tumors: Report from the International Society of Urologic Pathology consensus conference. *Am. J. Surg. Pathol.* **2014**, *38*, e35–e49. [PubMed]
13. Tanas Isikci, O.; He, H.; Grossmann, P.; Alaghehbandan, R.; Ulamec, M.; Michalova, K.; Pivovarcikova, K.; Montiel, D.P.; Ondic, O.; Daum, O.; et al. Low-grade spindle cell proliferation in clear cell renal cell carcinoma is unlikely to be an initial step in sarcomatoid differentiation. *Histopathology* **2018**, *72*, 804–813. [CrossRef] [PubMed]
14. Delahunt, B.; Srigley, J.R.; Egevad, L.; Montironi, R. International Society of Urological Pathology Grading and Other Prognostic Factors for Renal Neoplasia. *Eur. Urol.* **2014**, *66*, 795–798. [CrossRef] [PubMed]
15. Warren, A.Y.; Harrison, D. WHO/ISUP classification, grading and pathological staging of renal cell carcinoma: Standards and controversies. *World J. Urol.* **2018**, *36*, 1913–1926. [CrossRef]
16. Cheville, J.C.; Lohse, C.M.; Zincke, H.; Weaver, A.L.; Leibovich, B.C.; Frank, I.; Blute, M.L. Sarcomatoid Renal Cell Carcinoma. *Am. J. Surg. Pathol.* **2004**, *28*, 7. [CrossRef]
17. Adibi, M.; Thomas, A.Z.; Borregales, L.D.; Merrill, M.M.; Slack, R.S.; Chen, H.-C.; Sircar, K.; Murugan, P.; Tamboli, P.; Jonasch, E.; et al. Percentage of sarcomatoid component as a prognostic indicator for survival in renal cell carcinoma with sarcomatoid dedifferentiation. *Urol. Oncol.* **2015**, *33*, 427.e17–427.e23. [CrossRef]
18. Alevizakos, M.; Gaitanidis, A.; Nasioudis, D.; Msaouel, P.; Appleman, L.J. Sarcomatoid Renal Cell Carcinoma: Population-Based Study of 879 Patients. *Clin. Genitourin. Cancer* **2019**, *17*, e447–e453. [CrossRef]
19. Shuch, B.; Said, J.; LaRochelle, J.C.; Zhou, Y.; Li, G.; Klatte, T.; Pouliot, F.; Kabbinavar, F.F.; Belldegrun, A.S.; Pantuck, A.J. Histologic evaluation of metastases in renal cell carcinoma with sarcomatoid transformation and its implications for systemic therapy. *Cancer* **2010**, *116*, 616–624. [CrossRef]
20. Abel, E.J.; Culp, S.H.; Matin, S.F.; Tamboli, P.; Wallace, M.J.; Jonasch, E.; Tannir, N.M.; Wood, C.G. Percutaneous biopsy of primary tumor in metastatic renal cell carcinoma to predict high risk pathological features: Comparison with nephrectomy assessment. *J. Urol.* **2010**, *184*, 1877–1881. [CrossRef]
21. Jones, T.D.; Eble, J.N.; Wang, M.; MacLennan, G.T.; Jain, S.; Cheng, L. Clonal divergence and genetic heterogeneity in clear cell renal cell carcinomas with sarcomatoid transformation. *Cancer* **2005**, *104*, 1195–1203. [CrossRef] [PubMed]
22. Sircar, K.; Yoo, S.-Y.; Majewski, T.; Wani, K.; Patel, L.R.; Voicu, H.; Torres-Garcia, W.; Verhaak, R.G.W.; Tannir, N.; Karam, J.A.; et al. Biphasic components of sarcomatoid clear cell renal cell carcinomas are molecularly similar to each other, but distinct from non-sarcomatoid renal carcinomas. *J. Pathol. Clin. Res.* **2015**, *1*, 212–224. [CrossRef] [PubMed]
23. Bi, M.; Zhao, S.; Said, J.W.; Merino, M.J.; Adeniran, A.J.; Xie, Z.; Nawaf, C.B.; Choi, J.; Belldegrun, A.S.; Pantuck, A.J.; et al. Genomic characterization of sarcomatoid transformation in clear cell renal cell carcinoma. *Proc. Natl. Acad. Sci. USA* **2016**, *113*, 2170–2175. [CrossRef] [PubMed]
24. Wang, Z.; Kim, T.B.; Peng, B.; Karam, J.A.; Creighton, C.J.; Joon, A.Y.; Kawakami, F.; Trevisan, P.; Jonasch, E.; Chow, C.-W.; et al. Sarcomatoid renal cell carcinoma has a distinct molecular pathogenesis, driver mutation profile and transcriptional landscape. *Clin. Cancer Res.* **2017**, *23*, 6686–6696. [CrossRef]
25. Brannon, A.R.; Reddy, A.; Seiler, M.; Arreola, A.; Moore, D.T.; Pruthi, R.S.; Wallen, E.M.; Nielsen, M.E.; Liu, H.; Nathanson, K.L.; et al. Molecular Stratification of Clear Cell Renal Cell Carcinoma by Consensus Clustering Reveals Distinct Subtypes and Survival Patterns. *Genes Cancer* **2010**, *1*, 152–163. [CrossRef]
26. Pal, S.K.; He, M.; Tong, T.; Wu, H.; Liu, X.; Lau, C.; Wang, J.-H.; Warden, C.; Wu, X.; Signoretti, S.; et al. RNA-seq reveals aurora kinase-driven mTOR pathway activation in patients with sarcomatoid metastatic renal cell carcinoma. *Mol. Cancer Res. MCR* **2015**, *13*, 130–137. [CrossRef]

27. Malouf, G.G.; Ali, S.M.; Wang, K.; Balasubramanian, S.; Ross, J.S.; Miller, V.A.; Stephens, P.J.; Khayat, D.; Pal, S.K.; Su, X.; et al. Genomic Characterization of Renal Cell Carcinoma with Sarcomatoid Dedifferentiation Pinpoints Recurrent Genomic Alterations. *Eur. Urol.* **2016**, *70*, 348–357. [CrossRef]
28. The Cancer Genome Atlas Research Network Comprehensive molecular characterization of clear cell renal cell carcinoma. *Nature* **2013**, *499*, 43–49. [CrossRef]
29. Ricketts, C.J.; Cubas, A.A.D.; Fan, H.; Smith, C.C.; Lang, M.; Reznik, E.; Bowlby, R.; Gibb, E.A.; Akbani, R.; Beroukhim, R.; et al. The Cancer Genome Atlas Comprehensive Molecular Characterization of Renal Cell Carcinoma. *Cell Rep.* **2018**, *23*, 313–326.e5. [CrossRef]
30. Chen, Y.-B.; Xu, J.; Skanderup, A.J.; Dong, Y.; Brannon, A.R.; Wang, L.; Won, H.H.; Wang, P.I.; Nanjangud, G.J.; Jungbluth, A.A.; et al. Molecular analysis of aggressive renal cell carcinoma with unclassified histology reveals distinct subsets. *Nat. Commun.* **2016**, *7*, 13131. [CrossRef]
31. White, S.M.; Avantaggiati, M.L.; Nemazanyy, I.; Di Poto, C.; Yang, Y.; Pende, M.; Gibney, G.T.; Ressom, H.W.; Field, J.; Atkins, M.B.; et al. YAP/TAZ Inhibition Induces Metabolic and Signaling Rewiring Resulting in Targetable Vulnerabilities in NF2-Deficient Tumor Cells. *Dev. Cell* **2019**, *49*, 425–443.e9. [CrossRef] [PubMed]
32. Kawakami, F.; Sircar, K.; Rodriguez-Canales, J.; Fellman, B.M.; Urbauer, D.L.; Tamboli, P.; Tannir, N.M.; Jonasch, E.; Wistuba, I.I.; Wood, C.G.; et al. Programmed cell death ligand 1 and tumor-infiltrating lymphocyte status in patients with renal cell carcinoma and sarcomatoid dedifferentiation. *Cancer* **2017**, *123*, 4823–4831. [CrossRef] [PubMed]
33. Joseph, R.W.; Millis, S.Z.; Carballido, E.M.; Bryant, D.; Gatalica, Z.; Reddy, S.; Bryce, A.H.; Vogelzang, N.J.; Stanton, M.L.; Castle, E.P.; et al. PD-1 and PD-L1 Expression in Renal Cell Carcinoma with Sarcomatoid Differentiation. *Cancer Immunol. Res.* **2015**, *3*, 1303–1307. [CrossRef] [PubMed]
34. Flippot, R.; McGregor, B.A.; Flaifel, A.; Gray, K.P.; Signoretti, S.; Steinharter, J.A.; Van Allen, E.M.; Walsh, M.K.; Gundy, K.; Wei, X.X.; et al. Atezolizumab plus bevacizumab in non-clear cell renal cell carcinoma (NccRCC) and clear cell renal cell carcinoma with sarcomatoid differentiation (ccRCCsd): Updated results of activity and predictive biomarkers from a phase II study. *J. Clin. Oncol.* **2019**, *37*, 4583. [CrossRef]
35. Rini, B.I.; Motzer, R.J.; Powles, T.; McDermott, D.F.; Escudier, B.; Donskov, F.; Hawkins, R.E.; Bracarda, S.; Bedke, J.; De Giorgi, U.; et al. Atezolizumab (atezo) + bevacizumab (bev) versus sunitinib (sun) in pts with untreated metastatic renal cell carcinoma (mRCC) and sarcomatoid (sarc) histology: IMmotion151 subgroup analysis. *J. Clin. Oncol.* **2019**, *37*, 4512. [CrossRef]
36. 3Efficacy and biomarker analysis of patients (pts) with advanced renal cell carcinoma (aRCC) with sarcomatoid histology (sRCC): Subgroup analysis fr... Available online: https://oncologypro.esmo.org/Meeting-Resources/ESMO-2019-Congress/Efficacy-and-biomarker-analysis-of-patients-pts-with-advanced-renal-cell-carcinoma-aRCC-with-sarcomatoid-histology-sRCC-subgroup-analysis-from-the-phase-3-JAVELIN-Renal-101-trial-of-first-line-avelumab-plus-axitinib-A-Ax-vs-sunitinib-S (accessed on 30 September 2019).
37. Rini, B.I.; Powles, T.; Atkins, M.B.; Escudier, B.; McDermott, D.F.; Suarez, C.; Bracarda, S.; Stadler, W.M.; Donskov, F.; Lee, J.L.; et al. Atezolizumab plus bevacizumab versus sunitinib in patients with previously untreated metastatic renal cell carcinoma (IMmotion151): A multicentre, open-label, phase 3, randomised controlled trial. *Lancet* **2019**, *393*, 2404–2415. [CrossRef]
38. Samstein, R.M.; Lee, C.-H.; Shoushtari, A.N.; Hellmann, M.D.; Shen, R.; Janjigian, Y.Y.; Barron, D.A.; Zehir, A.; Jordan, E.J.; Omuro, A.; et al. Tumor mutational load predicts survival after immunotherapy across multiple cancer types. *Nat. Genet.* **2019**, *51*, 202–206. [CrossRef]
39. Bakouny, Z.; Vokes, N.; Gao, X.; Nassar, A.; Abou Alaiwi, S.; Flippot, R.; Bouchard, G.; Steinharter, J.A.; Nuzzo, P.; Pan, W.; et al. Efficacy of immune checkpoint inhibitors (ICI) and genomic characterization of sarcomatoid and/or rhabdoid (S/R) metastatic renal cell carcinoma (mRCC). *J. Clin. Oncol.* **2019**, *37*, 4514. [CrossRef]
40. Binnewies, M.; Roberts, E.W.; Kersten, K.; Chan, V.; Fearon, D.F.; Merad, M.; Coussens, L.M.; Gabrilovich, D.I.; Ostrand-Rosenberg, S.; Hedrick, C.C.; et al. Understanding the tumor immune microenvironment (TIME) for effective therapy. *Nat. Med.* **2018**, *24*, 541–550. [CrossRef]
41. Turajlic, S.; Litchfield, K.; Xu, H.; Rosenthal, R.; McGranahan, N.; Reading, J.L.; Wong, Y.N.S.; Rowan, A.; Kanu, N.; Bakir, M.A.; et al. Insertion-and-deletion-derived tumour-specific neoantigens and the immunogenic phenotype: A pan-cancer analysis. *Lancet Oncol.* **2017**, *18*, 1009–1021. [CrossRef]

42. Sharma, P.; Hu-Lieskovan, S.; Wargo, J.A.; Ribas, A. Primary, Adaptive and Acquired Resistance to Cancer Immunotherapy. *Cell* **2017**, *168*, 707–723. [CrossRef] [PubMed]
43. Golshayan, A.R.; George, S.; Heng, D.Y.; Elson, P.; Wood, L.S.; Mekhail, T.M.; Garcia, J.A.; Aydin, H.; Zhou, M.; Bukowski, R.M.; et al. Metastatic sarcomatoid renal cell carcinoma treated with vascular endothelial growth factor-targeted therapy. *J. Clin. Oncol. Off. J. Am. Soc. Clin. Oncol.* **2009**, *27*, 235–241. [CrossRef] [PubMed]
44. Haas, N.B.; Lin, X.; Manola, J.; Pins, M.; Liu, G.; McDermott, D.; Nanus, D.; Heath, E.; Wilding, G.; Dutcher, J. A phase II trial of doxorubicin and gemcitabine in renal cell carcinoma with sarcomatoid features: ECOG 8802. *Med. Oncol. Northwood Lond. Engl.* **2012**, *29*, 761–767. [CrossRef] [PubMed]
45. Maiti, A.; Nemati-Shafaee, M.; Msaouel, P.; Pagliaro, L.C.; Jonasch, E.; Tannir, N.M.; Shah, A.Y. Phase II Trial of Capecitabine, Gemcitabine, and Bevacizumab in Sarcomatoid Renal Cell Carcinoma. *Clin. Genitourin. Cancer* **2018**, *16*, e47–e57. [CrossRef] [PubMed]
46. Michaelson, M.D.; McKay, R.R.; Werner, L.; Atkins, M.B.; Van Allen, E.M.; Olivier, K.M.; Song, J.; Signoretti, S.; McDermott, D.F.; Choueiri, T.K. Phase 2 trial of sunitinib and gemcitabine in patients with sarcomatoid and/or poor-risk metastatic renal cell carcinoma. *Cancer* **2015**, *121*, 3435–3443. [CrossRef] [PubMed]
47. Motzer, R.J.; Tannir, N.M.; McDermott, D.F.; Arén Frontera, O.; Melichar, B.; Choueiri, T.K.; Plimack, E.R.; Barthélémy, P.; Porta, C.; George, S.; et al. Nivolumab plus Ipilimumab versus Sunitinib in Advanced Renal-Cell Carcinoma. *N. Engl. J. Med.* **2018**, *378*, 1277–1290. [CrossRef] [PubMed]
48. Rini, B.I.; Plimack, E.R.; Stus, V.; Gafanov, R.; Hawkins, R.; Nosov, D.; Pouliot, F.; Alekseev, B.; Soulières, D.; Melichar, B.; et al. Pembrolizumab plus Axitinib versus Sunitinib for Advanced Renal-Cell Carcinoma. *N. Engl. J. Med.* **2019**, *380*, 1116–1127. [CrossRef]
49. Rini, B.I.; Plimack, E.R.; Stus, V.; Gafanov, R.; Hawkins, R.; Nosov, D.; Pouliot, F.; Soulieres, D.; Melichar, B.; Vynnychenko, I.; et al. Pembrolizumab (pembro) plus axitinib (axi) versus sunitinib as first-line therapy for metastatic renal cell carcinoma (mRCC): Outcomes in the combined IMDC intermediate/poor risk and sarcomatoid subgroups of the phase 3 KEYNOTE-426 study. *J. Clin. Oncol.* **2019**, *37*, 4500. [CrossRef]
50. Gauci, M.-L.; Lanoy, E.; Champiat, S.; Caramella, C.; Ammari, S.; Aspeslagh, S.; Varga, A.; Baldini, C.; Bahleda, R.; Gazzah, A.; et al. Long-Term Survival in Patients Responding to Anti-Pd-1/Pd-L1 Therapy and Disease Outcome Upon Treatment Discontinuation. *Clin. Cancer Res.* **2019**, *25*, 946–956. [CrossRef]
51. First-Line Pembrolizumab (pembro) Monotherapy for Advanced Non-Clear Cell Renal Cell Carcinoma (nccRCC): Updated Follow-Up for KEYNOTE-427 Cohort B. Available online: https://oncologypro.esmo.org/Meeting-Resources/ESMO-2019-Congress/First-Line-Pembrolizumab-pembro-Monotherapy-for-Advanced-Non-Clear-Cell-Renal-Cell-Carcinoma-nccRCC-Updated-Follow-Up-for-KEYNOTE-427-Cohort-B (accessed on 30 September 2019).
52. Jung, H.-Y.; Fattet, L.; Yang, J. Molecular Pathways: Linking Tumor Microenvironment to Epithelial–Mesenchymal Transition in Metastasis. *Clin. Cancer Res. Off. J. Am. Assoc. Cancer Res.* **2015**, *21*, 962–968. [CrossRef]
53. Flippot, R.; Beinse, G.; Boilève, A.; Vibert, J.; Malouf, G.G. Long non-coding RNAs in genitourinary malignancies: A whole new world. *Nat. Rev. Urol.* **2019**, *16*, 484–504. [CrossRef] [PubMed]
54. Motzer, R.J.; Penkov, K.; Haanen, J.; Rini, B.; Albiges, L.; Campbell, M.T.; Venugopal, B.; Kollmannsberger, C.; Negrier, S.; Uemura, M.; et al. Avelumab plus Axitinib versus Sunitinib for Advanced Renal-Cell Carcinoma. *N. Engl. J. Med.* **2019**, *380*, 1103–1115. [CrossRef] [PubMed]
55. Rini, B.I.; Huseni, M.; Atkins, M.B.; McDermott, D.F.; Powles, T.B.; Escudier, B.; Banchereau, R.; Liu, L.-F.; Leng, N.; Fan, J.; et al. LBA31Molecular correlates differentiate response to atezolizumab (atezo) + bevacizumab (bev) vs sunitinib (sun): Results from a phase III study (IMmotion151) in untreated metastatic renal cell carcinoma (mRCC). *Ann. Oncol.* **2018**, *29*, mdy424-037. [CrossRef]
56. Bentebibel, S.-E.; Hurwitz, M.E.; Bernatchez, C.; Haymaker, C.; Hudgens, C.W.; Kluger, H.M.; Tetzlaff, M.T.; Tagliaferri, M.A.; Zalevsky, J.; Hoch, U.; et al. A First-in-Human Study and Biomarker Analysis of NKTR-214, a Novel IL2Rβγ-Biased Cytokine, in Patients with Advanced or Metastatic Solid Tumors. *Cancer Discov.* **2019**, *9*, 711–721. [CrossRef] [PubMed]
57. Flippot, R.; Escudier, B.; Albiges, L. Immune Checkpoint Inhibitors: Toward New Paradigms in Renal Cell Carcinoma. *Drugs* **2018**, *78*, 1443–1457. [CrossRef] [PubMed]

58. Theelen, W.S.M.E.; Peulen, H.M.U.; Lalezari, F.; van der Noort, V.; de Vries, J.F.; Aerts, J.G.J.V.; Dumoulin, D.W.; Bahce, I.; Niemeijer, A.-L.N.; de Langen, A.J.; et al. Effect of Pembrolizumab After Stereotactic Body Radiotherapy vs Pembrolizumab Alone on Tumor Response in Patients with Advanced Non–Small Cell Lung Cancer: Results of the PEMBRO-RT Phase 2 Randomized Clinical Trial. *JAMA Oncol.* **2019**, *5*, 1276–1282. [CrossRef] [PubMed]
59. Pal, S.K.; Ali, S.M.; Ross, J.; Choueiri, T.K.; Chung, J.H. Exceptional Response to Palbociclib in Metastatic Collecting Duct Carcinoma Bearing a CDKN2A Homozygous Deletion. *JCO Precis. Oncol.* **2017**, *1*, 1–5. [CrossRef]
60. Alldredge, J.K.; Eskander, R.N. EZH2 inhibition in ARID1A mutated clear cell and endometrioid ovarian and endometrioid endometrial cancers. *Gynecol. Oncol. Res. Pract.* **2017**, *4*, 17. [CrossRef]

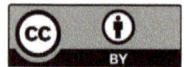

© 2019 by the authors. Licensee MDPI, Basel, Switzerland. This article is an open access article distributed under the terms and conditions of the Creative Commons Attribution (CC BY) license (http://creativecommons.org/licenses/by/4.0/).

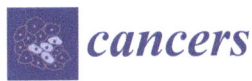

Review

Molecular Genetics of Renal Cell Tumors: A Practical Diagnostic Approach

Reza Alaghehbandan [1], Delia Perez Montiel [2], Ana Silvia Luis [3,4] and Ondrej Hes [5,*]

1. Department of Pathology, Faculty of Medicine, University of British Columbia, Royal Columbian Hospital, Vancouver, BC V3E 0G9, Canada; reza.alagh@gmail.com
2. Department of Pathology, Institute Nacional de Cancerologia, INCAN, Mexico DF 14080, Mexico; madeliapmg@yahoo.com.mx
3. Department of Pathology, Centro Hospitalar de Vila Nova de Gaia-Espinho, Vila Nova de Gaia, Cancer Biology and Epigenetics Group (CBEG), IPO Porto Research Center (CI-IPOP), Portuguese Oncology Institute of Porto (IPO Porto) & Porto Comprehensive Cancer Center (P.CCC), 4200-072 Porto, Portugal; anasilvialuis@gmail.com
4. Department of Microscopy, Institute of Biomedical Sciences Abel Salazar, University of Porto (ICBAS-UP), 4200-072 Porto, Portugal
5. Department of Pathology, Charles University in Prague, Faculty of Medicine in Plzen, 304 60 Pilsen, Czech Republic
* Correspondence: hes@biopticka.cz

Received: 1 December 2019; Accepted: 23 December 2019; Published: 30 December 2019

Abstract: Renal epithelial cell tumors are composed of a heterogeneous group of tumors with variable morphologic, immunohistochemical, and molecular features. A "histo-molecular" approach is now an integral part of defining renal tumors, aiming to be clinically and therapeutically pertinent. Most renal epithelial tumors including the new and emerging entities have distinct molecular and genetic features which can be detected using various methods. Most renal epithelial tumors can be diagnosed easily based on pure histologic findings with or without immunohistochemical examination. Furthermore, molecular-genetic testing can be utilized to assist in arriving at an accurate diagnosis. In this review, we presented the most current knowledge concerning molecular-genetic aspects of renal epithelial neoplasms, which potentially can be used in daily diagnostic practice.

Keywords: kidney; renal cell carcinoma; molecular genetic features; practical approach; review

1. Introduction

Renal cell tumors are one of the most extensively studied human neoplasms. A number of morphologic, immunohistochemical and molecular genetic features were described during the last 20 years, which have also led to recognition of new entities, expanding our knowledge and understanding of renal tumors.

"The Heidelberg classification of renal cell tumors" published in 1997 was the first classification integrating molecular genetic features as one of the diagnostic tools applicable to renal cell tumors [1]. This classification was further corroborated by the so-called UICC Rochester Classification [2], which later evolved through the 2004 World Health Organization (WHO) tumor classification [3], 2012 Vancouver ISUP (International Society of Urologic Pathology) consensus conference [4], and most recently the 2016 WHO blue book [5]. This "histo-molecular" approach is now an integral part of defining renal tumors and the emerging entities, aiming to be clinically and therapeutically pertinent. A summary of genetic tests and routinely used immunohistochemical examinations in daily practice is shown in Table 1. There have been many studies describing and examining molecular genetic changes of renal tumors. All these studies have shown that the molecular genetic changes are remarkably heterogeneous across the whole spectrum of renal cell carcinomas (RCCs) and other tumors and that molecular-genetic analysis cannot be used as a universal diagnostic tool.

In this review, we present the most current knowledge concerning molecular-genetic aspects of renal epithelial neoplasms, which potentially can be used in daily diagnostic practice. It is important to note that ISUP recommendations for molecular genetic testing of renal cell tumors will be published in the near future.

Table 1. Genetic tests and routinely used immunohistochemical examinations in renal cell tumors

Tumor Type	IHC	Mutation	Method
CCRCC	Carbonic Anhydrase (CA) IX, Vimentin	VHL (von Hippel Lindau) inactivation	Sequencing (NGS/classical)/methylation specific PCR (polymerase chain reaction)
MCRCNLMP	NS	VHL	NR
PRCC type 1 hereditary syndrome	CK7, AMACR	MET	Sequencing (NGS/classical)
PRCC type 1 conventional type	CK7, AMACR	Gain of 7,17	aCGH/FISH
PRCC type 2	NS	NS	
OPRCC	AMACR, Vimentin	KRAS	Sequencing (NGS/classical)
FH-deficient RCC	FH, 2SC	FH mutation/LOH analysis	Sequencing (NGS/classical)/fragment analysis
ChRCCC	CK7, CD117	NS	
"Hybrid" On/Ch tumors	NS	FLCN **	Sequencing (NGS/classical)
Oncocytoma	CK7, CD117	NS	
Clear cell PRCC	CK7, AMACR	VHL	Sequencing (NGS/classical)
MiT RCC	TFE3, Cathepsin K	TFE3, TFEB	FISH/NGS
MTSCC	AMACR, EMA	CNV pattern analysis	aCGH
TC-RCC	CK7, AMACR	CNV pattern analysis	aCGH
ACD-associated RCC	CK7, AMACR	NS	
RMC	INI1	SMARCB1	Sequencing (NGS/classical)
CDC	34betaE12, Ck7	NS	
SDH-deficient renal cell carcinoma	SDHB	SDHB	Sequencing (NGS, classical)/IHC

Clear cell renal cell carcinoma (CCRCC). Multilocular cystic renal cell neoplasm of low malignant potential (MCRCNLMP). Papillary RCC (PRCC). Oncocytic papillary RCC (OPRCC). "Hybrid" oncocytic/chromophobe tumors (Hybrid" On/Ch tumors). ** Diagnosis of Birt–Hogg–Dubé syndrome. (MTSCC) Mucinous tubular and spindle cell carcinoma. CNV (copy-number variation) Tubulocystic RCC (TC-RCC) Renal medullary carcinoma (RMC). Fluorescence in situ hybridization (FISH). Next-generation sequencing (NGS). Array comparative genome hybridization (aCGH). Not specific (NS). Immunohistochemistry (IHC). Not recommended (NR).

2. Clear Cell Renal Cell Carcinoma (CCRCC)

Clear cell renal cell carcinoma (CCRCC), the most common RCC, is typically composed of cells with clear cytoplasm and with a rich fine capillary network [5]. CCRCCs can also exhibit with eosinophilic cytoplasm and marked cellular pleomorphism. CCRCC cases mimicking clear cell papillary RCC are not infrequently found [6,7].

Chromosome 3p deletion has been described in CCRCC since the 80s [8], and was recognized as a characteristic genetic feature of this tumor in the Heidelberg classification [1], present in more than 90% of cases [9,10]. In parallel, *VHL* gene located on chromosome 3p was described as the most frequently mutated gene (50–75%) in CCRCC, and later found to be silenced by promoter methylation in 5–20% of cases [9,10]. Thus, the most frequent genetic alteration in CCRCC involves chromosome 3p deletion, *VHL* mutation and/or *VHL* promoter methylation, leading to *VHL* inactivation, an early and crucial event in sporadic CCRCC and in the familial cancer syndrome von Hippel–Lindau disease [9,11].

In addition to *VHL* located on chromosome 3p, there are other genes such the component of the SWI/SNF chromatin remodeling complex PBRM1 (26–33%), the histone modifying enzymes SETD2 (4–12%) and BAP1 (10%) being frequently reported in CCRCC [12–14].

Application in routine practice:

The presence of *VHL* mutation, chromosome 3p deletion or *VHL* promoter methylation is considered useful for the confirmation of CCRCC diagnosis in difficult cases (see following sections).

3. Multilocular Cystic Renal Cell Neoplasm of Low Malignant Potential (MCRCNLMP)

Multilocular cystic renal cell neoplasm of low malignant potential (MCRCNLMP) is a rare (<1%) renal tumor with an excellent prognosis, without recurrence or metastases described for bona fide cases [5]. Careful macroscopic evaluation and sampling are pivotal for the diagnosis, as the presence of solid nodules and/or cell clusters with expansive growth warrants a diagnosis of multicystic CCRCC [5]. MCRCNLMP, a low-grade tumor, had been considered a variant of CCRCC due to morphological similarities and analogous genetic features [15–17]. The most frequent genetic alterations in MCRCNLMP are identical to chromosome 3p deletion in 74% (14/19) of cases [17] and *VHL* mutation in 25% (3/12) of cases [18].

Interestingly, *KRAS* mutation was not found in small cohort of 12 MCRCNLMP cases, contrarily to codon 12 or codon 13 mutations identified in 12 CCRCC cases [19,20]. Of note, other studies that failed to identify *KRAS* mutation in CCRCC sequenced only codon 12 [21], codon 2 [22] or codons 1 and 2 [23], or used distinct methodology [24,25], which might have contributed to the conflicting results.

Application in routine practice:

Similar to CCRCC, chromosome 3p deletion and *VHL* mutation might be found in MCRCNLMP, but no specific genetic alterations have so far been identified. Careful macroscopic and microscopic evaluation is the gold standard for diagnosis.

4. Papillary Renal Cell Carcinoma (PRCC)

Papillary renal cell carcinoma (PRCC) is the second most common type of RCC, traditionally referred as tumor comprising of 15% of all RCCs [26]. According to the latest classification systems (WHO 2004, Vancouver ISUP Classification), it is classified into type 1 and type 2 PRCCs, which is also currently being used in the latest WHO 2016 classification. While PRCC type 1 seems to be a distinct and compact histo-molecular entity, the so-called type 2 appears to be, rather, composed of a group of tumors sharing papillary/tubulopapillary architecture with different molecular and genetic features [27]. In addition, there have recently been a number of subtypes/variants of papillary renal tumors (i.e., fumarate hydratase (FH)-deficient RCC, oncocytic PRCC), expanding the PRCC spectrum [27].

4.1. Type 1 Papillary RCC

The morphology of PRCC type 1 is well defined and in most cases would suffice for an accurate diagnosis in routine practice [5]. These tumors also have a distinct immunohistochemical profile, which can be further utilized in addition to basic hematoxylin and eosin (H&E) staining in the diagnostic workup [5].

The CNV (copy-number variation) pattern is relatively constant demonstrating polysomy or trisomy of chromosomes 7 or 17 as the most frequently referred changes. However, gains of chromosomes 3, 12, 16, and 20 (and less frequently gains of chromosomes 2, 4, 5, 6, 8, 13, and 18) have also been noted in these tumors. Of note, chromosomal losses have also been reported (chromosomes 1, 2, 4, 5, 7, 8, 9, 10, 11, 14, 15, 16, 18, 19, 20, 21, and 22) [28].

While mutations of *MET* are rarely referred for sporadic type 1 PRCC, it is commonly associated with hereditary papillary RCC syndrome. It should be noted that tumors occurring within hereditary papillary RCC syndrome are multiple otherwise typical PRCCs type 1 [29–31].

4.2. Type 2 Papillary RCC

"Type 2" papillary RCC is considered a controversial entity and currently by most authors deemed rather to represent multiple specific papillary renal neoplasms. Although gains of chromosomes 7 and 17 were reported to be the most frequently listed CNV changes for this subtype, the recent literature show that trisomy/polysomy 7/17 is not commonly associated with type 2 PRCC [28]. Based on a systematic review published recently, gains of chromosomes 12, 16 and 20 are also frequently reported in papillary RCC "Type 2" [28].

There are several genetic-based studies supporting the notion that the so-called "Type 2" PRCC is rather a group of tumors. Such tumors showed *CDKN2A* silencing, *SETD2* mutations, and increased expression of the NRF2 antioxidant response element pathway [27]. Of note, FH-deficient RCCs, a high grade PRCC which was previously categorized as PRCC "Type 2", have already been reclassified from Type 2 PRCC, owing to recent molecular and genetic studies on Type 2 PRCCs [27].

4.3. Oncocytic Papillary RCC/Papillary Renal Cell Neoplasm with Reverse Polarity

Oncocytic papillary RCC, the "third" variant/subtype of papillary RCC included in the WHO 2016 blue book [32–35], is a poorly understood papillary RCC entity composed of oncocytic neoplastic cells [26,36]. CNV pattern in these tumors is highly variable with at least 3 patterns being reported: (1) gains of chromosomes 7 and 17 [33–35], (2) gains of chromosomes 3 and 11, and (3) loss of chromosome Y in male patients as well as losses of chromosomes 1, 4, 14 and loss of chromosome X. Some these tumors have shown to have a copy number pattern identical to renal oncocytoma: disomic status of chromosomes 7 and 17, some with deletion of chromosome 14, deletion of 1p (locus 1p36) [37]. Saleeb et al. considered oncocytic PRCC as so-called "type 4" papillary RCC (oncocytic low-grade), [38]. Al-Obaidy et al. have proposed the term papillary renal cell neoplasm with reverse polarity at last for a part of the spectrum of oncocytic RCC with papillary architecture [39]. Interestingly, this tumor is characterized by frequent *KRAS* mutations [40].

4.4. Papillary RCC NOS: Other Variants

A number of unusual papillary RCC variants have recently been described such as solid, mucin secreting, biphasic squamoid, and Warthin-like, which potentially can create diagnostic challenges in routine practice [41–47]. It should be noted that all of these variants are defined mostly using morphologic features and that their molecular-genetic features are widely varied, as generally observed in papillary RCCs.

Application in routine practice:

PRCC type 1 is a distinct entity, demonstrating typical CNV of gain of 7, 17 and loss of the Y chromosome in male patients. PRCC type 2 is rather composed of a group of tumors without a consistent CNV pattern. Considering highly variable CNV patterns among PRCCs in general (except for type 1 PRCC), it is almost impossible to diagnose PRCC based on CNV or based on another molecular genetic methods only. In high grade papillary renal tumors, FH-deficient RCC should always be considered and ruled out using a combination of immunohistochemistry and *FH* mutation/LOH (loss of heterozygosity) analysis.

5. Chromophobe Renal Cell Carcinoma (ChRCC)

Molecular-genetic testing will not be required to make a diagnosis of typical chromophobe RCC (ChRCC) (classic or eosinophilic variants). In addition to classic and eosinophilic ChRCCs, there are several other variants which have been described in the literature including pigmented microcystic adenomatoid, multicystic variant, [48–51] ChRCC with neuroendocrine differentiation, [52–56] and renal oncocytoma-like variant [57]. With the exception of ChRCC with neuroendocrine features, it seems that such variability has no influence on biological behavior. However, ChRCC with neuroendocrine features is a more aggressive variant [52].

CNV in ChRCC is rather variable and as such would be challenging to utilize in routine practice. ChRCC is usually associated with multiple chromosomal losses including chromosomes Y, 1, 2, 6, 10, 13, 17, 21 [58,59]. However, multiple chromosomal gains (chromosomes 4, 7, 15, 19, and 20), or even diploid pattern have been described in otherwise typical CHRCCs [60–63].

Testing germline mutations in the novel tumor suppressor gene *FLCN* (folliculin) can be used to support the diagnosis of Birt–Hogg–Dubé syndrome, which predisposes to the so-called "hybrid" oncocytic/chromophobe tumors.

Application in routine practice:

Molecular genetic ancillary tests are not useful for diagnosing ChRCC in daily practice. However, *FLCN* gene analysis can be useful in "hybrid" oncocytic/chromophobe tumors in suspected cases.

6. Oncocytoma

Renal oncocytoma (RO) can mostly be diagnosed based on morphology, while in difficult cases immunohistochemical examination can be further utilized. Molecular genetic tests are rarely used to diagnose RO. There are 3 basic genetic patterns in ROs: (1) loss of chromosome 1 (in whole or in part) and loss of chromosome Y, (2) rearrangements of 11q13 (mostly translocation t(5;11)(q35;q13)), chromosome 14 deletion, and (3) a normal karyotype [64–69].

These patterns have led some authors to propose two or three dominant subtypes of RO, however the clinical utility of such categorization remains unclear [69,70]. It has recently been recognized that CCND1 (cyclin D1) is located on the 11q13 locus. There are several studies that have attempted to sub-classify ROs according to the CCND1 status [69–71]. Nonetheless, all these proposals have shown no clinical usefulness and utility in daily routine and differential diagnostic practice. Similar to ChRCCs, the most commonly used test is the analysis of the *FLCN* gene in a similar setting, such as in "hybrid" oncocytic/chromophobe tumors.

Application in routine practice:

Similar to ChRCCs, molecular-genetic ancillary tests are not very useful for ROs in daily practice. However, *FLCN* gene analysis in suspected cases of "hybrid" oncocytic/chromophobe tumors is useful.

7. Clear Cell Papillary Renal Cell Carcinoma (CCPRCC)

The diagnosis of typical clear cell papillary renal cell carcinoma (CCPRCC) is mostly based on the morphology and immunohistochemical profile. In typical cases with characteristic morphology, diffuse CK7 positivity, and strong cup-shaped positivity with CANH 9, molecular genetic testing is not necessary for the diagnosis of CCPRCC [72–74]. However, there are some cases of CCPRCCs which show more complex morphologic features and substantial overlap with other RCCs (i.e., CCRCC). Because CCPRCC is an indolent neoplasm (with few extremely rare exceptions), an accurate diagnosis is crucial for further management. We believe that in such instances, further analysis of the *VHL* gene is the most useful and valuable step in arriving at the correct diagnosis in routine practice [75]. In fact, analysis of 3p25 loss and *VHL* gene alterations (mutations and methylation status) together with morphology and immunohistochemical profile would allow us to correctly diagnose almost all such cases [75].

It is important to emphasis that CCPRCC has been described in patients with von Hippel–Lindau syndrome. In such cases, *VHL* germline mutation is an obvious finding and can't be helpful in differential diagnostic process.

Application in routine practice:

Majority of CCPRCC are diagnosed based on morphology and immunogistochemical profile. In challenging cases where the morphology and/or immunohistochemical profile are not typical of CCPRCC, genetic testing for *VHL* mutation/methylation and/or chromosome 3p loss are essential for rendering an accurate diagnosis of CCPRCC.

8. MiT Family Translocation-Associated Renal Cell Carcinoma

Renal tumors with *TFE3*, *TFEB*, and *MiTF* rearrangements are "classic" translocation-associated RCCs, being diagnosed based on a combination of morphologic, immunohistochemical, and molecular genetic analyses. RCC with *TFE3* rearrangements (Xp11.2) is the most common of all translocation-associated RCCs. Although morphologic features of translocation-associated RCCs are well described in the literature, recent studies have described morphologic variants associated with different fusion partners, which can in itself pose challenges to the diagnostic process. Some of these tumors are surprisingly similar in morphology to clear cell papillary RCC (*TFE3-NONO*). So far the following fusion partners for *TFE3* gene have been described: *ASPSCR1*, *PRCC*, *NONO*, *SFPQ*, *CLTC*, *PARP14*, *LUC7L3*, *KHSRP*, *DVL2*, *MED15*, *NEAT1*, *RBM10*, *KAT6A*, and *GRIPAP1* [76–84].

Although TFE3 translocation RCCs can show a diverse morphologic spectrum, certain morphologic features (i.e., high-grade cells with abundant clear/eosinophilic cytoplasm and papillary/nested architecture; psammomatous calcifications) can be suggestive of this entity. Immunohistochemical analysis may not be sufficient to confirm the diagnosis of TFE3 translocation RCC, and that in some cases further molecular genetic testing maybe indicated [85]. Fluorescence in situ hybridization (FISH) testing is usually used to confirm the diagnosis. It should be noted that in some fusion partners, FISH can produce false negative results [85,86]. Thus, NGS is more accurate, namely for cases, where fusion partner is beyond the reaches of probe or staying too close to *TFE3*.

TFEB or t(6;11) translocation RCC is much less common member of the MiT family RCCs. These tumors exhibit a typical biphasic morphologic feature composed of large epithelioid cells with clear/eosinophilic cytoplasm and a minor population of small eosinophilic cells that form rosette-like structures within basement membrane-like material. Immunohistochemically, these neoplasms express melanocytic markers (HMB45 and/or Melan A). Usually there is a fusion of *MALAT1* and *TFEB*, although other partners such as *COL21A1*, *CADM2*, and *KHDRBS2* have recently been described [27,87]. However, even in the group of *TFEB* or t(6;11) translocation RCC, there is morphologic variability and that not all cases follow a "classic" morphologic pattern with biphasic morphology (Figure 1).

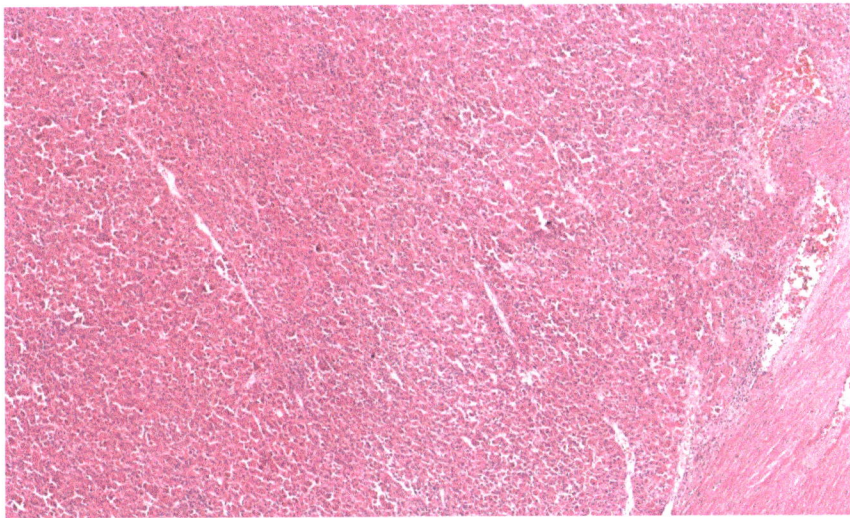

Figure 1. Some renal cell carcinomas (RCCs) with *TFEB* translocation lack typical morphology with pseudorosettes and rather show solid architecture. 4× magnification.

Recent studies have shown that amplification of the *TFEB* gene in TFEB or t(6;11) translocation RCCs can uncommonly occur and is associated with more aggressive clinical behavior with distant metastases (see *RCC* with *TFEB* amplification). It is worth noting that amplification of *TFEB* gene can rarely be found in various renal tumors, most of which are usually unclassified RCCs or translocation-like RCCs.

Application in routine practice:

Diagnosis of TFE3 translocation RCC should be considered in RCC with a mixture of clear cell and papillary features, psammoma bodies, abnormally voluminous cytoplasm, hyalinized stroma, or in a young/pediatric patient. Although positive immunohistochemical staining for TFE3 or TFEB proteins, melanocytic markers, or cathepsin K can be suggestive, molecular genetic testing is highly recommended for confirming the diagnosis. FISH for *TFE3* or *TFEB* rearrangement is a helpful diagnostic tool; however NGS is recommended in cases where false negative FISH can be expected (namely partners *RBM10*, *RBMX*, *GRIPAP1*, and *NONO*). In other words, when the morphology and/or immunohistochemical profile is suggestive of TFE3 translocation RCC, NGS analysis is recommended for confirmation. Amplification of *TFEB* gene seems to be a strong adverse prognostic indicator in TFEB translocation RCCs, however such cases are rare and less frequently encountered comparing with *TFEB* amplified RCCs (without *TFEB* break) its occurrence is rather rare.

9. Mucinous Tubular and Spindle Cell Carcinoma (MTSCC)

Mucinous tubular and spindle cell carcinoma (MTSCC) is usually a non-aggressive renal tumor with characteristic morphology. This neoplasm can resemble PRCC with overlapping morphologic and even immunohistochemical features [88–90]. In the past, studies reported variable CNV patterns for MTSCC, even sometimes resembling PRCC CNV pattern suggesting MTSCC to be a variant of PRCC type 1 [36,91]. However, recent studies have shown that MTSCCs typically have a CNV pattern with multiple chromosomal losses involving chromosomes 1, 4, 6, 8, 9, 13, 14, 15, and 22, without the gains of chromosomes 7 and 17 [92–95]. In cases where there is a morphologic overlap with PRCC (mostly type 1), CNV also shows overlapping features with frequent gains of chromosomes 7 and/or 17.

Application in routine practice:

MTSCC is an indolent and rare tumor with characteristic morphologic features that can be used in diagnosis in the vast majority of cases (with or without immunohistochemical studies). In difficult cases, CNV pattern analysis can be helpful. Tumors with features of PRCC, including gain of chromosome 7 or 17, should be classified as PRCC NOS.

10. Tubulocystic Renal Cell Carcinoma (TC-RCC)

Tubulocystic RCC (TC-RCC) is a relative new entity first officially included in the 2012 ISUP Vancouver Classification. Similar to MTSCC, TC-RCC has morphologic and immunohistochemical features that are frequently overlap with PRCC [36,96,97].

The genetic features of these tumors are variable with previous studies suggesting similar CNV patterns to that reported in type 1 PRCC (gain of chromosome 7 or 17 and loss of Y). However, more recent studies showed that gain of chromosomes 7 and 17 is not a typical CNV pattern in cases of TC-RCC where strict histo-diagnostic criteria are applied [96–98]. In fact, loss of chromosome 9 has been suggested as a characteristic feature of TC-RCC [99]. It should be noted that TC-RCC is a rare and indolent tumor that should not be confused with fumarate hydratase (FH)-deficient RCC, where the tumor shows a low grade tubulocystic pattern and with abrupt transition to high-grade infiltrative carcinoma. A similar situation exists in tumors with pure tubulocystic pattern and eosinophilic cells but with prominent macronucleoli. Such cases must be considered as potentially FH deficient RCCs and immunohistochemical/molecular-genetic examination of FH should be performed [100,101].

Application in routine practice:

TC-RCC should be diagnosed based on its strict histologic criteria, without mixed areas resembling PRCC. If CNV patterns show gains of chromosome 7 and 17, it is advised to best classify it as PRCC than TC RCC. RCCs with "Tubulocystic" features and high grade abrupt areas should raise the possibility of FH-deficient RCC and be further genetically tested for *FH* gene mutation/LOH.

11. Acquired Cystic Kidney Disease (ACD)-Associated Renal Cell Carcinoma

Acquired cystic kidney disease (ACD)-associated RCC is a relatively rare renal tumor. Its morphologic feature is relatively variable, as is its immunohistochemical profile. However several studies described gains of chromosomes 7 and 17, and other showed gain of chromosomes 3, 16, and Y [102–107].

Application in routine practice:

Currently there are no specific genetic alterations useful for routine practice in these tumors.

12. Renal Medullary Carcinoma

Renal medullary carcinoma is a rare, aggressive, and high grade renal tumor occurring mostly in African Americans with sickle cell trait or with other hemoglobinopathies. Within the differential diagnosis, collecting duct carcinoma, high-grade urothelial carcinoma and other high-grade RCCs should be always considered. [108] Medullary carcinoma is characterized by loss of the *SMARCB1* (INI-1) gene [109–111], which can also be detected immunohistochemically (following by positive OCT3/4 staining) [108,112–115]. In rare cases where alterations of *SMARCB1* gene or abnormal negative staining for the protein is documented in the absence of sickle trait, the term "RCC unclassified with medullary phenotype" has been proposed [116,117].

Application in routine practice:

High-grade renal tumors with histologic features suggestive of renal medullary carcinoma should be stained with SMARCB1. For cases with loss of SMARCB1 expression, molecular genetic testing of *SMARCB1* is useful. The result of immunohistochemical/genetic testing should be correlated with hematologic findings (i.e., sickle cell trait or other hemoglobinopathy). In situation, when RCCs with

SMARCB1 loss is encountered, and sickle trait or other hemoglobinopathies are absent, it is currently recommended to classify them as RCC unclassified with medullary phenotype.

13. Collecting Duct Carcinoma (CDC)

One of the most frequently misclassified renal tumors is still collecting duct carcinoma (CDC). Even nowadays, the diagnosis of CDC remains the diagnosis of exclusion. The following entities should be always be considered and excluded in such scenarios: FH-deficient RCC, high-grade urothelial carcinoma of renal pelvis, renal medullary carcinoma, and metastatic carcinoma from another organ.

Unfortunately, currently there is no characteristic molecular genetic feature or combination of features useful for differential diagnosis. Molecular genetic testing should be considered after excluding other entities in the differential diagnosis (i.e., FH-deficient RCC, renal medullary carcinoma).

Application in routine practice:

There is no specific molecular genetic test which can help to establish the diagnosis of CDC. FH-deficient RCC and renal medullary carcinoma should be always considered and diagnosis can be supported by genetic testing.

14. Succinate Dehydrogenase (SDH)-Deficient Renal Cell Carcinoma

Renal tumors associated with autosomal dominant germline mutations of *SDHA*, *SDHB*, *SDHC* and *SDHD* have recently been described. Such tumors are part of syndrome characterized by occurrence of renal carcinomas, paragangliomas/pheochromocytomas, gastrointestinal stromal tumors (GIST), and pituitary adenomas [118,119]. The majority of succinate dehydrogenase (SDH)-deficient RCCs demonstrate a characteristic morphology with solid alveolar architecture, eosinophilic cytoplasm with numerous intracytoplasmatic vacuoles (Figure 2). Cases with high grade features and overlapping morphology resembling CCRCC, PRCC or unclassified RCC have also been described. Immunohistochemical staining for SDHB is negative. Antibody against SDHB detects all 4 subgroups (*SDHA*, *SDHB*, *SDHC* and *SDHD*) deficiencies [118,119]. However, the interpretation of SDHB staining must be done with caution and an internal positive control should be present. SDH deficiency is almost always associated with germline SDH subunit mutation [118–121].

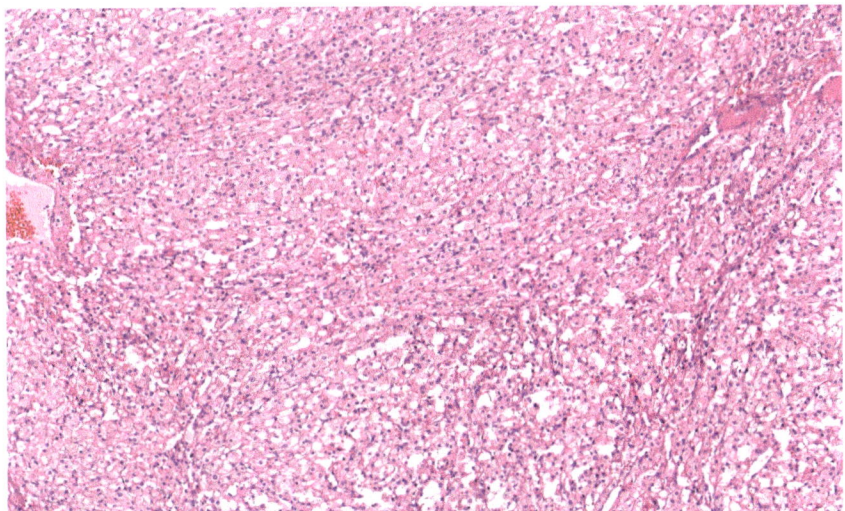

Figure 2. SDHB-deficient RCC with typical morphology-eosinophilic renal tumor with numerous vacuoles resembling texture of bubble wrap. 10× magnification.

Application in routine practice:

Suspected cases should be immunohistochemically stained for SDHB. Immunohistochemical staining for SDHB is negative in SDH-deficient cases. The vast majority of SDH-deficient RCCs are associated with germline mutation of the *SDHB* subunit. Genetic testing of *SDH* subunit mutation is not necessary, however in cases where the result of immunohistochemical examination is inconclusive, it is highly recommended.

15. Fumarate Hydratase (FH)-Deficient RCC and HLRCC (Hereditary Leiomyomatosis and Renal Cell Carcinoma)

FH-deficient RCC and hereditary leiomyomatosis and renal cell carcinoma associated RCC have been discussed extensively in the recent literature. Initially it was thought that these tumors are hereditary counterparts of the so-called "type 2" PRCC. Histologically, they show marked intratumoral heterogeneity with papillary, tubulocystic, solid or cribriform patterns, and usually the presence of large nuclei with deep red nucleoli (Figure 3A,B). However, no single or a combination of histologic features are diagnostic of FH-deficient RCCs/HLRCCs [101,108,122–128].

Immunohistochemically, FH-deficient RCCs show loss of staining for fumarate hydratase (FH) (sensitivity 80 to 90%) [101,108,123–129]. Positive immunohistochemical staining for 2SC (2-Succinocysteine) is supportive feature, however antibody for 2SC is not currently commercially available [123,125,129]. The CNV pattern is heterogeneous, no constant combination of changes has been disclosed so far and it is not possible to use it in differential diagnostic process [124].

Overall, in cases with suspected clinical and morphologic features (high-grade aggressive RCCs in young patients) FH-deficient RCCs/HLRCCs should be considered in the differential diagnostic workup. For screening, immunohistochemical staining with FH is useful, however cases where staining interpretation is not convincing or in suspected clinical settings it would be better to test for *FH* mutation/LOH.

Application in routine practice:

High-grade RCCs occurring in young patients exhibiting variable growth patterns and morphologic features should prompt the differential diagnosis of FH-deficient RCCs/HLRCCs. Immunohistochemically, FH can be helpful; however, it is not 100% specific, and as such analysis of *FH* mutation/LOH should be considered.

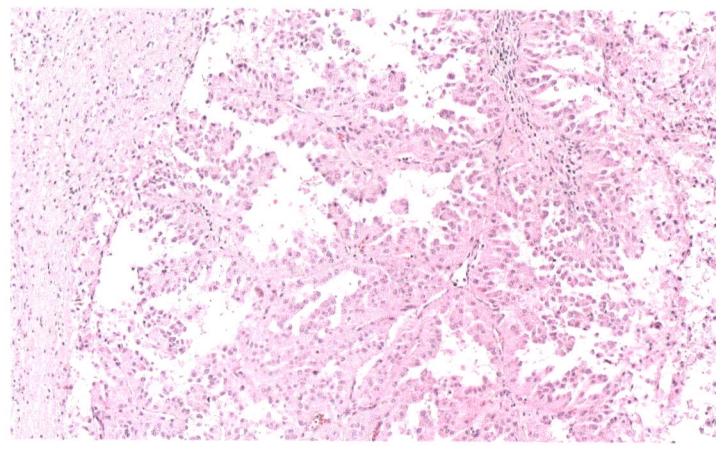

(A)

Figure 3. *Cont.*

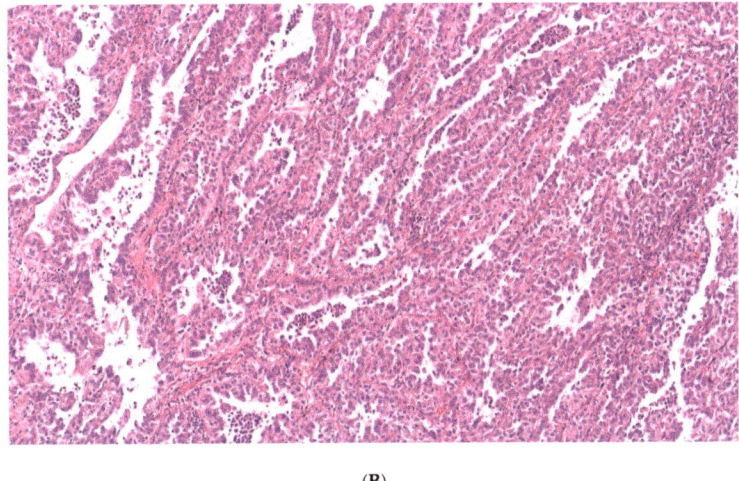

(B)

Figure 3. FH-deficient RCC: deep red macronucleoli can be prominent (**A**), however in some cases it is not easy to detect them (**B**). 4× magnification.

16. New but Perspective Renal Tumors

As mentioned earlier in the introduction, renal tumors are intensively studied and more new entities and variants are described every year. It is questionable whether all these variants will be regarded as established entities within future classifications or whether they will be reclassified as variants of some "traditional" renal tumors. Some of the published papers are recent without further corroboration by other studies, while others worked with a limited number of cases. More studies examining the ideas and hypotheses would be needed to allow including such entities in the future WHO classifications. In the following section we will briefly introduce such tumors. Majority of new entities will be covered in other reviews in this issue of *Cancers*.

16.1. Eosinophilic Solid and Cystic (ESC) RCC

Eosinophilic solid and cystic RCC (ESC-RCC) is a recently recognized entity, described in patients with TS (tuberous sclerosis) complex. Subsequently, identical tumors were described in patients without any relation to TS complex, mostly middle aged/elderly women [130,131]. These tumors have solid and cystic architecture, composed of neoplastic cells with voluminous cytoplasm showing basophilic stippling [132]. They are frequently positive for cytokeratin 20, which is highly unusual for any RCCs [132]. Both familiar and sporadic tumors have molecular alterations of *TSC1* or *TSC2* [133–137].

16.2. RCC with TSC/MTOR Gene Mutations

The molecular genetic revolution in the field of oncopathology has resulted in identifying more entities including a recently described subset of tumors harboring mutations of *TSC1*, *TSC2*, or *MTOR*, being recognized in sporadic patients as well as patients with tuberous sclerosis complex [130,131]. RCC with prominent smooth muscle (or sometimes referred as RCC with angioleiomyoma-like stroma), [130,138–142], tumors with oncocytic features named as HOT (high-grade oncocytic tumor) or descriptively as sporadic RCC with eosinophilic and vacuolated cytoplasm [143–145] are best known examples of this group.

16.3. TCEB1-Mutated RCC

These tumors are well-circumscribed, have predominantly tubular and papillary architecture, and have thick intersecting fibromuscular bands superficially resembling a renal angiomyoadenomatous tumor (RAT)-like morphology. They are distinct from both CCRCC and CCPRCC, harboring mutations of *TCEB1* but with no *VHL* gene abnormalities [24,138,140,146–148]. Given the limited data available on these tumors, it is rather early to assume concrete conclusions [146].

16.4. RCC with TFEB/6p21/VEGFA Amplification

RCC with *TFEB* rearrangement is a poorly understood entity, although such tumors have been described or briefly mentioned in several papers. The first systematic study summarizing knowledge about this group of tumors was published by Williamson at al. [149] in 2017. It appears that tumors from this group show amplification of chromosome 6p21 with changes in *TFEB* and *VEGFA* [149–156]. So far the described cases show variable morphology with shared positivity for melan-A and/or HMB45. Cathepsin K is usually positive [149,150]. RCC with *TFEB/6p21/VEGFA* amplification exhibit papillary architecture, however tumors resembling CCRCC or ChRCC were also documented. Molecular genetics usually disclose amplification of *TFEB/6p21/VEGFA*, while rearrangement of *TFEB* is usually not present. However, in one of the first cases authors pointed out that amplification of TFEB gene might be a marker of aggressive behavior showed both rearrangement and amplification [152] (Figure 4). Recent work shows that *TFEB* gene expression is increased in these tumors, although not as much as in *TFEB* translocation tumors, raising the possibility that other genes at the 6p21 locus, such as *VEGFA* or *CCND3* or other genes may be responsible for aggressive behavior [155].

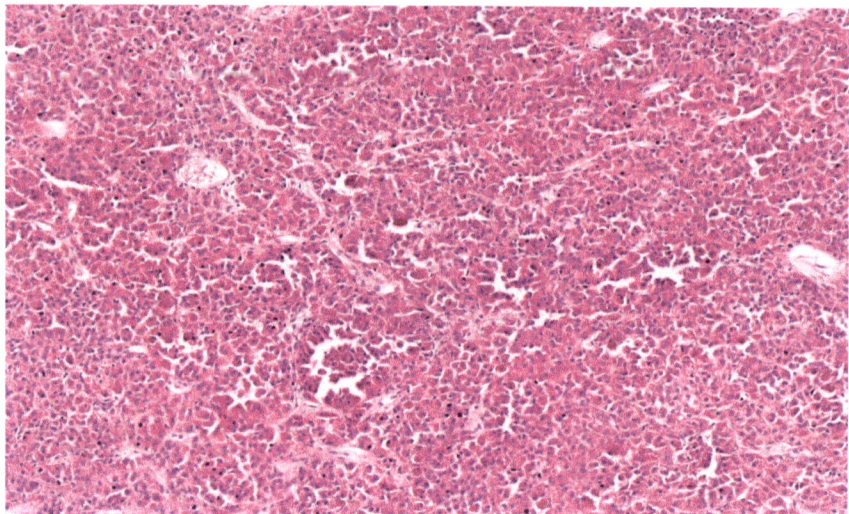

Figure 4. RCC with *TFEB* break and *TFEB* amplification. 4× magnification.

16.5. ALK-Rearranged RCC

Rearrangement of *ALK* has been described in various tumors, mostly in lymphomas, lung carcinomas, and thyroid carcinomas. In kidney, renal tumors with *ALK* rearrangement have also been rarely reported [157–174]. Histologically, they show a tubulopapillary or cribriform pattern with rhabdoid-like cell morphology in a myxoid/mucinous background (mostly interstitium). Fusion partners that have been identified in *ALK*-rearranged RCC are *TPM3, STRN, VCL, HOOK1, CLIP1*, and *KIF5B*. Some cases demonstrated highly surprising morphology, identical to metanephric adenoma or MTSCC [166].

17. Discussion

It is well-known that renal tumors are characterized by marked both intertumoral and intratumoral heterogeneity, which can play role in tumor evolution and hamper personalized therapeutic strategies. Molecular characterization of renal cell neoplasms has led to the identification of driver genes and specific molecular pathways. This comprehension along with the traditional histo-morphologic features has revolutionized the treatment approach and modalities in these tumors.

Imaging genomics, an emerging research field, has also created new opportunities for the diagnosis and prognosis of renal tumors. Of note, Cheng et al. [175] developed and examined an integrative genomics framework for constructing a prognostic model for clear cell renal cell carcinomas using both histopathologic images and genomic signatures. Similarly, Shao et al. [176] introduced ordinal multi-modal feature selection framework that simultaneously identified important features from both pathological images and multi-modal genomic data for the prognosis. It appears that such an integrative pathologic-genomics approach can help to better understand prognostic and hopefully therapeutic aspects of various renal tumors.

It should be noted that one of the main challenges in assessing the current literature on molecular-genetic characteristics of renal tumor is related to the heterogeneity of methodologies and definitions used in various studies. This is mainly due to the fact that our understating of renal neoplasms is evolving as the new molecular and technological advances are emerging such as NGS. Despite the limitations of the current literature, we are still able to draw the landscape of uniform histo-molecular renal entities.

18. Conclusions

Overall, most renal tumors can easily be diagnosed based on pure histologic findings with or without immunohistochemical examination. However, in selected cases, molecular-genetic testing can be utilized to assist in arriving at an accurate diagnosis.

Author Contributions: R.A.: literature search, first author D.P.M.: literature search, Table, A.S.L.: literature search, clear cell RCC and Multiloculasr Cystic Renal Cell Neoplasm of Low Malignant Potential section, O.H.: literature search, review design, photos. All authors have read and agreed to the published version of the manuscript.

Funding: This study was supported by the Charles University Research Fund (project number Q39) and by the grant of Ministry of Health of the Czech republic-Conceptual Development of Research Organization (Faculty Hospital in Plzen- FNPl 00669806).

Conflicts of Interest: The authors declare no conflict of interest.

References

1. Kovacs, G.; Akhtar, M.; Beckwith, B.J.; Bugert, P.; Cooper, C.S.; Delahunt, B.; Eble, J.N.; Fleming, S.; Ljungberg, B.; Medeiros, L.J.; et al. The Heidelberg classification of renal cell tumours. *J Pathol* **1997**, *183*, 131–133. [CrossRef]
2. Storkel, S.; Eble, J.N.; Adlakha, K.; Amin, M.; Blute, M.L.; Bostwick, D.G.; Darson, M.; Delahunt, B.; Iczkowski, K. Classification of renal cell carcinoma: Workgroup No. 1. Union Internationale Contre le Cancer (UICC) and the American Joint Committee on Cancer (AJCC). *Cancer* **1997**, *80*, 987–989. [CrossRef]
3. Eble, J.N.; Sauter, G.; Epstein, J.; Sesterhenn, I. *Pathology and Genetics of Tumours of the Urinary System and Male Genital Organs, WHO Classification of Tumours*, 3rd ed.; WHO: Geneva, Switzerland; IARC Press: Lyon, Switzerland, 2004; Volume 7.
4. Delahunt, B.; Srigley, J.R.; Montironi, R.; Egevad, L. Advances in renal neoplasia: Recommendations from the 2012 International Society of Urological Pathology Consensus Conference. *Urology* **2014**, *83*, 969–974. [CrossRef] [PubMed]
5. Moch, H.; Humphrey, P.A.; Ulbright, T.M.; Reuter, V.E. *WHO Classification of Tumours of the Urinary System and Male Genital Organs—WHO Classification of Tumours*, 4th ed.; WHO: Geneva, Switzerland; IARC Press: Lyon, Switzerland, 2016; Volume 8.

6. Petersson, F.; Grossmann, P.; Hora, M.; Sperga, M.; Montiel, D.P.; Martinek, P.; Gutierrez, M.E.; Bulimbasic, S.; Michal, M.; Branzovsky, J.; et al. Renal cell carcinoma with areas mimicking renal angiomyoadenomatous tumor/clear cell papillary renal cell carcinoma. *Hum. Pathol.* **2013**, *44*, 1412–1420. [CrossRef] [PubMed]
7. Somoracz, A.; Kuthi, L.; Micsik, T.; Jenei, A.; Hajdu, A.; Vrabely, B.; Raso, E.; Sapi, Z.; Bajory, Z.; Kulka, J.; et al. Renal Cell Carcinoma with Clear Cell Papillary Features: Perspectives of a Differential Diagnosis. *Pathol. Oncol. Res.* **2019**. [CrossRef]
8. Carroll, P.R.; Murty, V.V.; Reuter, V.; Jhanwar, S.; Fair, W.R.; Whitmore, W.F.; Chaganti, R.S. Abnormalities at chromosome region 3p12-14 characterize clear cell renal carcinoma. *Cancer Genet. Cytogenet.* **1987**, *26*, 253–259. [CrossRef]
9. Smits, K.M.; Schouten, L.J.; van Dijk, B.A.; Hulsbergen-van de Kaa, C.A.; Wouters, K.A.; Oosterwijk, E.; van Engeland, M.; van den Brandt, P.A. Genetic and epigenetic alterations in the von hippel-lindau gene: The influence on renal cancer prognosis. *Clin. Cancer Res.* **2008**, *14*, 782–787. [CrossRef]
10. Banks, R.E.; Tirukonda, P.; Taylor, C.; Hornigold, N.; Astuti, D.; Cohen, D.; Maher, E.R.; Stanley, A.J.; Harnden, P.; Joyce, A.; et al. Genetic and epigenetic analysis of von Hippel-Lindau (VHL) gene alterations and relationship with clinical variables in sporadic renal cancer. *Cancer Res.* **2006**, *66*, 2000–2011. [CrossRef]
11. Latif, F.; Tory, K.; Gnarra, J.; Yao, M.; Duh, F.M.; Orcutt, M.L.; Stackhouse, T.; Kuzmin, I.; Modi, W.; Geil, L.; et al. Identification of the von Hippel-Lindau disease tumor suppressor gene. *Science* **1993**, *260*, 1317–1320. [CrossRef]
12. Dalgliesh, G.L.; Furge, K.; Greenman, C.; Chen, L.; Bignell, G.; Butler, A.; Davies, H.; Edkins, S.; Hardy, C.; Latimer, C.; et al. Systematic sequencing of renal carcinoma reveals inactivation of histone modifying genes. *Nature* **2010**, *463*, 360–363. [CrossRef]
13. Guo, G.; Gui, Y.; Gao, S.; Tang, A.; Hu, X.; Huang, Y.; Jia, W.; Li, Z.; He, M.; Sun, L.; et al. Frequent mutations of genes encoding ubiquitin-mediated proteolysis pathway components in clear cell renal cell carcinoma. *Nat. Genet.* **2011**, *44*, 17–19. [CrossRef] [PubMed]
14. Varela, I.; Tarpey, P.; Raine, K.; Huang, D.; Ong, C.K.; Stephens, P.; Davies, H.; Jones, D.; Lin, M.L.; Teague, J.; et al. Exome sequencing identifies frequent mutation of the SWI/SNF complex gene PBRM1 in renal carcinoma. *Nature* **2011**, *469*, 539–542. [CrossRef] [PubMed]
15. Suzigan, S.; Lopez-Beltran, A.; Montironi, R.; Drut, R.; Romero, A.; Hayashi, T.; Gentili, A.L.; Fonseca, P.S.; deTorres, I.; Billis, A.; et al. Multilocular cystic renal cell carcinoma: A report of 45 cases of a kidney tumor of low malignant potential. *Am. J. Clin. Pathol.* **2006**, *125*, 217–222. [CrossRef] [PubMed]
16. Williamson, S.R.; Halat, S.; Eble, J.N.; Grignon, D.J.; Lopez-Beltran, A.; Montironi, R.; Tan, P.H.; Wang, M.; Zhang, S.; Maclennan, G.T.; et al. Multilocular cystic renal cell carcinoma: Similarities and differences in immunoprofile compared with clear cell renal cell carcinoma. *Am. J. Surg. Pathol.* **2012**, *36*, 1425–1433. [CrossRef] [PubMed]
17. Halat, S.; Eble, J.N.; Grignon, D.J.; Lopez-Beltran, A.; Montironi, R.; Tan, P.H.; Wang, M.; Zhang, S.; MacLennan, G.T.; Cheng, L. Multilocular cystic renal cell carcinoma is a subtype of clear cell renal cell carcinoma. *Mod. Pathol.* **2010**, *23*, 931–936. [CrossRef] [PubMed]
18. von Teichman, A.; Comperat, E.; Behnke, S.; Storz, M.; Moch, H.; Schraml, P. VHL mutations and dysregulation of pVHL- and PTEN-controlled pathways in multilocular cystic renal cell carcinoma. *Mod. Pathol.* **2011**, *24*, 571–578. [CrossRef] [PubMed]
19. Raspollini, M.R.; Castiglione, F.; Martignoni, G.; Cheng, L.; Montironi, R.; Lopez-Beltran, A. Unlike in clear cell renal cell carcinoma, KRAS is not mutated in multilocular cystic clear cell renal cell neoplasm of low potential. *Virchows Arch.* **2015**, *467*, 687–693. [CrossRef]
20. Raspollini, M.R.; Castiglione, F.; Cheng, L.; Montironi, R.; Lopez-Beltran, A. Synchronous clear cell renal cell carcinoma and multilocular cystic renal cell neoplasia of low malignant potential: A clinico-pathologic and molecular study. *Pathol. Res. Pr.* **2016**, *212*, 471–474. [CrossRef]
21. Szymanska, K.; Moore, L.E.; Rothman, N.; Chow, W.H.; Waldman, F.; Jaeger, E.; Waterboer, T.; Foretova, L.; Navratilova, M.; Janout, V.; et al. TP53, EGFR, and KRAS mutations in relation to VHL inactivation and lifestyle risk factors in renal-cell carcinoma from central and eastern Europe. *Cancer Lett.* **2010**, *293*, 92–98. [CrossRef]
22. Gattenlohner, S.; Etschmann, B.; Riedmiller, H.; Muller-Hermelink, H.K. Lack of KRAS and BRAF mutation in renal cell carcinoma. *Eur. Urol.* **2009**, *55*, 1490–1491. [CrossRef] [PubMed]

23. Bayrak, O.; Sen, H.; Bulut, E.; Cengiz, B.; Karakok, M.; Erturhan, S.; Seckiner, I. Evaluation of EGFR, KRAS and BRAF gene mutations in renal cell carcinoma. *J. Kidney Cancer VHL* **2014**, *1*, 40–45. [CrossRef] [PubMed]
24. Sato, Y.; Yoshizato, T.; Shiraishi, Y.; Maekawa, S.; Okuno, Y.; Kamura, T.; Shimamura, T.; Sato-Otsubo, A.; Nagae, G.; Suzuki, H.; et al. Integrated molecular analysis of clear-cell renal cell carcinoma. *Nat. Genet.* **2013**, *45*, 860–867. [CrossRef] [PubMed]
25. Cancer Genome Atlas Research, N. Comprehensive molecular characterization of clear cell renal cell carcinoma. *Nature* **2013**, *499*, 43–49. [CrossRef] [PubMed]
26. Delahunt, B.; Algaba, F.; Eble, J.; Cheville, J.; Amin, M.B.; Argani, P.; Martignoni, G.; Moch, H.; Srigley, J.R.; Tan, P.H.; et al. Papillary renal cell carcinoma. In *WHO Classification of Tumours of the Urinary System and Male Genital Organs*, 4th ed.; Moch, H., Humphrey, P.A., Ulbright, T.M., Reuter, V.E., Eds.; International Agency for Research on Cancer: Lyon, France, 2016; Volume 8, pp. 23–25.
27. Cancer Genome Atlas Research, N.; Linehan, W.M.; Spellman, P.T.; Ricketts, C.J.; Creighton, C.J.; Fei, S.S.; Davis, C.; Wheeler, D.A.; Murray, B.A.; Schmidt, L.; et al. Comprehensive Molecular Characterization of Papillary Renal-Cell Carcinoma. *N. Engl. J. Med.* **2016**, *374*, 135–145. [CrossRef]
28. Pitra, T.; Pivovarcikova, K.; Alaghehbandan, R.; Hes, O. Chromosomal numerical aberration pattern in papillary renal cell carcinoma: Review article. *Ann. Diagn. Pathol.* **2019**, *40*, 189–199. [CrossRef]
29. Zbar, B.; Tory, K.; Merino, M.; Schmidt, L.; Glenn, G.; Choyke, P.; Walther, M.M.; Lerman, M.; Linehan, W.M. Hereditary papillary renal cell carcinoma. *J. Urol.* **1994**, *151*, 561–566. [CrossRef]
30. Schmidt, L.; Duh, F.M.; Chen, F.; Kishida, T.; Glenn, G.; Choyke, P.; Scherer, S.W.; Zhuang, Z.; Lubensky, I.; Dean, M.; et al. Germline and somatic mutations in the tyrosine kinase domain of the MET proto-oncogene in papillary renal carcinomas. *Nat. Genet.* **1997**, *16*, 68–73. [CrossRef]
31. Dharmawardana, P.G.; Giubellino, A.; Bottaro, D.P. Hereditary papillary renal carcinoma type I. *Curr. Mol. Med.* **2004**, *4*, 855–868. [CrossRef]
32. Lefevre, M.; Couturier, J.; Sibony, M.; Bazille, C.; Boyer, K.; Callard, P.; Vieillefond, A.; Allory, Y. Adult papillary renal tumor with oncocytic cells: Clinicopathologic, immunohistochemical, and cytogenetic features of 10 cases. *Am. J. Surg. Pathol.* **2005**, *29*, 1576–1581. [CrossRef]
33. Han, G.; Yu, W.; Chu, J.; Liu, Y.; Jiang, Y.; Li, Y.; Zhang, W. Oncocytic papillary renal cell carcinoma: A clinicopathological and genetic analysis and indolent clinical course in 14 cases. *Pathol. Res. Pr.* **2017**, *213*, 1–6. [CrossRef]
34. Kunju, L.P.; Wojno, K.; Wolf, J.S., Jr.; Cheng, L.; Shah, R.B. Papillary renal cell carcinoma with oncocytic cells and nonoverlapping low grade nuclei: Expanding the morphologic spectrum with emphasis on clinicopathologic, immunohistochemical and molecular features. *Hum. Pathol.* **2008**, *39*, 96–101. [CrossRef] [PubMed]
35. Hes, O.; Brunelli, M.; Michal, M.; Cossu Rocca, P.; Hora, M.; Chilosi, M.; Mina, M.; Boudova, L.; Menestrina, F.; Martignoni, G. Oncocytic papillary renal cell carcinoma: A clinicopathologic, immunohistochemical, ultrastructural, and interphase cytogenetic study of 12 cases. *Ann. Diagn. Pathol.* **2006**, *10*, 133–139. [CrossRef] [PubMed]
36. Srigley, J.R.; Delahunt, B.; Eble, J.N.; Egevad, L.; Epstein, J.I.; Grignon, D.; Hes, O.; Moch, H.; Montironi, R.; Tickoo, S.K.; et al. The International Society of Urological Pathology (ISUP) Vancouver classification of renal neoplasia. *Am. J. Surg. Pathol.* **2013**, *37*, 1469–1489. [CrossRef] [PubMed]
37. Michalova, K.; Steiner, P.; Alaghehbandan, R.; Trpkov, K.; Martinek, P.; Grossmann, P.; Montiel, D.P.; Sperga, M.; Straka, L.; Prochazkova, K.; et al. Papillary renal cell carcinoma with cytologic and molecular genetic features overlapping with renal oncocytoma: Analysis of 10 cases. *Ann. Diagn. Pathol.* **2018**, *35*, 1–6. [CrossRef]
38. Saleeb, R.M.; Brimo, F.; Farag, M.; Rompre-Brodeur, A.; Rotondo, F.; Beharry, V.; Wala, S.; Plant, P.; Downes, M.R.; Pace, K.; et al. Toward Biological Subtyping of Papillary Renal Cell Carcinoma With Clinical Implications Through Histologic, Immunohistochemical, and Molecular Analysis. *Am. J. Surg. Pathol.* **2017**, *41*, 1618–1629. [CrossRef]
39. Al-Obaidy, K.I.; Eble, J.N.; Cheng, L.; Williamson, S.R.; Sakr, W.A.; Gupta, N.; Idrees, M.T.; Grignon, D.J. Papillary Renal Neoplasm with Reverse Polarity: A Morphologic, Immunohistochemical, and Molecular Study. *Am. J. Surg. Pathol.* **2019**, *43*, 1099–1111. [CrossRef]

40. Al-Obaidy, K.I.; Eble, J.N.; Nassiri, M.; Cheng, L.; Eldomery, M.K.; Williamson, S.R.; Sakr, W.A.; Gupta, N.; Hassan, O.; Idrees, M.T.; et al. Recurrent KRAS mutations in papillary renal neoplasm with reverse polarity. *Mod. Pathol.* **2019**. [CrossRef]
41. Marsaud, A.; Dadone, B.; Ambrosetti, D.; Baudoin, C.; Chamorey, E.; Rouleau, E.; Lefol, C.; Roussel, J.F.; Fabas, T.; Cristofari, G.; et al. Dismantling papillary renal cell carcinoma classification: The heterogeneity of genetic profiles suggests several independent diseases. *Genes Chromosomes Cancer* **2015**, *54*, 369–382. [CrossRef]
42. Pivovarcikova, K.; Peckova, K.; Martinek, P.; Montiel, D.P.; Kalusova, K.; Pitra, T.; Hora, M.; Skenderi, F.; Ulamec, M.; Daum, O.; et al. "Mucin"-secreting papillary renal cell carcinoma: Clinicopathological, immunohistochemical, and molecular genetic analysis of seven cases. *Virchows Arch.* **2016**, *469*, 71–80. [CrossRef]
43. Peckova, K.; Martinek, P.; Pivovarcikova, K.; Vanecek, T.; Alaghehbandan, R.; Prochazkova, K.; Montiel, D.P.; Hora, M.; Skenderi, F.; Ulamec, M.; et al. Cystic and necrotic papillary renal cell carcinoma: Prognosis, morphology, immunohistochemical, and molecular-genetic profile of 10 cases. *Ann. Diagn Pathol.* **2017**, *26*, 23–30. [CrossRef] [PubMed]
44. Ulamec, M.; Skenderi, F.; Trpkov, K.; Kruslin, B.; Vranic, S.; Bulimbasic, S.; Trivunic, S.; Montiel, D.P.; Peckova, K.; Pivovarcikova, K.; et al. Solid papillary renal cell carcinoma: Clinicopathologic, morphologic, and immunohistochemical analysis of 10 cases and review of the literature. *Ann. Diagn. Pathol.* **2016**, *23*, 51–57. [CrossRef] [PubMed]
45. Hes, O.; Condom Mundo, E.; Peckova, K.; Lopez, J.I.; Martinek, P.; Vanecek, T.; Falconieri, G.; Agaimy, A.; Davidson, W.; Petersson, F.; et al. Biphasic Squamoid Alveolar Renal Cell Carcinoma: A Distinctive Subtype of Papillary Renal Cell Carcinoma? *Am. J. Surg. Pathol.* **2016**, *40*, 664–675. [CrossRef] [PubMed]
46. Trpkov, K.; Athanazio, D.; Magi-Galluzzi, C.; Yilmaz, H.; Clouston, D.; Agaimy, A.; Williamson, S.R.; Brimo, F.; Lopez, J.I.; Ulamec, M.; et al. Biphasic papillary renal cell carcinoma is a rare morphological variant with frequent multifocality: A study of 28 cases. *Histopathology* **2018**, *72*, 777–785. [CrossRef]
47. Skenderi, F.; Ulamec, M.; Vanecek, T.; Martinek, P.; Alaghehbandan, R.; Foix, M.P.; Babankova, I.; Montiel, D.P.; Alvarado-Cabrero, I.; Svajdler, M.; et al. Warthin-like papillary renal cell carcinoma: Clinicopathologic, morphologic, immunohistochemical and molecular genetic analysis of 11 cases. *Ann. Diagn. Pathol.* **2017**, *27*, 48–56. [CrossRef] [PubMed]
48. Hes, O.; Vanecek, T.; Perez-Montiel, D.M.; Alvarado Cabrero, I.; Hora, M.; Suster, S.; Lamovec, J.; Curik, R.; Mandys, V.; Michal, M. Chromophobe renal cell carcinoma with microcystic and adenomatous arrangement and pigmentation–a diagnostic pitfall. Morphological, immunohistochemical, ultrastructural and molecular genetic report of 20 cases. *Virchows Arch.* **2005**, *446*, 383–393. [CrossRef] [PubMed]
49. Michal, M.; Hes, O.; Svec, A.; Ludvikova, M. Pigmented microcystic chromophobe cell carcinoma: A unique variant of renal cell carcinoma. *Ann. Diagn. Pathol.* **1998**, *2*, 149–153. [CrossRef]
50. Dundr, P.; Pesl, M.; Povysil, C.; Tvrdik, D.; Pavlik, I.; Soukup, V.; Dvoracek, J. Pigmented microcystic chromophobe renal cell carcinoma. *Pathol. Res. Pr.* **2007**, *203*, 593–597. [CrossRef] [PubMed]
51. Foix, M.P.; Dunatov, A.; Martinek, P.; Mundo, E.C.; Suster, S.; Sperga, M.; Lopez, J.I.; Ulamec, M.; Bulimbasic, S.; Montiel, D.P.; et al. Morphological, immunohistochemical, and chromosomal analysis of multicystic chromophobe renal cell carcinoma, an architecturally unusual challenging variant. *Virchows Arch.* **2016**, *469*, 669–678. [CrossRef]
52. Peckova, K.; Martinek, P.; Ohe, C.; Kuroda, N.; Bulimbasic, S.; Condom Mundo, E.; Perez Montiel, D.; Lopez, J.I.; Daum, O.; Rotterova, P.; et al. Chromophobe renal cell carcinoma with neuroendocrine and neuroendocrine-like features. Morphologic, immunohistochemical, ultrastructural, and array comparative genomic hybridization analysis of 18 cases and review of the literature. *Ann. Diagn. Pathol.* **2015**, *19*, 261–268. [CrossRef]
53. Parada, D.D.; Pena, K.B. Chromophobe renal cell carcinoma with neuroendocrine differentiation. *APMIS* **2008**, *116*, 859–865. [CrossRef]
54. Kuroda, N.; Tamura, M.; Hes, O.; Michal, M.; Gatalica, Z. Chromophobe renal cell carcinoma with neuroendocrine differentiation and sarcomatoid change. *Pathol. Int.* **2011**, *61*, 552–554. [CrossRef] [PubMed]
55. Mokhtar, G.A.; Al-Zahrani, R. Chromophobe renal cell carcinoma of the kidney with neuroendocrine differentiation: A case report with review of literature. *Urol. Ann.* **2015**, *7*, 383–386. [CrossRef] [PubMed]

56. Ohe, C.; Kuroda, N.; Matsuura, K.; Kai, T.; Moriyama, M.; Sugiguchi, S.; Terahata, S.; Hosaka, N.; Hes, O.; Michal, M.; et al. Chromophobe renal cell carcinoma with neuroendocrine differentiation/morphology: A clinicopathological and genetic study of three cases. *Hum. Pathol. Case Rep.* **2014**, *1*, 31–39. [CrossRef]
57. Kuroda, N.; Tanaka, A.; Yamaguchi, T.; Kasahara, K.; Naruse, K.; Yamada, Y.; Hatanaka, K.; Shinohara, N.; Nagashima, Y.; Mikami, S.; et al. Chromophobe renal cell carcinoma, oncocytic variant: A proposal of a new variant giving a critical diagnostic pitfall in diagnosing renal oncocytic tumors. *Med. Mol. Morphol.* **2013**, *46*, 49–55. [CrossRef]
58. Speicher, M.R.; Schoell, B.; du Manoir, S.; Schrock, E.; Ried, T.; Cremer, T.; Storkel, S.; Kovacs, A.; Kovacs, G. Specific loss of chromosomes 1, 2, 6, 10, 13, 17, and 21 in chromophobe renal cell carcinomas revealed by comparative genomic hybridization. *Am. J. Pathol.* **1994**, *145*, 356–364.
59. Paner, G.; Amin, M.B.; Moch, H.; Störkel, S. Chromophobe renal cell carcinoma. In *WHO Classification of Tumours of the Urinary System and Male Genital Organs*, 4th ed.; Moch, H., Humphrey, P.A., Ulbright, T.M., Reuter, V.E., Eds.; International Agency for Research on Cancer: Lyon, France, 2016; Volume 8, pp. 27–28.
60. Davis, C.F.; Ricketts, C.J.; Wang, M.; Yang, L.; Cherniack, A.D.; Shen, H.; Buhay, C.; Kang, H.; Kim, S.C.; Fahey, C.C.; et al. The somatic genomic landscape of chromophobe renal cell carcinoma. *Cancer Cell* **2014**, *26*, 319–330. [CrossRef]
61. Vieira, J.; Henrique, R.; Ribeiro, F.R.; Barros-Silva, J.D.; Peixoto, A.; Santos, C.; Pinheiro, M.; Costa, V.L.; Soares, M.J.; Oliveira, J.; et al. Feasibility of differential diagnosis of kidney tumors by comparative genomic hybridization of fine needle aspiration biopsies. *Genes Chromosomes Cancer* **2010**, *49*, 935–947. [CrossRef]
62. Sperga, M.; Martinek, P.; Vanecek, T.; Grossmann, P.; Bauleth, K.; Perez-Montiel, D.; Alvarado-Cabrero, I.; Nevidovska, K.; Lietuvietis, V.; Hora, M.; et al. Chromophobe renal cell carcinoma–chromosomal aberration variability and its relation to Paner grading system: An array CGH and FISH analysis of 37 cases. *Virchows Arch.* **2013**, *463*, 563–573. [CrossRef]
63. Tan, M.H.; Wong, C.F.; Tan, H.L.; Yang, X.J.; Ditlev, J.; Matsuda, D.; Khoo, S.K.; Sugimura, J.; Fujioka, T.; Furge, K.A.; et al. Genomic expression and single-nucleotide polymorphism profiling discriminates chromophobe renal cell carcinoma and oncocytoma. *BMC Cancer* **2010**, *10*, 196. [CrossRef]
64. Crotty, T.B.; Lawrence, K.M.; Moertel, C.A.; Bartelt, D.H., Jr.; Batts, K.P.; Dewald, G.W.; Farrow, G.M.; Jenkins, R.B. Cytogenetic analysis of six renal oncocytomas and a chromophobe cell renal carcinoma. Evidence that -Y, -1 may be a characteristic anomaly in renal oncocytomas. *Cancer Genet Cytogenet.* **1992**, *61*, 61–66. [CrossRef]
65. Fuzesi, L.; Gunawan, B.; Braun, S.; Boeckmann, W. Renal oncocytoma with a translocation t(9;11)(p23;q13). *J. Urol.* **1994**, *152*, 471–472. [CrossRef]
66. Paner, G.P.; Lindgren, V.; Jacobson, K.; Harrison, K.; Cao, Y.; Campbell, S.C.; Flanigan, R.C.; Picken, M.M. High incidence of chromosome 1 abnormalities in a series of 27 renal oncocytomas: Cytogenetic and fluorescence in situ hybridization studies. *Arch. Pathol. Lab. Med.* **2007**, *131*, 81–85. [CrossRef] [PubMed]
67. Lindgren, V.; Paner, G.P.; Omeroglu, A.; Campbell, S.C.; Waters, W.B.; Flanigan, R.C.; Picken, M.M. Cytogenetic analysis of a series of 13 renal oncocytomas. *J. Urol.* **2004**, *171*, 602–604. [CrossRef] [PubMed]
68. Picken, M.M.; Chyna, B.; Flanigan, R.C.; Lee, J.M. Analysis of chromosome 1p abnormalities in renal oncocytomas by loss of heterozygosity studies: Correlation with conventional cytogenetics and fluorescence in situ hybridization. *Am. J. Clin. Pathol.* **2008**, *129*, 377–382. [CrossRef] [PubMed]
69. Anderson, C.B.; Lipsky, M.; Nandula, S.V.; Freeman, C.E.; Matthews, T.; Walsh, C.E.; Li, G.; Szabolcs, M.; Mansukhani, M.M.; McKiernan, J.M.; et al. Cytogenetic analysis of 130 renal oncocytomas identify three distinct and mutually exclusive diagnostic classes of chromosome aberrations. *Genes Chromosomes Cancer* **2019**. [CrossRef] [PubMed]
70. Joshi, S.; Tolkunov, D.; Aviv, H.; Hakimi, A.A.; Yao, M.; Hsieh, J.J.; Ganesan, S.; Chan, C.S.; White, E. The Genomic Landscape of Renal Oncocytoma Identifies a Metabolic Barrier to Tumorigenesis. *Cell Rep.* **2015**, *13*, 1895–1908. [CrossRef]
71. Sukov, W.R.; Ketterling, R.P.; Lager, D.J.; Carlson, A.W.; Sinnwell, J.P.; Chow, G.K.; Jenkins, R.B.; Cheville, J.C. CCND1 rearrangements and cyclin D1 overexpression in renal oncocytomas: Frequency, clinicopathologic features, and utility in differentiation from chromophobe renal cell carcinoma. *Hum. Pathol.* **2009**, *40*, 1296–1303. [CrossRef]
72. Williamson, S.R.; Eble, J.N.; Cheng, L.; Grignon, D.J. Clear cell papillary renal cell carcinoma: Differential diagnosis and extended immunohistochemical profile. *Mod. Pathol.* **2013**, *26*, 697–708. [CrossRef]

73. Mantilla, J.G.; Antic, T.; Tretiakova, M.S. GATA-3 Is a Specific Marker for Clear Cell Papillary Renal Cell Carcinoma. *Mod. Pathol.* **2017**, *30*, 241A.
74. Martignoni, G.; Brunelli, M.; Segala, D.; Munari, E.; Gobbo, S.; Cima, L.; Borze, I.; Wirtanen, T.; Sarhadi, V.K.; Atanesyan, L.; et al. Validation of 34betaE12 immunoexpression in clear cell papillary renal cell carcinoma as a sensitive biomarker. *Pathology* **2017**, *49*, 10–18. [CrossRef]
75. Hes, O.; Comperat, E.M.; Rioux-Leclercq, N. Clear cell papillary renal cell carcinoma, renal angiomyoadenomatous tumor, and renal cell carcinoma with leiomyomatous stroma relationship of 3 types of renal tumors: A review. *Ann. Diagn. Pathol.* **2016**, *21*, 59–64. [CrossRef] [PubMed]
76. Gandhi, J.S.; Malik, F.; Amin, M.B.; Argani, P.; Bahrami, A. MiT family translocation renal cell carcinomas: A 15th anniversary update. *Histol. Histopathol.* **2019**, 18159. [CrossRef]
77. Argani, P.; Antonescu, C.R.; Illei, P.B.; Lui, M.Y.; Timmons, C.F.; Newbury, R.; Reuter, V.E.; Garvin, A.J.; Perez-Atayde, A.R.; Fletcher, J.A.; et al. Primary renal neoplasms with the ASPL-TFE3 gene fusion of alveolar soft part sarcoma: A distinctive tumor entity previously included among renal cell carcinomas of children and adolescents. *Am. J. Pathol.* **2001**, *159*, 179–192. [CrossRef]
78. Argani, P.; Lui, M.Y.; Couturier, J.; Bouvier, R.; Fournet, J.C.; Ladanyi, M. A novel CLTC-TFE3 gene fusion in pediatric renal adenocarcinoma with t(X;17)(p11.2;q23). *Oncogene* **2003**, *22*, 5374–5378. [CrossRef] [PubMed]
79. Argani, P.; Ladanyi, M. Renal carcinomas associated with Xp11.2 translocations / *TFE3* gene fusions. In *Pathology and Genetics of Tumours of the Urinary System and Male Genital Organs*, 1st ed.; Eble, J.N., Sauter, G., Epstein, J.I., Sesterhenn, I.A., Eds.; IARC Press: Lyon, France, 2004; pp. 37–38.
80. Argani, P.; Olgac, S.; Tickoo, S.K.; Goldfischer, M.; Moch, H.; Chan, D.Y.; Eble, J.N.; Bonsib, S.M.; Jimeno, M.; Lloreta, J.; et al. Xp11 translocation renal cell carcinoma in adults: Expanded clinical, pathologic, and genetic spectrum. *Am. J. Surg. Pathol.* **2007**, *31*, 1149–1160. [CrossRef] [PubMed]
81. Argani, P.; Hicks, J.; De Marzo, A.M.; Albadine, R.; Illei, P.B.; Ladanyi, M.; Reuter, V.E.; Netto, G.J. Xp11 translocation renal cell carcinoma (RCC): Extended immunohistochemical profile emphasizing novel RCC markers. *Am. J. Surg. Pathol.* **2010**, *34*, 1295–1303. [CrossRef]
82. Ellis, C.L.; Eble, J.N.; Subhawong, A.P.; Martignoni, G.; Zhong, M.; Ladanyi, M.; Epstein, I.I.; Netto, G.J.; Argani, P. Clinical heterogeneity of Xp11 translocation renal cell carcinoma: Impact of fusion subtype, age, and stage. *Mod. Pathol.* **2014**, *27*, 875–886. [CrossRef]
83. Argani, P. MiT family translocation renal cell carcinoma. *Semin. Diagn. Pathol.* **2015**, *32*, 103–113. [CrossRef]
84. Argani, P.; Zhong, M.; Reuter, V.E.; Fallon, J.T.; Epstein, J.I.; Netto, G.J.; Antonescu, C.R. TFE3-Fusion Variant Analysis Defines Specific Clinicopathologic Associations Among Xp11 Translocation Cancers. *Am. J. Surg. Pathol.* **2016**, *40*, 723–737. [CrossRef]
85. Hayes, M.; Peckova, K.; Martinek, P.; Hora, M.; Kalusova, K.; Straka, L.; Daum, O.; Kokoskova, B.; Rotterova, P.; Pivovarcikova, K.; et al. Molecular-genetic analysis is essential for accurate classification of renal carcinoma resembling Xp11.2 translocation carcinoma. *Virchows Arch.* **2015**, *466*, 313–322. [CrossRef]
86. Kato, I.; Furuya, M.; Baba, M.; Kameda, Y.; Yasuda, M.; Nishimoto, K.; Oyama, M.; Yamasaki, T.; Ogawa, O.; Niino, H.; et al. RBM10-TFE3 renal cell carcinoma characterised by paracentric inversion with consistent closely split signals in break-apart fluorescence in-situ hybridisation: Study of 10 cases and a literature review. *Histopathology* **2019**, *75*, 254–265. [CrossRef] [PubMed]
87. Malouf, G.G.; Su, X.; Yao, H.; Gao, J.; Xiong, L.; He, Q.; Comperat, E.; Couturier, J.; Molinie, V.; Escudier, B.; et al. Next-generation sequencing of translocation renal cell carcinoma reveals novel RNA splicing partners and frequent mutations of chromatin-remodeling genes. *Clin. Cancer Res.* **2014**, *20*, 4129–4140. [CrossRef] [PubMed]
88. Thway, K.; du Parcq, J.; Larkin, J.M.; Fisher, C.; Livni, N. Metastatic renal mucinous tubular and spindle cell carcinoma. Atypical behavior of a rare, morphologically bland tumor. *Ann. Diagn. Pathol.* **2012**, *16*, 407–410. [CrossRef] [PubMed]
89. Dhillon, J.; Amin, M.B.; Selbs, E.; Turi, G.K.; Paner, G.P.; Reuter, V.E. Mucinous tubular and spindle cell carcinoma of the kidney with sarcomatoid change. *Am. J. Surg. Pathol.* **2009**, *33*, 44–49. [CrossRef] [PubMed]
90. Bulimbasic, S.; Ljubanovic, D.; Sima, R.; Michal, M.; Hes, O.; Kuroda, N.; Persec, Z. Aggressive high-grade mucinous tubular and spindle cell carcinoma. *Hum. Pathol.* **2009**, *40*, 906–907. [CrossRef] [PubMed]

91. Paner, G.P.; Srigley, J.R.; Radhakrishnan, A.; Cohen, C.; Skinnider, B.F.; Tickoo, S.K.; Young, A.N.; Amin, M.B. Immunohistochemical analysis of mucinous tubular and spindle cell carcinoma and papillary renal cell carcinoma of the kidney: Significant immunophenotypic overlap warrants diagnostic caution. *Am J Surg. Pathol.* **2006**, *30*, 13–19. [CrossRef]
92. Ren, Q.; Wang, L.; Al-Ahmadie, H.A.; Fine, S.W.; Gopalan, A.; Sirintrapun, S.J.; Tickoo, S.K.; Reuter, V.E.; Chen, Y.B. Distinct Genomic Copy Number Alterations Distinguish Mucinous Tubular and Spindle Cell Carcinoma of the Kidney From Papillary Renal Cell Carcinoma With Overlapping Histologic Features. *Am. J. Surg. Pathol.* **2018**, *42*, 767–777. [CrossRef]
93. Peckova, K.; Martinek, P.; Sperga, M.; Montiel, D.P.; Daum, O.; Rotterova, P.; Kalusova, K.; Hora, M.; Pivovarcikova, K.; Rychly, B.; et al. Mucinous spindle and tubular renal cell carcinoma: Analysis of chromosomal aberration pattern of low-grade, high-grade, and overlapping morphologic variant with papillary renal cell carcinoma. *Ann. Diagn. Pathol.* **2015**, *19*, 226–231. [CrossRef]
94. Sadimin, E.T.; Chen, Y.B.; Wang, L.; Argani, P.; Epstein, J.I. Chromosomal abnormalities of high-grade mucinous tubular and spindle cell carcinoma of the kidney. *Histopathology* **2017**, *71*, 719–724. [CrossRef]
95. Cossu-Rocca, P.; Eble, J.N.; Delahunt, B.; Zhang, S.; Martignoni, G.; Brunelli, M.; Cheng, L. Renal mucinous tubular and spindle carcinoma lacks the gains of chromosomes 7 and 17 and losses of chromosome Y that are prevalent in papillary renal cell carcinoma. *Mod. Pathol.* **2006**, *19*, 488–493. [CrossRef]
96. Zhou, M.; Yang, X.J.; Lopez, J.I.; Shah, R.B.; Hes, O.; Shen, S.S.; Li, R.; Yang, Y.; Lin, F.; Elson, P.; et al. Renal tubulocystic carcinoma is closely related to papillary renal cell carcinoma: Implications for pathologic classification. *Am. J. Surg. Pathol.* **2009**, *33*, 1840–1849. [CrossRef] [PubMed]
97. Tran, T.; Jones, C.L.; Williamson, S.R.; Eble, J.N.; Grignon, D.J.; Zhang, S.; Wang, M.; Baldridge, L.A.; Wang, L.; Montironi, R.; et al. Tubulocystic renal cell carcinoma is an entity that is immunohistochemically and genetically distinct from papillary renal cell carcinoma. *Histopathology* **2016**, *68*, 850–857. [CrossRef] [PubMed]
98. Yang, X.J.; Zhou, M.; Hes, O.; Shen, S.; Li, R.; Lopez, J.; Shah, R.B.; Yang, Y.; Chuang, S.T.; Lin, F.; et al. Tubulocystic carcinoma of the kidney: Clinicopathologic and molecular characterization. *Am. J. Surg. Pathol.* **2008**, *32*, 177–187. [CrossRef]
99. Sarungbam, J.; Mehra, R.; Tomlins, S.A.; Smith, S.C.; Jayakumaran, G.; Al-Ahmadie, H.; Gopalan, A.; Sirintrapun, S.J.; Fine, S.W.; Zhang, Y.; et al. Tubulocystic renal cell carcinoma: A distinct clinicopathologic entity with a characteristic genomic profile. *Mod. Pathol.* **2019**, *32*, 701–709. [CrossRef] [PubMed]
100. Al-Hussain, T.O.; Cheng, L.; Zhang, S.; Epstein, J.I. Tubulocystic carcinoma of the kidney with poorly differentiated foci: A series of 3 cases with fluorescence in situ hybridization analysis. *Hum. Pathol.* **2013**, *44*, 1406–1411. [CrossRef] [PubMed]
101. Smith, S.C.; Trpkov, K.; Chen, Y.B.; Mehra, R.; Sirohi, D.; Ohe, C.; Cani, A.K.; Hovelson, D.H.; Omata, K.; McHugh, J.B.; et al. Tubulocystic Carcinoma of the Kidney With Poorly Differentiated Foci: A Frequent Morphologic Pattern of Fumarate Hydratase-deficient Renal Cell Carcinoma. *Am. J. Surg. Pathol.* **2016**, *40*, 1457–1472. [CrossRef]
102. Kuroda, N.; Ohe, C.; Mikami, S.; Hes, O.; Michal, M.; Brunelli, M.; Martignoni, G.; Sato, Y.; Yoshino, T.; Kakehi, Y.; et al. Review of acquired cystic disease-associated renal cell carcinoma with focus on pathobiological aspects. *Histol. Histopathol.* **2011**, *26*, 1215–1218. [CrossRef]
103. Kuroda, N.; Shiotsu, T.; Hes, O.; Michal, M.; Shuin, T.; Lee, G.H. Acquired cystic disease-associated renal cell carcinoma with gain of chromosomes 3, 7, and 16, gain of chromosome X, and loss of chromosome Y. *Med. Mol. Morphol.* **2010**, *43*, 231–234. [CrossRef]
104. Kuroda, N.; Tamura, M.; Hamaguchi, N.; Mikami, S.; Pan, C.C.; Brunelli, M.; Martignoni, G.; Hes, O.; Michal, M.; Lee, G.H. Acquired cystic disease-associated renal cell carcinoma with sarcomatoid change and rhabdoid features. *Ann. Diagn. Pathol.* **2011**, *15*, 462–466. [CrossRef]
105. Kuroda, N.; Yamashita, M.; Kakehi, Y.; Hes, O.; Michal, M.; Lee, G.H. Acquired cystic disease-associated renal cell carcinoma: An immunohistochemical and fluorescence in situ hybridization study. *Med. Mol. Morphol.* **2011**, *44*, 228–232. [CrossRef]
106. Cossu-Rocca, P.; Eble, J.N.; Zhang, S.; Martignoni, G.; Brunelli, M.; Cheng, L. Acquired cystic disease-associated renal tumors: An immunohistochemical and fluorescence in situ hybridization study. *Mod. Pathol.* **2006**, *19*, 780–787. [CrossRef] [PubMed]

107. Kuntz, E.; Yusenko, M.V.; Nagy, A.; Kovacs, G. Oligoarray comparative genomic hybridization of renal cell tumors that developed in patients with acquired cystic renal disease. *Hum. Pathol.* **2010**, *41*, 1345–1349. [CrossRef] [PubMed]

108. Ohe, C.; Smith, S.C.; Sirohi, D.; Divatia, M.; de Peralta-Venturina, M.; Paner, G.P.; Agaimy, A.; Amin, M.B.; Argani, P.; Chen, Y.B.; et al. Reappraisal of Morphologic Differences Between Renal Medullary Carcinoma, Collecting Duct Carcinoma, and Fumarate Hydratase-deficient Renal Cell Carcinoma. *Am. J. Surg. Pathol.* **2018**, *42*, 279–292. [CrossRef] [PubMed]

109. Jia, L.; Carlo, M.I.; Khan, H.; Nanjangud, G.J.; Rana, S.; Cimera, R.; Zhang, Y.; Hakimi, A.A.; Verma, A.K.; Al-Ahmadie, H.A.; et al. Distinctive mechanisms underlie the loss of SMARCB1 protein expression in renal medullary carcinoma: Morphologic and molecular analysis of 20 cases. *Mod. Pathol.* **2019**, *32*, 1329–1343. [CrossRef]

110. Calderaro, J.; Masliah-Planchon, J.; Richer, W.; Maillot, L.; Maille, P.; Mansuy, L.; Bastien, C.; de la Taille, A.; Boussion, H.; Charpy, C.; et al. Balanced Translocations Disrupting SMARCB1 Are Hallmark Recurrent Genetic Alterations in Renal Medullary Carcinomas. *Eur. Urol.* **2016**, *69*, 1055–1061. [CrossRef]

111. Carlo, M.I.; Chaim, J.; Patil, S.; Kemel, Y.; Schram, A.M.; Woo, K.; Coskey, D.; Nanjangud, G.J.; Voss, M.H.; Feldman, D.R.; et al. Genomic Characterization of Renal Medullary Carcinoma and Treatment Outcomes. *Clin. Genitourin. Cancer* **2017**, *15*, e987–e994. [CrossRef]

112. Calderaro, J.; Moroch, J.; Pierron, G.; Pedeutour, F.; Grison, C.; Maille, P.; Soyeux, P.; de la Taille, A.; Couturier, J.; Vieillefond, A.; et al. SMARCB1/INI1 inactivation in renal medullary carcinoma. *Histopathology* **2012**, *61*, 428–435. [CrossRef]

113. Liu, Q.; Galli, S.; Srinivasan, R.; Linehan, W.M.; Tsokos, M.; Merino, M.J. Renal medullary carcinoma: Molecular, immunohistochemistry, and morphologic correlation. *Am. J. Surg. Pathol.* **2013**, *37*, 368–374. [CrossRef]

114. Cheng, J.X.; Tretiakova, M.; Gong, C.; Mandal, S.; Krausz, T.; Taxy, J.B. Renal medullary carcinoma: Rhabdoid features and the absence of INI1 expression as markers of aggressive behavior. *Mod. Pathol.* **2008**, *21*, 647–652. [CrossRef]

115. Rao, P.; Tannir, N.M.; Tamboli, P. Expression of OCT3/4 in renal medullary carcinoma represents a potential diagnostic pitfall. *Am. J. Surg. Pathol.* **2012**, *36*, 583–588. [CrossRef]

116. Sirohi, D.; Smith, S.C.; Ohe, C.; Colombo, P.; Divatia, M.; Dragoescu, E.; Rao, P.; Hirsch, M.S.; Chen, Y.B.; Mehra, R.; et al. Renal cell carcinoma, unclassified with medullary phenotype: Poorly differentiated adenocarcinomas overlapping with renal medullary carcinoma. *Hum. Pathol.* **2017**, *67*, 134–145. [CrossRef] [PubMed]

117. Amin, M.B.; Smith, S.C.; Agaimy, A.; Argani, P.; Comperat, E.M.; Delahunt, B.; Epstein, J.I.; Eble, J.N.; Grignon, D.J.; Hartmann, A.; et al. Collecting duct carcinoma versus renal medullary carcinoma: An appeal for nosologic and biological clarity. *Am. J. Surg. Pathol.* **2014**, *38*, 871–874. [CrossRef] [PubMed]

118. Gill, A.J. Succinate dehydrogenase (SDH) and mitochondrial driven neoplasia. *Pathology* **2012**, *44*, 285–292. [CrossRef]

119. Gill, A.J. Succinate dehydrogenase (SDH)-deficient neoplasia. *Histopathology* **2018**, *72*, 106–116. [CrossRef]

120. Gill, A.J.; Benn, D.E.; Chou, A.; Clarkson, A.; Muljono, A.; Meyer-Rochow, G.Y.; Richardson, A.L.; Sidhu, S.B.; Robinson, B.G.; Clifton-Bligh, R.J. Immunohistochemistry for SDHB triages genetic testing of SDHB, SDHC, and SDHD in paraganglioma-pheochromocytoma syndromes. *Hum. Pathol.* **2010**, *41*, 805–814. [CrossRef] [PubMed]

121. van Nederveen, F.H.; Gaal, J.; Favier, J.; Korpershoek, E.; Oldenburg, R.A.; de Bruyn, E.M.; Sleddens, H.F.; Derkx, P.; Riviere, J.; Dannenberg, H.; et al. An immunohistochemical procedure to detect patients with paraganglioma and phaeochromocytoma with germline SDHB, SDHC, or SDHD gene mutations: A retrospective and prospective analysis. *Lancet Oncol.* **2009**, *10*, 764–771. [CrossRef]

122. Merino, M.J.; Linehan, W.M. Hereditary leiomyomatosis and renal cell carcinoma (HLRCC)-associated renal cell carcinoma. In *WHO Classification of Tumours of the Urinary System and Male Genital Organs*, 4th ed.; Moch, H., Humphrey, P.A., Ulbright, T.M., Reuter, V.E., Eds.; International Agency for Research on Cancer: Lyon, France, 2016; Volume 8, pp. 25–26.

123. Trpkov, K.; Hes, O.; Agaimy, A.; Bonert, M.; Martinek, P.; Magi-Galluzzi, C.; Kristiansen, G.; Luders, C.; Nesi, G.; Comperat, E.; et al. Fumarate Hydratase-deficient Renal Cell Carcinoma Is Strongly Correlated With Fumarate Hydratase Mutation and Hereditary Leiomyomatosis and Renal Cell Carcinoma Syndrome. *Am. J. Surg. Pathol.* **2016**, *40*, 865–875. [CrossRef]

124. Pivovarcikova, K.; Martinek, P.; Grossmann, P.; Trpkov, K.; Alaghehbandan, R.; Magi-Galluzzi, C.; Pane Foix, M.; Condom Mundo, E.; Berney, D.; Gill, A.; et al. Fumarate hydratase deficient renal cell carcinoma: Chromosomal numerical aberration analysis of 12 cases. *Ann. Diagn. Pathol.* **2019**, *39*, 63–68. [CrossRef] [PubMed]
125. Lau, H.D.; Chan, E.; Fan, A.C.; Kunder, C.A.; Williamson, S.R.; Zhou, M.; Idrees, M.T.; Maclean, F.M.; Gill, A.J.; Kao, C.S. A Clinicopathologic and Molecular Analysis of Fumarate Hydratase-Deficient Renal Cell Carcinoma in 32 Patients. *Am. J. Surg. Pathol.* **2019**. [CrossRef] [PubMed]
126. Shyu, I.; Mirsadraei, L.; Wang, X.; Robila, V.; Mehra, R.; McHugh, J.B.; Chen, Y.B.; Udager, A.M.; Gill, A.J.; Cheng, L.; et al. Clues to recognition of fumarate hydratase-deficient renal cell carcinoma: Findings from cytologic and limited biopsy samples. *Cancer Cytopathol.* **2018**. [CrossRef]
127. Chen, Y.B.; Brannon, A.R.; Toubaji, A.; Dudas, M.E.; Won, H.H.; Al-Ahmadie, H.A.; Fine, S.W.; Gopalan, A.; Frizzell, N.; Voss, M.H.; et al. Hereditary leiomyomatosis and renal cell carcinoma syndrome-associated renal cancer: Recognition of the syndrome by pathologic features and the utility of detecting aberrant succination by immunohistochemistry. *Am. J. Surg. Pathol.* **2014**, *38*, 627–637. [CrossRef] [PubMed]
128. Muller, M.; Guillaud-Bataille, M.; Salleron, J.; Genestie, C.; Deveaux, S.; Slama, A.; de Paillerets, B.B.; Richard, S.; Benusiglio, P.R.; Ferlicot, S. Pattern multiplicity and fumarate hydratase (FH)/S-(2-succino)-cysteine (2SC) staining but not eosinophilic nucleoli with perinucleolar halos differentiate hereditary leiomyomatosis and renal cell carcinoma-associated renal cell carcinomas from kidney tumors without FH gene alteration. *Mod. Pathol.* **2018**, *31*, 974–983. [CrossRef] [PubMed]
129. Harrison, W.J.; Andrici, J.; Maclean, F.; Madadi-Ghahan, R.; Farzin, M.; Sioson, L.; Toon, C.W.; Clarkson, A.; Watson, N.; Pickett, J.; et al. Fumarate Hydratase-deficient Uterine Leiomyomas Occur in Both the Syndromic and Sporadic Settings. *Am. J. Surg. Pathol.* **2016**, *40*, 599–607. [CrossRef] [PubMed]
130. Guo, J.; Tretiakova, M.S.; Troxell, M.L.; Osunkoya, A.O.; Fadare, O.; Sangoi, A.R.; Shen, S.S.; Lopez-Beltran, A.; Mehra, R.; Heider, A.; et al. Tuberous sclerosis-associated renal cell carcinoma: A clinicopathologic study of 57 separate carcinomas in 18 patients. *Am. J. Surg. Pathol.* **2014**, *38*, 1457–1467. [CrossRef] [PubMed]
131. Yang, P.; Cornejo, K.M.; Sadow, P.M.; Cheng, L.; Wang, M.; Xiao, Y.; Jiang, Z.; Oliva, E.; Jozwiak, S.; Nussbaum, R.L.; et al. Renal cell carcinoma in tuberous sclerosis complex. *Am. J. Surg. Pathol.* **2014**, *38*, 895–909. [CrossRef] [PubMed]
132. Trpkov, K.; Hes, O.; Bonert, M.; Lopez, J.I.; Bonsib, S.M.; Nesi, G.; Comperat, E.; Sibony, M.; Berney, D.M.; Martinek, P.; et al. Eosinophilic, Solid, and Cystic Renal Cell Carcinoma: Clinicopathologic Study of 16 Unique, Sporadic Neoplasms Occurring in Women. *Am. J. Surg. Pathol.* **2016**, *40*, 60–71. [CrossRef]
133. Mehra, R.; Vats, P.; Cao, X.; Su, F.; Lee, N.D.; Lonigro, R.; Premkumar, K.; Trpkov, K.; McKenney, J.K.; Dhanasekaran, S.M.; et al. Somatic Bi-allelic Loss of TSC Genes in Eosinophilic Solid and Cystic Renal Cell Carcinoma. *Eur. Urol.* **2018**, *74*, 483–486. [CrossRef]
134. Palsgrove, D.N.; Li, Y.; Pratilas, C.A.; Lin, M.T.; Pallavajjalla, A.; Gocke, C.; De Marzo, A.M.; Matoso, A.; Netto, G.J.; Epstein, J.I.; et al. Eosinophilic Solid and Cystic (ESC) Renal Cell Carcinomas Harbor TSC Mutations: Molecular Analysis Supports an Expanding Clinicopathologic Spectrum. *Am. J. Surg. Pathol.* **2018**, *42*, 1166–1181. [CrossRef]
135. Parilla, M.; Kadri, S.; Patil, S.A.; Ritterhouse, L.; Segal, J.; Henriksen, K.J.; Antic, T. Are Sporadic Eosinophilic Solid and Cystic Renal Cell Carcinomas Characterized by Somatic Tuberous Sclerosis Gene Mutations? *Am. J. Surg. Pathol.* **2018**, *42*, 911–917. [CrossRef]
136. Tretiakova, M.S. Eosinophilic solid and cystic renal cell carcinoma mimicking epithelioid angiomyolipoma: Series of 4 primary tumors and 2 metastases. *Hum. Pathol.* **2018**, *80*, 65–75. [CrossRef]
137. Li, Y.; Reuter, V.E.; Matoso, A.; Netto, G.J.; Epstein, J.I.; Argani, P. Re-evaluation of 33 'unclassified' eosinophilic renal cell carcinomas in young patients. *Histopathology* **2018**, *72*, 588–600. [CrossRef] [PubMed]
138. Williamson, S.R. Renal cell carcinomas with a mesenchymal stromal component: What do we know so far? *Pathology* **2019**, *51*, 453–462. [CrossRef]
139. Williamson, S.R.; Hornick, J.L.; Eble, J.N.; Gupta, N.S.; Rogers, C.G.; True, L.; Grignon, D.J.; Cheng, L. Renal cell carcinoma with angioleiomyoma-like stroma and clear cell papillary renal cell carcinoma: Exploring SDHB protein immunohistochemistry and the relationship to tuberous sclerosis complex. *Hum. Pathol.* **2018**, *75*, 10–15. [CrossRef] [PubMed]

140. Parilla, M.; Alikhan, M.; Al-Kawaaz, M.; Patil, S.; Kadri, S.; Ritterhouse, L.L.; Segal, J.; Fitzpatrick, C.; Antic, T. Genetic Underpinnings of Renal Cell Carcinoma With Leiomyomatous Stroma. *Am. J. Surg. Pathol.* **2019**, *43*, 1135–1144. [CrossRef] [PubMed]

141. Verkarre, V.; Mensah, A.; Leroy, X.; Sibony, M.; Vasiliu, V.; Comperat, E.; Richard, S.; Mejean, A. A Clinico-Pathologic Study of 17 Patients with Renal Cell Carcinoma Associated With Leiomyomatous Stroma Identifies a Strong Association With Tuberous Sclerosis. *Lab. Invest* **2015**, *95*, 266A.

142. Jia, L.; Jayakumaran, G.; Al-Ahmadie, H.; Fine, S.W.; Gopalan, A.; Sirintrapun, S.J.; Tickoo, S.; Reuter, V.; Cheng, Y.B. Expanding the Morphologic Spectrum of Sporadic Renal Cell Carcinoma (RCC) Harboring Somatic TSC or MTOR Alterations: Analysis of 8 Cases with Clear Cytoplasm and Leiomyomatous Stroma. *Mod. Pathol.* **2019**, *32*, 78–79.

143. Chen, Y.B.; Mirsadraei, L.; Jayakumaran, G.; Al-Ahmadie, H.A.; Fine, S.W.; Gopalan, A.; Sirintrapun, S.J.; Tickoo, S.K.; Reuter, V.E. Somatic Mutations of TSC2 or MTOR Characterize a Morphologically Distinct Subset of Sporadic Renal Cell Carcinoma with Eosinophilic and Vacuolated Cytoplasm. *Am. J. Surg. Pathol.* **2019**, *43*, 121–131. [CrossRef]

144. He, H.; Trpkov, K.; Martinek, P.; Isikci, O.T.; Maggi-Galuzzi, C.; Alaghehbandan, R.; Gill, A.J.; Tretiakova, M.; Lopez, J.I.; Williamson, S.R.; et al. "High-grade oncocytic renal tumor": Morphologic, immunohistochemical, and molecular genetic study of 14 cases. *Virchows Arch.* **2018**, *473*, 725–738. [CrossRef]

145. Trpkov, K.; Bonert, M.; Gao, Y.; Kapoor, A.; He, H.; Yilmaz, A.; Gill, A.J.; Williamson, S.R.; Comperat, E.; Tretiakova, M.; et al. High-grade oncocytic tumour (HOT) of kidney in a patient with tuberous sclerosis complex. *Histopathology* **2019**, *75*, 440–442. [CrossRef]

146. Hakimi, A.A.; Tickoo, S.K.; Jacobsen, A.; Sarungbam, J.; Sfakianos, J.P.; Sato, Y.; Morikawa, T.; Kume, H.; Fukayama, M.; Homma, Y.; et al. TCEB1-mutated renal cell carcinoma: A distinct genomic and morphological subtype. *Mod. Pathol.* **2015**, *28*, 845–853. [CrossRef]

147. Favazza, L.; Chitale, D.A.; Barod, R.; Rogers, C.G.; Kalyana-Sundaram, S.; Palanisamy, N.; Gupta, N.S.; Williamson, S.R. Renal cell tumors with clear cell histology and intact VHL and chromosome 3p: A histological review of tumors from the Cancer Genome Atlas database. *Mod. Pathol.* **2017**, *30*, 1603–1612. [CrossRef]

148. Hirsch, M.S.; Barletta, J.A.; Gorman, M.; Dal Cin, P. Renal Cell Carcinoma With Monosomy 8 and CAIX Expression: A Distinct Entity or Another Member or the Clear Cell Tubulopapillary RCC/RAT Family? *Mod. Pathol.* **2015**, *28*, 229A.

149. Williamson, S.R.; Grignon, D.J.; Cheng, L.; Favazza, L.; Gondim, D.D.; Carskadon, S.; Gupta, N.S.; Chitale, D.A.; Kalyana-Sundaram, S.; Palanisamy, N. Renal Cell Carcinoma With Chromosome 6p Amplification Including the TFEB Gene: A Novel Mechanism of Tumor Pathogenesis? *Am. J. Surg. Pathol.* **2017**, *41*, 287–298. [CrossRef]

150. Argani, P.; Reuter, V.E.; Zhang, L.; Sung, Y.S.; Ning, Y.; Epstein, J.I.; Netto, G.J.; Antonescu, C.R. TFEB-amplified Renal Cell Carcinomas: An Aggressive Molecular Subset Demonstrating Variable Melanocytic Marker Expression and Morphologic Heterogeneity. *Am. J. Surg. Pathol.* **2016**, *40*, 1484–1495. [CrossRef]

151. Gupta, S.; Johnson, S.H.; Vasmatzis, G.; Porath, B.; Rustin, J.G.; Rao, P.; Costello, B.A.; Leibovich, B.C.; Thompson, R.H.; Cheville, J.C.; et al. TFEB-VEGFA (6p21.1) co-amplified renal cell carcinoma: A distinct entity with potential implications for clinical management. *Mod. Pathol.* **2017**, *30*, 998–1012. [CrossRef]

152. Peckova, K.; Vanecek, T.; Martinek, P.; Spagnolo, D.; Kuroda, N.; Brunelli, M.; Vranic, S.; Djuricic, S.; Rotterova, P.; Daum, O.; et al. Aggressive and nonaggressive translocation t(6;11) renal cell carcinoma: Comparative study of 6 cases and review of the literature. *Ann. Diagn. Pathol.* **2014**, *18*, 351–357. [CrossRef]

153. Skala, S.L.; Xiao, H.; Udager, A.M.; Dhanasekaran, S.M.; Shukla, S.; Zhang, Y.; Landau, C.; Shao, L.; Roulston, D.; Wang, L.; et al. Detection of 6 TFEB-amplified renal cell carcinomas and 25 renal cell carcinomas with MITF translocations: Systematic morphologic analysis of 85 cases evaluated by clinical TFE3 and TFEB FISH assays. *Mod. Pathol.* **2018**, *31*, 179–197. [CrossRef]

154. Durinck, S.; Stawiski, E.W.; Pavia-Jimenez, A.; Modrusan, Z.; Kapur, P.; Jaiswal, B.S.; Zhang, N.; Toffessi-Tcheuyap, V.; Nguyen, T.T.; Pahuja, K.B.; et al. Spectrum of diverse genomic alterations define non-clear cell renal carcinoma subtypes. *Nat. Genet.* **2015**, *47*, 13–21. [CrossRef]

155. Gupta, S.; Argani, P.; Jungbluth, A.A.; Chen, Y.B.; Tickoo, S.K.; Fine, S.W.; Gopalan, A.; Al-Ahmadie, H.A.; Sirintrapun, S.J.; Sanchez, A.; et al. TFEB Expression Profiling in Renal Cell Carcinomas: Clinicopathologic Correlations. *Am. J. Surg. Pathol.* **2019**, *43*, 1445–1461. [CrossRef]

156. Andeen, N.K.; Qu, X.; Antic, T.; Tykodi, S.S.; Fang, M.; Tretiakova, M.S. Clinical Utility of Chromosome Genomic Array Testing for Unclassified and Advanced-Stage Renal Cell Carcinomas. *Arch. Pathol. Lab. Med.* **2019**, *143*, 494–504. [CrossRef]
157. Moch, H.; Amin, M.; Argani, P.; Cheville, J.; Delahunt, B.; Martignoni, G.; Srigley, J.; Tan, P.; Tickoo, S. Renal cell tumors. In *WHO Classification of Tumours of the Urinary System and Male Genital Organs*, 4th ed.; Moch, H., Humphrey, P.A., Ulbright, T.M., Reuter, V.E., Eds.; International Agency for Research on Cancer: Lyon, France, 2016; pp. 14–17.
158. Debelenko, L.V.; Raimondi, S.C.; Daw, N.; Shivakumar, B.R.; Huang, D.; Nelson, M.; Bridge, J.A. Renal cell carcinoma with novel VCL-ALK fusion: New representative of ALK-associated tumor spectrum. *Mod. Pathol.* **2011**, *24*, 430–442. [CrossRef]
159. Sugawara, E.; Togashi, Y.; Kuroda, N.; Sakata, S.; Hatano, S.; Asaka, R.; Yuasa, T.; Yonese, J.; Kitagawa, M.; Mano, H.; et al. Identification of anaplastic lymphoma kinase fusions in renal cancer: Large-scale immunohistochemical screening by the intercalated antibody-enhanced polymer method. *Cancer* **2012**, *118*, 4427–4436. [CrossRef]
160. Sukov, W.R.; Hodge, J.C.; Lohse, C.M.; Akre, M.K.; Leibovich, B.C.; Thompson, R.H.; Cheville, J.C. ALK alterations in adult renal cell carcinoma: Frequency, clinicopathologic features and outcome in a large series of consecutively treated patients. *Mod. Pathol.* **2012**, *25*, 1516–1525. [CrossRef] [PubMed]
161. Bodokh, Y.; Ambrosetti, D.; Kubiniek, V.; Tibi, B.; Durand, M.; Amiel, J.; Pertuit, M.; Barlier, A.; Pedeutour, F. ALK-TPM3 rearrangement in adult renal cell carcinoma: Report of a new case showing loss of chromosome 3 and literature review. *Cancer Genet.* **2018**, *221*, 31–37. [CrossRef] [PubMed]
162. Cajaiba, M.M.; Jennings, L.J.; George, D.; Perlman, E.J. Expanding the spectrum of ALK-rearranged renal cell carcinomas in children: Identification of a novel HOOK1-ALK fusion transcript. *Genes Chromosomes Cancer* **2016**, *55*, 814–817. [CrossRef] [PubMed]
163. Cajaiba, M.M.; Jennings, L.J.; Rohan, S.M.; Perez-Atayde, A.R.; Marino-Enriquez, A.; Fletcher, J.A.; Geller, J.I.; Leuer, K.M.; Bridge, J.A.; Perlman, E.J. ALK-rearranged renal cell carcinomas in children. *Genes Chromosomes Cancer* **2016**, *55*, 442–451. [CrossRef]
164. Hodge, J.C.; Pearce, K.E.; Sukov, W.R. Distinct ALK-rearranged and VCL-negative papillary renal cell carcinoma variant in two adults without sickle cell trait. *Mod. Pathol.* **2013**, *26*, 604–605. [CrossRef]
165. Jeanneau, M.; Gregoire, V.; Desplechain, C.; Escande, F.; Tica, D.P.; Aubert, S.; Leroy, X. ALK rearrangements-associated renal cell carcinoma (RCC) with unique pathological features in an adult. *Pathol. Res. Pr.* **2016**, *212*, 1064–1066. [CrossRef]
166. Kuroda, N.; Liu, Y.; Tretiakova, M.; Ulamec, M.; Takeuchi, K.; Przybycin, C.; Magi-Galluzzi, C.; Agaimy, A.; Yilmaz, A.; Trpkov, K.; et al. Clinicopathological Study of Seven Cases of ALK-positive Renal Tumor Identification of New Fusion Partners including CLIP1 and KIF5B Genes. *Mod. Pathol.* **2019**, *32*, 85.
167. Kuroda, N.; Sugawara, E.; Kusano, H.; Yuba, Y.; Yorita, K.; Takeuchi, K. A review of ALK-rearranged renal cell carcinomas with a focus on clinical and pathobiological aspects. *Pol. J. Pathol.* **2018**, *69*, 109–113. [CrossRef]
168. Kusano, H.; Togashi, Y.; Akiba, J.; Moriya, F.; Baba, K.; Matsuzaki, N.; Yuba, Y.; Shiraishi, Y.; Kanamaru, H.; Kuroda, N.; et al. Two Cases of Renal Cell Carcinoma Harboring a Novel STRN-ALK Fusion Gene. *Am. J. Surg. Pathol.* **2016**, *40*, 761–769. [CrossRef] [PubMed]
169. Lee, C.; Park, J.W.; Suh, J.H.; Nam, K.H.; Moon, K.C. ALK-Positive Renal Cell Carcinoma in a Large Series of Consecutively Resected Korean Renal Cell Carcinoma Patients. *Korean J. Pathol.* **2013**, *47*, 452–457. [CrossRef] [PubMed]
170. Marino-Enriquez, A.; Ou, W.B.; Weldon, C.B.; Fletcher, J.A.; Perez-Atayde, A.R. ALK rearrangement in sickle cell trait-associated renal medullary carcinoma. *Genes Chromosomes Cancer* **2011**, *50*, 146–153. [CrossRef]
171. Pal, S.K.; Bergerot, P.; Dizman, N.; Bergerot, C.; Adashek, J.; Madison, R.; Chung, J.H.; Ali, S.M.; Jones, J.O.; Salgia, R. Responses to Alectinib in ALK-rearranged Papillary Renal Cell Carcinoma. *Eur. Urol.* **2018**, *74*, 124–128. [CrossRef]
172. Smith, N.E.; Deyrup, A.T.; Marino-Enriquez, A.; Fletcher, J.A.; Bridge, J.A.; Illei, P.B.; Netto, G.J.; Argani, P. VCL-ALK renal cell carcinoma in children with sickle-cell trait: The eighth sickle-cell nephropathy? *Am. J. Surg. Pathol.* **2014**, *38*, 858–863. [CrossRef]
173. Thorner, P.S.; Shago, M.; Marrano, P.; Shaikh, F.; Somers, G.R. TFE3-positive renal cell carcinomas are not always Xp11 translocation carcinomas: Report of a case with a TPM3-ALK translocation. *Pathol. Res. Pr.* **2016**, *212*, 937–942. [CrossRef]

174. Yu, W.; Wang, Y.; Jiang, Y.; Zhang, W.; Li, Y. Genetic analysis and clinicopathological features of ALK-rearranged renal cell carcinoma in a large series of resected Chinese renal cell carcinoma patients and literature review. *Histopathology* **2017**, *71*, 53–62. [CrossRef]
175. Cheng, J.; Zhang, J.; Han, Y.; Wang, X.; Ye, X.; Meng, Y.; Parwani, A.; Han, Z.; Feng, Q.; Huang, K. Integrative Analysis of Histopathological Images and Genomic Data Predicts Clear Cell Renal Cell Carcinoma Prognosis. *Cancer Res.* **2017**, *77*, e91–e100. [CrossRef]
176. Shao, W.; Han, Z.; Cheng, J.; Cheng, L.; Wang, T.; Sun, L.; Lu, Z.; Zhang, J.; Zhang, D.; Huang, K. Integrative analysis of pathological images and multi-dimensional genomic data for early-stage cancer prognosis. *IEEE Trans. Med. Imaging* **2019**. [CrossRef]

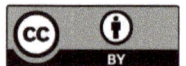

© 2019 by the authors. Licensee MDPI, Basel, Switzerland. This article is an open access article distributed under the terms and conditions of the Creative Commons Attribution (CC BY) license (http://creativecommons.org/licenses/by/4.0/).

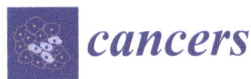

Review

Prognostic and Predictive Value of *PBRM1* in Clear Cell Renal Cell Carcinoma

Lucía Carril-Ajuria [1], María Santos [2], Juan María Roldán-Romero [2], Cristina Rodriguez-Antona [2,3,*] and Guillermo de Velasco [1,*]

[1] Department of Medical Oncology, University Hospital 12 de Octubre, 28041 Madrid, Spain; luciacarril@hotmail.com
[2] Hereditary Endocrine Cancer Group, Human Cancer Genetics Programme, Spanish National Cancer Research Centre (CNIO), 28029 Madrid, Spain; msantosr@cnio.es (M.S.); jmroldan@cnio.es (J.M.R.-R.)
[3] Centro de Investigación Biomédica en Red de Enfermedades Raras (CIBERER), 28029 Madrid, Spain
[*] Correspondence: crodriguez@cnio.es (C.R.-A.); gdevelasco.gdv@gmail.com (G.d.V.)

Received: 30 November 2019; Accepted: 15 December 2019; Published: 19 December 2019

Abstract: Renal cell carcinoma (RCC) is the most frequent kidney solid tumor, the clear cell RCC (ccRCC) being the major histological subtype. The probability of recurrence and the clinical behavior of ccRCC will greatly depend on the different clinical and histopathological features, already incorporated to different scoring systems, and on the genomic landscape of the tumor. In this sense, ccRCC has for a long time been known to be associated to the biallelic inactivation of Von Hippel-Lindau (*VHL*) gene which causes aberrant hypoxia inducible factor (HIF) accumulation. Recently, next generation-sequencing technologies have provided the bases for an in-depth molecular characterization of ccRCC, identifying additional recurrently mutated genes, such as *PBRM1* (≈40–50%), *SETD2* (≈12%), or *BAP1* (≈10%). *PBRM1*, the second most common mutated gene in ccRCC after *VHL*, is a component of the SWI/SNF chromatin remodeling complex. Different studies have investigated the biological consequences and the potential role of *PBRM1* alterations in RCC prognosis and as a drug response modulator, although some results are contradictory. In the present article, we review the current evidence on *PBRM1* as potential prognostic and predictive marker in both localized and metastatic RCC.

Keywords: polybromo-1; PBRM1; renal cell carcinoma; biomarker; prognosis; predictive role

---

1. Introduction

Kidney cancer is the 12th most frequent solid tumor worldwide with around 400,000 new cases and 175,000 deaths from renal cell carcinoma (RCC) estimated in 2018 [1]. RCC accounts for almost 90% of all kidney tumors, the clear cell (ccRCC) being the most common histologic subtype [2].

Approximately 70% of the RCC will present with localized disease, but around one third of them will relapse after surgical excision [3,4]. However, the probability of recurrence will depend greatly on different clinical and histopathological features, which have been incorporated to up to 20 different scoring systems characterized by substantial heterogeneity [5–7].

Regarding the molecular characteristics of RCC, the inactivation of the Von Hippel–Lindau (*VHL*) gene is by far the most common oncogenic driver event in ccRCC. *VHL* is an E3 ligase substrate that labels the transcription factors hypoxia inducible factor (HIF) 1alpha and HIF2alpha with ubiquitin for proteosomal degradation. The accumulation of HIF triggers the uncontrolled expression of angiogenesis promoting genes and gives rise to highly vascularized tumors [8].

Recent advances in next-generation sequencing (NGS) and their implementation in large cohort of cancer patients (e.g., The Cancer Genome Atlas (TCGA) projects), have led to the identification of additional genes frequently mutated in ccRCC, such as *PBRM1* (≈40–50%), *SETD2* (12%), *BAP1* (10%), and *KDM5C* (5%) [9–11]. These are genes coding for proteins participating in the regulation of chromatin remodeling and histone methylation. Although *VHL* is the initiating event in ccRCC, the acquisition of additional mutations, some in subclonal cancer cell populations, is a common characteristic during ccRCC tumor development and metastasis. In this context, multiregion sequencing-based studies have highlighted the potential relevance of *PBRM1* alterations for tumor growth and metastatic capacity, which are determinant for clinical outcome [10].

The advances in systemic therapy of advanced RCC (mRCC) in the last 20 years have been remarkable. This progress has led to a significant improvement in the median overall survival (OS), from 13 months in the cytokine therapy era to ≈30 months using combination of targeted therapies and immune checkpoint blockade [12–14]. Well established prognostic scoring systems for mRCC, such as the Memorial Sloan Kettering Cancer Center (MSKCC) or the International Metastatic RCC Database Consortium (IMDC), include clinical parameters such as performance status or time from diagnosis to treatment, as well as laboratory parameters [15]. However, other clinical variables which have a prognostic value in mRCC are not included in those models [16]. Likewise, in the current therapeutic context there is a need of updating the scoring systems with molecular parameters, to better personalize treatment strategies to achieve survival improvement and avoid unnecessary toxicities.

2. Bromodomain-Containing Protein BAF180 Function

The SWI/SNF complexes are multiprotein machineries able to mobilize nucleosomes and alter chromatin structure through the hydrolysis of ATP molecules. By controlling chromatin accessibility, these epigenetic remodeling complexes act as transcriptional regulators, mediating the binding of transcription factors, coactivators, and corepressors to target promoters and enhancers in the DNA. A wide variety of cellular functions are modulated by SWI/SNF complexes including the balance between self-renewal and cell differentiation, cell cycle, metabolism, and DNA repair processes [17]. SWI/SNF components are recurrently mutated across human malignancies. It is estimated that about 20% of all human tumors harbor alterations in genes encoding SWI/SNF complex subunits [18]. This mutation frequency is comparable to that observed for other canonical cancer genes such as *TP53*, *KRAS*, or *PTEN* [19]. Interestingly, mutations in particular SWI/SNF components are tumor type-dependent, which may indicate that these complexes carry out not only universal but also tissue-specific functions. For instance, *SMARCB1* is found mutated in almost 95% of malignant rhabdoid tumors and *PBRM1* is mutated in ≈40% of ccRCC [20]. Other components of the SWI/SNF complex, such as *ARID1A*, are highly mutated in several cancer types, but rarely altered in ccRCC (e.g., *ARID1A* is mutated in 49% of ovarian clear cell carcinomas, 39% of endometrial cancers, and only in 3% of ccRCC tumors).

The gene *PBRM1* encodes the bromodomain-containing protein BAF180 that serves as the DNA-targeting subunit of the pBAF SWI/SNF complex [21]. BAF180 harbors six bromodomains that bind acetylated residues on histone tails. These domains are capable of recognizing acetylating patterns and target the complete complex to specific chromatin regions. This protein is involved in various DNA repair mechanisms [22] and it is also important for cohesion between centromeres, which is necessary for maintaining genomic stability [23].

How mutations in the gene *PBRM1* promote carcinogenesis and tumor progression is still unknown. *PBRM1* is considered a tumor suppressor gene and this role is supported by in vitro experiments in ccRCC derived cell-lines, which show that *PBRM1* gene silencing results in increased proliferation, migration, and colony formation [20]. Consistently, Macher-Goeppinger et al. found that re-expression of *PBRM1* into A704 cells, that harbor a homozygous truncating mutation in this gene, results in diminished colony formation [24]. The role of *PBRM1* as tumor suppressor is also supported by the fact that ≈80% of the somatic mutations found in the gene result in loss of function (LOF) of the protein, not only in ccRCC but also in other tumor types, including breast and pancreatic cancers. Furthermore, BAF180 has been demonstrated to modulate the activity of p53 [24], inducing the transcription of some p53-targets such as p21 and repressing other such as 14–3-3σ (Figure 1). *PBRM1* inactivation can therefore disturb p53-dependent chromatin regulation and enable ccRCC tumors to escape from p53-mediated surveillance [25]. Even if *PBRM1* has mainly been described as a tumor suppressor gene, Murakami et al. recently demonstrated that its role may be context dependent, and that *PBRM1* may also act as an oncogene under specific conditions [26]. They showed that the inactivation of *PBRM1* in 786-O cells, a ccRCC cell line expressing BAF180, resulted in a reduction of cell survival and proliferation. This effect seemed to be dependent on HIF1α/HIF2α expression. In this regard, *PBRM1* acts as a coactivator of both transcription factors, which play opposite roles in established ccRCC tumors. In this particular context, HIF1α acts as a tumor suppressor gene [27], while HIF2α favors tumor development. In in vitro models in which both transcription factors are expressed, *PBRM1* showed tumor suppressive activity. By contrast, when HIF1α was not expressed, *PBRM1* induced expression of HIF2α oncogenic targets, which resulted in increased cell survival and proliferation. In summary, in ccRCC the function of *PBRM1* as a tumor-suppressor or oncogene is context dependent.

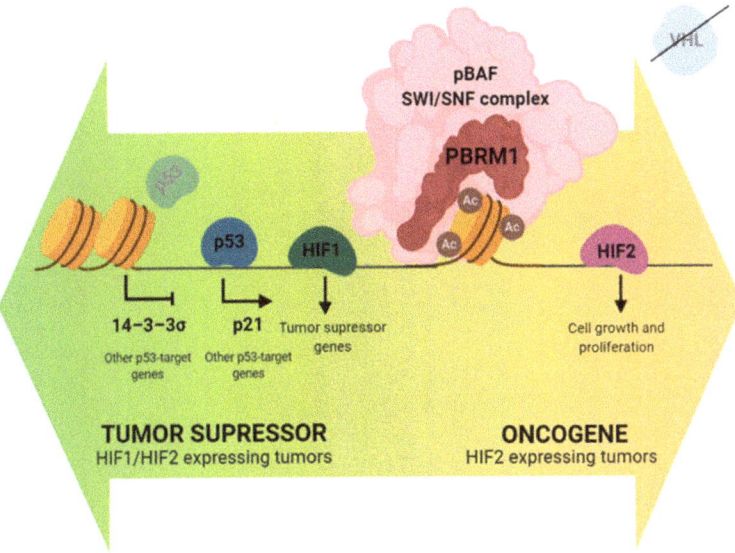

Figure 1. Role of *PBRM1* in established clear cell renal cell carcinoma (ccRCC) tumors.

3. *PBRM1* Mutations in Clear Cell Renal Cell Carcinoma

Hereditary cases of RCC account for 3–5% of all renal cancers. These cases are associated with RCC syndromes and are characterized by young age of onset and multi or bilateral tumors. They are related to mutations in specific susceptibility genes such as *VHL*, *MET*, *FLCN*, *FH*, and *SDHB*, which increase the risk of developing specific RCC subtypes [28,29]. Other minority inherited forms of RCC are associated with *BAP1* tumor predisposition syndrome and constitutional chromosome 3 translocations. Nevertheless, some cases of inherited RCC tumors are not explained by any of the genes mentioned above. Recently, a *PBRM1* mutational screening in a cohort of 35 French unrelated patients with a familial history of RCC revealed one patient with a germline *PBRM1* truncating mutation (p.Asp1333Glyfs). In the family there were three additional cases with ccRCC and the truncating mutation co-segregated with the disease [30]. To our knowledge, this case is the only familial form of RCC explained by a germline mutation in *PBRM1*. This finding could eventually support the inclusion of this gene in genetic screenings for RCC syndromes.

The somatic genomic landscape of ccRCC tumors is characterized by *VHL* inactivation, which is found altered in ≈90% of the cases. Inactivation is typically achieved through the loss of the chromosome arm 3p (encompassing the genes *VHL*, *PBRM1*, *BAP1*, and *SETD2*) in a process of unbalanced translocation followed by the somatic inactivation of the remaining *VHL* allele. However, even if *VHL* biallelic inactivation is a critical founder event, it is not sufficient for tumor development and additional mutations and epigenetic changes are necessary. Extensive sequencing projects by TCGA have identified *PBRM1* as the second most frequently altered gene in ccRCC (49% of explored cases, 163 point mutations, eight deep deletions, and one fusion in a total of 354 cases) [20,31] Even though ccRCC is the tumor type with the highest mutational rate in *PBRM1* in the TCGA Pan-Can Project [32], somatic *PBRM1* mutations were first described in breast cancer [29] and are also observed in other cancer types such as cholangiocarcinoma (22%) and uterine (10%). Notably, the high incidence of mutations in *PBRM1* in renal cancer seems to be limited to clear cell histology and mutations are rare or not observed in other renal cancer subtypes, such as papillary (4%) or chromophobe (0%). In agreement with its role as a tumor suppressor, most mutations observed in ccRCC are truncating (137 out of 163 mutations) while missense mutations are less frequent (23 out of 163). Mutations in *PBRM1* are found distributed along the entire gene, affecting Bromodomains, Bromo-Adjacent Homology (BAH) and High Mobility Group (HMG) domains, with some relevant hotspots of truncating mutations [33] (Figure 2). *PBRM1* gene (at 3p21.1) is also affected by copy number alterations, as a consequence of the characteristic chromosome 3p deletion in ccRCC tumors.

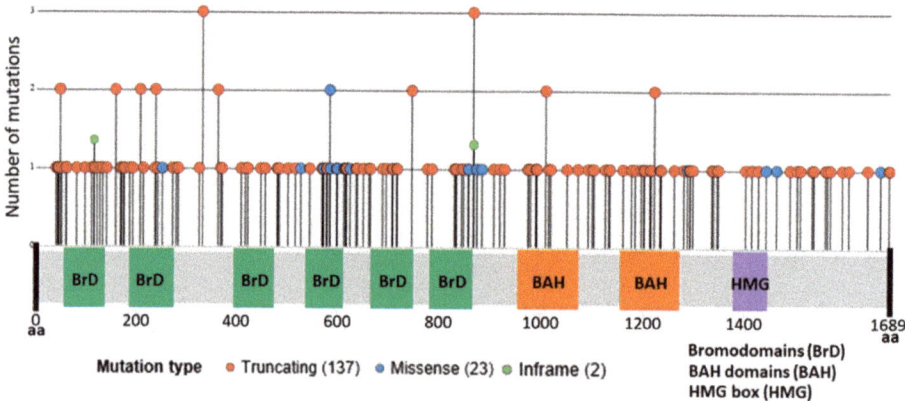

Figure 2. *PBRM1* mutations in clear cell RCC. From The Cancer Genome Atlas (TCGA) PanCancer Atlas Project.

Intratumoral heterogeneity (ITH) is a common feature of primary ccRCC tumors, leading to somatic point mutations and copy number alterations that are only present in a subset of tumor cells within the same tumor [10,34]. Multiregion sequencing showed that renal tumors are characterized by harboring only a small number of clonal mutations, shared by all tumor cells, and a majority of subclonal alterations found at varying frequencies across the tumor. Mutations in *PBRM1* are clonal in ≈75% of cases and subclonal in the remaining 25% of ccRCC primary tumors. Truncal *PBRM1* mutations define particular evolutionary trajectories in the tumor, that impact the prognosis and therapeutic response. Three out of the seven evolutionary patterns described in primary ccRCC tumors presented somatic mutations in *PBRM1* as a truncal event that precede subclonal mutations in *SETD2*, genes from the PI3K pathway or copy number alterations [35] (Figure 3). These three clonal *PBRM1* driven evolutionary patterns are enriched in tumors with high ITH and a large number of different subclones. Tumors following these evolutionary trajectories are characterized by a slow growth rate, are associated with advanced disease and with longer progression free survival (PFS). Consistently, Joseph RW et al. found that the loss of *PBRM1* expression in 1330 ccRCC tumor samples was associated with an increased risk of metastasis development, without an effect on OS [36]. Several studies have described mutual exclusivity between *PBRM1* and *BAP1* mutations in RCC primary tumors [37,38]. Still, truncal *PBRM1* mutations are observed in an additional ccRCC evolutionary subtype characterized by multiple driver clonal mutations in genes that include, in addition to *PBRM1*, *BAP1*, *SETD2*, or *PTEN*. These tumors have low ITH and high genomic instability and are associated with a rapid progression to multiple sites. *BAP1* clonal mutations are characteristic of an additional ccRCC evolutionary pattern that harbors a high genomic instability and a low ITH.

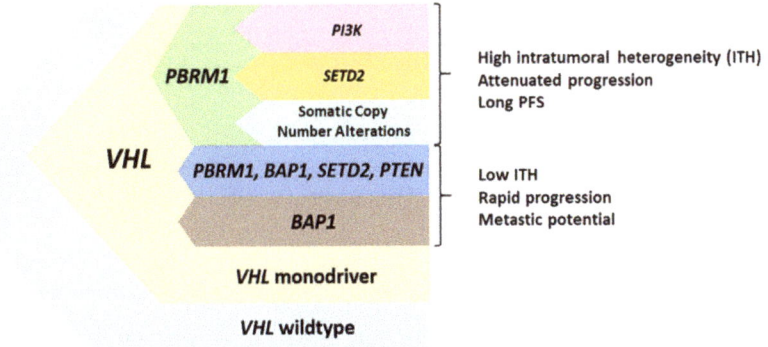

Figure 3. Branched clear cell RCC evolutionary model. Based on Turajlic et al. [35].

Turajlic et al. proposed that tumor clones with mutations in *PBRM1* are preferably selected for metastasis development [35]. However, mutations in additional genes seem to be needed for RCC progression [39]. Metastatic dissemination of primary tumors harboring *VHL* and *PBRM1* mutations as the two only clonal events, is mainly an attenuated process that leads to initial solitary or oligometastases. Metastatic potential in these ccRCC tumors is acquired gradually over time and it is limited to certain subpopulations in the primary tumor that act as a reservoir of metastases. Therefore, mutations in *PBRM1* are a key factor not only for primary tumor development but also for tumor metastatic dissemination, in which additional subclonal mutations, acquired after *PBRM1* loss, seem to play a decisive role. Detection of clonal and subclonal events in *PBRM1*, *SETD2*, PI3K pathway genes, together with somatic copy number alterations is therefore essential to establish a reliable map of the complexity of tumor progression driven by *PBRM1* loss.

4. Prognostic Value of *PBRM1* Mutations in Localized and Advanced Disease

Different studies have tried to elucidate the impact of *PBRM1* status in RCC but with controversial results [36,40–51]. Two small retrospective studies were conducted to compare the different prognostic implications of both *BAP1* and *PBRM1* mutations in localized ccRCC. The study conducted by Kapur et al. showed no survival differences depending on the *PBRM1* mutational status, but identified two molecular subgroups with different prognostic implications and different gene expression [40]. The *PBRM1*-mutant group showed superior median OS than the *BAP1*-mutant group (HR = 2.7; *PBRM1*-MT 10.6 months vs. *BAP1*-MT 4.6 months). Likewise, Gossage et al. reported worse relapse free survival (RFS) in those tumors carrying *BAP1* mutation when compared to *PBRM1* mutant tumors, although no differences in OS were found (Table 1) [41].

Table 1. Value of *BAP1* versus *PBRM1* in localized disease.

Author [Ref.]	Year	Country	Gender M(%)/F(%)	Age (y)	N	BAP1 MT(%)	PBRM1 MT(%)	Tech	Survival Efficacy Parameters	
									RFS (HR/ p)	OS (HR/ p)
Kapur [40]	2013	USA	80(55)/65(45)	62	145	21(14)	78(54)	NGS	NA	BAP1 MT: 4.6; PBRM1 MT: 10.6 (2.7/0.044)
Gossage [41]	2014	UK	83(63)/49(37)	62	132	14(11)	42(33)	NGS	BAP1 MT: 1.2 [a]; PBRM1 MT: 4.9 [a] (n.sp./0.059)	n.sp. (n.sp./NS)

M: male patients. F: female patients. Age: median age. y: years. N: number of patients. MT: mutant patients. Tech: Technique. NGS: next-generation sequencing. RFS: recurrence-free-survival in years. HR: hazard ratio. OS: overall survival in years. NS: non statistically significant. NA: not assessed. n.sp.: not specified. [a] 75th percentile for survival.

According to recent studies focused exclusively on *PBRM1* status as a prognostic factor, it seems that the *PBRM1* LOF is associated with a different prognostic value in localized and advanced disease.

4.1. Localized Disease

Most studies assessing the prognostic value of *PBRM1* in RCC have focused on localized disease. It is noteworthy that only one of these studies has included other histological subtypes aside from ccRCC [42]. The loss of *PBRM1* function has also been correlated with advanced tumor and clinical stage, as well as with more aggressive features, such as lymphovascular invasion and poor differentiation [42,43]. In a systematic review including seven studies (Table 2) *PBRM1* LOF in localized disease was associated with poor prognosis, both in terms of RFS and OS [44].

In 2013 the results obtained by Costa et al. showed that *PBRM1* LOF was associated with poor prognosis and worse 5 years RFS rates (*PBRM1* MT 66.7% vs. *PBRM1* WT 87.3%; $p = 0.048$) and worse 5 years disease-specific survival rates (DSS) (*PBRM1* MT 70.6% vs. *PBRM1* WT 89.7%; $p = 0.017$) [43]. Pawlowski et al. conducted a similar study but including different histological subtypes (227 clear cell, 40 papillary and 12 chromophobe). Their results confirmed that *PBRM1* LOF is more frequent in ccRCC than in other histological subtypes, and suggested that most of truncating mutations in ccRCC negatively affect *PBRM1* expression [42]. The study also showed an association of *PBRM1* LOF with late tumor stage and worse OS (*PBRM1* negative 80 months vs. *PBRM1* positive NR (not reached)). Conversely, a Korean article, which also demonstrated the independent prognostic value of *PBRM1* expression, suggested that the negative prognostic impact of *PBRM1* LOF was limited to lower-stage tumors (stage I/II; $p = 0.001$ for cancer specific survival (CSS)/PFS and not to higher-stage tumors (stage III/IV; $p > 0.05$), although most of the patients (≈76.6%) were stage I/II [45]. Hakimi et al. investigated the impact of *PBRM1* status in 609 patients with ccRCC from two different cohorts (MSKCC, $n = 188$ and TCGA, $n = 421$) showing no significant impact on CSS. However, the addition of *PBRM1* mutation to *BAP1* mutation, which did correlate with a poor prognosis, increased the risk of cancer death (HR 4.18) [46]. The largest study to date was conducted by the Mayo Clinic and included 1330 patients with ccRCC. *PBRM1* and *BAP1* expression were analyzed by immunohistochemistry (IHC) and they did not find significant differences in CSS according to *PBRM1* expression and adjusting by age [36]. The authors did find, however, a significantly higher risk of metastasis in *PBRM1* deficient tumors. The study was also able to define, with regards to the prognostic significance, four different ccRCC subtypes depending on *PBRM1* and *BAP1* status. Thus, there was a progressive worsening of both RFS and CSS from *PBRM1*+/*BAP1*+ to *PBRM1*-/*BAP1*+ to *PBRM1*+/*BAP1*- to *PBRM1*-/*BAP1*- [36].

Overall, it seems that in localized ccRCC, the loss of *PBRM1* function correlates with aggressive features and advanced stage, as well as with worse prognosis.

Table 2. Current evidence on *PBRM1* prognosis value.

Disease Type	Author [Ref.]	Year	Country	Gender M(%)/F(%)	Age (y)	N	PBRM1 -/Low (%)	Tech	Ab (Dilution)	PBRM1 Cut-off	Survival Efficacy Parameters RFS/PFS (HR/p)	OS/CSS (HR/p)
Loc	da Costa [43]	2013	Brazil	66(59)/46(41)	56	112	34(30)	IHC	PB1 Ab [b] (1:25)	Presence	PBRM1 -: 66.7% vs. PBRM1 +: 87.3% [d] (n.sp./0.048)	PBRM1 -: 70.6 vs. PBRM1 +: 89.7% [f] (n.sp./0.017)
	Hakimi [46]	2013	USA	408(67)/200(33)	61	609	198(33)	NGS	-	-	NA	n.sp. (n.sp./NS)
	Pawlowski [42]	2013	Switzerland	NA	NA	279	175(64) [a]	IHC	PB1Ab [c] (1:25)	>5%	NA	PBRM1 -: 80 vs. PBRM1 +: not reach (n.sp./0.025)
	Nam [45]	2015	Korea	485(74)/172(26)	NA	657	NA	IHC	PB1 Ab [c] (1:100)	>50%	PBRM1 LE: 109.5 vs. PBRM1 HE: 156.2 (n.sp./<0.001)	PBRM1 LE: 145.5 vs. PBRM1 HE: 171.7 (n.sp./<0.001)
	Joseph [36]	2016	USA	823(62)/435(33)	64	1330	674(51)	IHC	PB1 Ab [c]	Presence	PBRM1 -: higher mtx. risk (1.46/0.001)	n.sp. (n.sp/NS)
	Kim [52]	2017	Korea	244(70)/107(30)	54	351	208(59)	IHC	PB1 Ab	Score > 2	n.sp. (0.81/0.64)	n.sp. (1.86/0.1)
Loc and Mtx	Jiang [47]	2017	USA	118(74)/42(26)	60	160	49(31)	IHC	PB1 Ab [c] (1:50)	>5%	n.sp. (0.79/0.21)	n.sp. (0.42/2.45e-05)
	Carlo [49]	2017	USA	77(73)/28(27)	57	105	53(51)	NGS	-	-	PBRM1 MT: 12.0 vs. PBRM1 WT: 6.9 [e] (n.sp./0.01)	PBRM1 MT: not reach vs. PBRM1 WT: 36.3 (n.sp./0.12)
	Tennenbaum [50]	2017	USA	116(69)/51(31)	60	167	64(38)	NGS	-	-	NA	n.sp. (0.87/0.49)
Mtx	Kim [48]	2015	Korea	44(83)/9(17)	62	53	28(52)	IHC	PB1 Ab [c] (1:100)	Score >2.5	NA	PBRM1 LE: 46 vs. PBRM1 HE: 24 (n.sp./0.022)
	Voss [51]	2018	USA	279(74)/98(26)	61	357	160(45)	NGS	-	-	PBRM1 MT: 11.1 vs. PBRM1 WT: 8.2 (0.67/0.004)	PBRM1 MT: 35.5 vs. PBRM1 WT: 23.8 (0.63/0.002)

Loc: localized. Mtx: metastatic. M: male patients. F: female patients. Age: median age. y: years. N: number of patients. PBRM1 -: patients not expressing PBRM1. PBRM1 LE: patients with low PBRM1 expression. PBRM1 HE: patients with high PBRM1 expression. Tech: technology. Ab: antibody. IHC: immunohistochemistry. NGS: next-generation sequencing. RFS: recurrence-free survival in months. PFS: progression-free survival in months. OS: overall survival in months. CSS: cancer-specific-survival. MT: mutant patients. WT: wild-type patients. n.sp.: not specified. NA: not assessed. HR: hazard ratio. [a]: Out of the 175 patients negative for PBRM1 expression 155(68%) were clear cell, 16(40%) papillary and 4(30%) chromophobe histology. [b]: Anti-BAF180 antibody (Sigma-Aldrich, MO, USA). [c]: PB1/BAF180 antibody (Montgomery TX, Texas, USA). [d]: 5-year recurrence free survival rate. [e]: Time to treatment failure in months. [f]: 5-year cancer-specific survival rate.

4.2. Advanced Disease

There is less data on *PBRM1* role in advanced ccRCC compared to localized disease. The first study to assess the prognostic value of *PBRM1* expression in stage IV/recurrent RCC was a Korean study including a small population ($n = 53$) [48]. Patients were divided in two groups using 2.5 IHC score for *PBRM1* expression as the cut-off value. Patients with high expression of *PBRM1* in the tumor had a significantly worse OS than those with low *PBRM1* expression. (HR 2.29, $p = 0.039$), but there was not statistically significant difference when only the ccRCC subgroup was considered (HR 2.22, $p = 0.068$) [48]. Consistently, patients harboring tumors with high expression of *PBRM1* showed shorter OS when treated with both sunitinib and everolimus (low vs. high expression; OS 45.0 vs. 23.0 months, $p = 0.035$) [48]. However, the most robust data come from the study conducted by Voss et al. which included 357 advanced ccRCC patients (COMPARZ trial (training cohort), $n = 357$/RECORD3 trial (validation cohort), $n = 258$) [51]. They confirmed the prognostic role of *BAP1*, *TP53*, and *PBRM1* in metastatic renal cell carcinoma patients treated with tyrosine kinase inhibitors (TKI). Remarkably, *PBRM1* mutations were associated with a better prognosis, both in terms of PFS (HR 0.67, $p = 0.004$) and OS (HR 0.63, $p = 0.002$) [51], whereas *BAP1* mutations were associated with worse prognosis, and a significant worse OS (HR 1.51). Conversely, Tennenbaum et al. did not find an association between *PBRM1* mutational status (determined by NGS) and OS in 167 advanced ccRCC patients from the MSKCC and TCGA cohorts [50].

Other studies which included cohorts with both localized and advanced disease have shown contradictory results (Table 2) [47,49].

Overall, the studies published to date suggest that *PBRM1* LOF has a different role in localized and advanced disease, constituting a poor prognostic factor in localized disease and a good prognostic factor in advanced disease. The inactivation of *BAP1* and *PBRM1* mainly contribute to different pathways of tumor evolution, being almost mutually exclusive events conferring different prognosis. As suggested, ccRCC could be initiated by a focal mutation in *VHL* followed by 3p loss, predisposing to *BAP1* or *PBRM1* inactivation. The mutation of the remaining allele of *PBRM1* or *BAP1* would lead to tumorigenesis, and depending on which gene is mutated, to different tumor aggressiveness. In advanced RCC, *BAP1* mutation leads to a more aggressive disease and *PBRM1* mutation would be associated with a better prognosis [35].

5. Predictive Value of *PBRM1* Mutations

Antiangiogenics have constituted the cornerstone of mRCC systemic treatment for years. However, during the last years the treatment landscape of mRCC has rapidly changed with the development of new drugs, such as cabozantinib, a multikinase inhibitor, or immune-checkpoint inhibitors, as well as the investigation of different treatment combinations. With such a wide range of treatment options, efforts are now focused on identifying predictive biomarkers of response that will help to establish the best treatment sequence for each tumor and patient. There are studies that suggest the correlation of certain mutations with treatment outcomes [53–55]. According to some retrospective studies and preclinical data it seems that the mutational status of *PBRM1* could have a predictive role [48,56–58]

5.1. Targeted Therapy

Data on *PBRM1* predictive value for targeted therapy is scarce and mainly derive from retrospective studies (Table 3) [48,56], aside from the prospective IMMOTION150 trial [59]. According to the results of the IMMOTION150 study, molecular profiles, related with angiogenesis, immune infiltration, and myeloid inflammation, could constitute predictors of response to immunotherapy and antiangiogenics. Interestingly, the tumors with high angiogenesis were enriched for *PBRM1* mutations. In addition, when comparing the treatment outcomes, there was a clear benefit in sunitinib PFS, compared to atezolizumab monotherapy and to atezolizumab plus bevacizumab, in tumors with *PBRM1* mutations.

These results suggest an association between angiogenesis and *PBRM1* mutations, indicating that *PBRM1* mutated patients may benefit more from antiangiogenics than from immunotherapy.

Similarly, Fay et al. performed whole-exome sequencing in pretreatment specimens of 27 mRCC patients who had experienced an "extreme response" (extreme responders or primary refractory patients) to first line VEGF targeted therapy (sunitinib or pazopanib). In agreement with IMMOTION150 study, *PBRM1* mutations were significantly more frequent in patients benefiting from antiangiogenic treatment (54% vs. 7%, respectively) [60].

The retrospective study conducted by Kim et al. investigated the correlation of *PBRM1* expression and treatment outcomes in 53 clear cell mRCC patients [48]. Lines of therapy were not specified. High *PBRM1* expression correlated with worse outcomes in patients treated with either sunitinib or everolimus. When analyzing each drug separately, the effect of *PBRM1* expression was stronger in patients treated with everolimus (median PFS in low and high *PBRM1* expression groups was 3.0 months and 1.9 months, respectively; $p = 0.10$) although it did not reach statistical significance. *PBRM1* expression did not correlate with PFS in patients treated with sunitinib (low vs. high median PFS 7.3 vs. 9.0 months, $p = 0.83$).

Later on, Hsieh et al. investigated the association between *PBRM1* mutational status, analyzed by NGS, and treatment outcomes in 220 clear cell mRCC patients included in the RECORD3 trial [56]. The RECORD3 trial was a phase 2 randomized study comparing sunitinib with everolimus in the first line setting with a crossover design. In this study, patients harboring *PBRM1* mutation had better outcomes than those with *PBRM1* wild type tumors in the everolimus-sunitinib sequence group (MT vs. WT PFS 12.8 vs. 5.5 months; HR 0.53, $p = 0.004$), whereas no differences were seen in the sunitinib-everolimus sequence group ($p = 0.4$).

Table 3. Current evidence supporting *PBRM1* predictive value for everolimus in metastatic disease.

Author [Ref.]	Year	Country	Gender M(%)/F(%)	Age (y)	N	BAP1 MT (%)	PBRM1 MT (%)	Tech	Ab(Dilution)	PBRM1 Cut-off	Everolimus PFS PBRM1 MT or LE vs. PBRM1 WT or HE (HR/p)	Sunitinib PFS PBRM1 MT or LE vs. PBRM1 WT or HE (HR/p)
Hsieh [56]	2016	USA	168 (76)/52(24)	62	220	42(19)	101(46)	NGS	-	-	12.8 vs. 5.5 (0.53/0.004)	11.0 vs. 8.3 (0.79/0.4)
Kim [48]	2015	Korea	44(83)/9(17)	62	53	NA	25(47)	IHC	PB1 Ab [a] (1:100)	2.5	3.0 vs. 1.9 (NA/0.1)	7.3 vs. 9 (NA/0.8)

M: male patients. F: female patients. Age: median age. y: years. N: number of patients. MT: mutant patients. NA: not assessed. Tech: technique. NGS: next-generation sequencing. IHC: immunohistochemistry. PFS: progression-free-survival in months. HR: hazard ratio. NA: not assessed. [a] PB1/BAF180 AB Montgomery, TX.

5.2. Immunotherapy

Immune checkpoint inhibitors (ICI) have become a new standard of treatment in RCC. Therefore, there is a need to identify which patients will benefit most from ICI or antiangiogenics in order to better determine the treatment sequence and improve survival outcomes. Although PD-L1 expression is a well established biomarker of response to ICI in some tumors (e.g., non-small cell lung cancer), in RCC it is not useful [59,61,62]. Furthermore, neither the tumor mutational burden or the neoantigen expression have been shown to be suitable for patient selection [63].

The PBAF loss was shown in preclinical *in vivo* studies to increase sensitivity to T-cell mediated cytotoxicity compared to those with intact PBAF [64]. Recently, Miao et al. as part of a prospective trial (CA 209-009), analyzed by whole exome sequencing 35 pretreated tumors [57]. They tried to correlate the tumor genome profile with the clinical benefit from anti-PD1 therapy and discovered there was a correlation between *PBRM1* mutations and clinical benefit. However, when they tried to compare the type of tumor-immune microenvironment in ccRCC tumors according to the mutational status of *PBRM1*, in three different cohorts (TCGA, an independent cohort of untreated ccRCC tumors and patient tumors of their study), tumors harboring *PBRM1* mutations in all three cohorts showed a lower expression of immune inhibitory ligands than those with intact *PBRM1*.

More recently, a post hoc analysis of the CHECKMATE025 trial which compared nivolumab and sunitinib in ccRCC patients previously treated with antiangiogenics, analyzed the correlation between *PBRM1* status and outcomes (PFS and OS) across-treatment in 382 of the 803 patients included in the trial [58]. The results showed a significant correlation between *PRBM1* status and response to anti-PD1 therapy, with a significant benefit both in PFS and OS in those patients harboring *PBRM1* mutations (HR 0.67, 95% CI, 0.47–0.96; $p = 0.03$, and HR 0.65, 95% CI, 0.44–0.96; $p = 0.03$ respectively) compared to those with *PBRM1* wild type tumors. There was no evidence of an association between *PBRM1* status and clinical outcomes in the everolimus cohort [58].

On the other hand, as discussed above, in the clinical trial IMMOTION150 the group of tumors with high angiogenesis showed an enrichment in *PBRM1* mutations and these patients seemed to perform worse when treated with ICI alone (atezolizumab) than when treated with antiangiogenics alone (sunitinib) or in combination with immunotherapy (atezolizumab plus bevacizumab) [59].

Altogether, it seems that *PBRM1* mutations are associated with specific molecular tumor expression profiles, and that they may have a predictive role. However, its predictive value is still unclear and needs to be elucidated in future larger randomized trials.

6. Future Perspectives and Conclusions

Cancer is a combination of evolutionary inherited and environmental factors. Most recurrently mutated genes in RCC include *PBRM1*. Evolutionary information from the TRACERX study has shown that RCC tumors with *PBRM1* mutations may have a less aggressive behavior, however, additional events may be synergistic and confer a worse prognosis. This may support that *PBRM1* gene could have dual roles in oncogenesis under different cellular contexts (i.e., localized disease or metastatic disease). This duality in tumor suppressors genes (e.g., *TP53*) have been shown in other tumors [65]. For a gene with both oncogenic and tumor-suppressor potentials, it is possible that one single mutation event would unleash its oncogenic power and abolish its tumor-suppressor function. Theoretically, such mutation events would be easy to target. Indeed, systematic drug sensitivity analyses have proven drug vulnerabilities associated with loss of tumor suppressor genes. This could lead to expanding precision cancer medicine in tumors with a basis on mutations of tumor suppressor genes [66].

In summary, the definition of RCC genetic components that contribute to cancer development is an area of great interest, as it will help to understand cancer evolution and to generate better targeted therapies for the patients. *PBRM1*, the second most commonly mutated gene in ccRCC, seems to play a relevant role shaping tumor aggressiveness and pathway dependencies. This knowledge has important clinical implications and, together with additional genomic markers, will have the potential to personalize the clinical management of RCC patients.

Author Contributions: Conceptualization, C.R.-A. and G.d.V.; Methodology, L.C.-A., M.S. and J.M.R.-R.; Original Draft Preparation, all authors; Writing-Review & Editing, all authors; Supervision, C.R.-A. and G.d.V. All authors have read and agreed to the published version of the manuscript.

Funding: This research was funded by Agencia Estatal de Investigación, Ministerio de Ciencia, Innovación y Universidades, co-funded by the European Regional Development Fund ERDF (grant number RTI2018-095039-B-I00) and from the Carlos III Institute of Health, Ministry of Economy and Competitiveness (Spain), reference FSI17/1728.

Conflicts of Interest: Guillermo de Velasco reports consulting and advisory services and speaking/writing engagements from Pfizer, Novartis, Bayer, Roche, Ipsen, Astellas, Bristol-Myers Squibb, and MSD, and research fees from Ipsen, Roche, and Pfizer, outside the submitted work. Cristina Rodriguez-Antona reports research projects funded by Pfizer.

References

1. Ferlay, J.; Colombet, M.; Soerjomataram, I.; Mathers, C.; Parkin, D.M.; Piñeros, M.; Znaor, A.; Bray, F. Estimating the global cancer incidence and mortality in 2018: GLOBOCAN sources and methods. *Int. J. Cancer* **2019**, *144*, 1941–1953. [CrossRef]
2. Moch, H.; Cubilla, A.L.; Humphrey, P.A.; Reuter, V.E.; Ulbright, T.M. The 2016 WHO classification of tumors of the urinary system and male genital organs-part A: Renal, penile, and testicular tumors. *Eur. Urol.* **2016**, *70*, 93–105. [CrossRef]
3. TNM. Classification of Malignant Tumors, 8th Edition | Wiley [Internet]. Wiley.com. Available online: https://www.wiley.com/en-es/TNM+Classification+of+Malignant+Tumors%2C+8th+Edition-p-9781119263579 (accessed on 1 November 2019).
4. Janzen, N.K.; Kim, H.L.; Figlin, R.A.; Belldegrun, A.S. Surveillance after radical or partial nephrectomy for localized renal cell carcinoma and management of recurrent disease. *Urol. Clin. N. Am.* **2003**, *30*, 843–852. [CrossRef]
5. Meskawi, M.; Sun, M.; Trinh, Q.-D.; Bianchi, M.; Hansen, J.; Tian, Z.; Rink, M.; Ismail, S.; Shariat, S.F.; Montorsi, F.; et al. A review of integrated staging systems for renal cell carcinoma. *Eur. Urol.* **2012**, *62*, 303–314. [CrossRef]
6. Patard, J.-J.; Kim, H.L.; Lam, J.S.; Dorey, F.J.; Pantuck, A.J.; Zisman, A.; Ficarra, V.; Han, K.R.; Cindolo, L.; De La Taille, A.; et al. Use of the University of California Los Angeles integrated staging system to predict survival in renal cell carcinoma: An international multicenter study. *J. Clin. Oncol.* **2004**, *22*, 3316–3322. [CrossRef] [PubMed]
7. Leibovich, B.C.; Blute, M.L.; Cheville, J.C.; Lohse, C.M.; Frank, I.; Kwon, E.D.; Weaver, A.L.; Parker, A.S.; Zincke, H. Prediction of progression after radical nephrectomy for patients with clear cell renal cell carcinoma: A stratification tool for prospective clinical trials. *Cancer* **2003**, *97*, 1663–1671. [CrossRef] [PubMed]
8. Gnarra, J.R.; Tory, K.; Weng, Y.; Schmidt, L.; Wei, M.H.; Li, H.; Latif, F.; Liu, S.; Chen, F.; Duh, F.M.; et al. Mutations of the VHL tumor suppressor gene in renal carcinoma. *Nat. Genet.* **1994**, *7*, 85–90. [CrossRef] [PubMed]
9. Brugarolas, J. Molecular genetics of clear-cell renal cell carcinoma. *J. Clin. Oncol.* **2014**, *32*, 1968–1976. [CrossRef] [PubMed]
10. Gerlinger, M.; Horswell, S.; Larkin, J.; Rowan, A.J.; Salm, M.P.; Varela, I.; Fisher, R.; McGranahan, N.; Matthews, N.; Santos, C.R.; et al. Genomic architecture and evolution of clear renal cell carcinomas defined by multiregion sequencing. *Nat. Genet.* **2014**, *46*, 225–233. [CrossRef]
11. Linehan, W.M.; Ricketts, C.J. The Cancer Genome Atlas of renal cell carcinoma: Findings and clinical implications. *Nat. Rev. Urol.* **2019**, *16*, 539–552. [CrossRef]
12. Ljungberg, B.; Albiges, L.; Abu-Ghanem, Y.; Bensalah, K.; Dabestani, S.; Fernández-Pello, S.; Rachel, H.G.; Fabian, H.; Milan, H.; Markus, A.K.; et al. European association of urology guidelines on renal cell carcinoma: The 2019 update. *Eur. Urol.* **2019**, *75*, 799–810. [CrossRef] [PubMed]
13. Choueiri, T.K.; Motzer, R.J. Systemic therapy for metastatic renal-cell carcinoma. *N. Engl. J. Med.* **2017**, *376*, 354–366. [CrossRef] [PubMed]
14. de Velasco, G.; Bex, A.; Albiges, L.; Powles, T.; Rini, B.I.; Motzer, R.J.; Heng, D.Y.C.; Escudier, B. Sequencing and combination of systemic therapy in metastatic renal cell carcinoma. *Eur. Urol. Oncol.* **2019**, *2*, 505–514. [CrossRef]

15. Heng, D.Y.C.; Xie, W.; Regan, M.M.; Warren, M.A.; Golshayan, A.R.; Sahi, C.; Eigl, B.J.; Ruether, J.D.; Cheng, T.; North, S.; et al. Prognostic factors for overall survival in patients with metastatic renal cell carcinoma treated with vascular endothelial growth factor-targeted agents: Results from a large, multicenter study. *J. Clin. Oncol.* **2009**, *27*, 5794–5799. [CrossRef]
16. Graham, J.; Dudani, S.; Heng, D.Y.C. Prognostication in kidney cancer: Recent advances and future directions. *J. Clin. Oncol.* **2018**, *36*, 3567–3573. [CrossRef]
17. Hargreaves, D.C.; Crabtree, G.R. ATP-dependent chromatin remodeling: Genetics, genomics and mechanisms. *Cell Res.* **2011**, *21*, 396–420. [CrossRef]
18. Kadoch, C.; Hargreaves, D.C.; Hodges, C.; Elias, L.; Ho, L.; Ranish, J.; Crabtree, G.R. Proteomic and bioinformatic analysis of mammalian SWI/SNF complexes identifies extensive roles in human malignancy. *Nat. Genet.* **2013**, *45*, 592–601. [CrossRef]
19. Masliah-Planchon, J.; Bièche, I.; Guinebretière, J.-M.; Bourdeaut, F.; Delattre, O. SWI/SNF chromatin remodeling and human malignancies. *Annu. Rev. Pathol. Mech. Dis.* **2015**, *10*, 145–171. [CrossRef]
20. Varela, I.; Tarpey, P.; Raine, K.; Huang, D.; Ong, C.K.; Stephens, P.; Davies, H.; Jones, D.; Lin, M.L.; Teague, J.; et al. Exome sequencing identifies frequent mutation of the SWI/SNF complex gene PBRM1 in renal carcinoma. *Nature* **2011**, *469*, 539–542. [CrossRef]
21. Chowdhury, B.; Porter, E.G.; Stewart, J.C.; Ferreira, C.R.; Schipma, M.J.; Dykhuizen, E.C. PBRM1 regulates the expression of genes involved in metabolism and cell adhesion in renal clear cell carcinoma. *PLoS ONE* **2016**, *11*, e0153718. [CrossRef]
22. Kakarougkas, A.; Ismail, A.; Chambers, A.L.; Riballo, E.; Herbert, A.D.; Künzel, J.; Löbrich, M.; Jeggo, P.A.; Downs, J.A. Requirement for PBAF in transcriptional repression and repair at DNA breaks in actively transcribed regions of chromatin. *Mol. Cell* **2014**, *55*, 723–732. [CrossRef] [PubMed]
23. Brownlee, P.M.; Chambers, A.L.; Cloney, R.; Bianchi, A.; Downs, J.A. BAF180 promotes cohesion and prevents genome instability and aneuploidy. *Cell Rep.* **2014**, *6*, 973–981. [CrossRef] [PubMed]
24. Macher-Goeppinger, S.; Keith, M.; Tagscherer, K.E.; Singer, S.; Winkler, J.; Hofmann, T.G.; Pahernik, S.; Duensing, S.; Hohenfellner, M.; Kopitz, J.; et al. PBRM1 (BAF180) protein is functionally regulated by p53-induced protein degradation in renal cell carcinomas. *J Pathol.* **2015**, *237*, 460–471. [CrossRef]
25. Burrows, A.E.; Smogorzewska, A.; Elledge, S.J. Polybromo-associated BRG1-associated factor components BRD7 and BAF180 are critical regulators of p53 required for induction of replicative senescence. *Proc. Natl. Acad. Sci. USA* **2010**, *107*, 14280–14285. [CrossRef]
26. Murakami, A.; Wang, L.; Kalhorn, S.; Schraml, P.; Rathmell, W.K.; Tan, A.C.; Nemenoff, R.; Stenmark, K.; Jiang, B.H.; Reyland, M.E.; et al. Context-dependent role for chromatin remodeling component PBRM1/BAF180 in clear cell renal cell carcinoma. *Oncogenesis* **2017**, *6*, e287. [CrossRef]
27. Gordan, J.D.; Bertout, J.A.; Hu, C.-J.; Diehl, J.A.; Simon, M.C. HIF-2alpha promotes hypoxic cell proliferation by enhancing c-myc transcriptional activity. *Cancer Cell* **2007**, *11*, 335–347. [CrossRef]
28. Linehan, W.M.; Srinivasan, R.; Schmidt, L.S. The genetic basis of kidney cancer: A metabolic disease. *Nat. Rev. Urol.* **2010**, *7*, 277–285. [CrossRef]
29. Xia, W.; Nagase, S.; Montia, A.G.; Kalachikov, S.M.; Keniry, M.; Su, T.; Memeo, L.; Hibshoosh, H.; Parsons, R. BAF180 is a critical regulator of p21 induction and a tumor suppressor mutated in breast cancer. *Cancer Res.* **2008**, *68*, 1667–1674. [CrossRef]
30. Benusiglio, P.R.; Couvé, S.; Gilbert-Dussardier, B.; Deveaux, S.; Le Jeune, H.; Da Costa, M.; Fromont, G.; Memeteau, F.; Yacoub, M.; Coupier, I.; et al. A germline mutation in PBRM1 predisposes to renal cell carcinoma. *J. Med. Genet.* **2015**, *52*, 426–430. [CrossRef]
31. Ricketts, C.J.; De Cubas, A.A.; Fan, H.; Smith, C.C.; Lang, M.; Reznik, E.; Bowlby, R.; Gibb, E.A.; Akbani, R.; Beroukhim, R.; et al. The cancer genome atlas comprehensive molecular characterization of renal cell carcinoma. *Cell Rep.* **2018**, *23*, 313.e5–326.e5. [CrossRef]
32. Bailey, M.H.; Tokheim, C.; Porta-Pardo, E.; Sengupta, S.; Bertrand, D.; Weerasinghe, A.; Colaprico, A.; Wendl, M.C.; Kim, J.; Reardon, B.; et al. Comprehensive characterization of cancer driver genes and mutations. *Cell* **2018**, *173*, 371.e18–385.e18. [CrossRef]
33. cBioPortal for Cancer Genomics [Internet]. Available online: http://www.cbioportal.org/ (accessed on 27 November 2019).

34. Gerlinger, M.; Rowan, A.J.; Horswell, S.; Math, M.; Larkin, J.; Endesfelder, D.; Gronroos, E.; Martinez, P.; Matthews, N.; Stewart, A.; et al. Intratumor heterogeneity and branched evolution revealed by multiregion sequencing. *N. Engl. J. Med.* **2012**, *366*, 883–892. [CrossRef]
35. Turajlic, S.; Xu, H.; Litchfield, K.; Rowan, A.; Chambers, T.; Lopez, J.I.; Nicol, D.; O'Brien, T.; Larkin, J.; Horswell, S.; et al. Tracking cancer evolution reveals constrained routes to metastases: TRACERx renal. *Cell* **2018**, *173*, 581.e12–594.e12. [CrossRef]
36. Joseph, R.W.; Kapur, P.; Serie, D.J.; Parasramka, M.; Ho, T.H.; Cheville, J.C.; Frenkel, E.; Parker, A.S.; Brugarolas, J. Clear cell renal cell carcinoma subtypes identified by BAP1 and PBRM1 expression. *J. Urol.* **2016**, *195*, 180–187. [CrossRef]
37. Peña-Llopis, S.; Vega-Rubín-de-Celis, S.; Liao, A.; Leng, N.; Pavía-Jiménez, A.; Wang, S.; Yamasaki, T.; Zhrebker, L.; Sivanand, S.; Spence, P.; et al. BAP1 loss defines a new class of renal cell carcinoma. *Nat. Genet.* **2012**, *44*, 751–759. [CrossRef]
38. Peña-Llopis, S.; Christie, A.; Xie, X.-J.; Brugarolas, J. Cooperation and antagonism among cancer genes: The renal cancer paradigm. *Cancer Res.* **2013**, *73*, 4173–4179. [CrossRef]
39. Gu, Y.-F.; Cohn, S.; Christie, A.; McKenzie, T.; Wolff, N.; Do, Q.N.; Madhuranthakam, A.J.; Pedrosa, I.; Wang, T.; Dey, A.; et al. Modeling renal cell carcinoma in mice: Bap1 and Pbrm1 inactivation drive tumor grade. *Cancer Discov.* **2017**, *7*, 900–917. [CrossRef]
40. Kapur, P.; Peña-Llopis, S.; Christie, A.; Zhrebker, L.; Pavía-Jiménez, A.; Rathmell, W.K.; Xie, X.J.; Brugarolas, J. Effects on survival of BAP1 and PBRM1 mutations in sporadic clear-cell renal-cell carcinoma: A retrospective analysis with independent validation. *Lancet Oncol.* **2013**, *14*, 159–167. [CrossRef]
41. Gossage, L.; Murtaza, M.; Slatter, A.F.; Lichtenstein, C.P.; Warren, A.; Haynes, B.; Marass, F.; Roberts, I.; Shanahan, S.J.; Claas, A.; et al. Clinical and pathological impact of VHL, PBRM1, BAP1, SETD2, KDM6A, and JARID1c in clear cell renal cell carcinoma. *Genes Chromosomes Cancer* **2014**, *53*, 38–51. [CrossRef]
42. Pawłowski, R.; Mühl, S.M.; Sulser, T.; Krek, W.; Moch, H.; Schraml, P. Loss of PBRM1 expression is associated with renal cell carcinoma progression. *Int. J. Cancer* **2013**, *132*, E11–E17. [CrossRef]
43. da Costa, W.H.; Rezende, M.; Carneiro, F.C.; Rocha, R.M.; da Cunha, I.W.; Carraro, D.M.; Guimaraes, G.C.; de Cassio Zequi, S. Polybromo-1 (PBRM1), a SWI/SNF complex subunit is a prognostic marker in clear cell renal cell carcinoma. *BJU Int.* **2014**, *113*, E157–E163. [CrossRef]
44. Wang, Z.; Peng, S.; Guo, L.; Xie, H.; Wang, A.; Shang, Z.; Niu, Y. Prognostic and clinicopathological value of PBRM1 expression in renal cell carcinoma. *Clin. Chim. Acta* **2018**, *486*, 9–17. [CrossRef]
45. Nam, S.J.; Lee, C.; Park, J.H.; Moon, K.C. Decreased PBRM1 expression predicts unfavorable prognosis in patients with clear cell renal cell carcinoma. *Urol. Oncol.* **2015**, *33*, 340.e9–340.e16. [CrossRef]
46. Hakimi, A.A.; Ostrovnaya, I.; Reva, B.; Schultz, N.; Chen, Y.-B.; Gonen, M.; Liu, H.; Takeda, S.; Voss, M.H.; Tickoo, S.K.; et al. Adverse outcomes in clear cell renal cell carcinoma with mutations of 3p21 epigenetic regulators BAP1 and SETD2: A report by MSKCC and the KIRC TCGA research network. *Clin. Cancer Res.* **2013**, *19*, 3259–3267. [CrossRef]
47. Jiang, W.; Dulaimi, E.; Devarajan, K.; Parsons, T.; Wang, Q.; O'Neill, R.; Solomides, C.; Peiper, S.C.; Testa, J.R.; Uzzo, R.; et al. Intratumoral heterogeneity analysis reveals hidden associations between protein expression losses and patient survival in clear cell renal cell carcinoma. *Oncotarget* **2017**, *8*, 37423–37434. [CrossRef]
48. Kim, J.-Y.; Lee, S.-H.; Moon, K.C.; Kwak, C.; Kim, H.H.; Keam, B.; Kim, T.M.; Heo, D.S. The impact of PBRM1 expression as a prognostic and predictive marker in metastatic renal cell carcinoma. *J. Urol.* **2015**, *194*, 1112–1119. [CrossRef]
49. Carlo, M.I.; Manley, B.; Patil, S.; Woo, K.M.; Coskey, D.T.; Redzematovic, A.; Arcila, M.; Ladanyi, M.; Lee, W.; Chen, Y.B.; et al. Genomic alterations and outcomes with VEGF-targeted therapy in patients with clear cell renal cell carcinoma. *Kidney Cancer* **2017**, *1*, 49–56. [CrossRef]
50. Tennenbaum, D.M.; Manley, B.J.; Zabor, E.; Becerra, M.F.; Carlo, M.I.; Casuscelli, J.; Redzematovic, A.; Khan, N.; Arcila, M.E.; Voss, M.H.; et al. Genomic alterations as predictors of survival among patients within a combined cohort with clear cell renal cell carcinoma undergoing cytoreductive nephrectomy. *Urol. Oncol.* **2017**, *35*, 532.e7–532.e13. [CrossRef]
51. Voss, M.H.; Reising, A.; Cheng, Y.; Patel, P.; Marker, M.; Kuo, F.; Chan, T.A.; Choueiri, T.K.; Hsieh, J.J.; Hakimi, A.A.; et al. Genomically annotated risk model for advanced renal-cell carcinoma: A retrospective cohort study. *Lancet Oncol.* **2018**, *19*, 1688–1698. [CrossRef]

52. Kim, S.H.; Park, W.S.; Park, E.Y.; Park, B.; Joo, J.; Joung, J.Y.; Seo, H.K.; Lee, K.H.; Chung, J. The prognostic value of BAP1, PBRM1, pS6, PTEN, TGase2, PD-L1, CA9, PSMA, and Ki-67 tissue markers in localized renal cell carcinoma: A retrospective study of tissue microarrays using immunohistochemistry. *PLoS ONE* **2017**. [CrossRef]
53. Voss, M.H.; Hakimi, A.A.; Pham, C.G.; Brannon, A.R.; Chen, Y.-B.; Cunha, L.F.; Akin, O.; Liu, H.; Takeda, S.; Scott, S.N.; et al. Tumor genetic analyses of patients with metastatic renal cell carcinoma and extended benefit from mTOR inhibitor therapy. *Clin. Cancer Res.* **2014**, *20*, 1955–1964. [CrossRef]
54. Kwiatkowski, D.J.; Choueiri, T.K.; Fay, A.P.; Rini, B.I.; Thorner, A.R.; de Velasco, G.; Tyburczy, M.E.; Hamieh, L.; Albiges, L.; Agarwal, N.; et al. Mutations in TSC1, TSC2, and MTOR are associated with response to rapalogs in patients with metastatic renal cell carcinoma. *Clin. Cancer Res.* **2016**, *22*, 2445–2452. [CrossRef]
55. Ho, T.H.; Choueiri, T.K.; Wang, K.; Karam, J.A.; Chalmers, Z.; Frampton, G.; Elvin, J.A.; Johnson, A.; Liu, X.; Lin, Y.; et al. Correlation between molecular subclassifications of clear cell renal cell carcinoma and targeted therapy response. *Eur. Urol. Focus* **2016**, *2*, 204–209. [CrossRef]
56. Hsieh, J.J.; Chen, D.; Wang, P.I.; Marker, M.; Redzematovic, A.; Chen, Y.B.; Selcuklu, S.D.; Weinhold, N.; Bouvier, N.; Huberman, K.H.; et al. Genomic biomarkers of a randomized trial comparing first-line everolimus and sunitinib in patients with metastatic renal cell carcinoma. *Eur. Urol.* **2017**, *71*, 405–414. [CrossRef]
57. Miao, D.; Margolis, C.A.; Gao, W.; Voss, M.H.; Li, W.; Martini, D.J.; Norton, C.; Bossé, D.; Wankowicz, S.M.; Cullen, D.; et al. Genomic correlates of response to immune checkpoint therapies in clear cell renal cell carcinoma. *Science* **2018**, *359*, 801–806. [CrossRef]
58. Braun, D.A.; Ishii, Y.; Walsh, A.M.; Van Allen, E.M.; Wu, C.J.; Shukla, S.A.; Choueiri, T.K. Clinical validation of PBRM1 alterations as a marker of immune checkpoint inhibitor response in renal cell carcinoma. *JAMA Oncol.* **2019**, *5*, 1631–1633. [CrossRef]
59. McDermott, D.F.; Huseni, M.A.; Atkins, M.B.; Motzer, R.J.; Rini, B.I.; Escudier, B.; Fong, L.; Joseph, R.W.; Pal, S.K.; Reeves, J.A.; et al. Clinical activity and molecular correlates of response to atezolizumab alone or in combination with bevacizumab versus sunitinib in renal cell carcinoma. *Nat. Med.* **2018**, *24*, 749–757. [CrossRef]
60. Fay, A.P.; de Velasco, G.; Ho, T.H.; Van Allen, E.M.; Murray, B.; Albiges, L.; Signoretti, S.; Hakimi, A.A.; Stanton, M.L.; Bellmunt, J.; et al. Whole-exome sequencing in two extreme phenotypes of response to VEGF-targeted therapies in patients with metastatic clear cell renal cell carcinoma. *J. Natl. Compr. Cancer Netw. JNCCN* **2016**, *14*, 820–824. [CrossRef]
61. Motzer, R.J.; Tannir, N.M.; McDermott, D.F.; ArénFrontera, O.; Melichar, B.; Choueiri, T.K.; Plimack, E.R.; Barthélémy, P.; Porta, C.; George, S.; et al. Nivolumab plus ipilimumab versus sunitinib in advanced renal-cell carcinoma. *N. Engl. J. Med.* **2018**, *378*, 1277–1290. [CrossRef]
62. Motzer, R.J.; Escudier, B.; McDermott, D.F.; George, S.; Hammers, H.J.; Srinivas, S.; Tykodi, S.S.; Sosman, J.A.; Procopio, G.; Plimack, E.R.; et al. Nivolumab versus everolimus in advanced renal-cell carcinoma. *N. Engl. J. Med.* **2015**, *373*, 1803–1813. [CrossRef]
63. Maia, M.C.; Almeida, L.; Bergerot, P.G.; Dizman, N.; Pal, S.K. Relationship of tumor mutational burden (TMB) to immunotherapy response in metastatic renal cell carcinoma (mRCC). *J. Clin. Oncol.* **2018**, *36* (Suppl. 6), 662. [CrossRef]
64. Pan, D.; Kobayashi, A.; Jiang, P.; Ferrari de Andrade, L.; Tay, R.E.; Luoma, A.M.; Tsoucas, D.; Qiu, X.; Lim, K.; Rao, P.; et al. A major chromatin regulator determines resistance of tumor cells to T cell-mediated killing. *Science* **2018**, *359*, 770–775. [CrossRef]
65. Soussi, T.; Wiman, K.G. TP53: An oncogene in disguise. *Cell Death Differ.* **2015**, *22*, 1239–1249. [CrossRef]
66. Ding, H.; Zhao, J.; Zhang, Y.; Yu, J.; Liu, M.; Li, X.; Xu, L.; Lin, M.; Liu, C.; He, Z.; et al. Systematic analysis of drug vulnerabilities conferred by tumor suppressor loss. *Cell Rep.* **2019**, *27*, 3331.e6–3344.e6. [CrossRef]

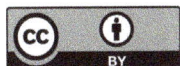 © 2019 by the authors. Licensee MDPI, Basel, Switzerland. This article is an open access article distributed under the terms and conditions of the Creative Commons Attribution (CC BY) license (http://creativecommons.org/licenses/by/4.0/).

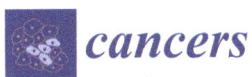

Review

The Interplay between Inflammation, Anti-Angiogenic Agents, and Immune Checkpoint Inhibitors: Perspectives for Renal Cell Cancer Treatment

Nicole Brighi [1], Alberto Farolfi [1,*], Vincenza Conteduca [1], Giorgia Gurioli [2], Stefania Gargiulo [2], Valentina Gallà [3], Giuseppe Schepisi [1], Cristian Lolli [1], Chiara Casadei [1] and Ugo De Giorgi [1]

[1] Medical Oncology Department, Istituto Scientifico Romagnolo per lo Studio e la Cura dei Tumori (IRST) IRCCS, 47014 Meldola, Italy; nicolebrighi@hotmail.com (N.B.); vincenza.conteduca@irst.emr.it (V.C.); giuseppe.schepisi@irst.emr.it (G.S.); cristian.lolli@irst.emr.it (C.L.); chiara.casadei@irst.emr.it (C.C.); ugo.degiorgi@irst.emr.it (U.D.G.)

[2] Bioscience Laboratory, Istituto Scientifico Romagnolo per lo Studio e la Cura dei Tumori (IRST) IRCCS, 47014 Meldola, Italy; giorgia.gurioli@irst.emr.it (G.G.); stefania.gargiulo.94@gmail.com (S.G.)

[3] Unit of Biostatistics and Clinical Trials, Istituto Scientifico Romagnolo per lo Studio e la Cura dei Tumori (IRST) IRCCS, 47014 Meldola, Italy; valentina.galla@irst.emr.it

* Correspondence: alberto.farolfi@irst.emr.it; Tel.: +39-0543739100; Fax: +39-0543739151

Received: 4 November 2019; Accepted: 1 December 2019; Published: 4 December 2019

Abstract: Treatment options for metastatic renal cell carcinoma (RCC) have been expanding in the last years, from the consolidation of several anti-angiogenic agents to the approval of immune checkpoint inhibitors (ICIs). The rationale for the use of immunomodulating agents derived from the observation that RCC usually shows a diffuse immune-cell infiltrate. ICIs target Cytotoxic T Lymphocytes Antigen 4 (CTLA-4), programmed death 1 (PD-1), or its ligand (PD-L1), showing promising therapeutic efficacy in RCC. PD-L1 expression is associated with poor prognosis; however, its predictive role remains debated. In fact, ICIs may be a valid option even for PD-L1 negative patients. The establishment of valid predictors of treatment response to available therapeutic options is advocated to identify those patients who could benefit from these agents. Both local and systemic inflammation contribute to tumorigenesis and development of cancer. The interplay of tumor-immune status and of cancer-related systemic inflammation is pivotal for ICI-treatment outcome, but there is an unmet need for a more precise characterization. To date, little is known on the role of inflammation markers on PD-1 blockade in RCC. In this paper, we review the current knowledge on the interplay between inflammation markers, PD-1 axis, and anti-angiogenic agents in RCC, focusing on biological rationale, implications for treatment, and possible future perspectives.

Keywords: kidney cancer; immunotherapy; renal cell; inflammation markers; programmed death-ligand 1; immune checkpoint inhibitors; prognostic factors; predictive factors

1. Introduction

Renal cell carcinoma (RCC) is the seventh most common type of cancer in men and the tenth in women in Western countries [1,2]. RCC incidence has been increasing in the last 30 years, at an annual rate of around 3%, but the figures are recently showing a tendency of plateauing [3]. At the time of diagnosis, 25% to 30% of patients present with metastatic disease associated with high mortality. However, when all stages of RCC are considered, mortality rates seem to have leveled [4]. In fact, the widespread use of noninvasive radiological techniques leads to frequent incidental detection of early and small kidney tumors, which are potentially curable.

For many years, treatments for advanced RCC were limited to interferon α (IFNα) and interleukin (IL)-2. After the cytokine era, two more categories of drugs became available, namely anti-angiogenic agents and mammalian target of rapamycin (mTOR) inhibitors. In the last years, immune-checkpoint inhibitors (ICIs) obtained indication at first as second-line treatment and are now available also as first-line treatment in metastatic RCC.

In this paper, we review the current knowledge on the interaction of inflammation and the PD-L1/PD-L1 axis in RCC, focusing on their possible role as prognostic and predictive factors in patients affected by these tumors and treated with ICIs or anti-angiogenic agents.

2. Anti-Angiogenic Agents in RCC Treatment

Anti-angiogenic agents, such as various tyrosine kinase inhibitors (TKIs) (i.e., sunitinib, axitinib, sorafenib, pazopanib, and lenvatinib), target multiple receptors for platelet-derived growth factor (PDGF-Rs) and vascular endothelial growth factor receptors (VEGFRs), which play a role in both tumor angiogenesis and tumor-cell proliferation. Similarly, bevacizumab, a recombinant humanized monoclonal antibody, blocks angiogenesis by inhibiting vascular endothelial growth factor A (VEGF-A). Also, the mesenchymal–epithelial transition (MET) and multityrosine kinases inhibitor cabozantinib is currently used in advanced RCC.

The use of these drugs resulted in improved outcomes, particularly for overall survival (OS) (sunitinib, pazopanib, and cabozantinib) and for progression-free survival (PFS) (sunitinib, axitinib, cabozantinib, sorafenib, and pazopanib) [5–12].

3. Immune Checkpoint Inhibitors in RCC Treatment

In recent years, therapeutic options for RCC have expanded, and the use of ICIs, has been approved. Nivolumab, targeting programmed-death receptor 1 (PD-1), and ipilimumab, directed against cytotoxic T lymphocytes antigen 4 (CTLA-4), are currently considered standard treatment options for RCC. The rationale for the use of these drugs lies in the inhibitory role on specific pathways related to the immune response, frequently hyperactivated by tumor-cell interaction. By inhibiting these pathways, ICIs reactivate an immune response against tumor cells. The high mutation load typical of RCC probably correlates with a high antigen expression and has led to the testing of these drugs at different stages of the disease. CheckMate 025 was a large phase III clinical trial, comparing nivolumab (PD-1 inhibitor) to everolimus in patients with locally advanced or metastatic RCC, progressed after treatment with at least one VEGF/VEGFR inhibitor. The study showed an OS benefit in patients treated with nivolumab. Furthermore, the immunotherapy-treated cohort had a higher overall response rate (ORR) compared to everolimus, with a considerable rate of long-lasting responses [13]. Due to these satisfactory results, ICIs are being tested in earlier settings (adjuvant and neo-adjuvant) and are now also available as first-line treatment [14,15].

In fact, another large phase III study has demonstrated that the combination of ipilimumab and nivolumab was superior to sunitinib in intermediate- and poor-risk patients when used as first-line treatment. In this population, the association of the two ICIs improved OS, as well as response rate, with a complete response rate of about 10% [15].

Furthermore, following the mounting evidence of the interaction between angiogenesis and immune escape, several trials have been designed and conducted to evaluate the role of the association of ICIs with antiangiogenic agents as first-line treatment (see Table 1) or further.

For example, the IMmotion150 study, a phase II trial, evaluated the use of atezolizumab (an anti-PD-L1 inhibitor) plus bevacizumab compared to atezolizumab alone or sunitinib as first-line treatment for locally advanced and metastatic RCC. The study showed that patients treated with the association of atezolizumab and bevacizumab had a longer PFS compared to atezolizumab (6.1 months) and sunitinib arms; furthermore, a higher percentage ORR was reported in the combination arm. Interesting results were observed in patients with PD-L1 positive expression (≥1%), achieving a longer PFS (14.7 months) and higher ORR (46%) in the atezolizumab monotherapy arm [16].

Two recent phase III trials (JAVELIN Renal 101 and KEYNOTE-426) investigated the role of the association of ICIs and TKIs and showed better outcomes in patients treated respectively with the association of avelumab plus axitinib or pembrolizumab plus axitinib compared to sunitinib in previously untreated advanced RCC [17,18].

COSMIC-313 (NCT 03937219) is a multicenter, randomized, controlled phase III trial that evaluates the combination of cabozantinib/placebo plus nivolumab and ipilimumab in previously untreated intermediate- and poor-risk RCC.

The interplay of inflammatory mediators and pathways related to immune response is extremely complex, and its role is pivotal both for RCC tumorigenesis and for treatment response.

Table 1. First-line trials in advanced renal cell carcinoma, combining anti-angiogenic agents and immune checkpoint inhibitors.

Trial Name	Trial Phase	Agents	No. of Patients	mPFS (Months)	Overall Response Rate	Ref.
Checkmate 016	I	Nivolumab + sunitinib	33	48.9	52%	[19]
Checkmate 016	I	Nivolumab + pazopanib	20	31.4	45%	[19]
NCT02133742	Ib	Axitinib + pembrolizumab	52	15.1	71%	[20]
NCT00372853	I	Tremelimumab + sunitinib	28	NA	76%	[21]
KEYNOTE-018	I/II	Pazopanib + pembrolizumab	10	NA	60%	[22]
IMmotion150	II	Bevacizumab + atezolizumab vs. atezolizumab vs. sunitinib	305	11.7	NA	[16]
IMmotion151	III	Bevacizumab + atezolizumab vs. sunitinib	101 (ongoing)	NA	32% (ongoing)	[23]
JAVELIN Renal 100	Ib	Axitinib + avelumab	55	NA	58%	[24]
JAVELIN Renal 101	III	Axitinib + avelumab vs. sunitinib	886	13.8	51%	[17]
CLEAR	III	Lenvatinib + everolimus or pembrolizumab vs. sunitinib	Ongoing	NA	NA	[25]
KEYNOTE-426	III	Axitinib + pembrolizumab vs. sunitinib	Ongoing	NA	NA	[18]
Checkmate 9ER	III	Nivolumab + cabozantinib vs. sunitinib	Ongoing	NA	NA	[26]
COSMIC-313	III	Nivolumab + ipilimumab + cabozantinib vs. nivolumab + ipilimumab + placebo	Ongoing	NA	NA	NA

Abbreviations: mPFS = median progression-free survival, NA = not available, Ref. = reference.

4. Inflammation and Cancer and the PD-1/PD-L1 Axis

The potential relation between cancer and inflammation was originally proposed by Virchow in the 19th century [27]. In the following years, the pivotal role of inflammation in mediating tumorigenesis, progression, and metastasis of cancer has progressively been unraveled and recognized [28,29].

It has been observed that systemic inflammation damages the immune response, allowing tumor cells to escape from immune surveillance. Cancer immune surveillance is a fundamental host-defense process to inhibit carcinogenesis. However, cancer cells can progressively adapt to escape from immune-mediated rejection, through the process of "immune editing", resulting from a selective pressure on the tumor microenvironment, leading to tumor progression [30].

The role of systemic inflammation, and particularly of all the leucocytes cells, in aiding tumoral immune escape is mediated by the inhibition of apoptosis, promotion of genomic instability and tumoral invasion, angiogenesis, and metastatic spread through different processes [27,28,31].

Neutrophils can be recruited by the tumor through the production of cancer-related chemokines and cytokines (e.g., IL-6 and TNF). Neutrophils are involved in the proliferation, invasion, and metastatic spread of tumor cells, also inducing drug resistance [30,32].

A lower level of lymphocytes, which is frequently observed in systemic inflammation, is frequently related to low levels of CD4+ T cells, resulting in less-effective immune surveillance. On the other hand, tumor-associated macrophages (TAMs), deriving from monocytes, can promote invasion, proliferation, and angiogenesis of tumor cells, thus favoring cancer spread and metastases formation [28,30].

Cyclooxygenase-2 (COX-2) is involved in the conversion of arachidonic acid to prostaglandin H2, an important precursor of prostacyclin, which is expressed widely in inflammation and in tumors. In RCC, COX-2 expression is present in the majority of the tumors and correlates with a worse stage and grade and poorer outcomes [33–35].

Epidemiological data demonstrate that the use of nonsteroidal anti-inflammatory drugs (NSAIDs), including long-term use of aspirin, decreases incidence, metastasis, and mortality risk in several cancers [36–40]. The antitumoral effect of NSAIDs is thought to be related mainly to the inhibition of COX-2, but COX-independent mechanisms have also been observed [41]. NSAIDs have been shown to inhibit tumor growth by inducing cancer-cell apoptosis and inhibiting the Wnt/β-catenin signaling pathway [42]. NSAIDs may therefore inhibit the development of early malignant lesions and cause regression of tumors in animal models of colorectal cancers and a decrease in recurrence rates of adenomas [43–45]. In RCC, NSAIDs (but not aspirin) have been implicated as a risk factor for RCC development [46,47]. In the setting of metastatic RCC, a retrospective analysis on 4736 patients included in several phase II and phase III trials concluded that NSAIDs do not confer a survival advantage in mRCC patients [48].

Taking into account the paramount importance of inflammation in cancer development, the role of IL-1 as potential mediator for tumoral angiogenesis and metastatic spread is being investigated in various preclinical models. Two recent studies showed that IL-1b promotes the stem-cell properties of gastric cancer cells, through activation of the phosphoinositide 3-kinase pathway [49] and the IL-1b/IL-6 network is highly expressed in human colorectal cancer, reinforcing the possible correlation of the inflammatory mediators with cancer progression [50].

Canakinumab is a human monoclonal antibody against interleukin-1b. Canakinumab has been proven to significantly reduce atherosclerosis and other cardiometabolic diseases related to inflammation (diabetes, stroke, and chronic kidney disease) [51]. Interestingly, a significant reduction in the incidence of lung cancer in patients treated with higher doses of canakinumab was observed. However, no significant decrease in the rate of other primary cancers was observed in the canakinumab group, as compared with the placebo.

Currently, to investigate the role of this drug on renal cell cancer, an early phase I trial (SPARC-1, NCT04028245) is enrolling patients to be treated with the association of canakinumab and spartalizumab (an anti-PD1 monoclonal antibody) as neoadjuvant treatment before radical nephrectomy.

The role of PD-1/PD-L1 axis in mediating tumor escape from the immune system has been widely investigated in the last years. Under normal conditions, the immune system can recognize cancer cells and induce apoptosis mediated by T-cell activation. The PD-1/PD-L1 pathway is an adaptive immune resistance mechanism used by cancer cells in response to the host immune-related antitumor activity. PD-L1 is overexpressed in tumor cells or in its microenvironment, and it binds to PD-1 receptors on the activated T cells, resulting in the inhibition of cytotoxic T cells and tumor escape.

Human PD-1 is a type I transmembrane glycoprotein of the CD28/CTLA-4 immune checkpoint receptor family; its ligands are PD-L1 and PD-L2 [52,53]. PD-1 is expressed in hematopoietic tissues and cells, including T cells, B cells, NK cells, monocytes/macrophages, and dendritic cells [54]. PD-1 expression is rapidly induced consequently to T- or B-cell antigen stimulation, or upon lymphoid-cell activation conditions. The expression pattern of PD-L1 is wider, displaying both constitutive and inducible expression in lymphoid, myeloid, and endothelial cells [55]. PD-L1 expression is high in many human cancers, both in the tumor-infiltrating immune cells and in the tumor cells [53,56]. In RCC patients, PD-1 is highly expressed on the surface of both activated tumor-infiltrating immune cells and peripheral blood cells [57].

The main effect of PD-1/PD-L1 interaction at the base of immune evasion is the negative signaling on the antigen receptor complexes, resulting in the trigger of the reversal of CD3-complex tyrosine phosphorylation and the decline in cytokine production and lymphocyte proliferation [58]. In addition,

PD-L1 also plays protumorigenic roles in cancer cells by binding to its receptors in hematopoietic cells, which results in activation of proliferative- and survival-signaling pathways, leading to subsequent tumor progression [59].

PD 1/PD-L1 and CTLA 4 inhibitors can target specific pathways related to immune-response hyperactivated by tumor-cell interaction. By inhibition of these targets, ICIs could reactivate a specific immune response against tumor cells. Agents targeting the PD-1/PD-L1 axis increase the proliferation and cytolytic activity of T cells, resulting in durable ORR [53].

It has been demonstrated that there is a synergistic effect of ICIs and anti-angiogenic agents (Figure 1). Besides their direct inhibitory effect on angiogenesis, anti-angiogenic agents can reverse tumor-related immune suppression through several mechanisms, such as the decrease of immunosuppressive cells (MDSCs, regulatory T cells) and cytokines (TGFβ and IL-10) and the direct inhibiting interaction on PD-1 on T cells [60]. Thus, the use of a combination of these agents and ICIs has a strong biological rationale and is currently the object of many clinical and preclinical research studies.

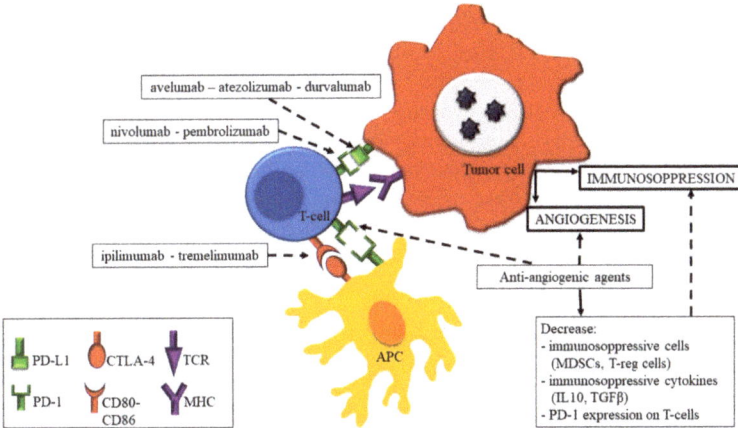

Figure 1. The synergistic effect of anti-angiogenetic agents and immune checkpoint inhibitors on tumor-derived angiogenesis and immunosuppression (dotted line: inhibiting action, continuous line: activating action). Abbreviations: APC = antigen-presenting cell; PD-L1 = programmed death-ligand 1; PD-1; programmed death 1; CTLA-4 = cytotoxic T lymphocyte antigen 4; TCR = T-cell receptor; MHC = major histocompatibility complex; MDSCs = myeloid-derived suppressor cells.

5. Inflammation as Prognostic Factor

Prognostic factors for localized RCC include anatomical, histological, clinical, and molecular features. Tumor stage (as per TNM staging) and Fuhrman nuclear grade are the strongest independent prognostic factors for localized RCC. However, the use of integrated systems (such as the UCLA Integrated Staging System (UISS); the Stage, Size, Grade and Necrosis (SSIGN) system; or other nomograms) combining multiple independent prognostic factors results in higher accuracy [61–64]. These tools have been widely used in clinical practice, to guide decision making. Several molecular and genetic markers have been investigated as potential prognostic factors for RCC: Von Hippel Lindau (VHL) gene alterations, hypoxia-induced factor 1 alpha (HIF-1a), mTOR, ribosomal protein S6 and phosphatase PTEN, Ki-67, levels of carbonic anhydrase 9 (CAIX), and matrix metalloproteinase 2 and 9 [64]. However, their role on determining prognosis is still controversial and only for investigational use. In the metastatic setting, the classical anatomical factors (stage, size, perinephric fat, and venous or adrenal invasion) used as prognostic factors in localized RCC have a very limited prognostic role. In fact, the prognostic role of the primary tumor on prognosis disappears when the tumor becomes metastatic. Some metastases features have been proved to be reliable prognostic factors. For example, the resectability of metastases is currently considered an independent prognostic factor, regardless of the anatomic site [65,66]. The presence of multiple resectable pulmonary lesions with nodal involvement is associated with worse prognosis. Bone and spinal metastases are associated with poor outcomes, similarly to the presence of multiple brain metastases [67–69].

Regarding the role of histology as prognostic factor in metastatic RCC, the histological subtype and the presence of sarcomatoid component have prognostic significance. Sarcomatoid differentiation is clearly associated with very poor prognosis [70].

As for clinical criteria, performance status (assessed either by Karnofsky index or Eastern Cooperative Oncology Group (ECOG) scale) is the most important clinical prognostic factor in metastatic RCC, regardless of the class of the type of treatment [71–73]. Other significant clinical prognostic variables are presence or absence of previous nephrectomy, time from nephrectomy to treatment, and time from diagnosis to treatment [64,73].

Additionally, low hemoglobin, elevated lactate dehydrogenase, corrected serum calcium, and inflammatory markers have been historically described as significant prognosticators [74–76]. The International Metastatic Renal-Cell Carcinoma Database Consortium (IMDC) model, one of the most-used indexes in clinical practice, efficaciously stratifies patients into three risk groups combining several clinical parameters (anemia, neutrophilia, thrombocytosis, hypercalcemia, Karnofsky performance status and time from diagnosis to treatment) [77].

Increasing evidence is showing the existence of a complex interplay between several inflammation factors and the prognosis of patients with various types of cancers, including RCC [10,30]. The biological rationale lies in the concept that local immune response and systemic inflammation play an important role in the initiation, development, and progression of cancer. Inflammatory cells, such as neutrophils, monocytes, and lymphocytes, promote the intravasation of neoplastic cells in the circulation system, allowing the growth of distant metastases. This mechanism is thought to be one of the reasons contributing to patients' poor outcomes [78,79]. In clinical practice, systemic inflammation is easily evaluated by peripheral blood counts of immune and inflammatory cells and acute-phase proteins such as C-reactive protein (CRP). Several inflammation markers or inflammation indexes have been identified. Inflammation indexes combine and integrate conventional inflammatory parameters and have been proved to be potential prognostic values in several studies focusing on various types of cancer [79–83].

Serum CRP is produced in hepatocytes; its production is regulated by inflammation-associated cytokines (IL-6 and IL-1b). These cytokines are produced in various cells, including inflammatory cells and cancer cells. Thus, serum CRP concentration might be elevated due to hepatic stimulation by cancer-cell-derived inflammatory cytokines [84].

Elevation of CRP is associated with poorer survival in patients with cancer [85,86]. CRP dosing is easily reproducible, inexpensive, and has good sensitivity. Several studies have shown that CRP can be considered a good prognostic factors both in localized and metastatic RCC, with a significant association between high CRP and worse outcomes [87–90]. One of the greatest limits of CRP as a prognosticator is the lack of a specific cutoff, due to the different values used in the available studies.

The most promising indexes identified so far are the neutrophil to lymphocyte ratio (NLR), the platelet to lymphocyte ratio (PLR), the prognostic nutritional index (PNI), the systemic immune-inflammation index (SII), and the systemic inflammation response index (SIRI).

Neutrophils, lymphocytes, and macrophages have been implicated in promoting neoplastic angiogenesis and metastases diffusion, but they are also thought to be involved in the formation of premetastatic niches and in primary and acquired drug resistance [91].

NLR, defined as the absolute neutrophil count divided by the absolute lymphocyte count, is probably the most-studied prognostic index. An increased NLR is associated with poor prognosis in several tumors such as breast, lung, pancreatic, colorectal, gastric, urothelial, prostate, ovarian, and kidney cancers [91–93]. Neutrophils are known to be able to aid the proliferation and survival of malignant cells, promoting angiogenesis and metastasis. Conversely, lymphocytes suppress tumor growth and invasion through their cytolytic activity. Taken together, patients with high NLR have a relative lymphopenia, and this may result in a poor immune response and worse outcomes. In RCC, lymphopenia in preoperative blood count has been associated with poor prognosis, and in elderly patients with RCC treated with sunitinib [94,95]. A large number of study and several meta-analyses have reported that increased NLR is associated with poor prognosis in RCC [93,96–111].

Baum et al. reported that NLR ≥ 4 was associated with a shorter OS as compared to RCC patients with NLR < 4 [112].

SII (defined as platelets*neutrophils/lymphocytes) combines these three parameters and has already been proved to be significantly associated with prognosis in hepatocellular carcinoma and in colorectal cancer [85,113]. Due to high levels of neutrophils and platelets and low levels of lymphocytes, a higher SII usually indicates a stronger inflammatory and a weaker immune response in patients. It may be associated with invasion and metastasis of tumor cells, and hence leads to poor survival.

In a recent retrospective series by Lolli et al., SII was identified as being a reliable parameter both as prognostic and predictive factor in RCC patients treated with sunitinib. Baseline SII values were independent factors for PFS and OS [114]. However, not all studies agree on the prognostic value of SII. To shed light on this issue, a recent metanalysis investigated the significance of SII in determining the prognosis of patients affected by several kinds of cancers [115]. The metanalysis confirmed that elevated SII indicates poor prognosis and may be considered a cost-effective prognostic biomarker. However, of the 15 papers included in the analysis, only one was based on RCC patients [114]. Therefore, the clinical significance of SII as prognostic factor should be further evaluated. Glasgow Prognostic Score (GPS), or its modified version (mGPS), is an index based on the combination of serum CRP and albumin. GPS and mGPS are considered a measure of systemic inflammation, representing the immune response and nutritional status of patients. Many studies have shown the independent prognostic value of GPS/mGPS in various types of cancers [116–118]. GPS/mGPS has the advantage of using a specific cutoff value, allowing comparison among studies.

In RCC, metastatic patients are reported as presenting an elevated GPS/mGPS compared to non-metastatic patients. Several studies showed a significant association between elevated GPS/mGPS and worse prognosis [119–123].

Platelet count has also been shown to be related to prognosis in RCC [77,124]. Platelet-to-lymphocyte ratio (PLR) is defined as the platelet count divided by the lymphocyte count. It is an easily acquirable and cheap marker. Higher PLR was significantly associated with worse outcomes in different types of cancers [99,125,126]. However, most studies regarding RCC failed to confirm the prognostic value of PLR in this setting [125,127,128].

PNI has been introduced as a simple and reproducible biomarker, reflecting the nutritional and immunological status of cancer patients. PNI is a combination of serum albumin and peripheral blood lymphocyte count. High values of PNI are associated with a good prognosis in cancer patients [84]. Studies evaluating the prognostic value of PNI in patients with RCC are few but confirm these results [129–135].

Recently, the determination of SIRI index (defined as neutrophils x monocytes/lymphocytes) has been determined to be a reliable prognostic factor in different kinds of tumors [136–138].

Besides aiding immune surveillance evasion, metastatic adhesion of cancer cells, and tumor angiogenesis by the production of proangiogenic factors, neutrophils can secrete large amounts of reactive oxygen species and nitric oxide, leading to T-cell disorders. Tumor-associated macrophages derive from circulating monocytes, which can be recruited to the tumor tissue and promote the growth and migration of the tumor. Another role of tumor-associated macrophages is to induce the apoptosis of activated T cells, resulting in the formation of new tumor vessels. Peripheral monocyte counts may reflect the level of tumor-associated macrophages, and higher monocyte counts are considered negative markers for tumors. Lymphocytes are crucial components of the immune system, serving as the main defense against cancer cells. They inhibit tumor progression by releasing cytokines such as interferon-γ and tumor necrosis factor-α [139]. Downregulation of peripheral lymphocytes causes an impairment of anticancer immunity and increases tumor-cell dissemination. The index SIRI combines these aforementioned cell types and reflects the complex interplay between immune and inflammatory cells in the tumor microenvironment [79].

In RCC, the potential prognostic value of SIRI has been evaluated in several studies, but the results are largely controversial.

Chen et al. investigated the role of SIRI in 414 patients and with an independent validation cohort of 168 patients with localized or locally advanced RCC who received radical or partial nephrectomy, suggesting that SIRI might be a better prognostic predictor than PLR, NLR, MLR, and MSKCC score [30].

Overall, inflammation markers and derived indexes as prognostic factors are easily measurable, reproducible, cheap, and thus advantageous.

However, some limitations need to be taken into account. One of these includes cutoff values that have not been clearly determined yet, thus strongly limiting their usefulness in the management of patients. Further studies are indeed needed to allow the use of these tools in clinical practice.

Several recent studies and meta-analyses have shown that PD-L1 expression correlates with clinical–pathological prognostic factors in RCC, such as the WHO/ISUP grade, presence of necrosis and sarcomatoid features, tumor size, and TNM stage [140,141].

Furthermore, many studies in RCC have suggested that patients with intratumoral high PD-L1 expression exhibited aggressive behavior and are related to poor outcomes, with an increased risk of cancer-related death [142–146].

However, it is known that RCC is a very heterogeneous disease, and PD-L1 expression might vary within primary tumor and between primary neoplasm and metastases, greatly limiting the value of this biomarker [147]. Another pitfall related to PD-L1 expression evaluation is the use of various antibodies in clinical practice that causes a lack of standardization and, consequently, difficulties in comparing studies' results. In Table 2, we report phase II and phase III trials evaluating various ICI regimens, along with the characteristics of the several PD-L1 antibody clones and different cutoffs used.

In addition to PD-L1 expression, identification of the lymphocyte density in the tumor microenvironment as a prognostic biomarker could facilitate detecting patients who could benefit from the checkpoint blockade [148].

Table 2. Characteristics of PD-L1 antibody clones and cutoffs used in phase II and phase III trials evaluating various ICI regimens. Cutoffs are indicated as the percentage of PD-L1 positive cells at immunohistochemistry (where not otherwise indicated).

Trial Name	ICI	PD-L1 Antibody Clone	Developer	Cutoff	Reference
Checkmate 025	Nivolumab	Not reported	Dako	PD-L1 ≥ 1% vs. <1% and ≥5% vs. <5%	[13]
Checkmate 214	Ipilimumab, nivolumab	28-8	Dako	PD-L1 ≥ 1% vs. <1%	[15]
IMMotion 150	Atezolizumab	SP142	Ventana	PD-L1 < 1% or absent (IC 0), ≥1% to <5% (IC 1), ≥5% to <10% (IC 2), or ≥10% (IC3)	[16]
IMMotion 151	Atezolizumab	SP142	Ventana	PD-L1 < 1% vs. ≥1%	[23]
Javelin Renal 101	Avelumab	SP263	Ventana	PD-L1 ≥ 1%	[17]
CLEAR	Pembrolizumab	Not reported	Not reported	Not reported	[25]
KEYNOTE-426	Pembrolizumab	22C3	Agilent Technologies	Combined positive score (PD-L1+ cell no. divided by tumor cell no., multiplied by 100)> or <1	[18]
Checkmate 9ER	Nivolumab	Not reported	Not reported	Not reported	[26]

Abbreviations: ICIs = immune checkpoint inhibitors, PD-L1 = programmed death-ligand 1.

6. Inflammation as Predictive Factor

The clinical scenario of the treatment of RCC has changed dramatically in recent years due to the development, after the cytokine era, of molecular-targeted agents at first and subsequently of ICIs.

The availability of effective treatments represents a challenge for clinicians, who need valid tools to predict response to therapy and patients' prognosis.

However, the search for predictive markers has not led to satisfactory results yet, and robust biomarkers for the several available classes of treatments are still lacking.

When cytokine-based immunotherapy was the only available treatment for RCC, the French group of Immunotherapy validated a prognostic model based on performance status, metastases features, time from diagnosis to treatment, hemoglobin level, neutrophil absolute count, and other biological parameters related to inflammation. This model was developed to predict the outcome of RCC patients after cytokine-based treatment, stratifying three prognostic groups (good, intermediate, and poor risk) with different median OS [149].

In the era of molecular-targeted treatments, several studies reported no association of various biomarkers with the outcome of patients treated with sunitinib, pazopanib, and everolimus. Similarly, cMET expression did not result as a good predictor for cabozantinib treatment [150].

Ongoing studies are evaluating the role of several potential markers of the VHL pathway or the mTOR pathway, such as the VEGF gene family, CAIX, VEGFRs, PDGFRs, VHL and pAkt, PTEN, p27, and pS6 [151–153]. However, to date, no valid biomarker has been identified in this setting.

As for the use of predictive systems combining several independent variables (such as the classification of the French group of immunotherapy for predicting outcomes after cytokines treatment, or the model by Choueiri et al., focusing on prognosis after anti-angiogenic treatments), the predictive accuracy of available models in the metastatic setting is inferior to those developed for localized RCC [72,149].

Motzer et al. developed a nomogram to predict PFS after first-line treatment with sunitinib. The model included several clinical parameters, such as hemoglobin levels, platelet count > 400,000/uL, corrected serum calcium levels, alkaline phosphatase and lactate dehydrogenase levels, ECOG performance, prior nephrectomy, number and site of metastases, and time from diagnosis to treatment [73].

Shin et al. demonstrated that PD-L1 expression is significantly related to poor response to VEGF-TKI; in addition, PD-L1 is independently associated with shorter survival in metastatic RCC patients after VEGF-TKI treatment [154]. Hara et al. also showed that positive expression of immune-checkpoint-associated molecules, including PD-1, PD-L1, and PD-L2, is related to poor outcomes in metastatic RCC patients who received TKIs as first-line systemic therapy [140]. A retrospective study by Ueda et al. reported that PD-1 expression is not only a prognostic indicator for poor OS in patients with metastatic RCC receiving molecular targeted therapies [141].

In the last years, with the advent of the ICI era, systemic inflammatory status has been proved to be associated with clinical outcomes in the treatment for RCC [155–157].

Some studies have tried to identify the role of CRP in patients treated with molecular-targeted agents: Patient with the deepest decreases of CRP after treatment had a significantly better outcome [89,90]. The NLR has also been evaluated as a possible predictive marker for molecular-targeted agents. Park et al. showed that a lower post-treatment NLR and larger reduction in NLR after sunitinib treatment were significantly associated with better responses in patients with advanced RCC [107].

If inflammation-related biomarkers may be considered good prognostic factors, their role as predictive factor has not been established yet, particularly in the setting of ICIs. In fact, studies on the correlation of inflammatory markers and response to immunotherapy are few, mostly with a retrospective nature and with very small cohorts of patients.

A recent meta-analysis aimed to study the effectiveness of NLR as a predictive factor in patients receiving ICIs. Although the meta-analysis included relatively few studies on different cancer types, the results suggest that NLR is a potentially useful predictive tool [158].

In a retrospective series on 42 patients by Jeyakumar et al., the role of NLR as predictor of ORR, PFS, and OS in mRCC patients treated with ICIs was evaluated. The authors demonstrated that baseline NLR < 3 was an independent predictor of longer PFS and OS in patients treated with ICIs [159].

In another recent series by the same authors, NLR > 4 was associated with shorter OS and PFS in 57 patients receiving ICIs for RCC or urothelial carcinomas [160].

Bilen et al., in a retrospective series on 38 patients, observed that low baseline NLR was associated with longer PFS and OS in patients with metastatic RCC who received nivolumab therapy. Notably, they used a cutoff value of 5.5 for NLR, which was different from the prior studies [161].

A study by Lalani et al. on 142 patients treated with ICIs in any line confirmed that patients with a higher baseline NLR had a worse prognosis and reported that NLR decrease ≥25% during ICI treatment was significantly associated with improved outcomes (both PFS and OS) [162].

These results suggest that NLR can be considered an attractive, cost-effective biomarker that can easily be measured from routine laboratory data.

However, due to the retrospective nature and the small cohorts of patients included in these studies, the results need to be interpreted with caution and need validation, possibly through larger population and prospective trials. It is also clear that a valid cutoff value has not been identified yet and the values defining elevated NLR are different in each of these studies.

The role of predictive factors of ICI treatment in metastatic RCC patients was evaluated in a large Italian retrospective study, collecting data from a prospective cohort of 389 patients enrolled in the Italian Expanded Access Program (EAP) who were treated with nivolumab [162].

The authors report that patients with a high SII (≥1375) had a significantly shorter OS and that, at multivariate analysis, SII seemed to be superior to NLR in predicting outcomes. Furthermore, SII changes at three months after treatment started predicted survival [163].

To our knowledge, studies on other inflammation-related biomarkers (e.g., PLR, SIRI, PNI, and GPS) during ICI treatments are lacking but eagerly awaited.

Tumor-associated PD-L1 expression has been proposed as a potential predictive biomarker for PD-1 pathway expression in many cancer types, although it is limited by the abovementioned pitfalls. A recent meta-analysis evaluated PD-1 and PD-L1 inhibitors' efficacy compared to other treatments in patients with different tumors (mainly lung cancer, but also RCC, melanoma, head/neck cancer, and urothelial cancer) classified in two groups according to PD-L1 expression. PD-L1 expression resulted as a very unsatisfactory predictor because ICIs were beneficial in both groups [164].

The CheckMate 025 phase III trial evaluated nivolumab (3 mg/kg every 2 weeks) versus everolimus (10 mg daily). The trial included 821 patients with previously treated metastatic RCC [13].

The median OS was 25 months in the nivolumab group and 19.6 months in the everolimus group; PFS was not different among the two groups.

Interestingly, PD-L1-positive patients had worse outcomes in both treatment arms. Moreover, nivolumab showed clinical benefit both in PD-L1-positive and PD-L1-negative patients.

On the opposite side, patients with positive PD-L1 expression were reported to have more clinical benefit from ICIs both in the Immotion150 trial and Checkmate 214 [15,16].

The first study evaluated the use of atezolizumab plus bevacizumab versus atezolizumab plus sunitinib in untreated metastatic RCC [16].

In Checkmate, 214 treatment-naive advanced or metastatic RCC were treated with nivolumab plus ipilimumab or sunitinib [15]. In the combination arm, patients reported higher ORR in intermediate/poor risk patients. Of note, patients with intermediate/poor risk disease and PD-L1 expression ≥1% had higher ORR and PFS when treated with an ICI combination compared to sunitinib, while patients with favorable category of risk (showing lower PD-L1 expression) displayed a longer PFS and a higher ORR if treated with sunitinib.

Two recent phase III trials have focused on the association between ICIs and axitinib, exploring also the possible role of PD-L1 on treatment outcomes [17,18]. Axitinib showed clinical activity and an acceptable safety profile as first-line treatment of metastatic RCC in a phase III trial, in which it was compared to sorafenib [165].

The phase III JAVELIN Renal 101 trial reported that patients with PD-L1 positive, advanced RCC receiving first-line avelumab plus axitinib had significantly better outcomes than those treated with sunitinib. Interestingly, better PFS and ORR were observed in the avelumab plus axitinib, regardless of PD-L1 expression [17].

In the KEYNOTE-426 3 trial, treatment with pembrolizumab plus axitinib resulted in significantly longer OS and PFS, as well as a higher ORR, compared to sunitinib in previously untreated patients with advanced RCC. Similarly to the JAVELIN Renal 101 trial results [17], the benefit of pembrolizumab plus axitinib was observed in both PD-L1 expression subgroups (<1 and ≥1) and defined according to the combined positive score (defined as the number of PD-L1–positive cells, such as tumor cells, lymphocytes, and macrophages, divided by the total number of tumor cells, multiplied by 100) [18].

In a recent study by Tatli-Dogan et al., PD-L1 expression was reported to be associated with high HIF-2α expression (suggesting a possible regulation of PD-L1 by HIF-2α) and dense lymphocytic infiltration. The authors suggest that these parameters could be used as predictive factors and these patients could benefit from PD-L1-targeted therapy [148].

Particular considerations have to be made for nonclear cell RCC (ncc-RCC) histotypes.

When considering the PD1 axis as prognostic factor, a study by Abbas et al. on patients undergoing radical renal tumor surgery reported that neither PD-1 positive tumor-infiltrating mononuclear cells or intratumoral PD-L1 expression seemed to significantly impact tumor aggressiveness or clinical outcome in ncc-RCC specimens [166]. Therefore, these cannot be considered good prognosticators.

Although it has been observed that PD-L1 is expressed on tumors of ncc-RCC and sarcomatoid RCC, its role in predicting response to ICI treatments is not clear yet.

Data on the activity of ICIs in patients with ncc-RCC, such as papillary, chromophobe, medullary, Xp11.2 translocation, collecting duct carcinomas, and unclassified carcinomas, or patients with sarcomatoid/rhabdoid differentiation, are limited, due to the diversity of this population and the small numbers in each subset, with consequent low representation in clinical trials.

In a recent pooled analysis on 43 patients with metastatic ncc-RCC or with clear cell cancer with >20% sarcomatoid or rhabdoid differentiation treated with a PD1 or PD-L1 targeting agent (either as monotherapy or in association), the overall response rate was 31% in treatment-naive patients [167]. Patients with RCC with sarcomatoid and/or rhabdoid differentiation and papillary RCC experienced higher ORR, while no patient with chromophobe RCC or unclassified carcinomas responded. The median OS was 12.9 months, and a 12-month OS rate was 64%.

In particular, it has been demonstrated that RCC with a sarcomatoid differentiation may express PD1 and PD-L1 at higher rates than clear cell RCC, and, thus, ICIs have shown initial promising efficacy in this population [168].

A retrospective exploratory analysis from CheckMate 214 showed an impressive efficacy in patients with intermediate/poor risk RCC with sarcomatoid features treated with nivolumab plus ipilimumab versus sunitinib. A higher proportion of patients with sarcomatoid RCC had baseline tumor PD-L1 expression ≥ 1% compared to the CheckMate214 intention-to-treat population (47% vs. 26%, respectively) [15,169].

Furthermore, it has been observed that PD-L1 may play a key role in the biology of Xp11.2 translocation RCC. In fact, in a study by Choueiri, 30% of patients had PD-L1 positivity in tumor cells, and 90% harbored PD-L1+ tumor-infiltrating mononuclear cells. Similarly, in collecting duct carcinoma, 20% of patients expressed PD-L1 on tumor cells [170]. Therefore, these features could represent an important therapeutic target for these histotypes, for which few therapeutic options are currently available.

It is clear that the role of PD-L1 expression as predictive factor is still controversial and under great debate. Further studies are needed to assess whether and how this biomarker will be able to become a valid and robust prognosticator and clinical tool.

7. Future Perspectives

In the fast-changing and stimulating scenario of immunotherapy for RCC treatment, several molecules are being investigated as potential targets, beyond the already consolidated PD-1 and CTLA-4. Among the most promising molecules, a mention has to be made on chemokine receptors, the V-domain immunoglobulin-containing suppressor of T-cell activation (VISTA), the soluble lymphocyte-activation gene-3 (LAG-3), OX40 (CD134) and the B and T lymphocyte attenuator (BTLA) [171,172].

In this situation of growing complexity, it seems clear that the sole assessment of PD-1/PD-L1 expression cannot reflect tumor dynamicity.

Besides PD-L1 expression, T-cell density in pretreated samples, T-cell receptor clonality, mutational or neoantigen burden, immunogen signatures, assessment of peripheral T-cell populations, and multiplex IHC with assessment of tumor and immune-cell phenotypes are currently under investigation [173,174]. Combining these strategies in order to evaluate the immune status of the tumor microenvironment will probably result in the identification of more effective biomarkers.

Fundamental will be the identification of different cellular profiles combined with the genetic architecture of RCC, in order to achieve a precision medicine approach and to guide treatment decision among anti-angiogenic agents, ICIs, or a combination of these. For example, VHL and PBRM1 mutant tumors, which have been shown to be associated with both an immune profile and an angiogenic signature, would probably benefit most from a combination treatment [175,176]. In contrast, loss of BAP1, proved to be associated with decreased angiogenic signaling, would probably benefit mostly from ICI treatment [177]. The choice between the combination and sequencing approach will also be essential to improve outcomes for RCC patients.

Therefore, foreseeing the paramount importance of identifying tumor microenvironment changes during the course of different treatments, avoiding the clinical impact of repeated multiple biopsies, the identification of valid biomarkers either on circulating tumor cells or exosomes will become mandatory in the next future [178].

This will be a fundamental process to allow the optimization of treatment choice in cancer patients.

8. Conclusions

The interplay between tumor immune status and cancer-related systemic inflammation is crucial for the outcome of RCC treatment with ICIs. However, to date, there is a great unmet need for a more precise characterization of the role of systemic inflammation and inflammatory mediators, both as prognostic and predictive factors of response to these drugs.

It is unquestionably accepted that immunotherapy has profoundly changed the outcomes of patients affected by RCC and is representing an unparalleled revolution. However, in a scenario with several available therapeutic options, future researches will have to shed light on how to best tailor treatments depending on every patient's specific biological and clinical features.

Due to the availability of multiple options, the sequencing of agents is becoming a daily challenge. The identification of biomarkers to guide therapeutic choices in RCC is advocated. This will help clinicians optimize the selection of treatments, avoiding the exposure to the adverse events related to therapies with predictable low likelihood of clinical benefit, also resulting in better, more cost-effective clinical management.

Due to the paramount importance of the complex interplay among immunological status and immunotherapy, the identification of validated and reproducible biomarkers associated with tumor immune status will be essential to improve the clinical management and, consequently, the outcomes for these patients.

Author Contributions: Conceptualization, N.B., A.F., and U.D.G.; methodology, N.B., A.F., and U.D.G.; formal analysis, N.B. and U.D.G.; resources, N.B., A.F., G.G., S.G., V.G., G.S., C.L., C.C., and U.D.G.; writing—original draft preparation, N.B., A.F., and U.D.G.; writing—review and editing, N.B., G.G., S.G., V.G., G.S., C.L., V.C., and U.D.G.; visualization, N.B. and G.S.; supervision, U.D.G. and V.C.

Funding: This research received no external funding.

Conflicts of Interest: V.C. has received speaker honoraria or travel support from Astellas, Janssen-Cilag, and Sanofi-Aventis, and has received a consulting fee from Bayer. U.D.G. has served as consultant/advisory board member for Astellas, Bayer, BMS, Ipsen, Janssen, Merck, Pfizer, Sanofi, and has received travel support from BMS, Ipsen, Janssen, and Pfizer, and has received research funding from AstraZeneca, Roche, and Sanofi (Inst). No potential conflicts of interest were disclosed by the other authors.

References

1. Siegel, R.L.; Miller, K.D.; Jemal, A. Cancer statistics, 2016. *CA Cancer J. Clin.* **2016**, *66*, 7–30. [CrossRef]
2. Ljunberg, B.; Campbell, S.C.; Cho, H.Y.; Jacqmin, D.; Lee, J.E.; Weikert, S.; Kiemeney, L.A. The epidemiology of renal cell carcinoma. *Eur. Urol.* **2011**, *60*, 615–621. [CrossRef] [PubMed]
3. Chow, W.H.; Dong, L.M.; Devesa, S.S. Epidemiology and risk factors for kidney cancer. *Nat. Rev. Urol.* **2010**, *7*, 245–257. [CrossRef] [PubMed]
4. Escudier, B.; Porta, C.; Schmidinger, M.; Rioux-Leclercq, N.; Bex, A.; Khoo, V.; Grünwald, V.; Gillessen, S.; Horwich, A. ESMO Guidelines Committee. Renal cell carcinoma: ESMO Clinical Practice Guidelines for diagnosis, treatment and follow up. *Ann. Oncol.* **2019**, *30*, 706–720. [CrossRef] [PubMed]
5. De Lisi, D.; De Giorgi, U.; Lolli, C.; Schepisi, G.; Conteduca, V.; Menna, C.; Tonini, G.; Santini, D.; Farolfi, A. Lenvatinib in the management of metastatic renal cell carcinoma: A promising combination therapy? *Expert Opin. Drug Metab. Toxicol.* **2018**, *14*, 461–467. [CrossRef] [PubMed]
6. Motzer, R.J.; Hutson, T.E.; Tomczak, P.; Michaelson, M.D.; Bukowski, R.M.; Rixe, O.; Oudard, S.; Negrier, S.; Szczylik, C.; Kim, S.T.; et al. Sunitinib versus interferon alfa in metastatic renal-cell carcinoma. *N. Engl. J. Med.* **2007**, *356*, 115–124. [CrossRef] [PubMed]
7. Motzer, R.J.; Hutson, T.E.; Cella, D.; Reeves, J.; Hawkins, R.; Guo, J.; Nathan, P.; Staehler, M.; de Souza, P.; Merchan, J.R.; et al. Pazopanib versus sunitinib in metastatic renal-cell carcinoma. *N. Engl. J. Med.* **2013**, *369*, 722–731. [CrossRef] [PubMed]
8. Choueiri, T.K.; Escudier, B.; Powles, T.; Tannir, N.M.; Mainwaring, P.N.; Rini, B.I.; Hammers, H.J.; Donskov, F.; Roth, B.J.; Peltola, K.; et al. METEOR investigators. Cabozantinib versus everolimus in advanced renal-cell carcinoma. *N. Engl. J. Med.* **2015**, *373*, 1814–1823. [CrossRef]
9. Motzer, R.J.; Escudier, B.; Tomczak, P.; Hutson, T.E.; Michaelson, M.D.; Negrier, S.; Oudard, S.; Gore, M.E.; Tarazi, J.; Hariharan, S.; et al. Axitinib versus sorafenib as second-line treatment for advanced renal cell carcinoma: Overall survival analysis and updated results from a randomised phase 3 trial. *Lancet Oncol.* **2013**, *14*, 552–562. [CrossRef]
10. Motzer, R.J.; Escudier, B.; Oudard, S.; Hutson, T.E.; Porta, C.; Bracarda, S.; Grünwald, V.; Thompson, J.A.; Figlin, R.A.; Hollaender, N.; et al. RECORD-1 Study Group. Phase 3 trial of everolimus for metastatic renal cell carcinoma: Final results and analysis of prognostic factors. *Cancer* **2010**, *116*, 4256–4265. [CrossRef]
11. Escudier, B.; Eisen, T.; Stadler, W.M.; Szczylik, C.; Oudard, S.; Staehler, M.; Negrier, S.; Chevreau, C.; Desai, A.A.; Rolland, F.; et al. Sorafenib for treatment of renal cell carcinoma: Final efficacy and safety results of the phase III treatment approaches in renal cancer global evaluation trial. *J. Clin. Oncol.* **2009**, *27*, 3312–3318. [CrossRef] [PubMed]
12. Motzer, R.J.; Hutson, T.E.; Glen, H.; Michaelson, M.D.; Molina, A.; Eisen, T.; Jassem, J.; Zolnierek, J.; Maroto, J.P.; Mellado, B.; et al. Lenvatinib, everolimus, and the combination in patients with metastatic renal cell carcinoma: A randomised, phase 2, open-label, multicentre trial. *Lancet Oncol.* **2015**, *16*, 1473–1482. [CrossRef]
13. Motzer, R.J.; Escudier, B.; McDermott, D.F.; George, S.; Hammers, H.J.; Srinivas, S.; Tykodi, S.S.; Sosman, J.A.; Procopio, G.; Plimack, E.R.; et al. CheckMate025 Investigators. Nivolumab versus everolimus in advanced renal cell carcinoma. *N. Engl. J. Med.* **2015**, *373*, 1803–1813. [CrossRef] [PubMed]
14. Massari, F.; Di Nunno, V.; Ciccarese, C.; Graham, J.; Porta, C.; Comito, F.; Cubelli, M.; Iacovelli, R.; Heng, D.Y.C. Adjuvant therapy in renal cell carcinoma. *Cancer Treat Rev.* **2017**, *60*, 152–157. [CrossRef]
15. Motzer, R.J.; Tannir, N.M.; McDermott, D.F.; Arén Frontera, O.; Melichar, B.; Choueiri, T.K.; Plimack, E.R.; Barthélémy, P.; Porta, C.; George, S.; et al. CheckMate 214 Investigators. Nivolumab plus ipilimumab versus sunitinib in advanced renal-cell carcinoma. *N. Engl. J. Med.* **2018**, *378*, 1277–1290. [CrossRef]
16. Atkins, M.B.; McDermott, D.F.; Powles, T.; Motzer, J.R.; Rini, B.I.; Fong, L.; Joseph, R.W.; Pal, S.K.; Sznol, M.; Hainsworth, J.D.; et al. IMmotion150: A phase II trial in untreated metastatic renal cell carcinoma (mRCC)

patients (pts) of atezolizumab (atezo) and bevacizumab (bev) vs and following atezo or sunitinib (sun). *J. Clin. Oncol.* **2017**, *35*, 4505. [CrossRef]

17. Motzer, R.J.; Penkov, K.; Haanen, J.; Rini, B.; Albiges, L.; Campbell, M.T.; Venugopal, B.; Kollmannsberger, C.; Negrier, S.; Uemura, M.; et al. Avelumab plus Axitinib versus Sunitinib for Advanced Renal-Cell Carcinoma. *N. Engl. J. Med.* **2019**, *380*, 1103–1115. [CrossRef]

18. Rini, B.I.; Plimack, E.R.; Stus, V.; Gafanov, R.; Hawkins, R.; Nosov, D.; Pouliot, F.; Alekseev, B.; Soulières, D.; Melichar, B.; et al. KEYNOTE-426 Investigators. Pembrolizumab plus Axitinib versus Sunitinib for Advanced Renal-Cell Carcinoma. *N. Engl. J. Med.* **2019**, *380*, 1116–1127. [CrossRef]

19. Amin, A.; Plimack, E.R.; Infante, J.R.; Ernstoff, M.S.; Rini, B.I.; McDermott, D.F.; Knox, J.J.; Pal, S.K.; Voss, M.H.; Sharma, P.; et al. Nivolumab (anti-PD-1; BMS-936558, ONO-4538) in combination with sunitinib or pazopanib in patients (pts) with metastatic renal cell carcinoma (mRCC). *J. Clin. Oncol.* **2014**, *32*, 5010. [CrossRef]

20. Atkins, M.B.; Plimack, E.R.; Puzanov, I.; Fishman, M.N.; McDermott, D.F.; Cho, D.C.; Vaishampayan, U.; George, S.; Olencki, T.E.; Tarazi, J.C.; et al. Axitinib in combination with pembrolizumab in patients with advanced renal cell cancer: A non-randomised, open-label, dose-finding and dose-expansion phase 1b trial. *Lancet Oncol.* **2018**, *19*, 405–415. [CrossRef]

21. Rini, B.I.; Stein, M.; Shannon, P.; Eddy, S.; Tyler, A.; Stephenson, J.J., Jr.; Catlett, L.; Huang, B.; Healey, D.; Gordon, M. Phase 1 dose-escalation trial of tremelimumab plus sunitinib in patients with metastatic renal cell carcinoma. *Cancer* **2011**, *117*, 758–767. [CrossRef] [PubMed]

22. Chowdhury, S.; McDermott, D.F.; Voss, M.H.; Hawkins, R.E.; Aimone, P.; Voi, M.; Isabelle, N.; Wu, Y.; Infante, J.R. A phase I/II study to assess the safety and efficacy of pazopanib and pembrolizumab in patients with advanced renal cell carcinoma. *J. Clin. Oncol.* **2017**, *35*, 4506. [CrossRef]

23. Rini, B.I.; Powles, T.; Atkins, M.B.; Escudier, B.; McDermott, D.F.; Suarez, C.; Bracarda, S.; Stadler, W.M.; Donskov, F.; Lee, J.L.; et al. Atezolizumab plus bevacizumab versus sunitinib in patients with previously untreated metastatic renal cell carcinoma (IMmotion151): A multicentre, open-label, phase 3, randomised controlled trial. *Lancet* **2019**, *15*, 2404–2415. [CrossRef]

24. Choueiri, T.K.; Larkin, J.M.; Oya, M.; Thistlethwaite, F.C.; Martignoni, M.; Nathan, P.D.; Powles, T.; McDermott, D.F.; Robbins, P.B.; Chism, D.D.; et al. First-line avelumab + axitinib therapy in patients with advanced renal cell carcinoma: Results from a phase Ib trial. *J. Clin. Oncol.* **2017**, *35* (Suppl. 15), 35. [CrossRef]

25. Grünwald, V.; Powles, T.; Choueiri, T.K.; Hutson, T.E.; Porta, C.; Eto, M.; Sternberg, C.N.; Rha, S.Y.; He, C.S.; Dutcus, C.E.; et al. Lenvatinib plus everolimus or pembrolizumab versus sunitinib in advanced renal cell carcinoma: Study design and rationale. *Future Oncol.* **2019**, *15*, 929–941. [CrossRef]

26. Choueiri, T.K.; Apolo, A.B.; Powles, T.; Escudier, B.; Aren, O.R.; Shah, A.; Kessler, E.R.; Hsieh, J.J.; Zhang, J.; Simsek, B.; et al. A phase 3, randomized, open-label study of nivolumab combined with cabozantinib vs sunitinib in patients with previously untreated advanced or metastatic renal cell carcinoma (RCC. CheckMate 9ER). *J. Clin. Oncol.* **2018**, *36* (Suppl. 15), TPS4598. [CrossRef]

27. Balkwill, F.; Mantovani, A. Inflammation and cancer: Back to Virchow? *Lancet* **2001**, *357*, 539–545. [CrossRef]

28. Mantovani, A.; Allavena, P.; Sica, A.; Balkwill, F. Cancer-related inflammation. *Nature* **2008**, *454*, 436–444. [CrossRef]

29. Coussens, L.M.; Werb, Z. Inflammation and cancer. *Nature* **2002**, *420*, 860–867. [CrossRef]

30. Chen, Z.; Wang, K.; Lu, H.; Xue, D.; Fan, M.; Zhuang, Q.; Yin, S.; He, X.; Xu, R. Systemic inflammation response index predicts prognosis in patients with clear cell renal cell carcinoma: A propensity score-matched analysis. *Cancer Manag. Res.* **2019**, *18*, 909–919. [CrossRef]

31. Elinav, E.; Nowarski, R.; Thaiss, C.A.; Hu, B.; Jin, C.; Flavell, R.A. Inflammation-induced cancer: Crosstalk between tumours, immune cells and microorganisms. *Nat. Rev. Cancer* **2013**, *13*, 759–771. [CrossRef] [PubMed]

32. Diakos, C.I.; Charles, K.A.; McMillan, D.C.; Clarke, S.J. Cancer-related inflammation and treatment effectiveness. *Lancet Oncol.* **2014**, *15*, e493–e503. [CrossRef]

33. Li, J.F.; Chu, Y.W.; Wang, G.M.; Zhu, T.Y.; Rong, R.M.; Hou, J.; Xu, M. The prognostic value of peritumoral regulatory T cells and its correlation with intratumoral cyclooxygenase-2 expression in clear cell renal cell carcinoma. *BJU Int.* **2009**, *103*, 399–405. [CrossRef] [PubMed]

34. Sozen, S.; Gurocak, S.; Erdem, O.; Acar, C.; Kordan, Y.; Akyol, G.; Alkibay, T. Cyclooxygenase-2 expression: Does it have a probable role in tumorigenesis mechanisms of renal cell carcinoma? *Int. Urol. Nephrol.* **2009**, *40*, 295–301. [CrossRef] [PubMed]
35. Tuna, B.; Yorukoglu, K.; Gurel, D.; Mungan, U.; Kirkali, Z. Significance of COX-2 expression in human renal cell carcinoma. *Urology* **2004**, *64*, 1116–1120. [CrossRef] [PubMed]
36. Muscat, J.E.; Chen, S.Q.; Richie, J.P., Jr.; Altorki, N.K.; Citron, M.; Olson, S.; Neugut, A.I.; Stellman, S.D. Risk of lung carcinoma among users of nonsteroidal antiinflammatory drugs. *Cancer* **2003**, *97*, 1732–1736. [CrossRef]
37. Rothwell, P.M.; Wilson, M.; Price, J.F.; Belch, J.F.; Meade, T.W.; Mehta, Z. Effect of daily aspirin on risk of cancer metastasis: A study of incident cancers during randomised controlled trials. *Lancet* **2012**, *379*, 1591–1601. [CrossRef]
38. Rothwell, P.M.; Wilson, M.; Elwin, C.E.; Norrving, B.; Algra, A.; Warlow, C.P.; Meade, T.W. Long-term effect of aspirin on colorectal cancer incidence and mortality: 20-year follow-up of five randomised trials. *Lancet* **2010**, *376*, 1741–1750. [CrossRef]
39. Vidal, A.C.; Howard, L.E.; Moreira, D.M.; Castro-Santamaria, R.; Andriole, G.L.; Freedland, S.J. Aspirin, NSAIDs, and risk of prostate cancer: Results from the REDUCE study. *Clin. Cancer Res.* **2015**, *21*, 756–762. [CrossRef]
40. Ruder, E.H.; Laiyemo, A.O.; Graubard, B.I.; Hollenbeck, A.R.; Schatzkin, A.; Cross, A.J. Non-steroidal anti-inflammatory drugs and colorectal cancer risk in a large, prospective cohort. *Am. J. Gastroenterol.* **2011**, *106*, 1340–1350. [CrossRef]
41. Janssen, A.; Maier, T.J.; Schiffmann, S.; Coste, O.; Seegel, M.; Geisslinger, G.; Grösch, S. Evidence of COX-2 independent induction of apoptosis and cell cycle block in human colon carcinoma cells after S- or R-ibuprofen treatment. *Eur. J. Pharmacol.* **2006**, *540*, 24–33. [CrossRef] [PubMed]
42. Gurpinar, E.; Grizzle, W.E.; Piazza, G.A. NSAIDs inhibit tumorigenesis, but how? *Clin. Cancer Res.* **2014**, *20*, 1104–1113. [CrossRef] [PubMed]
43. Reddy, B.S.; Hirose, Y.; Lubet, R.; Steele, V.; Kelloff, G.; Paulson, S.; Seibert, K.; Rao, C.V. Chemoprevention of colon cancer by specific cyclooxygenase-2 inhibitor, celecoxib, administered during different stages of carcinogenesis. *Cancer Res.* **2000**, *60*, 293–297. [PubMed]
44. Steele, V.E.; Rao, C.V.; Zhang, Y.; Patlolla, J.; Boring, D.; Kopelovich, L.; Juliana, M.M.; Grubbs, C.J.; Lubet, R.A. Chemopreventive efficacy of naproxen and nitric oxide-naproxen in rodent models of colon, urinary bladder, and mammary cancers. *Cancer Prev. Res. (Phila)* **2009**, *2*, 951–956. [CrossRef]
45. Steinbach, G.; Lynch, P.M.; Phillips, R.K.; Wallace, M.H.; Hawk, E.; Gordon, G.B.; Wakabayashi, N.; Saunders, B.; Shen, Y.; Fujimura, T.; et al. The effect of celecoxib, a cyclooxygenase-2 inhibitor, in familial adenomatous polyposis. *N. Engl. J. Med.* **2000**, *342*, 1946–1952. [CrossRef]
46. Cho, E.; Curhan, G.; Hankinson, S.E.; Kantoff, P.; Atkins, M.B.; Stampfer, M.; Choueiri, T.K. Prospective evaluation of analgesic use and risk of renal cell cancer. *Arch. Intern. Med.* **2011**, *171*, 1487–1493. [CrossRef]
47. Choueiri, T.K.; Je, Y.; Cho, E. Analgesic use and the risk of kidney cancer: A meta-analysis of epidemiologic studies. *Int. J. Cancer* **2014**, *134*, 384–396. [CrossRef]
48. Hamieh, L.; Moreira, R.B.; Lin, X.; Simantov, R.; Choueiri, T.K.; McKay, R.R. Impact of Aspirin and Non-Aspirin Nonsteroidal Anti-Inflammatory Drugs on Outcomes in Patients with Metastatic Renal Cell Carcinoma. *Kidney Cancer* **2018**, *2*, 37–46. [CrossRef]
49. Yu, A.; Wang, Y.; Bian, Y.; Chen, L.; Guo, J.; Shen, W.; Chen, D.; Liu, S.; Sun, X. IL-1b promotes the nuclear translocation of S100A4 protein in gastric cancer cells MGC803 and the cell's stemlike properties through PI3K pathway. *J. Cell. Biochem.* **2018**, *119*, 8163–8173. [CrossRef]
50. Cui, G.; Yuan, A.; Sun, Z.; Zheng, W.; Pang, Z. IL-1b/IL-6 network in the tumor microenvironment of human colorectal cancer. *Pathol. Res. Pract.* **2018**, *214*, 986–992. [CrossRef]
51. Ridker, P.; Everett, B.; Thuren, T.; MacFadyen, J.G.; Chang, W.H.; Ballantyne, C.; Fonseca, F.; Nicolau, J.; Koenig, W.; Anker, S.D.; et al. Antiinflammatory therapy with canakinumab for atherosclerotic disease. *N. Engl. J. Med.* **2017**, *377*, 1119–1131. [CrossRef] [PubMed]
52. Ding, H.; Wu, X.; Gao, W. PD-L1 is expressed by human renal tubular epithelial cells and suppresses T cell cytokine synthesis. *Clin. Immunol.* **2005**, *115*, 184–191. [CrossRef] [PubMed]

53. Nunes-Xavier, C.E.; Angulo, J.C.; Pulido, R.; López, J.A. A Critical Insight into the Clinical Translation of PD-1/PD-L1 Blockade Therapy in Clear Cell Renal Cell Carcinoma. *Curr. Urol. Rep.* **2019**, *20*, 1. [CrossRef] [PubMed]
54. Yao, H.; Wang, H.; Li, C.; Fang, J.Y.; Xu, J. Cancer cell-intrinsic PD-1 and implications in combinatorial immunotherapy. *Front. Immunol.* **2018**, *9*, 1774. [CrossRef] [PubMed]
55. Keir, M.E.; Butte, M.J.; Freeman, G.J.; Sharpe, A.H. PD-1 and its ligands in tolerance and immunity. *Ann. Rev. Immunol.* **2008**, *26*, 677–704. [CrossRef] [PubMed]
56. Gibbons-Johnson, R.M.; Dong, H. Functional expression of programmed death-ligand 1 (B7-H1) by immune cells and tumor cells. *Front. Immunol.* **2017**, *8*, 961. [CrossRef] [PubMed]
57. Thompson, R.H.; Dong, H.; Lohse, C.M.; Leibovich, B.C.; Blute, M.L.; Cheville, J.C.; Kwon, E.D. PD-1 is expressed by tumor-infiltrating immune cells and is associated with poor outcome for patients with renal cell carcinoma. *Clin. Cancer Res.* **2007**, *13*, 1757–1761. [CrossRef]
58. Freeman, G.J.; Long, A.J.; Iwai, Y.; Bourque, K.; Chernova, T.; Nishimura, H.; Fitz, L.J.; Malenkovich, N.; Okazaki, T.; Byrne, M.C.; et al. Engagement of the PD-1 immunoinhibitory receptor by a novel B7 family member leads to negative regulation of lymphocyte activation. *J. Exp. Med.* **2000**, *192*, 1027–1034. [CrossRef]
59. Dong, P.; Xiong, Y.; Yue, J.; Hanley, S.J.B.; Watari, H. Tumor-intrinsic PD-L1 signaling in cancer initiation, development and treatment: Beyond immune evasion. *Front. Oncol.* **2018**, *8*, 385. [CrossRef]
60. Tartour, E.; Pere, H.; Maillere, B.; Terme, M.; Merillon, N.; Taieb, J.; Sandoval, F.; Quintin-Colonna, F.; Lacerda, K.; Karadimou, A.; et al. Angiogenesis and immunity: A bidirectional link potentially relevant for the monitoring of antiangiogenic therapy and the development of novel therapeutic combination with immunotherapy. *Cancer Metastasis Rev.* **2011**, *30*, 83–95. [CrossRef]
61. Frank, I.; Blute, M.L.; Cheville, J.C.; Lohse, C.M.; Weaver, A.L.; Zincke, H. An outcome prediction model for patients with clear cell renal cell carcinoma treated with radical nephrectomy based on tumor stage, size, grade and necrosis: The SSIGN score. *J. Urol.* **2002**, *168*, 2395–2400. [CrossRef]
62. Kattan, M.W.; Reuter, V.; Motzer, R.J.; Katz, J.; Russo, P. A postoperative prognostic nomogram for renal cell carcinoma. *J. Urol.* **2001**, *166*, 63–67. [CrossRef]
63. Karakiewicz, P.I.; Briganti, A.; Chun, F.K.; Trinh, Q.D.; Perrotte, P.; Ficarra, V.; Cindolo, L.; De la Taille, A.; Tostain, J.; Mulders, P.F.; et al. Multi-institutional validation of a new renal cancer-specific survival nomogram. *J. Clin. Oncol.* **2007**, *25*, 1316–1322. [CrossRef] [PubMed]
64. Volpe, A.; Patard, J.J. Prognostic factors in renal cell carcinoma. *World J. Urol.* **2010**, *28*, 319–327. [CrossRef]
65. Eggener, S.E.; Yossepowitch, O.; Kundu, S.; Motzer, R.J.; Russo, P. Risk score and metastasectomy independently impact prognosis of patients with recurrent renal cell carcinoma. *J. Urol.* **2008**, *180*, 873–878. [CrossRef]
66. Kavolius, J.P.; Mastorakos, D.P.; Pavlovich, C.; Russo, P.; Burt, M.E.; Brady, M.S. Resection of metastatic renal cell carcinoma. *J. Clin. Oncol.* **1998**, *16*, 2261–2266. [CrossRef]
67. Pfannschmidt, J.; Hoffmann, H.; Muley, T.; Krysa, S.; Trainer, C.; Dienemann, H. Prognostic factors for survival after pulmonary resection of metastatic renal cell carcinoma. *Ann. Thorac. Surg.* **2002**, *74*, 1653–1657. [CrossRef]
68. Kuruvath, S.; Naidu, S.; Bhattacharyya, M.; Benjamin, J.C.; O'Donovan, D.G. Spinal metastasis from renal cell carcinoma, 31 years following nephrectomy-case report. *Clin. Neuropathol.* **2007**, *26*, 176–179. [CrossRef]
69. Shuch, B.; La Rochelle, J.C.; Klatte, T.; Riggs, S.B.; Liu, W.; Kabbinavar, F.F.; Pantuck, A.J.; Belldegrun, A.S. Brain metastasis from renal cell carcinoma: Presentation, recurrence, and survival. *Cancer* **2008**, *113*, 1641–1648. [CrossRef]
70. Mian, B.M.; Bhadkamkar, N.; Slaton, J.W.; Pisters, P.W.; Daliani, D.; Swanson, D.A.; Pisters, L.L. Prognostic factors and survival of patients with sarcomatoid renal cell carcinoma. *J. Urol.* **2002**, *167*, 65–70. [CrossRef]
71. De Reijke, T.M.; Bellmunt, J.; van Poppel, H.; Marreaud, S.; Aapro, M. EORTC-GU group expert opinion on metastatic renal cell cancer. *Eur. J. Cancer.* **2009**, *45*, 765–773. [CrossRef] [PubMed]
72. Choueiri, T.K.; Garcia, J.A.; Elson, P.; Khasawneh, M.; Usman, S.; Golshayan, A.R.; Baz, R.C.; Wood, L.; Rini, B.I.; Bukowski, R.M. Clinical factors associated with outcome in patients with metastatic clear-cell renal cell carcinoma treated with vascular endothelial growth factor-targeted therapy. *Cancer* **2007**, *110*, 543–550. [CrossRef] [PubMed]

73. Motzer, R.J.; Bukowski, R.M.; Figlin, R.A.; Hutson, T.E.; Michaelson, M.D.; Kim, S.T.; Baum, C.M.; Kattan, M.W. Prognostic nomogram for sunitinib in patients with metastatic renal cell carcinoma. *Cancer* **2008**, *113*, 1552–1558. [CrossRef] [PubMed]
74. Negrier, S.; Gomez, F.; Douillard, J.Y.; Ravaud, A.; Chevreau, C.; Buclon, M.; Perol, D.; Lasset, C.; Escudier, B.; d'Immunothérapie, G.F. Prognostic factors of response or failure of treatment in patients with metastatic renal carcinomas treated by cytokines: A report from the Groupe Francais d'Immunotherapie. *World J. Urol.* **2005**, *23*, 161–165. [CrossRef] [PubMed]
75. Motzer, R.J.; Mazumdar, M.; Bacik, J.; Berg, W.; Amsterdam, A.; Ferrara, J. Survival and prognostic stratification of 670 patients with advanced renal cell carcinoma. *J. Clin. Oncol.* **1999**, *17*, 2530–2540. [CrossRef] [PubMed]
76. Motzer, R.J.; Bacik, J.; Schwartz, L.H.; Reuter, V.; Russo, P.; Marion, S.; Mazumdar, M. Prognostic factors for survival in previously treated patients with metastatic renal cell carcinoma. *J. Clin. Oncol.* **2004**, *22*, 454–463. [CrossRef]
77. Heng, D.Y.; Xie, W.; Regan, M.M.; Harshman, L.C.; Bjarnason, G.A.; Vaishampayan, U.N.; Mackenzie, M.; Wood, L.; Donskov, F.; Tan, M.H.; et al. External validation and comparison with other models of the International Metastatic Renal-Cell Carcinoma Database Consortium prognostic model: A population-based study. *Lancet Oncol.* **2013**, *14*, 141–148. [CrossRef]
78. Hanahan, D.; Weinberg, R.A. Hallmarks of cancer: The next generation. *Cell* **2011**, *144*, 646–674. [CrossRef]
79. Li, S.; Xu, H.; Wang, W.; Gao, H.; Li, H.; Zhang, S.; Xu, J.; Zhang, W.; Xu, S.; Li, T.; et al. The systemic inflammation response index predicts survival and recurrence in patients with resectable pancreatic ductal adenocarcinoma. *Cancer Manag. Res.* **2019**, *11*, 3327–3337. [CrossRef]
80. Viers, B.R.; Boorjian, S.A.; Frank, I.; Tarrell, R.F.; Thapa, P.; Karnes, R.J.; Thompson, R.H.; Tollefson, M.K. Pretreatment neutrophil-to-lymphocyte ratio is associated with advanced pathologic tumor stage and increased cancer-specific mortality among patients with urothelial carcinoma of the bladder undergoing radical cystectomy. *Eur. Urol.* **2014**, *66*, 1157–1164. [CrossRef]
81. Grilz, E.; Posch, F.; Konigsbrugge, O.; Schwarzinger, I.; Lang, I.M.; Marosi, C.; Pabinger, I.; Ay, C. Association of platelet-to-lymphocyte ratio and neutrophil-to-lymphocyte ratio with the risk of thromboembolism and mortality in patients with cancer. *Thromb. Haemost.* **2018**, *118*, 1875–1884. [CrossRef] [PubMed]
82. Pinato, D.J.; North, B.V.; Sharma, R. A novel, externally validated inflammation-based prognostic algorithm in hepatocellular carcinoma: The prognostic nutritional index (PNI). *Br. J. Cancer* **2012**, *106*, 1439–1445. [CrossRef] [PubMed]
83. Hu, B.; Yang, X.R.; Xu, Y.; Sun, Y.F.; Sun, C.; Guo, W.; Zhang, X.; Wang, W.M.; Qiu, S.J.; Zhou, J.; et al. Systemic immune-inflammation index predicts prognosis of patients after curative resection for hepatocellular carcinoma. *Clin. Cancer Res.* **2014**, *20*, 6212–6222. [CrossRef] [PubMed]
84. Ohno, Y. Role of systemic inflammatory response markers in urological malignancy. *Int. J. Urol.* **2019**, *26*, 31–47. [CrossRef]
85. Mahmoud, F.A.; Rivera, N.I. The role of C-reactive protein as a prognostic indicator in advanced cancer. *Curr. Oncol. Rep.* **2002**, *4*, 250–255. [CrossRef]
86. Køstner, A.H.; Kersten, C.; Lowenmark, T.; Ydsten, K.A.; Peltonen, R.; Isoniemi, H.; Haglund, C.; Gunnarsson, U.; Isaksson, B. The prognostic role of systemic inflammation in patients undergoing resection of colorectal liver metastases: C-reactive protein (CRP) is a strong negative prognostic biomarker. *J. Surg. Oncol.* **2016**, *114*, 895–899. [CrossRef]
87. De Martino, M.; Klatte, T.; Seemann, C.; Waldert, M.; Haitel, A.; Schatzl, G.; Remzi, M.; Weibl, P. Validation of serum C-reactive protein (CRP) as an independent prognostic factor for disease-free survival in patients with localised renal cell carcinoma (RCC). *BJU Int.* **2013**, *111*, E348–E353. [CrossRef]
88. Komai, Y.; Saito, K.; Sakai, K.; Morimoto, S. Increased preoperative serum C reactive protein level predicts a poor prognosis in patients with localized renal cell carcinoma. *BJU Int.* **2007**, *99*, 77–80. [CrossRef]
89. Yasuda, Y.; Saito, K.; Yuasa, T.; Uehara, S.; Kawamura, N.; Yokoyama, M.; Ishioka, J.; Matsuoka, Y.; Yamamoto, S.; Okuno, T.; et al. Early response of C-reactive protein as a predictor of survival in patients with metastatic renal cell carcinoma treated with tyrosine kinase inhibitors. *Int. J. Clin. Oncol.* **2017**, *22*, 1081–1086. [CrossRef]

90. Teishima, J.; Kobatake, K.; Shinmei, S.; Inoue, S.; Hayashi, T.; Ohara, S.; Mita, K.; Hasegawa, Y.; Maruyama, S.; Kajiwara, M.; et al. The effect of kinetics of C-reactive protein in the prediction of overall survival in patients with metastatic renal cell carcinoma treated with tyrosine kinase inhibitor. *Urol. Oncol.* **2017**, *35*, E1–E7. [CrossRef]
91. Hu, K.; Lou, L.; Ye, J.; Zhang, S. Prognostic role of the neutrophil-lymphocyte ratio in renal cell carcinoma: A meta-analysis. *BMJ Open* **2015**, *8*, E006404. [CrossRef] [PubMed]
92. Farolfi, A.; Petrone, M.; Scarpi, E.; Gallà, V.; Greco, F.; Casanova, C.; Longo, L.; Cormio, G.; Orditura, M.; Bologna, A.; et al. Inflammatory Indexes as Prognostic and Predictive Factors in Ovarian Cancer Treated with Chemotherapy Alone or Together with Bevacizumab. A Multicenter, Retrospective Analysis by the MITO Group (MITO 24). *Target. Oncol.* **2018**, *13*, 469–479. [CrossRef] [PubMed]
93. Templeton, A.J.; McNamara, M.G.; Šeruga, B.; Vera-Badillo, F.E.; Aneja, P.; Ocaña, A.; Leibowitz-Amit, R.; Sonpavde, G.; Knox, J.J.; Tran, B.; et al. Prognostic role of neutrophil-to-lymphocyte ratio in solid tumors: A systematic review and meta-analysis. *J. Natl. Cancer Inst.* **2014**, *106*, dju124. [CrossRef] [PubMed]
94. Saroha, S.; Uzzo, R.G.; Plimack, E.R.; Ruth, K.; Al-Saleem, T. Lymphopenia is an independent predictor of inferior outcome in clear cell renal carcinoma. *J. Urol.* **2013**, *189*, 454–461. [CrossRef]
95. De Giorgi, U.; Rihawi, K.; Aieta, M.; Lo Re, G.; Sava, T.; Masini, C.; Baldazzi, V.; De Vincenzo, F.; Camerini, A.; Fornarini, G.; et al. Lymphopenia and clinical outcome of elderly patients treated with sunitinib for metastatic renal cell cancer. *J. Geriatr. Oncol.* **2014**, *5*, 156–163. [CrossRef]
96. Grimes, N.; Tyson, M.; Hannan, C.; Mulholland, C. A systematic review of the prognostic role of hematologic scoring systems in patients with renal cell carcinoma undergoing nephrectomy with curative intent. *Clin. Genitourin. Cancer* **2016**, *14*, 271–276. [CrossRef]
97. Boissier, R.; Campagna, J.; Branger, N.; Karsenty, G.; Lechevallier, E. The prognostic value of the neutrophil-lymphocyte ratio in renal oncology: A review. *Urol. Oncol.* **2017**, *35*, 135–141. [CrossRef]
98. Li, X.; Ma, X.; Tang, L.; Wang, B.; Chen, L.; Zhang, F.; Zhang, X. Prognostic value of neutrophil-to-lymphocyte ratio in urothelial carcinoma of the upper urinary tract and bladder: A systematic review and meta-analysis. *Oncotarget* **2016**, *8*, 62681–62692. [CrossRef]
99. Hu, H.; Yao, X.; Xie, X.; Wu, X.; Zheng, C.; Xia, W.; Ma, S. Prognostic value of preoperative NLR, dNLR, PLR and CRP in surgical renal cell carcinoma patients. *World J. Urol.* **2017**, *35*, 261–270. [CrossRef]
100. Fukuda, H.; Takagi, T.; Kondo, T.; Shimizu, S.; Tanabe, K. Predictive value of inflammation-based prognostic scores in patients with metastatic renal cell carcinoma treated with cytoreductive nephrectomy. *Oncotarget* **2018**, *9*, 14296–14305. [CrossRef]
101. Ohno, Y.; Nakashima, J.; Ohori, M.; Hatano, T.; Tachibana, M. Pretreatment neutrophil-to-lymphocyte ratio as an independent predictor of recurrence in patients with nonmetastatic renal cell carcinoma. *J. Urol.* **2010**, *184*, 873–878. [CrossRef] [PubMed]
102. Pichler, M.; Hutterer, G.C.; Stojakovic, T.; Mannweiler, S.; Pummer, K.; Zigeuner, R. High plasma fibrinogen level represents an independent negative prognostic factor regarding cancer-specific, metastasis-free, as well as overall survival in a European cohort of non-metastatic renal cell carcinoma patients. *Br. J. Cancer* **2013**, *109*, 1123–1129. [CrossRef] [PubMed]
103. De Martino, M.; Pantuck, A.J.; Hofbauer, S.; Waldert, M.; Shariat, S.F.; Belldegrun, A.S.; Klatte, T. Prognostic impact of preoperative neutrophil-to-lymphocyte ratio in localized nonclear cell renal cell carcinoma. *J. Urol.* **2013**, *190*, 1999–2004. [CrossRef] [PubMed]
104. Jeyakumar, G.; Kim, S.; Bumma, N.; Landry, C.; Silski, C.; Suisham, S.; Dickow, B.; Heath, E.; Fontana, J.; Vaishampayan, U. Neutrophil lymphocyte ratio and duration of prior anti-angiogenic therapy as biomarkers in metastatic RCC receiving immune checkpoint inhibitor therapy. *J. Immunother. Cancer* **2017**, *5*, 82. [CrossRef]
105. Zhang, T.; Zhu, J.; George, D.J.; Nixon, A.B. Metastatic clear cell renal cell carcinoma: Circulating biomarkers to guide antiangiogenic and immune therapies. *Urol. Oncol.* **2016**, *34*, 510–518. [CrossRef]
106. Santoni, M.; Buti, S.; Conti, A.; Porta, C.; Procopio, G.; Sternberg, C.N.; Bracarda, S.; Basso, U.; De Giorgi, U.; Rizzo, M.; et al. Prognostic significance of host immune status in patients with late relapsing renal cell carcinoma treated with targeted therapy. *Target. Oncol.* **2015**, *10*, 517–522. [CrossRef]
107. Park, Y.H.; Ku, J.H.; Kwak, C.; Kim, H.H. Post-treatment neutrophil-to-lymphocyte ratio in predicting prognosis in patients with metastatic clear cell renal cell carcinoma receiving sunitinib as first line therapy. *Springerplus* **2014**, *3*, 243. [CrossRef]

108. Cetin, B.; Berk, V.; Kaplan, M.A.; Afsar, B.; Tufan, G.; Ozkan, M.; Isikdogan, A.; Benekli, M.; Coskun, U.; Buyukberber, S. Is the pretreatment neutrophil to lymphocyte ratio an important prognostic parameter in patients with metastatic renal cell carcinoma? *Clin. Genitourin. Cancer* **2013**, *11*, 141–148. [CrossRef]
109. Santoni, M.; De Giorgi, U.; Iacovelli, R.; Conti, A.; Burattini, L.; Rossi, L.; Burgio, S.L.; Berardi, R.; Muzzonigro, G.; Cortesi, E.; et al. Pre-treatment neutrophil-to-lymphocyte ratio may be associated with the outcome in patients treated with everolimus for metastatic renal cell carcinoma. *Br. J. Cancer.* **2013**, *109*, 1755–1759. [CrossRef]
110. Keizman, D.; Ish-Shalom, M.; Huang, P.; Eisenberger, M.A.; Pili, R.; Hammers, H.; Carducci, M.A. The association of pre-treatment neutrophil to lymphocyte ratio with response rate, progression free survival and overall survival of patients treated with sunitinib for metastatic renal cell carcinoma. *Eur. J. Cancer* **2012**, *48*, 202–208. [CrossRef]
111. Ohno, Y.; Nakashima, J.; Ohori, M.; Tanaka, A.; Hashimoto, T.; Gondo, T.; Hatano, T.; Tachibana, M. Clinical variables for predicting metastatic renal cell carcinoma patients who might not benefit from cytoreductive nephrectomy: Neutrophil-to-lymphocyte ratio and performance status. *Int. J. Clin. Oncol.* **2014**, *19*, 139–145. [CrossRef] [PubMed]
112. Baum, Y.S.; Patil, D.; Huang, J.H.; Spetka, S.; Torlak, M.; Nieh, P.T.; Alemozaffar, M.; Ogan, K.; Master, V.A. Elevated preoperative neutrophil-to-lymphocyte ratio may be associated with decreased overall survival in patients with metastatic clear cell renal cell carcinoma undergoing cytoreductive nephrectomy. *Asian J. Urol.* **2016**, *3*, 20–25. [CrossRef] [PubMed]
113. Passardi, A.; Scarpi, E.; Cavanna, L.; Dall'Agata, M.; Tassinari, D.; Leo, S.; Bernardini, I.; Gelsomino, F.; Tamberi, S.; Brandes, A.A.; et al. Inflammatory indexes as predictors of prognosis and bevacizumab efficacy in patients with metastatic colorectal cancer. *Oncotarget* **2016**, *7*, 33210–33219. [CrossRef] [PubMed]
114. Lolli, C.; Basso, U.; Derosa, L.; Scarpi, E.; Sava, T.; Santoni, M.; Crabb, S.J.; Massari, F.; Aieta, M.; Conteduca, V.; et al. Systemic immune-inflammation index predicts the clinical outcome in patients with metastatic renal cell cancer treated with sunitinib. *Oncotarget* **2016**, *7*, 54564–54571. [CrossRef] [PubMed]
115. Zhong, J.H.; Huang, D.H.; Chen, Z.Y. Prognostic role of systemic immune-inflammation index in solid tumors: A systematic review and meta-analysis. *Oncotarget* **2017**, *8*, 75381–75388. [CrossRef] [PubMed]
116. Forrest, L.M.; McMillan, D.C.; McArdle, C.S.; Angerson, W.J.; Dunlop, D.J. Evaluation of cumulative prognostic scores based on the systemic inflammatory response in patients with inoperable non-small-cell lung cancer. *Br. J. Cancer* **2003**, *89*, 1028–1030. [CrossRef] [PubMed]
117. Proctor, M.J.; Talwar, D.; Balmar, S.M.; O'Reilly, D.S.; Foulis, A.K.; Horgan, P.G.; Morrison, D.S.; McMillan, D.C. The relationship between the presence and site of cancer, an inflammation-based prognostic score and biochemical parameters. Initial results of the Glasgow Inflammation Outcome Study. *Br. J. Cancer* **2010**, *103*, 870–876. [CrossRef]
118. McMillan, D.C.; Crozier, J.E.M.; Canna, K.; Angerson, W.J.; McArdle, C.S. Evaluation of an inflammation-based prognostic score (GPS) in patients undergoing resection for colon and rectal cancer. *Int. J. Colorectal Dis.* **2007**, *22*, 881–886. [CrossRef]
119. Tsujino, T.; Komura, K.; Matsunaga, T.; Yoshikawa, Y.; Takai, T.; Uchimoto, T.; Saito, K.; Tanda, N.; Oide, R.; Minami, K.; et al. Preoperative measurement of the modified Glasgow prognostic score predicts patient survival in non-metastatic renal cell carcinoma prior to nephrectomy. *Ann. Surg. Oncol.* **2017**, *24*, 2787–27893. [CrossRef]
120. Cho, D.S.; Kim, S.I.; Choo, S.H.; Jang, S.H.; Ahn, H.S.; Kim, S.J. Prognostic significance of modified Glasgow prognostic score in patients with non-metastatic clear cell renal cell carcinoma. *Scand. J. Urol.* **2016**, *50*, 186–191. [CrossRef]
121. Lucca, I.; De Martino, M.; Hofbauer, S.L.; Zamani, N.; Shariat, S.F.; Klatte, T. Comparison of the prognostic value of pretreatment measurements of systemic inflammatory response in patients undergoing curative resection of clear cell renal cell carcinoma. *World J. Urol.* **2015**, *33*, 2045–2052. [CrossRef] [PubMed]
122. Lamb, G.W.A.; Aitchison, M.; Ramsey, S.; Housley, S.L.; McMillan, D.C. Clinical utility of the Glasgow prognostic score in patients undergoing curative nephrectomy for renal clear cell cancer: Basis of new prognostic scoring systems. *Br. J. Cancer* **2012**, *106*, 279–283. [CrossRef] [PubMed]
123. Ramsey, S.; Lamb, G.W.A.; Aitchison, M.; Graham, J.; McMillan, D.C. Evaluation of an inflammation-based prognostic score in patients with metastatic renal cancer. *Cancer* **2007**, *109*, 205–212. [CrossRef] [PubMed]

124. Heng, D.Y.; Xie, W.; Regan, M.M.; Warren, M.A.; Golshayan, A.R.; Sahi, C.; Eigl, B.J.; Ruether, J.D.; Cheng, T.; North, S.; et al. Prognostic factors for overall survival in patients with metastatic renal cell carcinoma treated with vascular endothelial growth factor-targeted agents: Results from a large, multicenter study. *J. Clin. Oncol.* **2009**, *27*, 5794–5799. [CrossRef]

125. Ishihara, H.; Kondo, T.; Yoshida, K.; Omae, K.; Takagi, T.; Iizuka, J.; Tanabe, K. Effect of systemic inflammation of survival in patients with metastatic renal cell carcinoma receiving second line molecular-targeted therapy. *Clin. Genitourin. Cancer* **2017**, *15*, 495–501. [CrossRef]

126. Kang, M.; Jeong, C.W.; Kwak, C.; Kim, H.H.; Ku, J.H. Preoperative neutrophil-lymphocyte ratio can significantly predict mortality outcomes in patients with non-muscle invasive bladder cancer undergoing transurethral resection of bladder tumor. *Oncotarget* **2017**, *8*, 12891–12901. [CrossRef]

127. Rausch, S.; Kruck, S.; Walter, K.; Stenzl, A.; Bedke, J. Metastasectomy for metastatic renal cell carcinoma in the era of modern systemic treatment: C-reactive protein is an independent predictor of overall survival. *Int. J. Urol* **2016**, *23*, 916–921. [CrossRef]

128. Gunduz, S.; Mutlu, H.; Tural, D.; Yıldız, Ö.; Uysal, M.; Coskun, H.S.; Bozcuk, H. Platelet to lymphocyte ratio as a new prognostic for patients with metastatic renal cell cancer. *Asia Pac. J. Clin. Oncol* **2015**, *11*, 288–292. [CrossRef]

129. Kang, M.; Chang, C.T.; Sung, H.H.; Jeon, H.G.; Jeong, B.C.; Seo, S.I.; Jeon, S.S.; Choi, H.Y.; Lee, H.M. Prognostic significance of pre- to postoperative dynamics of the prognostic nutritional index for patients with renal cell carcinoma who underwent radical nephrectomy. *Ann. Surg. Oncol.* **2017**, *24*, 4067–4075. [CrossRef]

130. Peng, D.; He, Z.S.; Li, X.S.; Tang, Q.; Zhang, L.; Yang, K.W.; Yu, X.T.; Zhang, C.J.; Zhou, L.Q. Prognostic value of inflammatory and nutritional scores in renal cell carcinoma after nephrectomy. *Clin. Genitourin. Cancer* **2017**, *15*, 582–590. [CrossRef]

131. Kwon, W.A.; Kim, S.; Kim, S.H.; Joung, J.Y.; Seo, H.K.; Lee, K.H.; Chung, J. Pretreatment prognostic nutritional index is an independent predictor of survival in patients with metastatic renal cell carcinoma treated with targeted therapy. *Clin. Genitourin. Cancer* **2017**, *15*, 100–111. [CrossRef] [PubMed]

132. Broggi, M.S.; Patil, D.; Baum, Y.; Nieh, P.T.; Alemozaffar, M.; Pattaras, J.G.; Ogan, K.; Master, V.A. Onodera's prognostic nutritional index as an independent prognostic factor in clear cell renal cell carcinoma. *Urology* **2016**, *96*, 99–105. [CrossRef] [PubMed]

133. Jeon, H.G.; Choi, D.K.; Sung, H.H.; Jeong, B.C.; Seo, S.I.; Jeon, S.S.; Choi, H.Y.; Lee, H.M. Preoperative prognostic nutritional index is a significant predictor of survival in renal cell carcinoma patients undergoing nephrectomy. *Ann. Surg. Oncol.* **2016**, *23*, 321–327. [CrossRef] [PubMed]

134. Hofbauer, S.L.; Pantuck, A.J.; de Martino, M.; Lucca, I.; Haitel, A.; Shariat, S.F.; Belldegrun, A.S.; Klatte, T. The preoperative prognostic nutritional index is an independent predictor of survival in patients with renal cell carcinoma. *Urol. Oncol.* **2015**, *33*, E1–E7. [CrossRef] [PubMed]

135. Huang, J.; Yuan, Y.; Wang, Y.; Chen, Y.; Kong, W.; Xue, W.; Chen, H.; Zhang, J.; Huang, Y. Preoperative prognostic nutritional index is a significant predictor of survival in patients with localized upper tract urothelial carcinoma after radical nephroureterectomy. *Urol. Oncol.* **2017**, *35*, E1–E71. [CrossRef]

136. Qi, Q.; Zhuang, L.; Shen, Y.; Geng, Y.; Yu, S.; Chen, H.; Liu, L.; Meng, Z.; Wang, P.; Chen, Z. A novel systemic inflammation response index (SIRI) for predicting the survival of patients with pancreatic cancer after chemotherapy. *Cancer* **2016**, *122*, 2158–2167. [CrossRef]

137. Geng, Y.; Zhu, D.; Wu, C.; Wu, J.; Wang, Q.; Li, R.; Jiang, J.; Wu, C. A novel systemic inflammation response index (SIRI) for predicting postoperative survival of patients with esophageal squamous cell carcinoma. *Int. Immunopharmacol.* **2018**, *65*, 503–510. [CrossRef]

138. Li, S.; Lan, X.; Gao, H.; Li, Z.; Chen, L.; Wang, W.; Song, S.; Wang, Y.; Li, C.; Zhang, H.; et al. Systemic Inflammation Response Index (SIRI), cancer stem cells and survival of localised gastric adenocarcinoma after curative resection. *J. Cancer Res. Clin. Oncol.* **2017**, *143*, 2455–2468. [CrossRef]

139. Ferrone, C.; Dranoff, G. Dual roles for immunity in gastrointestinal cancers. *J. Clin. Oncol.* **2010**, *28*, 4045–4051. [CrossRef]

140. Hara, T.; Miyake, H.; Fujisawa, M. Expression pattern of immune check-point associated molecules in radical nephrectomy specimens as a prognosticator in patients with metastatic renal cell carcinoma treated with tyrosine kinase inhibitors. *Urol. Oncol.* **2017**, *35*, 363–369. [CrossRef]

141. Ueda, K.; Suekane, S.; Kurose, H.; Chikui, K.; Nakiri, M.; Nishihara, K.; Matsuo, M.; Kawahara, A.; Yano, H.; Igawa, T. Prognostic value of PD-1 and PD-L1 expression in patients with metastatic clear cell renal cell carcinoma. *Urol. Oncol.* **2018**, *36*, E9-499. [CrossRef] [PubMed]
142. Choueiri, T.K.; Figueroa, D.J.; Fay, A.P.; Signoretti, S.; Liu, Y.; Gagnon, R.; Deen, K.; Carpenter, C.; Benson, P.; Ho, T.H.; et al. Correlation of PD-L1 tumor expression and treatment outcomes in patients with renal cell carcinoma receiving sunitinib or pazopanib: Results from COMPARZ, a randomized controlled trial. *Clin. Cancer Res.* **2015**, *21*, 1071–1077. [CrossRef] [PubMed]
143. Thompson, R.H.; Gillett, M.D.; Cheville, J.C.; Lohse, C.M.; Dong, H.; Webster, W.S.; Chen, L.; Zincke, H.; Blute, M.L.; Leibovich, B.C.; et al. Costimulatory molecule B7-H1 in primary and metastatic clear cell renal cell carcinoma. *Cancer* **2005**, *104*, 2084–2091. [CrossRef] [PubMed]
144. Thompson, R.H.; Kuntz, S.M.; Leibovich, B.C.; Dong, H.; Lohse, C.M.; Webster, W.S.; Sengupta, S.; Frank, I.; Parker, A.S.; Zincke, H.; et al. Tumor B7-H1 is associated with poor prognosis in renal cell carcinoma patients with long-term follow up. *Cancer Res.* **2006**, *66*, 3381–3385. [CrossRef] [PubMed]
145. Xu, F.; Xu, L.; Wang, Q.; An, G.; Feng, G.; Liu, F. Clinicopathological and prognostic value of programmed death ligand-1 (PD-L1) in renal cell carcinoma: A meta-analysis. *Int. J. Clin. Exp. Med.* **2015**, *8*, 14595–14603. [PubMed]
146. Leite, K.R.; Reis, S.T.; Junior, J.P.; Zerati, M.; Gomes Dde, O.; Camara-Lopes, L.H.; Srougi, M. PD-L1 expression in renal cell carcinoma clear cell type is related to unfavorable prognosis. *Diagn. Pathol.* **2015**, *10*, 189. [CrossRef]
147. Callea, M.; Albiges, L.; Gupta, M.; Cheng, S.C.; Genega, E.M.; Fay, A.P.; Song, J.; Carvo, I.; Bhatt, R.S.; Atkins, M.B.; et al. Differential expression of PD-L1 between primary and metastatic sites in clear-cell renal cell carcinoma. *Cancer Immunol. Res.* **2015**, *3*, 1158–1164. [CrossRef]
148. Tatli Dogan, H.; Kiran, M.; Bilgin, B.; Kiliçarslan, A.; Sendur, M.A.N.; Yalçin, B.; Ardiçoglu, A.; Atmaca, A.F.; Gumuskaya, B. Prognostic significance of the programmed death ligand 1 expression in clear cell renal cell carcinoma and correlation with the tumor microenvironment and hypoxia inducible factor expression. *Diagn. Pathol.* **2018**, *13*, 60. [CrossRef]
149. Negrier, S.; Escudier, B.; Gomez, F.; Douillard, J.Y.; Ravaud, A.; Chevreau, C.; Buclon, M.; Pérol, D.; Lasset, C. Prognostic factors of survival and rapid progression in 782 patients with metastatic renal carcinomas treated by cytokines: A report from the Groupe Francais d'Immunotherapie. *Ann. Oncol.* **2002**, *13*, 1460–1468. [CrossRef]
150. Ruiz-Morales, J.M.; Heng, D.Y. Cabozantinib in the treatment of advanced renal cell carcinoma: Clinical trial evidence and experience. *Ther. Adv. Urol.* **2016**, *8*, 338–347. [CrossRef]
151. Deprimo, S.E.; Bello, C.L.; Smeraglia, J.; Baum, C.M.; Spinella, D.; Rini, B.I.; Michaelson, M.D.; Motzer, R.J. Circulating protein biomarkers of pharmacodynamic activity of sunitinib in patients with metastatic renal cell carcinoma: Modulation of VEGF and VEGF-related proteins. *J. Transl. Med.* **2007**, *5*, 32. [CrossRef] [PubMed]
152. Pantuck, A.J.; Seligson, D.B.; Klatte, T.; Yu, H.; Leppert, J.T.; Moore, L.; O'Toole, T.; Gibbons, J.; Belldegrun, A.S.; Figlin, R.A. Prognostic relevance of the mTOR pathway in renal cell carcinoma: Implications for molecular patient selection for targeted therapy. *Cancer* **2007**, *109*, 2257–2267. [CrossRef] [PubMed]
153. Cho, D.; Signoretti, S.; Dabora, S.; Regan, M.; Seeley, A.; Mariotti, M.; Youmans, A.; Polivy, A.; Mandato, L.; McDermott, D.; et al. Potential histologic and molecular predictors of response to temsirolimus in patients with advanced renal cell carcinoma. *Clin. Genitourin. Cancer* **2007**, *5*, 379–385. [CrossRef] [PubMed]
154. Shin, S.J.; Jeon, Y.K.; Cho, Y.M.; Lee, J.L.; Chung, D.H.; Park, J.Y.; Go, H. The association between PD-L1 expression and the clinical outcomes to vascular endothelial growth factor-targeted therapy in patients with metastatic clear cell renal cell carcinoma. *Oncologist* **2015**, *20*, 1253–1260. [CrossRef]
155. Byun, S.S.; Hwang, E.C.; Kang, S.H.; Hong, S.H.; Chung, J.; Kwon, T.G.; Kim, H.H.; Kwak, C.; Kim, Y.J.; Lee, W.K. Age-dependent prognostic value of body mass index for non-metastatic clear cell renal cell carcinoma: A large multicenter retrospective analysis. *J. Surg. Oncol.* **2018**, *118*, 199–205. [CrossRef]
156. Komura, K.; Inamoto, T.; Black, P.C.; Koyama, K.; Katsuoka, Y.; Watsuji, T.; Azuma, H. Prognostic significance of body mass index in Asian patients with localized renal cell carcinoma. *Nutr. Cancer* **2011**, *63*, 908–915. [CrossRef]
157. Ramsey, S. The role of the systemic inflammatory response as a biomarker in immunotherapy for renal cell cancer. *Mol. Diagn. Ther.* **2009**, *13*, 277–281. [CrossRef]

158. Sacdalan, D.B.; Lucero, J.A.; Sacdalan, D.L. Prognostic utility of baseline neutrophil-to-lymphocyte ratio in patients receiving immune checkpoint inhibitors: A review and meta-analysis. *OncoTargets Ther.* **2018**, *11*, 955–965. [CrossRef]
159. Jeyakumar, G.; Bumma, N.; Kim, S.H.; Landry, C.; Kim, H.; Silski, C.; Suisham, S.; Dickow, B.; Heath, E.I.; Fontana, J.A.; et al. Neutrophil lymphocyte ratio (NLR) as a clinical biomarker predictive of outcomes with immune checkpoint inhibitor therapy in genitourinary cancers. *J. Clin. Oncol.* **2017**, *35* (Suppl. 6S). [CrossRef]
160. Bilen, M.A.; Dutcher, G.M.A.; Liu, Y.; Ravindranathan, D.; Kissick, H.T.; Carthon, B.C.; Kucuk, O.; Harris, W.B.; Master, V.A. Association Between Pretreatment Neutrophil-to-Lymphocyte Ratio and Outcome of Patients with Metastatic Renal-Cell Carcinoma Treated with Nivolumab. *Clin. Genitour. Cancer* **2018**, *16*, e563–e575. [CrossRef]
161. Lalani, A.K.; Wanling, X.; Martini, D.J.; Steinharter, J.A.; Norton, C.K.; Krajewski, K.M.; Duquette, A.; Bossé, D.; Bellmunt, J.; Van Allen, E.M.; et al. Change in neutrophil-to-lymphocyte ratio (NLR) in response to immune checkpoint blockade for metastatic renal cell carcinoma. *J. Immunother. Cancer* **2018**, *6*, 5. [CrossRef] [PubMed]
162. De Giorgi, U.; Cartenì, G.; Giannarelli, D.; Basso, U.; Galli, L.; Cortesi, E.; Caserta, C.; Pignata, S.; Sabbatini, R.; Bearz, A.; et al. Safety and efficacy of nivolumab for metastatic renal cell carcinoma: Real-world results from an expanded access programme. *BJU Int.* **2019**, *123*, 98–105. [CrossRef] [PubMed]
163. De Giorgi, U.; Procopio, G.; Giannarelli, D.; Sabbatini, R.; Bearz, A.; Buti, S.; Basso, U.; Mitterer, M.; Ortega, C.; Bidoli, P.; et al. Association of Systemic Inflammation Index and Body Mass Index With Survival in Patients With Renal Cell Cancer Treated With Nivolumab. *Clin. Cancer Res.* **2019**, *25*, 3839–3846. [CrossRef] [PubMed]
164. Shen, X.; Zhao, B. Efficacy of PD-1 or PD-L1 inhibitors and PD-L1expression status in cancer: Meta-analysis. *BMJ* **2018**, *362*, 3529. [CrossRef]
165. Hutson, T.E.; Lesovoy, V.; Al-Shukri, S.; Stus, V.P.; Lipatov, O.N.; Bair, A.H.; Rosbrook, B.; Chen, C.; Kim, S.; Vogelzang, N.J. Axitinib versus sorafenib as first-line therapy in patients with metastatic renal-cell carcinoma: A randomised open-label phase 3 trial. *Lancet Oncol.* **2013**, *14*, 1287–1294. [CrossRef]
166. Abbas, M.; Steffens, S.; Bellut, M.; Becker, J.U.; Großhennig, A.; Eggers, H.; Wegener, G.; Kuczyk, M.A.; Kreipe, H.H.; Grünwald, V.; et al. Do programmed death 1 (PD-1) and its ligand (PD-L1) play a role in patients with non-clear cell renal cell carcinoma? *Med. Oncol.* **2016**, *33*, 59. [CrossRef]
167. McKay, R.R.; Bossè, D.; Xie, W.; Wankowicz, S.A.M.; Flaifel, A.; Brandao, R.; Lalani, A.A.; Martini, D.J.; Wei, X.X.; Braun, D.A.; et al. The clinical activity of PD-1/PD-L1 inhibitors in metastatic non-clear cell renal cell carcinoma. *Cancer Immunol. Res.* **2018**, *6*, 758–765. [CrossRef]
168. Joseph, R.W.; Millis, S.Z.; Carballido, E.M.; Bryant, D.; Gatalica, Z.; Reddy, S.; Bryce, A.H.; Vogelzang, N.J.; Stanton, M.L.; Castle, E.P.; et al. PD-1 and PD-L1 expression in Renal Cell Carcinoma with Sarcomatoid Differentiation. *Cancer Immunol. Res.* **2015**, *3*, 1303–1307. [CrossRef]
169. McDermott, D.F.; Choueiri, T.K.; Motzer, R.J.; Aren, O.R.; George, S.; Powles, T.; Donskov, F.; Harrison, M.R.; Rodriguez Cid, R.R.; Ishii, Y.; et al. CheckMate 214 post-hoc analyses of nivolumab plus ipilimumab or sunitinib in IMDC intermediate/poor-risk patients with previously untreated advanced renal cell carcinoma with sarcomatoid features. *J. Clin. Oncol.* **2019**, *37* (Suppl. 15), 4513. [CrossRef]
170. Choueiri, T.K.; Fay, A.P.; Gray, K.P.; Callea, M.; Ho, T.H.; Albiges, L.; Bellmunt, J.; Song, J.; Carvo, I.; Lampron, M.; et al. PD-L1 expression in nonclear-cell renal cell carcinoma. *Ann. Oncol.* **2014**, *25*, 2178–2184. [CrossRef]
171. Montironi, R.; Santoni, M.; Cheng, L.; Lopez-Beltran, A.; Massari, F.; Matrana, M.R.; Moch, H.; Scarpelli, M. An overview of emerging immunotargets of genitourinary tumors. *Curr. Drug Targets* **2016**, *17*, 750–756. [CrossRef] [PubMed]
172. Slovin, S.F. The need for immune biomarkers for treatment prognosis and response in genitourinary malignancies. *Biomark. Med.* **2017**, *11*, 1149–1159. [CrossRef] [PubMed]
173. Gibney, G.T.; Weiner, L.M.; Atkins, M.B. Predictive biomarkers for checkpoint inhibitor-based immunotherapy. *Lancet Oncol.* **2016**, *17*, e542–e551. [CrossRef]
174. Wang, T.; Lu, R.; Kapur, P.; Jaiswal, B.S.; Hannan, R.; Zhang, Z.; Pedrosa, I.; Luke, J.J.; Zhang, H.; Goldstein, L.D.; et al. An empirical approach leveraging tumorgrafts to dissect the tumor microenvironment in Renal Cell Carcinoma identifies missing link to prognostic inflammatory factors. *Cancer Discov.* **2018**, *8*, 1142–1155. [CrossRef] [PubMed]

175. Turajlic, S.; Swanton, C.; Boshoff, C. Kidney Cancer: The next decade. *J. Exp. Med.* **2018**, *215*, 2477–2479. [CrossRef] [PubMed]
176. Turajlic, S.; Xu, H.; Litchfield, K.; Rowan, A.; Chambers, T.; Lopez, J.I.; Nicol, D.; O'Brien, T.; Larkin, J.; Horswell, S.; et al. Tracking Cancer Evolution Reveals Constrained Routes to Metastases: TRACERx Renal. *Cell* **2018**, *173*, 581–594. [CrossRef] [PubMed]
177. Voss, M.H.; Chen, D.; Markeret, M.; Voss, M.H.; Chen, D.; Marker, M.; Xu, J.; Patel, P.; Han, X.; Hsieh, J.; et al. Tumor genomic analysis for 128 renal cell carcinoma (RCC) patients receiving first-line everolimus: Correlation between outcome and mutations status in MTOR, TSC1, and TSC2. *J. Clin. Oncol.* **2017**, *35*, 484. [CrossRef]
178. Tartari, F.; Santoni, M.; Burattini, L.; Mazzanti, P.; Onofri, A.; Berardi, R. Economic sustainability of anti-PD-1 agents nivolumab and pembrolizumab in cancer patients: Recent insights and future challenges. *Cancer Treat. Rev.* **2016**, *48*, 20–24. [CrossRef]

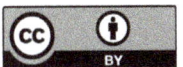 © 2019 by the authors. Licensee MDPI, Basel, Switzerland. This article is an open access article distributed under the terms and conditions of the Creative Commons Attribution (CC BY) license (http://creativecommons.org/licenses/by/4.0/).

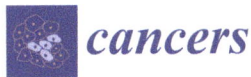

Review

The Changing Therapeutic Landscape of Metastatic Renal Cancer

Javier C. Angulo [1],* and Oleg Shapiro [2]

[1] Departamento Clínico, Facultad de Ciencias Biomédicas, Universidad Europea de Madrid, Hospital Universitario de Getafe, Carretera de Toledo km 12.5, Getafe, 28043 Madrid, Spain
[2] SUNY Upstate Medical University, Upstate University Hospital, Syracuse, NY 13210, USA
* Correspondence: javier.angulo@salud.madrid.org

Received: 23 July 2019; Accepted: 19 August 2019; Published: 22 August 2019

Abstract: The practising clinician treating a patient with metastatic clear cell renal cell carcinoma (CCRCC) faces a difficult task of choosing the most appropriate therapeutic regimen in a rapidly developing field with recommendations derived from clinical trials. NCCN guidelines for kidney cancer initiated a major shift in risk categorization and now include emerging treatments in the neoadjuvant setting. Updates of European Association of Urology clinical guidelines also include immune checkpoint inhibition as the first-line treatment. Randomized trials have demonstrated a survival benefit for ipilimumab and nivolumab combination in the intermediate and poor-risk group, while pembrolizumab plus axitinib combination is recommended not only for unfavorable disease but also for patients who fit the favorable risk category. Currently vascular endothelial growth factor (VEGF) targeted therapy based on tyrosine kinase inhibitors (TKI), sunitinib and pazopanib is the alternative regimen for patients who cannot tolerate immune checkpoint inhibitors (ICI). Cabozantinib remains a valid alternative option for the intermediate and high-risk group. For previously treated patients with TKI with progression, nivolumab, cabozantinib, axitinib, or the combination of ipilimumab and nivolumab appear the most plausible alternatives. For patients previously treated with ICI, any VEGF-targeted therapy, not previously used in combination with ICI therapy, seems to be a valid option, although the strength of this recommendation is weak. The indication for cytoreductive nephrectomy (CN) is also changing. Neoadjuvant systemic therapy does not add perioperative morbidity and can help identify non-responders, avoiding unnecessary surgery. However, the role of CN should be investigated under the light of new immunotherapeutic interventions. Also, markers of response to ICI need to be identified before the optimal selection of therapy could be determined for a particular patient.

Keywords: renal cell carcinoma; immune checkpoint inhibitors; tyrosine kinase inhibitors; efficacy; toxicity; cytoreductive nephrectomy

1. Immune Checkpoint Inhibition in Renal Cancer

The ability to evade immune surveillance and programmed cell death characterize kidney cancer cells. Some tumors express biomarkers to prevent or elude an immune response, which is crucial in not allowing cells with damaged genetic load to proliferate. Cellular damage causes cell division arrest, so the cell can repair itself, and cell death is induced if repair is not possible to avoid the development of a malignant cell line. Restoring the ability of the immune system to function through its various checkpoints is mandatory. In this scenario, T-regulatory cells play a significant role in regulating the immune response to what the body recognizes as foreign [1,2]. Targeting immune checkpoints in clear cell renal cell carcinoma (CCRCC) is being extensively analyzed currently [3–5]. The pitfalls of the clinical translation of PD-1/PD-L1 blockade have also been critically reviewed [6–8].

CTLA-4 (CD15) is found on T-cells and if activated, results in the inhibition of T-cell function. Ipilimumab, investigated in patients who previously received IL-2, induced autoimmune events. Of patients with a sustained response, 30% had an autoimmune event [9]. Tremelimumab has also been evaluated in patients with metastatic (CRRCC) in association with sunitinib, a vascular endothelial growth factor (VEGF) inhibitor, and durable response was confirmed in 43% of the cases [10].

PD-1 (PDCD1) is a type I transmembrane glycoprotein receptor, part of the CD28/CTLA-4 immune checkpoint receptor family, expressed on peripheral blood mononuclear cells and activated tumor-infiltrating mononuclear immune cells and responsible for the down-regulation of T-cells. PD-1 is monomeric and contains a single immunoglobulin-like variable (IgV) domain in its N-terminal extracellular region, which mediates PD-1 binding to its ligands PD-L1 and PD-L2 [11,12]. The PD-1 intracellular region contains two immunoreceptor tyrosine-based regulatory structures that experience tyrosine phosphorylation and are responsible for the binding to the SH2-domain-containing tyrosine phosphatases PTPN6 (SHP1) and PTPN11 (SHP2), thus inhibiting T and B cell antigen receptor-mediated signaling [13]. A serum soluble variant of PD-1 has been found, although its relevance in CCRCC remains to be determined [8].

PD-1 ligand PD-L1 (CD274) is another type I transmembrane glycoprotein, part of the B7 family of immune checkpoint proteins [14]. PD-L1 expression correlates with VHL inactivation and HIF-2α expression [15,16], and carries bad prognosis for patients with CCRCC [17,18]. PD-L2 (PDCD1LG2) is another PD-1 ligand, a closely related protein to PD-L1. Both PD-1 ligands are expressed in kidney epithelial cells under normal conditions and upregulated by inflammation [19]. A serum soluble PD-L1 associated with tumor aggressiveness has been detected in patients with CCRCC [20].

Ipilimumab and nivolumab are monoclonal antibodies targeting the immune checkpoint proteins CTLA-4 and PD-1, respectively. PD-1 acts as a negative regulator of T-cell activity by binding to PD-L1 on either antigen-presenting or tumor cells, causing the inhibition of T-cell anti-neoplastic responses. CTLA-4 acts as a negative regulator of T-cell activation by binding to the B7 ligand CD80, and CD86 expressed on antigen-presenting cells, thus preventing the interaction between CD28 and the B7 ligands. Nivolumab binds to PD-1 and blocks the inhibitory signaling of the PD-1/PD-L1 interaction. Ipilimumab binds to CTLA-4 and blocks the inhibitory signaling of the CTLA-4/B7 interaction (Figure 1).

Nivolumab was approved by the FDA in 2015 as second-line therapy for mCCRCC after the results of the Phase 3 Checkmate-025 trial (NCT01668784) were published. The trial revealed superiority in overall survival in the nivolumab group compared to the everolimus group. Shortly thereafter, treatment with nivolumab monotherapy became the standard of care for patients who progressed after initial treatment with a VEGF inhibitor. After the Checkmate-214 trial (NCT02231749) results came to light in 2018, the combination of nivolumab plus ipilimumab was approved as first-line therapy for intermediate and poor-risk patients [21], thus totally changing the therapeutic landscape of advanced CCRCC. A better knowledge of the immunology of T-cell activation is leading to the establishment of immune checkpoint inhibition (ICI), and the beginning of a new era in the treatment paradigm of patients with advanced CCRCC, using monoclonal antibodies to block the inhibition of T-cell activation.

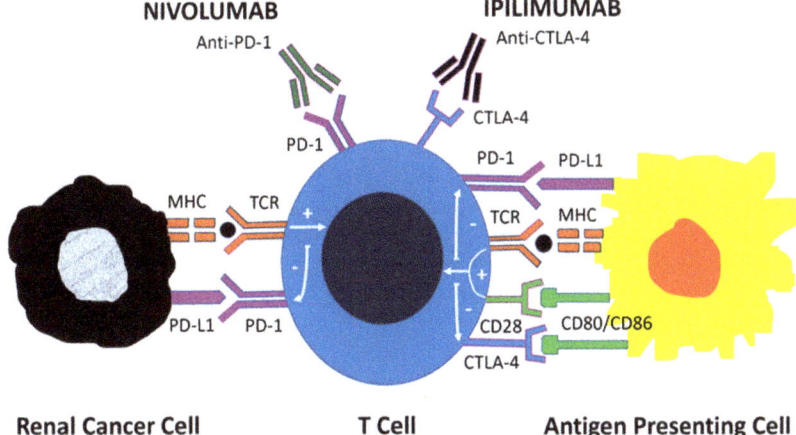

Figure 1. Mechanisms of action of immune checkpoint inhibitors. PD-1 acts as a negative regulator of T-cell activity by binding to PD-L1 on tumor cells and antigen-presenting cells, leading to downstream signaling that inhibits the antitumor T-cell response. CTLA-4 also negatively regulates T-cell activation by binding to B7 ligands CD80 and CD86 on antigen-presenting cells, thus preventing the co-stimulatory interaction between CD28 and B7 ligands. The monoclonal antibodies Nivolumab and Ipilimumab target the immune checkpoint proteins PD-1 and CTLA-4, respectively. Nivolumab blocks the inhibitory signal of the PD1: PD-L1 interaction while Ipilimumab blocks the inhibitory signal of the CTLA-4: B7 interaction.

2. The New Paradigm to Treat Metastatic Renal Cancer

Systemic therapy is the mainstay of treatment in patients with mCRRCC. The last 15 years saw a revolution in therapy based on VEGF-inhibition and immune checkpoint inhibition (ICI). Trials have shown a durable response in patients and an increase in the overall survival. The drastic change in the treatment paradigm happened in 2007 once the tyrosine kinase inhibitor (TKI), sunitinib, a potent VEGF inhibitor, proved superior to interferon-alfa in the treatment of metastatic clear cell renal cell carcinoma [22,23]. In 2015, another important trial showed nivolumab, the programmed cell death 1 (PD-1) receptor inhibitory signal blocker, to be superior to everolimus. This allowed immunotherapy to become the standard of care as second-line therapy for metastatic CCRCC [24].

Advances in risk group stratification were a major catalyst needed for the evolution of treatments and better interpretation of trial data. Original risk group categories were proposed by the Memorial Sloan Kettering Cancer Center (MSKCC) in the era of interferon-alpha and were widely used until very recently. This classification consists of five prognosis predicting factors, including time from the initial diagnosis to the start of systemic therapy, Karnofsky performance status, hemoglobin, serum calcium, and lactate dehydrogenase [25]. A similar classification system was proposed by Heng et al., taking into account neutrophil and platelet counts [26]. Accumulation of risk factors define favorable (0 positive factors), intermediate (1–2 factors), and high-risk (3 or more factors) groups. The International Metastatic Renal Cell Carcinoma Database Consortium (IMDC) validated Heng's criteria in patients treated with first, or second-line VEGF targeted therapy, making it applicable to a more contemporary cohort of patients [27].

The Checkmate-214 trial (NCT02231749) looked at the combination nivolumab plus imilimumab versus sunitinib in mCRRCC. The risk categories were defined as "good" (favorable) and "bad" (intermediate/poor) in the trial. The results revealed that in the metastatic setting, the combination of nivolumab plus ipilimumab demonstrated obvious superiority in the treatment-naïve patients with intermediate and poor-risk mCRRCC (objective response rate (ORR) 42% vs. 29%; $p < 0.0001$). Interestingly, the combination of nivolumab plus ipilimumab did not demonstrate superiority for favorable-risk disease (ORR 39% vs. 50%; $p = 0.14$). Paradoxically, there was a noticeable trend towards improvement in the progression-free survival with sunitinib versus the combination therapy (25.1% vs. 15.3%; $p < 0.0001$) [21,28,29]. Subsequently, the National Comprehensive Cancer Network (NCCN) Guidelines for metastatic kidney cancer have adopted the combination of ipilimumab plus nivolumab as the first-line therapy in the intermediate and poor-risk groups [30]. The tolerability of this combination immunotherapy was acceptable, despite the fact that more patients discontinued the therapy as compared to the sunitinib arm (24% vs. 12%). The most frequently seen grade 3–4 immune-related adverse effects (AEs) were diarrhea, hepatitis, and hypophysitis. Almost 60% of the patients with AEs required corticosteroids to manage their symptoms [21,29].

Further, the shift in first-line management of metastatic RCC has occurred as the results of the Keynote-426 trial (NCT02853331) became available. Pembrolizumab plus axitinib were shown to be superior to sunitinib regardless of the risk groups (ORR 59% vs. 35%; $p < 0.001$), with an acceptable safety profile [31]. Furthermore, the Javelin Renal-101 trial (NCT02684006) revealed avelumab plus axitinib to be more efficacious than sunitinib (ORR 51% vs. 25%). The Hazard Ratio (HR) for progression to death was 0.50 (95% CI 0.26–0.97) for favorable, 0.64 (0.47–0.88) for intermediate and 0.53 (0.30–0.93) for poor International Metastatic Renal Cell Carcinoma Database Consortium (IMDC) risk groups [32]. These trials cemented the strategy of using combined immune checkpoint and VEGF inhibition in patients with previously untreated metastatic CRRCC. This treatment paradigm has found its way into the NCCN and European Urological Association guidelines (Table 1) [30,33].

Table 1. Treatment recommendations for first-line and second-line therapy of metastatic clear cell renal cell carcinoma according to the Updated European Association of Urology Guidelines on Renal Cell Carcinoma.

Risk Group/Previous Treatments	Evidence-Based Standard (Level of Evidence)	Alternative Options (Level of Evidence)
IMDC favorable risk	PEMBROLIZUMAB/AXITINIB (1b)	SUNITINIB [1] (1b) PAZOPANIB [1] (1b)
IMDC intermediate and poor-risk groups	PEMBROLIZUMAB/AXITINIB (1b) IPILIMUMAB/ NIVOLUMAB (1b)	CABOZANTINIB (2a) SUNITINIB [1] (1b) PAZOPANIB [1] (1b)
Second-line prior TKI	NIVOLUMAB (1b) CABOZANTINIB (1b)	AXITINIB [1] (2b)
Second-line prior ICI	Any VEGF targeted therapy not previously used in combination with ICI [4]	

[1] Alternative options with no overall survival benefit proven are specially recommended in patients who cannot tolerate or do not have access to immune checkpoint inhibitors; IMDC: International Metastatic Renal Cell Carcinoma Database Consortium; TKI: Tyrosine kinase inhibitors; ICI: Immune checkpoint inhibitors; VEGF: Vascular endothelial growth factor; Oxford Level of Evidence: 1b (based on at least one randomized controlled phase III trial), 2a (based on at least one randomized controlled phase II trial), 2b (subgroup analysis of a randomized controlled phase III trial), 4 (expert opinion).

The IMmotion151 trial (NCT02420821) evaluated the programmed death-ligand 1 (PD-L1) blocker atezolizumab and VEGF-A inhibitor bevacizumab, compared to sunitinib as first-line therapy. Interim analysis has confirmed the combination of monoclonal antibodies prolonged progression-free survival in the PD-L1 positive patients (HR = 0.74; 95% CI 0.57–0.96; $p = 0.02$), but not in the overall population [34]. Two additional Phase III trials investigating different combination strategies, such as cabozantinib plus nivolumab compared to sunitinib (Checkmate-9ER, NCT01984242), and lenvatinib plus pembrolizumab compared to lenvatinib plus everolimus or sunitinib (Clear, NCT02811861) have not matured as of yet (Table 2).

Table 2. Efficacy results of Phase III clinical trials comparing immune checkpoint inhibitors in combination strategies with single-agent sunitinib.

Combination	Control Arm	Clinical Trial	Primary Endpoints	Results Reported
Ipilimumab + Nivolumab	Sunitinib	CheckMate-214 NCT02231749	ORR, OS, PFS	Intermediate, poor-risk disease: ORR: 42% vs. 29% ($p < 0.0001$) OS: Not reached vs. 26.6 mo ($p < 0.0001$) PFS: 8.2 vs. 8.3 mo ($p = 0.001$) Favorable risk disease: ORR: 39% vs. 50% ($p = 0.14$) OS: Not reached vs. Not reached ($p = 0.44$) PFS: 13.9 vs. 19.9 mo ($p = 0.189$)
Pembrolizumab + Axitinib	Sunitinib	Keynote-426 NCT02853331	OS, PFS	OS: 89.9 vs. 78.3 at 12 mo ($p < 0.0001$) PFS: 15.1 vs. 11.1 mo ($p < 0.0001$)
Avelumab + Axitinib	Sunitinib	Javelin Renal-101 NCT02684006	OS, PFS in PD-L1(+)	OS: Not yet reported PFS: 13.8 vs. 7.2 mo ($p < 0.0001$)
Atezolizumab + Becacizumab	Sunitinib	IMmotion-151 NCT02420821	ORR, OS, PFS in PD-L1(+)	ORR: 43% vs. 35% OS: Not yet reported PFS: 11.2 vs. 7.7 mo ($p = 0.02$)
Lenvatinib + Pembrolizumab	Lenvatinib + Everolimus or Sunitinib	Clear NCT02811861	PFS	PFS: Not yet reported
Cabozantinib + Nivolumab	Sunitinib	CheckMate-9ER NCT03141177	PFS	PFS: Not yet reported

ORR: Overall Response Rate; OS: Overall Survival; PFS: Progression-Free Survival; mo: months.

Combination treatments have shown improved response rates comparing to single-agent therapy with sunitinib and have replaced VEGF-targeted therapy as the standard first-line treatment in good and intermediate-risk groups. Interestingly, combination therapies have replaced the mammalian targets of rapamycin (mTOR) inhibitors, such as temsirolimus and everolimus, which were used for treatment-naïve poor-risk patients and patients treated with VEGF-TKI agents, respectively. However, the toxicity of newer treatment strategies using ICI should be carefully balanced to that of monotherapies. Treating physicians and investigators should take into consideration the incidence of treatment-related grade 3–4 adverse events (AEs) and treatment discontinuation due to these events, before optimal individualized therapy for mCRRCC is decided.

The overall toxicity profile of ICI differs from that of traditional therapies, and a better understanding of the AEs and their optimal management is critical for practising physicians [35]. A systematic review revealed 80% of patients receiving ICI, experienced AE patients with grade 3–4 AEs constitute 20% of the cohort, and less than 10% have to discontinue treatment due to adverse events [36]. Immune-related AEs (irAEs) are due to treatment and most commonly affect the skin (rash, pruritus) 30%, liver (elevated AST and ALT) 20%, gastrointestinal tract (diarrhea) 15%, endocrine system (hypothyroidism) 12%, kidneys (elevated creatinine) 7%, and lungs (pneumonitis) (5%). The most common grade 3–4 irAEs involve the liver. Interestingly, there were no deaths due to AEs reported in the trials reviewed [36].

Most trials and pooled analysis of ICI therapy suggest irAEs may occur anytime from weeks to years after the start of therapy, even after therapy cessation. However, the majority take place within the first year of treatment and resolve with the appropriate therapy [37]. Systemic corticosteroids are the mainstay of treatment for immune complications, but anti-TNF-α can also be used for refractory irAEs [38]. The use of systemic immunosuppressants does not seem to negatively impact the therapeutic effects of ICI therapy [36,37].

Patients who cannot tolerate ICI therapy can alternatively receive VEGF-TKI-based therapy. In these patients, sunitinib and pazopanib appear to be the optimal regimen in the favorable group, and cabozantinib remains a valid option for the intermediate and high-risk groups. However, as ICI is increasingly utilized as the front-line therapy for mCCRCC, limited data exist on the response rates and survival of patients treated with second-line VEGFR-TKI-based therapy. Antitumor activity and tolerance of TKI monotherapy after failed ICI seems comparable to historical data for the first-line TKI regimen [39].

3. Current Role of Multikinase Inhibitor Monotherapy

The introduction of VEGF receptor inhibitors, sorafenib and sunitinib in 2005 started a revolution in the management of mCCRCC. These therapies produced response rates of 40% in the front-line setting and progression-free survival estimates in the range of 9 and 12 months [40,41]. Salvage therapy involved treatment with mTOR inhibitor everolimus, but the response rate with this intervention was only modest [42], this created a void in the salvage therapy space. This led to the evolution of other salvage regimens such as multitargeted kinases and immunotherapy [29].

Cabozantinib, a multikinase inhibitor, was approved by the FDA in 2016 for patients with advanced kidney cancer that were formerly treated with one or more antiangiogenic drugs. The drug is a potent inhibitor of MET and VEGF receptor 2, but also of other receptor tyrosine kinases (RET, KIT, AXL and FLT3) [43,44]. It was the first medication that showed a statistical improvement in the three endpoints of clinical efficacy: response rate, progression-free survival, and overall survival. Meteor trial (NCT01865747), which ran concurrently with Checkmate-025, compared cabozantinib and everolimus. Cabozantinib improved progression-free survival (HR 0.51, 95% CI 0.41–0.62) and ORR (17% vs. 3%). The median overall survival was 21.4 months for cabozantinib versus 16.5 months for everolimus (HR 0.66; 95% CI 0.53–0.83). Grade 3–4 AEs occurred in 39% of the cabozantinib group and 40% of patients treated with everolimus. Most common grade 3–4 AEs were hypertension 15%, diarrhea 13%, fatigue 11%, hand-foot syndrome 8%, anemia 6%, and hypomagnesemia 5%. The dose reduction is effective to manage toxicities in this patient population and was required in 60% of the affected cohort in the Meteor trial [45–47]. The Cabosun trial (NCT01835158) compared cabozantinib to sunitinib. Unlike Checkmate-214 trial, no patients in the good-risk group by the IMDC criteria were included. Progression-free survival was 8.6 months for cabozantinib and 5.3 months for sunitinib (HR 0.66; 95% CI 0.46–0.95). The overall survival was higher with cabozantinib (30.3 vs. 21.8 months), but the difference did not reach statistical significance (HR 0.80; 95% CI 0.50-1.26) [48]. Since cabozantinib and nivolumab were developed in the same timeframe, there are no studies looking at the optimal sequencing of these agents. The current dogma tells us that patients who have prolonged clinical benefit with initial anti-VEGF therapy and demonstrated tolerability to this therapy are likely to benefit from cabozantinib as second-line treatment at progression [49]. Still, real-world data indicate comparable overall survival and time to treatment failure for nivolumab and cabozantinib. Therefore, both are reasonable therapeutic options in patients experiencing progression after initial first-line VEGF-TKI agents [50].

The Axis trial (NCT00678392) compared the efficacy and safety of axitinib versus sorafenib as second-line treatment. The overall survival did not differ between the two groups, but the progression-free survival was longer for axitinib (HR 0.656; 95% CI 0.552–0.779). Common grade 3–4 AEs were hypertension (17%), diarrhea (11%) and fatigue (10%) in axitinib-treated patients and hand-foot syndrome (17%), hypertension (12%) and diarrhea (8%) in sorafenib-treated patients [51]. These data allowed axitinib to become another second-line treatment option after first-line TKIs sunitinib, sorafenib, or pazopanib [52]. Optimal sequence and selection of nivolumab, cabozantinib, and axitinib remain undefined [53]. The reimbursement landscape differs around the world and often limits treatment options [54].

4. Cytoreductive Nephrectomy in the Era of Immunotherapy

Based on retrospective data, traditional treatment of mCCRCC includes a combination of VEGF-TKI-targeted therapy and cytoreductive nephrectomy (CN). This approach has recently become a matter of debate as new data suggest the lack of survival benefit for patients undergoing CN. A recent meta-analysis evaluating the efficacy and safety of perioperative sunitinib in patients with metastatic and advanced renal cancer revealed superior response rate, overall survival, and progression-free survival [55]. The randomized controlled study, Carmena (NCT00930033), has failed to show that CN plus sunitinib is superior to sunitinib alone in terms of overall survival (HR 0.89; 95% CI 0.71–1.10). Non-inferiority of targeted therapy alone was demonstrated. Also, CN was associated with a significant risk of perioperative mortality and morbidity. However, among many limitations of this study was the selection of many poor-risk patients for cytoreductive nephrectomy, who were unlikely to benefit from surgical intervention anyway. Based on these results, CN should be re-considered in many poor and intermediate-risk patients. Most good-risk patients would still likely benefit from cytoreductive nephrectomy [56,57].

Surtime (NCT01099423) compared immediate surgery versus neoadjuvant sunitinib followed by surgery. The progression-free rate at 28 weeks was not improved in patients treated with neoadjuvant sunitinib (43% vs. 42%; $p = 0.61$); however, more patients received sunitinib, and CN could be avoided in those with progressive disease [58]. In summary, neoadjuvant sunitinib may identify patients who are non-responders to systemic therapy, in whom CN could be safely avoided without affecting the outcome. Conversely, a minimally invasive approach and sometimes nephron-sparing surgery could be performed in selected patients [59,60].

As stated above, the superiority of nivolumab and ipilimumab over sunitinib has led to a paradigm shift in the first-line treatment of intermediate and poor-risk patients. Unfortunately, the role of CN in the setting of a novel immunotherapy is unknown and should be investigated [61]. One out of five patients entering Checkmate-214 and demonstrating a survival benefit with ICI had their primary tumor in place. That means the role of CN needs to be better defined in the era of immunotherapy.

5. The Need for New Markers in the Era of Immunotherapy

Treatment options for mCCRCC are evolving, with an increase in combination treatments being approved and new immunotherapies on the horizon. We must remember that RCC is a very heterogeneous tumor and that challenges the identification of biomarkers for this disease [62,63]. We do not know whether liquid biopsy and other emerging molecular technologies could help solve this problem [64]. What is more, it is difficult to isolate markers predictive of treatment response in a fast-changing therapeutic environment. Single-cell sequencing methods, novel PD-L1 tracer-based imaging modalities, ex vivo tumor spheroids for the creation of tumor immunograms, and immuno-PET are some of the most likely translational approaches to predict treatment responses in the immunotherapy era [65,66]. Future directions include next-generation sequencing of circulating tumor DNA and the study of the gut microbiome [67]. Of course, efforts to identify biomarkers evaluating early therapeutic efficacy could be of help to optimize the length of time for effective treatment in each line [68].

ICI targeting the PD-1/PD-L1 interaction and the activation of CTLA-4 via B7-1 or B7-2 are changing the therapeutic landscape in renal cancer. In the CheckMate 214 trial, patients with PD-L1 levels ≥1% before treatment had an ORR of 58% versus 25% after receiving nivoliumab plus ipilimumab versus sunitinib, respectively, and lower levels of PD-L1 expression were correlated with a more favorable risk [67]. However, the real prognostic value of PD-1, PD-L1, and CTLA-4 remains unclear as these biomarkers have been evaluated in clinical trials, but a clear definition of which is the most appropriate cannot be defined at present (Table 3) [67].

Table 3. Protein expression of immunological markers and their clinical significance in clinical trials.

Markers on Immunohistochemistry	Significance
PD-1 Positive in TIMC	Higher grade, OS
PD-L1 Positive in Tumor Cells	Histologic variant, high grade
PD-L1 Positive in TIMC	Histologic variant
CTLA-4 ≥ 2% in TIMC	OS, CSS
PD-1 in TIMC Positive and CTLA-4 in TIMC ≥2%	Histologic variant, High-grade, High-stage, OS, CSS

TIMC: Tumor-infiltrating mononuclear cells; OS: Overall survival; CSS: Cancer specific survival.

In metastatic disease, PD-L1 expression in tumor cells or in tumor-infiltrating mononuclear cells (TIMC) has been the most studied biomarker for the prediction of a response to PD-1/PD-L1 checkpoint inhibition therapy [69,70]. Response rates are better in PD-L1 positive tumors, but there is also a significant response in PD-L1 negative ones. Therefore, PD-L1 expression is not a good predictive marker itself, and thereof cannot be used to assign therapy in a particular patient [24,71,72]. Also, the role of CTLA-4 expression in TIMC has been underused in the evaluation of response markers to ICI [72].

Many issues are responsible for failure to develop predictive biomarkers for ICI therapy, including dynamic expression, and the aforementioned heterogeneity within the primary tumor, as well as between primary and metastatic sites. Unfortunately, the pattern of PD-L1 expression differs within areas of the same tumor [6,7], and the identification largely depends on the sampling extent and more precisely on the number of blocks evaluated by immunohistochemistry. A possible explanation for the response to anti-PD-L1 therapy in some patients with PD-L1 negative CCRCC might be inappropriate sampling. PD-L1 immunostaining with monoclonal antibodies recognizing different epitopes also increases the level of uncertainty in the interpretation of the results. Furthermore, the reactivity of different antibodies may also be affected by PD-L1 post-translational modifications [8,73]. Finally, PD-L2 expression either on tumor cells or tumor-infiltrating lymphocytes might partly explain the response to anti-PD-1 therapy in PD-L1-negative CCRCC patients [74]. Another controversial issue that needs to be addressed is the variability in the interpretation of immunohistochemical staining and the evaluation of these findings in daily practice [8].

It is an undeniable paradox that in a disease such as mCCRCC in which all present and future treatment strategies are targeted, a targeted approach for immunotherapy is not currently used [29]. The rationale for the selection of patients that will respond to ICI and those in which treatment resistance could be expected will allow a deeper understanding of ICI at the individual patient level, not only in clinical trials but also in clinical practice. Then, and only then, immunotherapy will make a huge impact on patients with metastatic kidney cancer.

6. Conclusions

Under the light of randomized clinical trials ICI is becoming the first-line treatment of mCCRCC. Survival benefit has been demonstrated for pembrolizumab plus axitinib combination for all risk groups and for ipilimumab and nivolumab combination in the intermediate and poor-risk groups. Sunitinib and pazopanib stand as the alterative options for all risk groups and cabozantinib for the intermediate and high-risk group as well. The indication for CN is also changing and its current role should also be investigated under the light of new immunotherapies. Unfortunately, optimal markers of response to ICI have not yet been identified either.

Author Contributions: J.C.A. and O.S. have made substantial contributions to the conception of the work, analysis and interpretation of the data, draft, and revision of the work, and have approved the submitted version.

Funding: This research received no external funding.

Conflicts of Interest: The authors declare no conflict of interest.

References

1. Kotecha, R.R.; Motzer, R.J.; Voss, M.H. Towards individualized therapy for metastatic renal cell carcinoma. *Nat. Rev. Clin. Oncol.* **2019**. [CrossRef]
2. Lecis, D.; Sangaletti, S.; Colombo, M.P.; Chiodoni, C. Immune checkpoint ligand reverse signaling: Looking back to go forward in cancer therapy. *Cancers* **2019**, *11*, 624. [CrossRef]
3. Chang, A.J.; Zhao, L.; Zhu, Z.; Boulanger, K.; Xiao, H.; Wakefield, M.R.; Bai, Q.; Fang, Y. The Past, Present and Future of Immunotherapy for Metastatic Renal Cell Carcinoma. *Anticancer Res.* **2019**, *39*, 2683–2687. [CrossRef]

4. Labriola, M.K.; Batich, K.A.; Zhu, J.; McNamara, M.A.; Harrison, M.R.; Armstrong, A.J.; George, D.J.; Zhang, T. Immunotherapy is changing first-line treatment of metastatic renal-cell carcinoma. *Clin. Genitourin. Cancer* **2019**, *17*, e513–e521. [CrossRef]
5. Osawa, T.; Takeuchi, A.; Kojima, T.; Shinohara, N.; Eto, M.; Nishiyama, H. Overview of current and future systemic therapy for metastatic renal cell carcinoma. *Jpn. J. Clin. Oncol.* **2019**, *49*, 395–403. [CrossRef]
6. López, J.I.; Pulido, R.; Cortés, J.M.; Angulo, J.C.; Lawrie, C.H. Potential impact of PD-L1 (SP-142) immunohistochemical heterogeneity in clear cell renal cell carcinoma immunotherapy. *Pathol. Res. Pract.* **2018**, *214*, 1110–1114. [CrossRef]
7. López, J.I.; Pulido, R.; Lawrie, C.H.; Angulo, J.C. Loss of PD-L1 (SP-142) expression characterizes renal vein tumor thrombus microenvironment in clear cell renal cell carcinoma. *Ann. Diagn. Pathol.* **2018**, *34*, 89–93. [CrossRef]
8. Nunes-Xavier, C.E.; Angulo, J.C.; Pulido, R.; López, J.I.A. Critical insight into the clinical translation of PD-1/PD-L1 blockade therapy in clear cell renal cell carcinoma. *Curr. Urol. Rep.* **2019**, *20*, 1. [CrossRef]
9. Yang, J.C.; Hughes, M.; Kammula, U.; Royal, R.; Sherry, R.M.; Topalian, S.L.; Suri, K.B.; Levy, C.; Allen, T.; Mavroukakis, S.; et al. Ipilimumab (anti-CTLA4 antibody) causes regression of metastatic renal cell cancer associated with enteritis and hypophysitis. *J. Immunother.* **2007**, *30*, 825–830. [CrossRef]
10. Rini, B.I.; Stein, M.; Shannon, P.; Eddy, S.; Tyler, A.; Stephenson, J.J., Jr.; Catlett, L.; Huang, B.; Healey, D.; Gordon, M. Phase 1 dose-escalation trial of tremelimumab plus sunitinib in patients with metastatic renal cell carcinoma. *Cancer* **2011**, *117*, 758–767. [CrossRef]
11. Freeman, G.J.; Long, A.J.; Iwai, Y.; Bourque, K.; Chernova, T.; Nishimura, H.; Fitz, L.J.; Malenkovich, N.; Okazaki, T.; Byrne, M.C.; et al. Engagement of the PD-1 immunoinhibitory receptor by a novel B7 family member leads to negative regulation of lymphocyte activation. *J. Exp. Med.* **2000**, *192*, 1027–1034. [CrossRef]
12. Greenwald, R.J.; Freeman, G.J.; Sharpe, A.H. The B7 family revisited. *Annu. Rev. Immunol.* **2005**, *23*, 515–548. [CrossRef]
13. Dong, Y.; Sun, Q.; Zhang, X. PD-1 and its ligands are important immune checkpoints in cancer. *Oncotarget* **2017**, *8*, 2171–2186. [CrossRef]
14. Escors, D.; Gato-Canas, M.; Zuazo, M.; Arasanz, H.; García-Granda, M.J.; Vera, R.; Kochan, G. The intracelular signalosome of PD-L1 in cancer cells. *Signal. Transduct. Target. Ther.* **2018**, *3*, 26. [CrossRef]
15. Messai, Y.; Gad, S.; Noman, M.Z.; le Teuff, G.; Couve, S.; Janji, B.; Kammerer, S.F.; Rioux-Leclerc, N.; Hasmim, M.; Ferlicot, S.; et al. Renal cell carcinoma programmed death-ligand 1, a new direct target of hypoxia-inducible factor-2 alpha, is regulated by von Hippel-Lindau gene mutation status. *Eur. Urol.* **2016**, *70*, 623–632. [CrossRef]
16. Tatli Dogan, H.; Kiran, M.; Bilgin, B.; Kiliçarslan, A.; Sendur, M.A.N.; Yalçin, B.; Ardiçoglu, A.; Atmaca, A.F.; Gumuskaya, B. Prognostic significance of the programmed death ligand 1 expression in clear cell renal cell carcinoma and correlation with the tumor microenvironment and hypoxia-inducible factor expression. *Diagn. Pathol.* **2018**, *13*, 60. [CrossRef]
17. Iacovelli, R.; Nolè, F.; Verri, E.; Renne, G.; Paglino, C.; Santoni, M.; Cossu Rocca, M.; Giglione, P.; Aurilio, G.; Cullurà, D.; et al. Prognostic Role of PD-L1 Expression in Renal Cell Carcinoma. A Systematic Review and Meta-Analysis. *Target. Oncol.* **2016**, *11*, 143–148. [CrossRef]
18. Wang, Z.; Peng, S.; Xie, H.; Guo, L.; Cai, Q.; Shang, Z.; Jiang, N.; Niu, Y. Prognostic and clinicopathological significance of PD-L1 in patients with renal cell carcinoma: A meta-analysis based on 1863 individuals. *Clin. Exp. Med.* **2018**, *18*, 165–175. [CrossRef]
19. Latchman, Y.; Wood, C.R.; Chernova, T.; Chaudhary, D.; Borde, M.; Chernova, I.; Iwai, Y.; Long, A.J.; Brown, J.A.; Nunes, R.; et al. PD-L2 is a second ligand for PD-1 and inhibits T cell activation. *Nature Immunol.* **2001**, *2*, 261–268. [CrossRef]
20. Frigola, X.; Inman, B.A.; Lohse, C.M.; Krco, C.J.; Cheville, J.C.; Thompson, R.H.; Leibovich, B.; Blute, M.L.; Dong, H.; Kwon, E.D. Identification of a soluble form of B7-H1 that retains immunosuppressive activity and is associated with aggressive renal cell carcinoma. *Clin. Cancer Res.* **2011**, *17*, 1915–1923. [CrossRef]
21. Motzer, R.J.; Tannir, N.M.; McDermott, D.F.; Arén Frontera, O.; Melichar, B.; Choueiri, T.K.; Plimack, E.R.; Barthélémy, P.; Porta, C.; George, S.; et al. CheckMate 214 Investigators. Nivolumab plus ipilimumab versus sunitinib in advanced renal-cell carcinoma. *N. Engl. J. Med.* **2018**, *378*, 1277–1290. [CrossRef]

22. Motzer, R.J.; Hutson, T.E.; Tomczak, P.; Michaelson, M.D.; Bukowski, R.M.; Rixe, O.; Oudard, S.; Negrier, S.; Szczylik, C.; Kim, S.T.; et al. Sunitinib versus interferon alfa in metastatic renal-cell carcinoma. *N. Engl. J. Med.* **2007**, *356*, 115–124. [CrossRef]
23. Motzer, R.J.; Hutson, T.E.; Tomczak, P.; Michaelson, M.D.; Bukowski, R.M.; Oudard, S.; Negrier, S.; Szczylik, C.; Pili, R.; Bjarnason, G.A.; et al. Overall survival and updated results for sunitinib compared with interferon alfa in patients with metastatic renal cell carcinoma. *J. Clin. Oncol.* **2009**, *27*, 3584–3590. [CrossRef]
24. Motzer, R.J.; Escudier, B.; McDermott, D.F.; George, S.; Hammers, H.J.; Srinivas, S.; Tykodi, S.S.; Sosman, J.A.; Procopio, G.; Plimack, E.R.; et al. CheckMate 025 Investigators. Nivolumab versus everolimus in advanced renal-cell carcinoma. *N. Engl. J. Med.* **2015**, *373*, 1803–1813. [CrossRef]
25. Motzer, R.J.; Bacik, J.; Murphy, B.A.; Russo, P.; Mazumdar, M. Interferon-alfa as a comparative treatment for clinical trials of new therapies against advanced renal cell carcinoma. *J. Clin. Oncol.* **2002**, *20*, 289–296. [CrossRef]
26. Heng, D.Y.; Xie, W.; Regan, M.M.; Warren, M.A.; Golshayan, A.R.; Sahi, C.; Eigl, B.J.; Ruether, J.D.; Cheng, T.; North, S.; et al. Prognostic factors for overall survival in patients with metastatic renal cell carcinoma treated with vascular endothelial growth factor-targeted agents: Results from a large, multicenter study. *J. Clin. Oncol.* **2009**, *27*, 5794–5799. [CrossRef]
27. Ko, J.J.; Choueiri, T.K.; Rini, B.I.; Lee, J.L.; Kroeger, N.; Srinivas, S.; Harshman, L.C.; Knox, J.J.; Bjarnason, G.A.; MacKenzie, M.J.; et al. First-, second-, third-line therapy for mRCC: Benchmarks for trial design from the IMDC. *Br. J. Cancer.* **2014**, *110*, 1917–1922. [CrossRef]
28. Gao, X.; McDermott, D.F. Ipilimumab in combination with nivolumab for the treatment of renal cell carcinoma. *Expert Opin. Biol. Ther.* **2018**, *18*, 947–957. [CrossRef]
29. Salgia, N.J.; Dara, Y.; Bergerot, P.; Salgia, M.; Pal, S.K. The changing landscape of management of metastatic renal cell carcinoma: Current treatment options and future directions. *Curr. Treat. Options Oncol.* **2019**, *20*, 41. [CrossRef]
30. Jonasch, E. NCCN Guidelines Updates: Management of Metastatic Kidney Cancer. *J. Natl. Compr. Cancer Netw.* **2019**, *17*, 587–589.
31. Rini, B.I.; Plimack, E.R.; Stus, V.; Gafanov, R.; Hawkins, R.; Nosov, D.; Pouliot, F.; Alekseev, B.; Soulières, D.; Melichar, B.; et al. KEYNOTE-426 Investigators. Pembrolizumab plus axitinib versus sunitinib for advanced renal-cell carcinoma. *N. Engl. J. Med.* **2019**, *380*, 1116–1127. [CrossRef]
32. Motzer, R.J.; Penkov, K.; Haanen, J.; Rini, B.; Albiges, L.; Campbell, M.T.; Venugopal, B.; Kollmannsberger, C.; Negrier, S.; Uemura, M.; et al. Avelumab plus axitinib versus sunitinib for advanced renal-cell carcinoma. *N. Engl. J. Med.* **2019**, *380*, 1103–1115. [CrossRef]
33. Albiges, L.; Powles, T.; Staehler, M.; Bensalah, K.; Giles, R.H.; Hora, M.; Kuczyk, M.A.; Lam, T.B.; Ljungberg, B.; Marconi, L.; et al. Updated European Association of Urology Guidelines on renal cell carcinoma: Immune checkpoint inhibition is the new backbone in first-line treatment of metastatic clear-cell renal cell carcinoma. *Eur. Urol.* **2019**. [CrossRef]
34. Rini, B.I.; Powles, T.; Atkins, M.B.; Escudier, B.; McDermott, D.F.; Suarez, C.; Bracarda, S.; Stadler, W.M.; Donskov, F.; Lee, J.L.; et al. IMmotion151 Study Group. Atezolizumab plus bevacizumab versus sunitinib in patients with previously untreated metastatic renal cell carcinoma (IMmotion151): A multicentre, open-label, phase 3, randomised controlled trial. *Lancet* **2019**, *393*, 2404–2415. [CrossRef]
35. Costa, R.; Carneiro, B.A.; Agulnik, M.; Rademaker, A.W.; Pai, S.G.; Villaflor, V.M.; Cristofanilli, M.; Sosman, J.A.; Giles, F.J. Toxicity profile of approved anti-PD-1 monoclonal antibodies in solid tumors: A systematic review and meta-analysis of randomized clinical trials. *Oncotarget* **2017**, *8*, 8910–8920. [CrossRef]
36. Ornstein, M.C.; Garcia, J.A. Toxicity of checkpoint inhibition in advanced RCC: A systematic review. *Kidney Cancer* **2017**, *1*, 133–141. [CrossRef]
37. Weber, J.S.; Hodi, F.S.; Wolchok, J.D.; Topalian, S.L.; Schadendorf, D.; Larkin, J.; Sznol, M.; Long, G.V.; Li, H.; Waxman, I.M.; et al. Safety profile of nivolumab monotherapy: A pooled analysis of patients with advanced melanoma. *J. Clin. Oncol.* **2017**, *35*, 785–792. [CrossRef]
38. Haanen, J.B.A.G.; Carbonnel, F.; Robert, C.; Kerr, K.M.; Peters, S.; Larkin, J.; Jordan, K.; ESMO Guidelines Committee. Management of toxicities from immunotherapy: ESMO Clinical Practice Guidelines for diagnosis, treatment and follow-up. *Ann. Oncol.* **2017**, *28*, iv119–iv142. [CrossRef]

39. Shah, A.Y.; Kotecha, R.R.; Lemke, E.A.; Chandramohan, A.; Chaim, J.L.; Msaouel, P.; Xiao, L.; Gao, J.; Campbell, M.T.; Zurita, A.J.; et al. Outcomes of patients with metastatic clear-cell renal cell carcinoma treated with second-line VEGFR-TKI after first-line immune checkpoint inhibitors. *Eur. J. Cancer.* **2019**, *114*, 67–75. [CrossRef]
40. Escudier, B.; Eisen, T.; Stadler, W.M.; Szczylik, C.; Oudard, S.; Siebels, M.; Negrier, S.; Chevreau, C.; Solska, E.; Desai, A.A.; et al. TARGET Study Group. Sorafenib in advanced clear-cell renal-cell carcinoma. *N. Engl. J. Med.* **2007**, *356*, 125–134. [CrossRef]
41. Strumberg, D. Sorafenib for the treatment of renal cancer. *Expert Opin. Pharmacother.* **2012**, *13*, 407–419. [CrossRef] [PubMed]
42. Motzer, R.J.; Escudier, B.; Oudard, S.; Hutson, T.E.; Porta, C.; Bracarda, S.; Grünwald, V.; Thompson, J.A.; Figlin, R.A.; Hollaender, N.; et al. RECORD-1 Study Group. Efficacy of everolimus in advanced renal cell carcinoma: A double-blind, randomised, placebo-controlled phase III trial. *Lancet* **2008**, *372*, 449–456. [CrossRef]
43. Yakes, F.M.; Chen, J.; Tan, J.; Yamaguchi, K.; Shi, Y.; Yu, P.; Qian, F.; Chu, F.; Bentzien, F.; Cancilla, B.; et al. Cabozantinib (XL184), a novel MET and VEGFR2 inhibitor, simultaneously suppresses metastasis, angiogenesis, and tumor growth. *Mol. Cancer Ther.* **2011**, *10*, 2298–2308. [CrossRef] [PubMed]
44. Abdelaziz, A.; Vaishampayan, U. Cabozantinib for renal cell carcinoma: Current and future paradigms. *Curr. Treat. Options Oncol.* **2017**, *18*, 18. [CrossRef] [PubMed]
45. Choueiri, T.K.; Escudier, B.; Powles, T.; Mainwaring, P.N.; Rini, B.I.; Donskov, F.; Hammers, H.; Hutson, T.E.; Lee, J.L.; Peltola, K.; et al. METEOR Investigators. Cabozantinib versus everolimus in advanced renal-cell carcinoma. *N. Engl. J. Med.* **2015**, *373*, 1814–1823. [CrossRef] [PubMed]
46. Choueiri, T.K.; Escudier, B.; Powles, T.; Tannir, N.M.; Mainwaring, P.N.; Rini, B.I.; Hammers, H.J.; Donskov, F.; Roth, B.J.; Peltola, K.; et al. METEOR investigators. Cabozantinib versus everolimus in advanced renal cell carcinoma (METEOR): Final results from a randomised, open-label, phase 3 trial. *Lancet Oncol.* **2016**, *17*, 917–927. [CrossRef]
47. Cella, D.; Escudier, B.; Tannir, N.M.; Powles, T.; Donskov, F.; Peltola, K.; Schmidinger, M.; Heng, D.Y.C.; Mainwaring, P.N.; Hammers, H.J.; et al. Quality of Life Outcomes for Cabozantinib Versus Everolimus in Patients with Metastatic Renal Cell Carcinoma: METEOR Phase III Randomized Trial. *J. Clin. Oncol.* **2018**, *36*, 757–764. [CrossRef]
48. Choueiri, T.K.; Halabi, S.; Sanford, B.L.; Hahn, O.; Michaelson, M.D.; Walsh, M.K.; Feldman, D.R.; Olencki, T.; Picus, J.; Small, E.J.; et al. Cabozantinib versus sunitinib as initial targeted therapy for patients with metastatic renal cell carcinoma of poor or intermediate risk: The Alliance A031203 CABOSUN trial. *J. Clin. Oncol.* **2017**, *35*, 591–597. [CrossRef]
49. Bersanelli, M.; Leonardi, F.; Buti, S. Spotlight on cabozantinib for previously untreated advanced renal cell carcinoma: Evidence to date. *Cancer Manag. Res.* **2018**, *10*, 3773–3780. [CrossRef]
50. Stukalin, I.; Wells, J.C.; Graham, J.; Yuasa, T.; Beuselinck, B.; Kollmansberger, C.; Ernst, D.S.; Agarwal, N.; Le, T.; Donskov, F.; et al. Real-world outcomes of nivolumab and cabozantinib in metastatic renal cell carcinoma: Results from the International Metastatic Renal Cell Carcinoma Database Consortium. *Curr. Oncol* **2019**, *26*, e175–e179. [CrossRef]
51. Motzer, R.J.; Escudier, B.; Tomczak, P.; Hutson, T.E.; Michaelson, M.D.; Negrier, S.; Oudard, S.; Gore, M.E.; Tarazi, J.; Hariharan, S.; et al. Axitinib versus sorafenib as second-line treatment for advanced renal cell carcinoma: Overall survival analysis and updated results from a randomised phase 3 trial. *Lancet Oncol.* **2013**, *14*, 552–562. [CrossRef]
52. Kondo, T. Treatment overview. In *Renall Cell Carcinoma. Molecular Features and Therapeutic Updates*; Mototsugu, O., Ed.; Springer: Tokyo, Japan, 2017; pp. 177–208.
53. Bracarda, S.; Bamias, A.; Casper, J.; Negrier, S.; Sella, A.; Staehler, M.; Tarazi, J.; Felici, A.; Rosbrook, B.; Jardinaud-Lopez, M.; et al. Is axitinib still a valid option for mRCC in the second-line setting? Prognostic factor analyses from the AXIS trial. *Clin. Genit. Cancer* **2019**, *17*, e689–e703. [CrossRef] [PubMed]
54. Schey, C.; Meier, G.; Pan, J. Metastatic renal cell cancer: An analysis of reimbursement decisions. *Adv. Ther.* **2019**, *36*, 1266–1278. [CrossRef] [PubMed]

55. Jin, H.; Zhang, J.; Shen, K.; Hao, J.; Feng, Y.; Yuan, C.; Zhu, Y.; Ma, X. Efficacy and safety of perioperative appliance of sunitinib in patients with metastatic or advanced renal cell carcinoma: A systematic review and meta-analysis. *Medicine* **2019**, *98*, e15424. [CrossRef] [PubMed]
56. Méjean, A.; Ravaud, A.; Thezenas, S.; Colas, S.; Beauval, J.B.; Bensalah, K.; Geoffrois, L.; Thiery-Vuillemin, A.; Cormier, L.; Lang, H.; et al. Sunitinib alone or after nephrectomy in metastatic renal-cell carcinoma. *N. Engl. J. Med.* **2018**, *379*, 417–427. [CrossRef]
57. Bex, A.; Albiges, L.; Ljungberg, B.; Bensalah, K.; Dabestani, S.; Giles, R.H.; Hofmann, F.; Hora, M.; Kuczyk, M.A.; Lam, T.B.; et al. Updated European Association of Urology Guidelines for cytoreductive nephrectomy in patients with synchronous metastatic clear-cell renal cell carcinoma. *Eur. Urol.* **2018**, *74*, 805–809. [CrossRef]
58. Bex, A.; Mulders, P.; Jewett, M.; Wagstaff, J.; van Thienen, J.V.; Blank, C.U.; van Velthoven, R.; Del Pilar Laguna, M.; Wood, L.; van Melick, H.H.E.; et al. Comparison of immediate vs. deferred cytoreductive nephrectomy in patients with synchronous metastatic renal cell carcinoma receiving sunitinib: The SURTIME randomized clinical trial. *JAMA Oncol.* **2019**, *5*, 164–170. [CrossRef]
59. Larcher, A.; Wallis, C.J.D.; Bex, A.; Blute, M.L.; Ficarra, V.; Mejean, A.; Karam, J.A.; Van Poppel, H.; Pal, S.K. Individualised indications for cytoreductive nephrectomy: Which criteria define the optimal candidates? *Eur. Urol. Oncol.* **2019**, *2*, 365–378. [CrossRef]
60. Ghali, F.; Patel, S.H.; Derweesh, I.H. Current status of immunotherapy for localized and locally advanced renal cell carcinoma. *J. Oncol.* **2019**, *2019*, 7309205. [CrossRef]
61. Powles, T.; Albiges, L.; Staehler, M.; Bensalah, K.; Dabestani, S.; Giles, R.H.; Hofmann, F.; Hora, M.; Kuczyk, M.A.; Lam, T.B.; et al. Updated European Association of Urology Guidelines recommendations for the treatment of first-line metastatic clear cell renal cancer. *Eur. Urol.* **2018**, *73*, 311–315. [CrossRef]
62. López, J.I.; Cortés, J.M. Multisite tumor sampling: A new tumor selection method to enhance intratumor heterogeneity detection. *Hum. Pathol.* **2017**, *64*, 1–6. [CrossRef] [PubMed]
63. López-Fernández, E.; López, J.I. The impact of tumor eco-evolution in renal cell carcinoma sampling. *Cancers* **2018**, *10*, 485. [CrossRef] [PubMed]
64. Cimadamore, A.; Gasparrini, S.; Massari, F.; Santoni, M.; Cheng, L.; Lopez-Beltran, A.; Scarpelli, M.; Montironi, R. Emerging molecular technologies in renal cell carcinoma: Liquid Biopsy. *Cancers* **2019**, *11*, 196. [CrossRef] [PubMed]
65. Bakouny, Z.; Flippot, R.; Braun, D.A.; Lalani, A.A.; Choueiri, T.K. State of the future: Translational approaches in renal cell carcinoma in the immunotherapy era. *Eur. Urol. Focus* **2019**. [CrossRef] [PubMed]
66. Vento, J.; Mulgaonkar, A.; Woolford, L.; Nham, K.; Christie, A.; Bagrodia, A.; de Leon, A.D.; Hannan, R.; Bowman, I.; McKay, R.M.; et al. PD-L1 detection using 89Zr-atezolizumab immuno-PET in renal cell carcinoma tumorgrafts from a patient with favorable nivolumab response. *J. Immunother. Cancer* **2019**, *7*, 144. [CrossRef] [PubMed]
67. Adashek, J.J.; Salgia, M.M.; Posadas, E.M.; Figlin, R.A.; Gong, J. Role of biomarkers in prediction of response to therapeutics in metastatic renal-cell carcinoma. *Clin. Genitourin Cancer* **2019**, *17*, e454–e460. [CrossRef] [PubMed]
68. Chen, V.J.; Hernandez-Meza, G.; Agrawal, P.; Zhang, C.A.; Xie, L.; Gong, C.L.; Hoerner, C.R.; Srinivas, S.; Oermann, E.K.; Fan, A.C. Time on therapy for at least three months correlates with overall survival in metastatic renal cell carcinoma. *Cancers* **2019**, *11*, 1000. [CrossRef]
69. Ribas, A.; Tumeh, P.C. The future of cancer therapy: Selecting patients likely to respond to PD1/L1 blockade. *Clin. Cancer Res.* **2014**, *20*, 4982–4984. [CrossRef]
70. Zhu, J.; Armstrong, A.J.; Friedlander, T.W.; Kim, W.; Pal, S.K.; George, D.J.; Zhang, T. Biomarkers of immunotherapy in urothelial and renal cell carcinoma: PD-L1, tumor mutational burden, and beyond. *J. Immunother. Cancer* **2018**, *6*, 4. [CrossRef]
71. Gandini, S.; Massi, D.; Mandalà, M. PD-L1 expression in cancer patients receiving anti PD-1/PD-L1 antibodies: A systematic review and meta-analysis. *Crit. Rev. Oncol. Hematol.* **2016**, *100*, 88–98. [CrossRef]
72. Kahlmeyer, A.; Stöhr, C.G.; Hartmann, A.; Goebell, P.J.; Wullich, B.; Wach, S.; Taubert, H.; Erlmeier, F. Expression of PD-1 and CTLA-4 are negative prognostic markers in renal cell carcinoma. *J. Clin. Med.* **2019**, *8*, 743. [CrossRef] [PubMed]

73. Horita, H.; Law, A.; Hong, S.; Middleton, K. Identifying regulatory posttranslational modifications of PD-L1: A focus on monoubiquitinaton. *Neoplasia* **2017**, *19*, 346–353. [CrossRef] [PubMed]
74. Shin, S.J.; Jeon, Y.K.; Kim, P.J.; Cho, Y.M.; Koh, J.; Chung, D.H.; Go, H. Clinicopathologic analysis of PD-L1 and PD-L2 expression in renal cell carcinoma: Association with oncogenic proteins status. *Ann. Surg. Oncol.* **2016**, *23*, 694–702. [CrossRef] [PubMed]

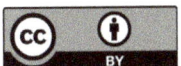

© 2019 by the authors. Licensee MDPI, Basel, Switzerland. This article is an open access article distributed under the terms and conditions of the Creative Commons Attribution (CC BY) license (http://creativecommons.org/licenses/by/4.0/).

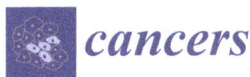

Review

MiT Family Translocation Renal Cell Carcinoma: from the Early Descriptions to the Current Knowledge

Anna Caliò [1], Diego Segala [2], Enrico Munari [3], Matteo Brunelli [1] and Guido Martignoni [1,2,*]

[1] Department of Diagnostic and Public Health, Section of Pathology, University of Verona, Verona 37134, Italy
[2] Department of Pathology, Pederzoli Hospital, Peschiera del Garda 37019, Italy
[3] Department of Pathology, Sacro Cuore Hospital, Negrar 37024, Italy
* Correspondence: guido.martignoni@univr.it

Received: 13 July 2019; Accepted: 30 July 2019; Published: 3 August 2019

Abstract: The new category of MiT family translocation renal cell carcinoma has been included into the World Health Organization (WHO) classification in 2016. The MiT family translocation renal cell carcinoma comprises Xp11 translocation renal cell carcinoma harboring *TFE3* gene fusions and t(6;11) renal cell carcinoma harboring *TFEB* gene fusion. At the beginning, they were recognized in childhood; nevertheless, it has been demonstrated that these neoplasms can occur in adults as well. In the nineties, among Xp11 renal cell carcinoma, *ASPL*, *PRCC*, and *SFPQ* (*PSF*) were the first genes recognized as partners in *TFE3* rearrangement. Recently, many other genes have been identified, and a wide spectrum of morphologies has been described. For this reason, the diagnosis may be challenging based on the histology, and the differential diagnosis includes the most common renal cell neoplasms and pure epithelioid PEComa/epithelioid angiomyolipoma of the kidney. During the last decades, many efforts have been made to identify immunohistochemical markers to reach the right diagnosis. To date, staining for PAX8, cathepsin K, and melanogenesis markers are the most useful identifiers. However, the diagnosis requires the demonstration of the chromosomal rearrangement, and fluorescent in situ hybridization (FISH) is considered the gold standard. The outcome of Xp11 translocation renal cell carcinoma is highly variable, with some patients surviving decades with indolent disease and others dying rapidly of progressive disease. Despite most instances of t(6;11) renal cell carcinoma having an indolent clinical course, a few published cases demonstrate aggressive behavior. Recently, renal cell carcinomas with *TFEB* amplification have been described in connection with t(6;11) renal cell carcinoma. Those tumors appear to be associated with a more aggressive clinical course. For the aggressive cases of MiT family translocation carcinoma, the optimal therapy remains to be determined; however, new target therapies seem to be promising, and the search for predictive markers is mandatory.

Keywords: MiT family translocation renal cell carcinoma; Xp11 translocation renal cell carcinoma; t(6;11) translocation renal cell carcinoma; FISH; TFE3; TFEB; TFEB-amplified renal cell carcinoma

1. Xp11 Translocation Renal Cell Carcinoma

Xp11 translocation renal cell carcinoma is a distinctive subtype of renal cell carcinoma, characterized by several chromosomal translocations involving the *TFE3* gene, located on chromosome Xp11.2. In these tumors, the *TFE3* transcription factor gene is fused by translocation to one of several other genes [1–9]:

- t(X;1) (p11.2;q21.2) gene *PRCC*
- t(X;17) (p11.2;q25) gene *ASPL* (*ASPSCR1*)
- t(X;1) (p11.2;p34) gene *SFPQ* (*PSF*)
- t(X;17) (p11.2;q23) gene *CLTC*

- t(X;3) (p11.2;q21) gene *PARP14*
- t(X;10) (11.2;q23) unknown gene
- t(X;17) (p11.2;q21.33) gene *LUC7L3*
- t(X;19) (p11.2;q13.3) gene *KHSRP*
- t(X;17) (p11.2;p13) gene *DVL2*
- t(X;22) (p11.2;q11.21) gene *MED15*
- t(X;6) (p11.2;q25.3) gene *ARIDB*
- t(X;5) (p11.2;q31.2) gene *MATR3*
- t(X;1) (p11.2;p31.1) gene *FUBP1*
- t(X;11) (p11.2;q13.1) gene *NEAT1*
- t(X;10) (p11.2;q22.2) gene *KAT6B*
- inv (X) (p11.2;q12) gene *NONO* (p54*nrb*)
- inv(X) (p11.2;p11.3) gene *RBM10*
- inv(X) (p11.23;p11.23) il gene *GRIPAP1*

The three most common Xp11 translocation renal cell carcinomas are those bearing the t(X;1) (p11.2;q21) which fuses the *PRCC* and *TFE3* genes, the t(X;17) (p11.2;q25) which fuses the *ASPL* and *TFE3* genes, and the t(X;1) (p11.2;p34) which fuses the *SFPQ (PSF)* and *TFE3* genes [10]. Interestingly, t(X;17) renal cell carcinoma or alveolar soft part sarcoma harbor the same *ASPL-TFE3* fusion gene [11]. However, the translocation is balanced in t(X;17) renal cell carcinoma and unbalanced in alveolar soft part sarcoma, which presumably explains the clinical and morphological differences. The function of chimeric TFE3 fusion proteins can also vary, which may explain the different histological features observed in this tumor entity of renal cell carcinoma.

1.1. Clinical Features

Xp11 translocation renal cell carcinoma comprises 20–75% of renal cell carcinomas in childhood [12] and 1–4% of adult renal cell carcinomas (calculated excluding patients younger than 18 years old) with an average age of onset of 40 years (Figure 1). The incidence of Xp11 translocation renal cell carcinoma in adults may be underestimated, likely for the morphological overlap with more common adult renal cell carcinoma subtypes, such as clear cell and papillary renal cell carcinoma. Considering an overall of 403 genetically confirmed Xp11 translocation renal cell carcinomas described in the literature, there is a slight female predominance (F:M ratio, 1.6:1). Clinically, there are no particular features typically presented. As other renal cell carcinomas, roughly one-third of all tumors are asymptomatic, often accidentally discovered. Prior exposure to cytotoxic chemotherapy has been reported as a risk factor [13].

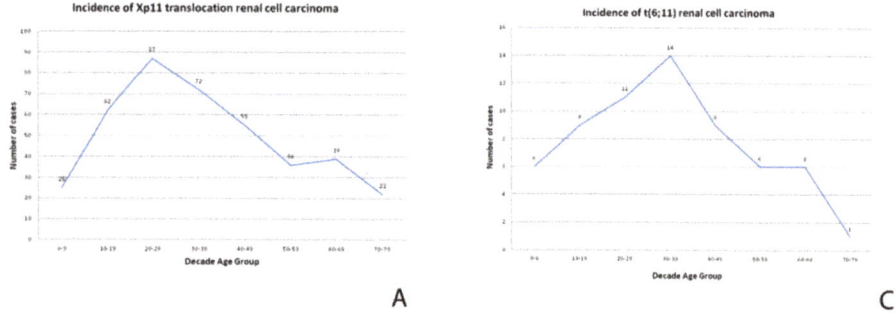

Figure 1. *Cont.*

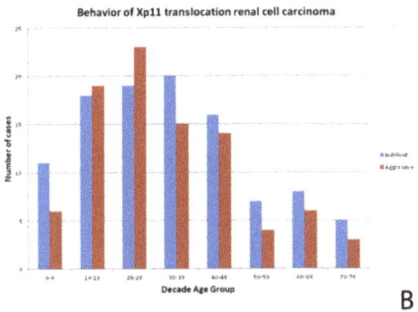 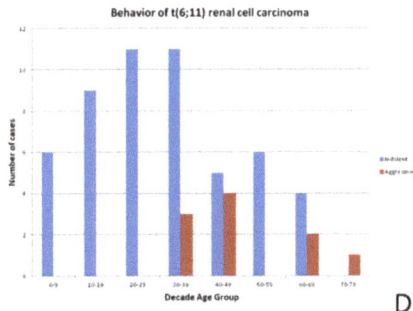

Figure 1. A chart showing the incidence (number of patients with tumors divided by the number of patients in the age group) of Xp11 translocation renal cell carcinomas (**A**) and t(6;11) renal cell carcinoma (**C**) at different ages. A chart showing the clinical behavior of Xp11 translocation renal cell carcinomas (**B**) and t(6;11) renal cell carcinoma (**D**) at different ages.

1.2. Pathologic Features

1.2.1. Gross Findings

They usually present as solitary cortical masses characterized by tan-yellow cut surfaces with foci of hemorrhage and necrosis and occasionally focal cystic degeneration. Although there is no specific macroscopic appearance of Xp11 translocation renal cell carcinoma, they do not share the macroscopic features of clear cell renal cell carcinoma.

1.2.2. Microscopic Features

Histologically, Xp11 translocation renal cell carcinomas are characterized by heterogeneous architectural and cytologic features, mimicking almost all subtypes of renal cell carcinoma [10,14]. The most distinctive morphologic pattern is the presence of a papillary architecture composed of epithelioid clear cells. However, different architectures have been reported, such as solid, nested, trabecular, and microcystic pattern. More frequently, tumor cells demonstrate voluminous clear to eosinophilic cytoplasm (Figure 2). The nuclei may show variability in size and are generally large with a prominent eosinophilic nucleolus (typically G3 by ISUP/WHO 2016) [1]. Psammoma bodies are often present.

1.2.3. Immunohistochemical Features and Fluorescent in Situ Hybridization (FISH) Analysis

Like other subtypes of renal cell carcinoma, Xp11 translocation renal cell carcinomas are positive for PAX8. Vimentin and cytokeratin 7 (CK7) are typically negative. Staining for CD10 and alpha-methylacyl-CoA racemase (AMACR) is generally reported. In one-third of all cases, Xp11 translocation renal cell carcinoma focally express melanogenic markers such as Melan-A and HMB45. Staining for cathepsin K is observed in a subset of Xp11 translocation renal cell carcinomas (approximately 50%) (Figure 2). Interestingly, PRCC-TFE3 renal cell carcinoma is labelled more frequently for cathepsin K than ASPL-TFE3 renal cell carcinoma [15,16]. TFE3 immunostaining, initially considered as the most sensitive and specific marker, should be cautiously used due to the not infrequent false-positive and false-negative results [17]. For this reason, the identification of the *TFE3* rearrangement by FISH assays on formalin-fixed and paraffin-embedded tissue sections is currently the gold standard to reach the correct diagnosis [17–19]. Of course, a reliable interpretation requires a univocal cut-off. However, different thresholds have been used to demonstrate the occurrence of translocation. A positive result was considered when >10%, >15%, or >20% of the neoplastic nuclei showed split signals. Nevertheless, an extensive review of previously reported cases of Xp11 translocation renal cell carcinoma in which it has been reported that the frequency of split signals in each case showed a high frequency of split signals (>40%). It is important to keep in mind that the FISH assay is unable to detect subtle *TFE3* gene inversions, such as those that result in the *RBM10-TFE3* gene fusion [20]. In the experience of the authors, minimally split fluorescent signals in which fluorescent signals were separated by a signal diameter or less were observed in few cases [21]. Recently, it has been argued whether *TFE3* gene rearrangement is the key event in tumorigenesis [22–24]. In our practice, the fraction of cells showing the translocation is commonly high, supporting the idea that it is the main driver event in tumorigenesis.

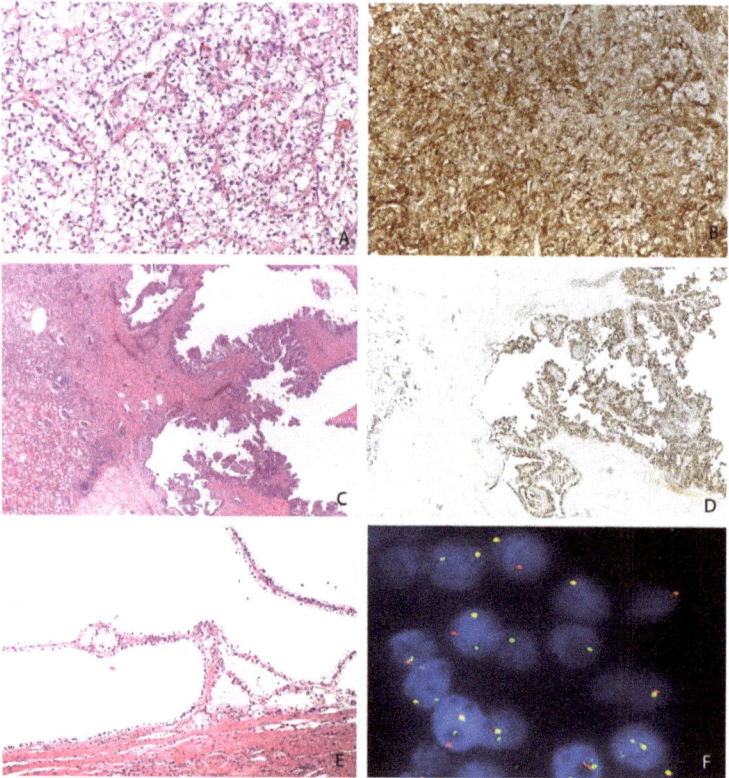

Figure 2. Different morphologies of Xp11 translocation renal cell carcinomas: resembling a clear cell renal cell carcinoma (Magnification: 200×) (**A**), showing a papillary (Magnification: 25×) (**C**) or cystic (Magnification: 100×) (**E**) pattern. An example of strong and diffuse expression of cathepsin K (Magnification: 200×) (**B**), the nuclear positivity of PAX8 (Magnification: 25×) (**D**), and the demonstration of *TFE3* gene rearrangement by FISH (Magnification: 1000×) (**F**).

1.3. Differential Diagnosis

Due to the wide spectrum of morphologies observed in Xp11 translocation renal cell carcinomas, the differential diagnosis is challenging, and it is important to consider these carcinomas in all unusual renal cell carcinomas occurring, especially in children and young adults [1]. Several neoplasms can be confused with Xp11 translocation renal cell carcinoma, mainly clear cell and papillary renal cell carcinomas. In this setting, cathepsin K is the most reliable immunohistochemical marker. Of note, as previously stated, immunolabelling for cathepsin K is observed in roughly half of all Xp11 translocation renal cell carcinomas. Other immunohistochemical markers may be helpful based on the differential diagnosis. CD10 is expressed in almost all Xp11 translocation renal cell carcinomas in analogy to clear cell renal cell carcinomas. However, carbonic anhydrase IX is usually negative or only focally present in Xp11 translocation renal cell carcinomas and positive in clear cell renal cell carcinomas, suggesting the usefulness of this marker in this particular differential diagnosis. On the other hand, AMACR (Alpha-methylacyl-CoA racemase) is frequently positive in Xp11 translocation renal cell carcinomas, as well as in papillary renal cell carcinomas, but CK7 is typically negative in Xp11 translocation renal cell carcinomas and positive in papillary renal cell carcinomas. Clear cell papillary renal cell carcinomas may be another tricky differential diagnosis [25]. Those tumors usually label for CK7 and GATA3, both not expressed in Xp11 translocation renal cell carcinomas. Finally, it is important to remember less frequent tumors, such as pure epithelioid PEComa/epithelioid angiomyolipoma. In those cases, PAX8 and CD68 (PG-M1) are extremely useful (see differential diagnosis of t(6;11) renal cell carcinomas).

1.4. Prognosis and Treatment

The outcome of Xp11 translocation renal cell carcinoma is highly variable, from indolent to rapidly aggressive behavior [12,26,27]. Overall, Xp11 translocation renal cell carcinoma has a worse prognosis than papillary renal cell carcinoma and there is a similar prognosis for clear cell renal cell carcinoma [28]. Although several studies have claimed that Xp11 translocation renal cell carcinomas in children have a relatively indolent course, the review of the literature (Figure 1) shows a high percentage of aggressive cases in young adults. Among Xp11 translocation renal cell carcinoma, patients with ASPL-TFE3 fusion seem to have a worse prognosis and more frequently lymph node metastasis, but it is still unclear whether the fusion partner plays a prognostic role [28,29]. Considering an overall 403 genetically confirmed Xp11 translocation renal cell carcinomas described in the literature, 47% of cases (91 of 194 tumors with available follow up) behaved aggressively. When aggressive and non-aggressive cases are compared, we observe that recurrences or metastases occurred within 24 months from the surgery. It is worth noting that sarcomatoid or rhabdoid de-differentiation have never been reported. There is no statistical difference of age between aggressive and non-aggressive cases. As expected, a larger tumor size ($p < 0.0001$) correlates with aggressive behavior. Interestingly, the presence of necrosis, but not nucleolar grade, correlates with aggressiveness, the same prognostic characteristics reported in chromophobe renal cell carcinoma.

With regard to the treatment, the optimal therapy for MiT family translocation renal cell carcinoma remains to be determined. For localized tumors, including patients with positive regional lymph nodes, surgery is the treatment of choice. For patients with hematogenous metastases, several attempts of therapy have been tried based on the treatment of clear cell renal cell carcinoma. Therapies targeting vascular endothelial growth factor receptor, immunotherapy, mTOR inhibitors, and target therapies for the MET signaling pathway are possible options [30–34]. Unfortunately, to date there is no data regarding predictive markers to choose the best therapy for an individual patient. In the past few years, the efficacy of Cabozantinib, a tyrosine kinase inhibitor with activity against c-MET, AXL, and vascular endothelial growth factor receptor 2, has been proven for the treatment of metastatic clear cell renal cell carcinomas [35,36] and recently for non-clear cell histologies [37]. Moreover, whole genome DNA and RNA sequencing studies have recently been reported on a small number of cases [10,38], providing the activity of other pathways which may present other potential targets for novel therapies [38].

2. t(6;11) Renal Cell Carcinoma

t(6;11) renal cell carcinoma is an extremely rare variant and accounts for 0.02% of all renal carcinomas. Although the initial description was in children [39], t(6;11) renal cell carcinoma may occur in adults. The t(6;11) translocation fuses the gene for *TFEB*, located on chromosome 6, with Alpha (*MALAT1*), a gene of unknown function, resulting in overexpression of TFEB.

2.1. Clinical Features

The t(6;11) renal cell carcinomas are less common than the Xp11 renal cell carcinomas; approximately 60 cases are documented in the literature, the majority of which in children and adolescents. However, it has been demonstrated that these neoplasms can occur in adults as well. The mean age of presentation is 34 years (Figure 1), with a wide reported range of 3–77 years. Conversely to Xp11 translocation renal cell carcinomas, in t(6;11) renal cell carcinoma there is no gender predominance (F:M ratio, 0.75:1). The tumor is usually an incidental finding. Similar to Xp11 translocation renal cell carcinoma, a subset of cases has occurred in patients who have received cytotoxic chemotherapy for other reasons.

2.2. Pathologic Features

2.2.1. Gross Findings

As Xp11 translocation renal cell carcinoma, t(6;11) renal cell carcinoma does not have a distinctive gross appearance.

2.2.2. Microscopic Features

Histologically, t(6;11) renal cell carcinoma has been classically characterized by a distinctive biphasic morphology with larger epithelioid cells and smaller cells clustered around eosinophilic spheres formed by basement membrane material (Figure 3) [1,40]. However, several reports have shown a broad range of morphology in molecularly confirmed t(6;11) renal cell carcinomas [41]. Papillary and tubulocystic architectures, clear cell and oncocytoma-like features, and diffuse hyalinization with thick-walled blood vessels are some of the unusual pathological features described [1]. The cells typically show nucleolar grade G2 and G3 by ISUP/WHO 2016 [42].

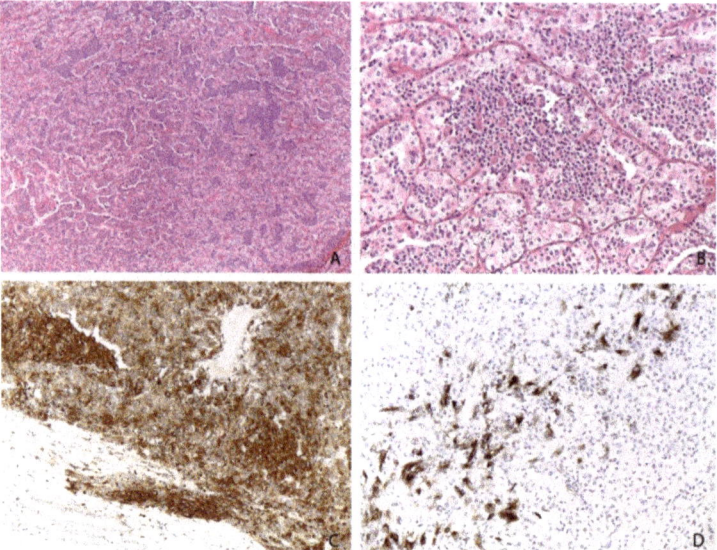

Figure 3. The most common morphology of t(6;11) renal cell carcinoma with larger epithelioid cells and smaller cells clustered around eosinophilic spheres formed by basement membrane material (**A**, Magnification: 25×; **B**, Magnification: 200×). Almost all cases are positive for cathepsin K (Magnification: 200×) (**C**) and HMB45 (Magnification: 200×) (**D**).

2.2.3. Immunohistochemical Features and FISH Analysis

Immunohistochemically, most t(6;11) renal cell carcinomas express PAX8, supporting renal tubular differentiation and melanogenesis markers, such as HMB-45 and Melan-A. Cathepsin K is overexpressed in almost all t(6;11) renal cell carcinomas [43,44]. Staining for TFEB was considered highly sensitive and specific for this tumor. However, the results can be inconsistent among laboratories, mainly because of technical factors such as fixation time and differences in the methods of antigen retrieval. Like Xp11 translocation renal cell carcinomas, the identification of the rearrangement by FISH analysis is the gold standard for the diagnosis [45]. As previously discussed for Xp11 translocation renal cell carcinomas, it is of paramount importance to define a proper cut-off to establish the occurrence of *TFEB* rearrangement, even in t(6;11) renal cell carcinoma, when the frequency of split signals is high (>38%). Although less frequently than in Xp11 translocation renal cell carcinoma, we observed minimally split fluorescent signals.

2.3. Differential Diagnosis

The wide spectrum of morphology results in several differential diagnoses including Xp11 translocation renal cell carcinoma, pure epithelioid PEComa/epithelioid angiomyolipoma, and other more common types of renal cell carcinoma [46–48]. Among them, pure epithelioid PEComa/epithelioid angiomyolipoma is the most challenging diagnosis in clinical practice [42]. Indeed, the two entities share the immunohistochemical expression of melanogenesis markers and cathepsin K, and both are often negative for cytokeratin. PAX8 immunoreactivity and CD68 (PG-M1) negativity supports the diagnosis of t(6;11) renal cell carcinoma, whereas pure epithelioid PEComa/epithelioid angiomyolipoma is PAX8 negative and CD68 (PG-M1) positive [42].

2.4. Prognosis and Treatment

Most instances of t(6;11) renal cell carcinoma have an indolent clinical course. An aggressive behavior is observed in roughly 17% of the cases (11 of 64 tumors with available follow up). Larger masses ($p = 0.04$) and older patients ($p = 0.007$) seem to be parameters correlated with aggressiveness. It should be noted that hematogenous metastases seem to be more common than nodal metastases. To date, there are no well-established prognostic markers to predict the biological behavior. However, it is possible that an increase in the copy number of the *TFEB* gene region in t(6;11) renal cell carcinoma may predict an aggressive clinical course [42,49]. The radical surgery remains the best therapeutic strategy. Because of the rarity of this tumor, no information regarding neoadjuvant or adjuvant therapies are available. Since these neoplasms have demonstrated the capacity to recur, follow-up examinations are important for these patients.

3. Renal Cell Carcinoma with *TFEB* Amplification

More recently, renal cell carcinomas with *TFEB* amplification have been described and appear to be associated with a poor outcome [50–55]. *TFEB* amplification in renal cell carcinoma can occur independently of or in association with *TFEB* rearrangement [50,55]. *TFEB* gene rearrangement or amplification increases TFEB expression which causes the subsequent expression of immunohistochemical markers such as cathepsin K, Melan-A, and HMB45 [43]. Nevertheless, *TFEB*-amplified renal cell carcinomas are different from t(6;11) renal cell carcinomas [50]. First, they typically occur in older patients (mean 65 years) compared to unamplified t(6;11) renal cell carcinoma (mean age 34 years). Second, their morphology is usually high grade and less typical than the biphasic appearance of t(6;11) renal cell carcinoma (Figure 4). Third, melanogenic marker expression is less reliable: while all cases have expressed Melan-A, roughly half of the cases express cathepsin K and HMB45, usually positive in t(6;11) renal cell carcinoma. Fourth, TFEB amplified renal cell carcinomas typically have a poor outcome while t(6;11) renal cell carcinomas are usually indolent. Of note, it has been demonstrated that renal cell carcinomas showing *TFEB* amplification harbor concurrent vascular endothelial growth factor A (*VEGFA*) gene amplification [52,55]. This is may be due to the proximity of those two genes, which are both located on the short arm of chromosome 6. With regard to the treatment, Gupta et al. hypothesized the possible usefulness of VEGFR-targeted therapy in a few cases of renal cell carcinomas with *TFEB/VEGFA* coamplification [52].

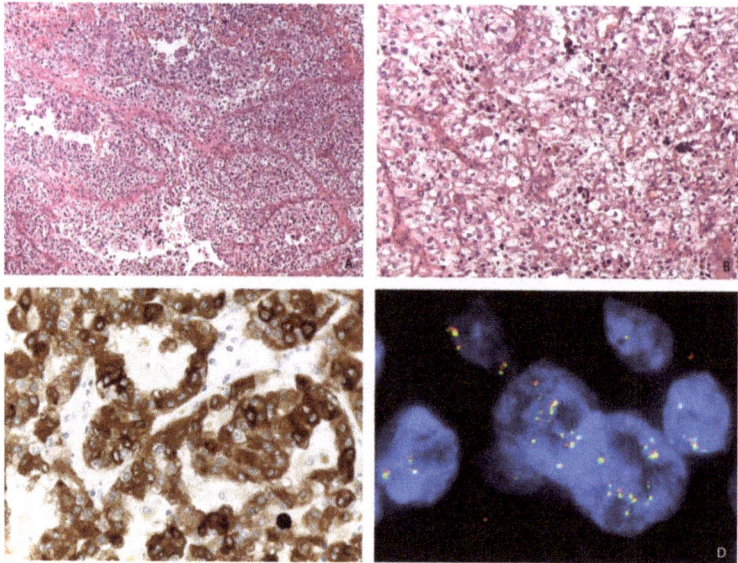

Figure 4. A high-grade renal cell carcinoma (**A**, Magnification: 50×; **B**, Magnification: 200×) expressing Melan-A (Magnification: 400×) (**C**) and showing *TFEB* gene amplification by FISH (Magnification: 1000×) (**D**).

4. Comparison of Xp11 Translocation Renal Cell Carcinoma and t(6;11) Renal Cell Carcinoma

As illustrated in Table 1, Xp11 translocation renal cell carcinoma and t(6;11) renal cell carcinoma differ in several ways. Xp11 translocation renal cell carcinoma seems to occur in patients younger than t(6;11) renal cell carcinoma; with a slight female predominance and a more frequently aggressive clinical course. Conversely to Xp11 translocation renal cell carcinoma, the immunohistochemical analysis of t(6;11) renal cell carcinoma is more consistent, showing the overexpression of cathepsin K and melanogenesis makers in almost all cases.

Table 1. Main differences between Xp11 translocation renal cell carcinoma and t(6;11) renal cell carcinoma.

Parameter	Xp11 Translocation RCC	t(6;11) RCC
Clinical		
Age distribution	peak: 20–29 years	peak: 30–39 years
Gender	F:M ratio, 1.6:1	F:M ratio, 0.75:1
Behavior	aggressive in 47% of cases	aggressive in 17% of cases
Morphology		
features	broad spectrum	usually biphasic
Immunohistochemistry		
Cathepsin K	47% positive	94% positive
Melan-A	39% positive	91% positive
HMB45	32% positive	83% positive

RCC: renal cell carcinoma; F: female; M: male.

5. Conclusions

On the basis of their clinical, immunohistochemical, and molecular similarities, the last WHO classification grouped Xp11 translocation renal cell carcinoma and t(6;11) renal cell carcinoma together under the name "MiT family translocation renal cell carcinoma". However, among them there are few differences, mainly in morphology and clinical behavior. For those reasons, we suggest to keep the distinction in the clinical practice. Overall, this review emphasizes that MiT family translocation renal cell carcinoma is a distinctive entity and therefore stresses the importance of recognizing it as a specific category of renal cell carcinoma to properly identify these cases in future clinical trials looking for effective therapies.

Funding: This research received no external funding.

Conflicts of Interest: The authors declare no conflict of interest.

References

1. Argani, P. MiT family translocation renal cell carcinoma. *Semin. Diagn. Pathol.* **2015**, *32*, 103–113. [CrossRef] [PubMed]
2. Xia, Q.Y.; Wang, X.T.; Ye, S.B.; Wang, X.; Li, R.; Shi, S.S.; Fang, R.; Zhang, R.S.; Ma, H.H.; Lu, Z.F.; et al. Novel gene fusion of PRCC-MITF defines a new member of MiT family translocation renal cell carcinoma: Clinicopathological analysis and detection of the gene fusion by RNA sequencing and FISH. *Histopathology* **2018**, *72*, 786–794. [CrossRef] [PubMed]
3. Xia, Q.Y.; Wang, X.T.; Zhan, X.M.; Tan, X.; Chen, H.; Liu, Y.; Shi, S.S.; Wang, X.; Wei, X.; Ye, S.B.; et al. Xp11 Translocation Renal Cell Carcinomas (RCCs) With RBM10-TFE3 Gene Fusion Demonstrating Melanotic Features and Overlapping Morphology With t(6;11) RCC: Interest and Diagnostic Pitfall in Detecting a Paracentric Inversion of TFE3. *Am. J. Surg. Pathol.* **2017**, *41*, 663–676. [CrossRef] [PubMed]
4. Xia, Q.Y.; Wang, Z.; Chen, N.; Gan, H.L.; Teng, X.D.; Shi, S.S.; Wang, X.; Wei, X.; Ye, S.B.; Li, R.; et al. Xp11.2 translocation renal cell carcinoma with NONO-TFE3 gene fusion: Morphology, prognosis, and potential pitfall in detecting TFE3 gene rearrangement. *Mod. Pathol.* **2017**, *30*, 416–426. [CrossRef] [PubMed]
5. Wang, X.T.; Xia, Q.Y.; Ni, H.; Ye, S.B.; Li, R.; Wang, X.; Shi, S.S.; Zhou, X.J.; Rao, Q. SFPQ/PSF-TFE3 renal cell carcinoma: A clinicopathologic study emphasizing extended morphology and reviewing the differences between SFPQ-TFE3 RCC and the corresponding mesenchymal neoplasm despite an identical gene fusion. *Hum. Pathol.* **2017**, *63*, 190–200. [CrossRef] [PubMed]
6. Antic, T.; Taxy, J.B.; Alikhan, M.; Segal, J. Melanotic Translocation Renal Cell Carcinoma With a Novel ARID1B-TFE3 Gene Fusion. *Am. J. Surg. Pathol.* **2017**, *41*, 1576–1580. [CrossRef]
7. Argani, P.; Zhong, M.; Reuter, V.E.; Fallon, J.T.; Epstein, J.I.; Netto, G.J.; Antonescu, C.R. TFE3-Fusion Variant Analysis Defines Specific Clinicopathologic Associations Among Xp11 Translocation Cancers. *Am. J. Surg. Pathol.* **2016**, *40*, 723–737. [CrossRef] [PubMed]
8. Pivovarcikova, K.; Grossmann, P.; Alaghehbandan, R.; Sperga, M.; Michal, M.; Hes, O. TFE3-Fusion Variant Analysis Defines Specific Clinicopathologic Associations Amog Xp11 Translocation Cancers. *Am. J. Surg. Pathol.* **2017**, *41*, 138–140. [CrossRef]
9. Pei, J.; Cooper, H.; Flieder, D.B.; Talarchek, J.N.; Al-Saleem, T.; Uzzo, R.G.; Dulaimi, E.; Patchefsky, A.S.; Testa, J.R.; Wei, S. NEAT1-TFE3 and KAT6A-TFE3 renal cell carcinomas, new members of MiT family translocation renal cell carcinoma. *Mod. Pathol.* **2019**. [CrossRef]
10. Wang, X.T.; Xia, Q.Y.; Ye, S.B.; Wang, X.; Li, R.; Fang, R.; Shi, S.S.; Zhang, R.S.; Tan, X.; Chen, J.Y.; et al. RNA sequencing of Xp11 translocation-associated cancers reveals novel gene fusions and distinctive clinicopathologic correlations. *Mod. Pathol.* **2018**, *31*, 1346–1360. [CrossRef]
11. Argani, P.; Antonescu, C.R.; Illei, P.B.; Lui, M.Y.; Timmons, C.F.; Newbury, R.; Reuter, V.E.; Garvin, A.J.; Perez-Atayde, A.R.; Fletcher, J.A.; et al. Primary renal neoplasms with the ASPL-TFE3 gene fusion of alveolar soft part sarcoma: A distinctive tumor entity previously included among renal cell carcinomas of children and adolescents. *Am. J. Pathol.* **2001**, *159*, 179–192. [CrossRef]

12. Sukov, W.R.; Hodge, J.C.; Lohse, C.M.; Leibovich, B.C.; Thompson, R.H.; Pearce, K.E.; Wiktor, A.E.; Cheville, J.C. TFE3 rearrangements in adult renal cell carcinoma: Clinical and pathologic features with outcome in a large series of consecutively treated patients. *Am. J. Surg. Pathol.* **2012**, *36*, 663–670. [CrossRef] [PubMed]
13. Argani, P.; Lae, M.; Ballard, E.T.; Amin, M.; Manivel, C.; Hutchinson, B.; Reuter, V.E.; Ladanyi, M. Translocation carcinomas of the kidney after chemotherapy in childhood. *J. Clin. Oncol.* **2006**, *24*, 1529–1534. [CrossRef] [PubMed]
14. Hayes, M.; Peckova, K.; Martinek, P.; Hora, M.; Kalusova, K.; Straka, L.; Daum, O.; Kokoskova, B.; Rotterova, P.; Pivovarcikova, K.; et al. Molecular-genetic analysis is essential for accurate classification of renal carcinoma resembling Xp11.2 translocation carcinoma. *Virchows Arch.* **2015**, *466*, 313–322. [CrossRef] [PubMed]
15. Argani, P.; Hicks, J.; De Marzo, A.M.; Albadine, R.; Illei, P.B.; Ladanyi, M.; Reuter, V.E.; Netto, G.J. Xp11 translocation renal cell carcinoma (RCC): Extended immunohistochemical profile emphasizing novel RCC markers. *Am. J. Surg. Pathol.* **2010**, *34*, 1295–1303. [CrossRef] [PubMed]
16. Martignoni, G.; Gobbo, S.; Camparo, P.; Brunelli, M.; Munari, E.; Segala, D.; Pea, M.; Bonetti, F.; Illei, P.B.; Netto, G.J.; et al. Differential expression of cathepsin K in neoplasms harboring TFE3 gene fusions. *Mod. Pathol.* **2011**, *24*, 1313–1319. [CrossRef] [PubMed]
17. Green, W.M.; Yonescu, R.; Morsberger, L.; Morris, K.; Netto, G.J.; Epstein, J.I.; Illei, P.B.; Allaf, M.; Ladanyi, M.; Griffin, C.A.; et al. Utilization of a TFE3 break-apart FISH assay in a renal tumor consultation service. *Am. J. Surg. Pathol.* **2013**, *37*, 1150–1163. [CrossRef]
18. Kim, S.H.; Choi, Y.; Jeong, H.Y.; Lee, K.; Chae, J.Y.; Moon, K.C. Usefulness of a break-apart FISH assay in the diagnosis of Xp11.2 translocation renal cell carcinoma. *Virchows Arch.* **2011**, *459*, 299–306. [CrossRef]
19. Rao, Q.; Williamson, S.R.; Zhang, S.; Eble, J.N.; Grignon, D.J.; Wang, M.; Zhou, X.J.; Huang, W.; Tan, P.H.; Maclennan, G.T.; et al. TFE3 break-apart FISH has a higher sensitivity for Xp11.2 translocation-associated renal cell carcinoma compared with TFE3 or cathepsin K immunohistochemical staining alone: Expanding the morphologic spectrum. *Am. J. Surg. Pathol.* **2013**, *37*, 804–815. [CrossRef]
20. Argani, P.; Zhang, L.; Reuter, V.E.; Tickoo, S.K.; Antonescu, C.R. RBM10-TFE3 Renal Cell Carcinoma: A Potential Diagnostic Pitfall Due to Cryptic Intrachromosomal Xp11.2 Inversion Resulting in False-negative TFE3 FISH. *Am. J. Surg. Pathol.* **2017**, *41*, 655–662. [CrossRef]
21. Kato, I.; Furuya, M.; Baba, M.; Kameda, Y.; Yasuda, M.; Nishimoto, K.; Oyama, M.; Yamasaki, T.; Ogawa, O.; Niino, H.; et al. RBM10-TFE3 Renal Cell Carcinoma Characterized by Paracentric Inversion with Consistent Closely Split Signals in Break-apart Fluorescence in situ Hybridization: Study of Ten Cases and a Literature Review. *Histopathology* **2019**. [CrossRef] [PubMed]
22. Chou, A.; Hes, O.; Turchini, J.; Trpkov, K.; Gill, A.J. Do significant TFE3 gene rearrangements occur in succinate dehydrogenase-deficient renal cell carcinoma? Borderline FISH results should be interpreted with caution. *Mod. Pathol.* **2017**, *30*, 1507–1508. [CrossRef] [PubMed]
23. Williamson, S.R.; Grignon, D.J.; Calio, A.; Stohr, B.A.; Eble, J.N.; Cheng, L. Reply to Chou et al. 'Do significant TFE3 gene rearrangements occur in succinate dehydrogenase deficient renal cell carcinoma? Borderline FISH results should be interpreted with caution'. *Mod. Pathol.* **2017**, *30*, 1509–1511. [CrossRef] [PubMed]
24. Calio, A.; Grignon, D.J.; Stohr, B.A.; Williamson, S.R.; Eble, J.N.; Cheng, L. Renal cell carcinoma with TFE3 translocation and succinate dehydrogenase B mutation. *Mod. Pathol.* **2017**, *30*, 407–415. [CrossRef] [PubMed]
25. Parihar, A.; Tickoo, S.K.; Kumar, S.; Arora, V.K. Xp11 translocation renal cell carcinoma morphologically mimicking clear cell-papillary renal cell carcinoma in an adult patient: Report of a case expanding the morphologic spectrum of Xp11 translocation renal cell carcinomas. *Int. J. Surg Pathol* **2015**, *23*, 234–237. [CrossRef] [PubMed]
26. Pan, C.C.; Sung, M.T.; Huang, H.Y.; Yeh, K.T. High chromosomal copy number alterations in Xp11 translocation renal cell carcinomas detected by array comparative genomic hybridization are associated with aggressive behavior. *Am. J. Surg. Pathol.* **2013**, *37*, 1116–1119. [CrossRef] [PubMed]
27. Meyer, P.N.; Clark, J.I.; Flanigan, R.C.; Picken, M.M. Xp11.2 translocation renal cell carcinoma with very aggressive course in five adults. *Am. J. Surg. Pathol.* **2007**, *128*, 70–79. [CrossRef]
28. Ellis, C.L.; Eble, J.N.; Subhawong, A.P.; Martignoni, G.; Zhong, M.; Ladanyi, M.; Epstein, J.I.; Netto, G.J.; Argani, P. Clinical heterogeneity of Xp11 translocation renal cell carcinoma: Impact of fusion subtype, age, and stage. *Mod. Pathol.* **2014**, *27*, 875–886. [CrossRef]

29. Camparo, P.; Vasiliu, V.; Molinie, V.; Couturier, J.; Dykema, K.J.; Petillo, D.; Furge, K.A.; Comperat, E.M.; Lae, M.; Bouvier, R.; et al. Renal translocation carcinomas: Clinicopathologic, immunohistochemical, and gene expression profiling analysis of 31 cases with a review of the literature. *Am. J. Surg. Pathol.* **2008**, *32*, 656–670. [CrossRef]
30. Choueiri, T.K.; Lim, Z.D.; Hirsch, M.S.; Tamboli, P.; Jonasch, E.; McDermott, D.F.; Dal Cin, P.; Corn, P.; Vaishampayan, U.; Heng, D.Y.; et al. Vascular endothelial growth factor-targeted therapy for the treatment of adult metastatic Xp11.2 translocation renal cell carcinoma. *Cancer* **2010**, *116*, 5219–5225. [CrossRef]
31. Malouf, G.G.; Camparo, P.; Oudard, S.; Schleiermacher, G.; Theodore, C.; Rustine, A.; Dutcher, J.; Billemont, B.; Rixe, O.; Bompas, E.; et al. Targeted agents in metastatic Xp11 translocation/TFE3 gene fusion renal cell carcinoma (RCC): A report from the Juvenile RCC Network. *Ann. Oncol.* **2010**, *21*, 1834–1838. [CrossRef] [PubMed]
32. Damayanti, N.P.; Budka, J.A.; Khella, H.W.Z.; Ferris, M.W.; Ku, S.Y.; Kauffman, E.; Wood, A.C.; Ahmed, K.; Chintala, V.N.; Adelaiye-Ogala, R.; et al. Therapeutic Targeting of TFE3/IRS-1/PI3K/mTOR Axis in Translocation Renal Cell Carcinoma. *Clin. Cancer Res.* **2018**, *24*, 5977–5989. [CrossRef] [PubMed]
33. Chang, K.; Qu, Y.; Dai, B.; Zhao, J.Y.; Gan, H.; Shi, G.; Zhu, Y.; Shen, Y.; Zhu, Y.; Zhang, H.; et al. PD-L1 expression in Xp11.2 translocation renal cell carcinoma: Indicator of tumor aggressiveness. *Sci. Rep.* **2017**, *7*, 2074. [CrossRef] [PubMed]
34. Tsuda, M.; Davis, I.J.; Argani, P.; Shukla, N.; McGill, G.G.; Nagai, M.; Saito, T.; Lae, M.; Fisher, D.E.; Ladanyi, M. TFE3 fusions activate MET signaling by transcriptional up-regulation, defining another class of tumors as candidates for therapeutic MET inhibition. *Cancer Res.* **2007**, *67*, 919–929. [CrossRef] [PubMed]
35. Choueiri, T.K.; Escudier, B.; Powles, T.; Tannir, N.M.; Mainwaring, P.N.; Rini, B.I.; Hammers, H.J.; Donskov, F.; Roth, B.J.; Peltola, K.; et al. Cabozantinib versus everolimus in advanced renal cell carcinoma (METEOR): Final results from a randomised, open-label, phase 3 trial. *Lancet Oncol.* **2016**, *17*, 917–927. [CrossRef]
36. Choueiri, T.K.; Halabi, S.; Sanford, B.L.; Hahn, O.; Michaelson, M.D.; Walsh, M.K.; Feldman, D.R.; Olencki, T.; Picus, J.; Small, E.J.; et al. Cabozantinib Versus Sunitinib As Initial Targeted Therapy for Patients With Metastatic Renal Cell Carcinoma of Poor or Intermediate Risk: The Alliance A031203 CABOSUN Trial. *J. Clin. Oncol.* **2017**, *35*, 591–597. [CrossRef] [PubMed]
37. Martinez Chanza, N.; Xie, W.; Asim Bilen, M.; Dzimitrowicz, H.; Burkart, J.; Geynisman, D.M.; Balakrishnan, A.; Bowman, I.A.; Jain, R.; Stadler, W.; et al. Cabozantinib in advanced non-clear-cell renal cell carcinoma: A multicentre, retrospective, cohort study. *Lancet Oncol.* **2019**. [CrossRef]
38. Malouf, G.G.; Su, X.; Yao, H.; Gao, J.; Xiong, L.; He, Q.; Comperat, E.; Couturier, J.; Molinie, V.; Escudier, B.; et al. Next-generation sequencing of translocation renal cell carcinoma reveals novel RNA splicing partners and frequent mutations of chromatin-remodeling genes. *Clin. Cancer Res.* **2014**, *20*, 4129–4140. [CrossRef]
39. Argani, P.; Hawkins, A.; Griffin, C.A.; Goldstein, J.D.; Haas, M.; Beckwith, J.B.; Mankinen, C.B.; Perlman, E.J. A distinctive pediatric renal neoplasm characterized by epithelioid morphology, basement membrane production, focal HMB45 immunoreactivity, and t(6;11) (p21.1;q12) chromosome translocation. *Am. J. Pathol.* **2001**, *158*, 2089–2096. [CrossRef]
40. Petersson, F.; Vanecek, T.; Michal, M.; Martignoni, G.; Brunelli, M.; Halbhuber, Z.; Spagnolo, D.; Kuroda, N.; Yang, X.; Cabrero, I.A.; et al. A distinctive translocation carcinoma of the kidney; "rosette forming," t(6;11), HMB45-positive renal tumor: A histomorphologic, immunohistochemical, ultrastructural, and molecular genetic study of 4 cases. *Hum. Pathol.* **2012**, *43*, 726–736. [CrossRef]
41. Williamson, S.R.; Eble, J.N.; Palanisamy, N. Sclerosing TFEB-rearrangement renal cell carcinoma: A recurring histologic pattern. *Hum. Pathol.* **2017**, *62*, 175–179. [CrossRef] [PubMed]
42. Calio, A.; Brunelli, M.; Segala, D.; Pedron, S.; Tardanico, R.; Remo, A.; Gobbo, S.; Meneghelli, E.; Doglioni, C.; Hes, O.; et al. t(6;11) renal cell carcinoma: A study of seven cases including two with aggressive behavior, and utility of CD68 (PG-M1) in the differential diagnosis with pure epithelioid PEComa/epithelioid angiomyolipoma. *Mod. Pathol.* **2018**, *31*, 474–487. [CrossRef] [PubMed]
43. Martignoni, G.; Pea, M.; Gobbo, S.; Brunelli, M.; Bonetti, F.; Segala, D.; Pan, C.C.; Netto, G.; Doglioni, C.; Hes, O.; et al. Cathepsin-K immunoreactivity distinguishes MiTF/TFE family renal translocation carcinomas from other renal carcinomas. *Mod. Pathol.* **2009**, *22*, 1016–1022. [CrossRef] [PubMed]
44. Martignoni, G.; Bonetti, F.; Chilosi, M.; Brunelli, M.; Segala, D.; Amin, M.B.; Argani, P.; Eble, J.N.; Gobbo, S.; Pea, M. Cathepsin K expression in the spectrum of perivascular epithelioid cell (PEC) lesions of the kidney. *Mod. Pathol.* **2012**, *25*, 100–111. [CrossRef] [PubMed]

45. Argani, P.; Lae, M.; Hutchinson, B.; Reuter, V.E.; Collins, M.H.; Perentesis, J.; Tomaszewski, J.E.; Brooks, J.S.; Acs, G.; Bridge, J.A.; et al. Renal carcinomas with the t(6;11) (p21;q12): Clinicopathologic features and demonstration of the specific alpha-TFEB gene fusion by immunohistochemistry, RT-PCR, and DNA PCR. *Am. J. Surg. Pathol.* **2005**, *29*, 230–240. [CrossRef] [PubMed]
46. Argani, P.; Yonescu, R.; Morsberger, L.; Morris, K.; Netto, G.J.; Smith, N.; Gonzalez, N.; Illei, P.B.; Ladanyi, M.; Griffin, C.A. Molecular confirmation of t(6;11) (p21;q12) renal cell carcinoma in archival paraffin-embedded material using a break-apart TFEB FISH assay expands its clinicopathologic spectrum. *Am. J. Surg. Pathol.* **2012**, *36*, 1516–1526. [CrossRef]
47. Smith, N.E.; Illei, P.B.; Allaf, M.; Gonzalez, N.; Morris, K.; Hicks, J.; Demarzo, A.; Reuter, V.E.; Amin, M.B.; Epstein, J.I.; et al. t(6;11) renal cell carcinoma (RCC): Expanded immunohistochemical profile emphasizing novel RCC markers and report of 10 new genetically confirmed cases. *Am. J. Surg. Pathol.* **2014**, *38*, 604–614. [CrossRef]
48. Rao, Q.; Zhang, X.M.; Tu, P.; Xia, Q.Y.; Shen, Q.; Zhou, X.J.; Shi, Q.L. Renal cell carcinomas with t(6;11) (p21;q12) presenting with tubulocystic renal cell carcinoma-like features. *Int. J. Clin. Exp. Pathol.* **2013**, *6*, 1452–1457.
49. Peckova, K.; Vanecek, T.; Martinek, P.; Spagnolo, D.; Kuroda, N.; Brunelli, M.; Vranic, S.; Djuricic, S.; Rotterova, P.; Daum, O.; et al. Aggressive and nonaggressive translocation t(6;11) renal cell carcinoma: Comparative study of 6 cases and review of the literature. *Ann. Diagn. Pathol* **2014**, *18*, 351–357. [CrossRef]
50. Argani, P.; Reuter, V.E.; Zhang, L.; Sung, Y.S.; Ning, Y.; Epstein, J.I.; Netto, G.J.; Antonescu, C.R. TFEB-amplified Renal Cell Carcinomas: An Aggressive Molecular Subset Demonstrating Variable Melanocytic Marker Expression and Morphologic Heterogeneity. *Am. J. Surg. Pathol.* **2016**, *40*, 1484–1495. [CrossRef]
51. Williamson, S.R.; Grignon, D.J.; Cheng, L.; Favazza, L.; Gondim, D.D.; Carskadon, S.; Gupta, N.S.; Chitale, D.A.; Kalyana-Sundaram, S.; Palanisamy, N. Renal Cell Carcinoma With Chromosome 6p Amplification Including the TFEB Gene: A Novel Mechanism of Tumor Pathogenesis? *Am. J. Surg. Pathol.* **2016**. [CrossRef] [PubMed]
52. Gupta, S.; Johnson, S.H.; Vasmatzis, G.; Porath, B.; Rustin, J.G.; Rao, P.; Costello, B.A.; Leibovich, B.C.; Thompson, R.H.; Cheville, J.C.; et al. TFEB-VEGFA (6p21.1) co-amplified renal cell carcinoma: A distinct entity with potential implications for clinical management. *Mod. Pathol.* **2017**, *30*, 998–1012. [CrossRef] [PubMed]
53. Skala, S.L.; Xiao, H.; Udager, A.M.; Dhanasekaran, S.M.; Shukla, S.; Zhang, Y.; Landau, C.; Shao, L.; Roulston, D.; Wang, L.; et al. Detection of 6 TFEB-amplified renal cell carcinomas and 25 renal cell carcinomas with MITF translocations: Systematic morphologic analysis of 85 cases evaluated by clinical TFE3 and TFEB FISH assays. *Mod. Pathol.* **2018**, *31*, 179–197. [CrossRef] [PubMed]
54. Mendel, L.; Ambrosetti, D.; Bodokh, Y.; Ngo-Mai, M.; Durand, M.; Simbsler-Michel, C.; Delhorbe, M.; Amiel, J.; Pedeutour, F. Comprehensive study of three novel cases of TFEB-amplified renal cell carcinoma and review of the literature: Evidence for a specific entity with poor outcome. *Genes Chromosomes Cancer* **2018**, *57*, 99–113. [CrossRef] [PubMed]
55. Calio, A.; Brunelli, M.; Segala, D.; Pedron, S.; Doglioni, C.; Argani, P.; Martignoni, G. VEGFA amplification/increased gene copy number and VEGFA mRNA expression in renal cell carcinoma with TFEB gene alterations. *Mod. Pathol.* **2019**, *32*, 258–268. [CrossRef] [PubMed]

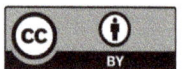

© 2019 by the authors. Licensee MDPI, Basel, Switzerland. This article is an open access article distributed under the terms and conditions of the Creative Commons Attribution (CC BY) license (http://creativecommons.org/licenses/by/4.0/).

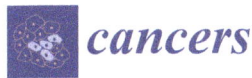

Brief Report

Hypertonicity-Affected Genes Are Differentially Expressed in Clear Cell Renal Cell Carcinoma and Correlate with Cancer-Specific Survival

Siarhei Kandabarau [1,2], Janna Leiz [3,4], Knut Krohn [5], Stefan Winter [1,2], Jens Bedke [6,7], Matthias Schwab [1,7,8,9], Elke Schaeffeler [1,2,9] and Bayram Edemir [3,*]

1. Dr. Margarete Fischer-Bosch Institute of Clinical Pharmacology, 70376 Stuttgart, Germany; Siarhei.Kandabarau@ikp-stuttgart.de (S.K.); Stefan.Winter@ikp-stuttgart.de (S.W.); matthias.schwab@ikp-stuttgart.de (M.S.); elke.schaeffeler@ikp-stuttgart.de (E.S.)
2. University of Tübingen, 72074 Tübingen, Germany
3. Department of Medicine, Hematology and Oncology, Martin Luther University Halle-Wittenberg, 06120 Halle (Saale), Germany; janna.leiz@mdc-berlin.de
4. Max Delbrück Center for Molecular Medicine (MDC), 13125 Berlin, Germany
5. Core Unit DNA–Technologien, Medizinische Fakultät, Universität Leipzig, 04103 Leipzig, Germany; krok@medizin.uni-leipzig.de
6. Department of Urology, University Hospital Tübingen, 72076 Tübingen, Germany; jens.bedke@med.uni-tuebingen.de
7. German Cancer Consortium (DKTK) and German Cancer Research Center (DKFZ), 69120 Heidelberg, Germany
8. Departments of Clinical Pharmacology, Pharmacy and Biochemistry, University Tübingen, 72076 Tübingen, Germany
9. iFIT Cluster of Excellence EXC 2180, University of Tübingen, 72076 Tübingen, Germany
* Correspondence: bayram.edemir@uk-halle.de; Tel.: +49-345-557-4890; Fax: +49-345-557-2950

Received: 29 November 2019; Accepted: 13 December 2019; Published: 18 December 2019

Abstract: The heterogeneity of renal cell carcinoma (RCC) subtypes reflects the cell type of origin in the nephron, with consequences for therapy and prognosis. The transcriptional cues that determine segment-specific gene expression patterns are poorly understood. We recently showed that hypertonicity in the renal medulla regulates nephron-specific gene expression. Here, we analyzed a set of 223 genes, which were identified in the present study by RNA-Seq to be differentially expressed by hypertonicity, for the prediction of cancer-specific survival (CSS). Cluster analyses of these genes showed discrimination between tumor and non-tumor samples of clear cell RCC (ccRCC). Refinement of this gene signature to a four-gene score (OSM score) through statistical analyses enabled prediction of CSS in ccRCC patients of The Cancer Genome Atlas (TCGA) ($n = 436$) in univariate (HR = 4.1; 95% CI: 2.78–6.07; $p = 4.39 \times 10^{-13}$), and multivariate analyses including primary tumor (T); regional lymph node (N); distant metastasis (M); grading (G)($p = 2.3 \times 10^{-5}$). The OSM score could be validated in an independent ccRCC study ($n = 52$) in univariate (HR = 1.29; 95% CI = 1.05–1.59; $p = 0.011$) and multivariate analyses ($p = 0.016$). Cell culture experiments using RCC cell lines demonstrated that the expression of the tumor suppressor *ELF5* could be restored by hypertonicity. The innovation of our novel gene signature is that these genes are physiologically regulated only by hypertonicity, thereby providing the possibility to be targeted for therapy.

Keywords: gene signature; renal cancer; survival prediction

1. Introduction

The kidney's anatomy and histology consists of different renal cell types located at defined parts of the kidneys, reflected in the complexity of renal function. This is also reflected by the heterogeneity of renal cell carcinoma (RCC) subtypes [1]. The main subtypes are clear cell (ccRCC), papillary (pRCC) and chromophobe (chRCC) renal cell carcinoma [2]. Although several targeted therapies are currently applied, survival rates—especially for metastatic RCC—are still low and innovative treatment strategies are needed [2].

Comprehensive studies carried out by The Cancer Genome Atlas (TCGA) provided further insight into the evolution and origin of RCC, for example, by identifying gene signatures that enable discrimination between the RCC subtypes or define the cell type of origin. Moreover, it was found to be possible to predict clinical outcome in ccRCC patients based on gene expression similarity to the proximal tubule of the nephron, which is the presumed origin of ccRCC [3]. Recently, another study analyzed the impact of different gene expression profiles on RCC ontogeny [1]. The authors were able to identify gene expression programs that were specific for a distinct nephron segment and were also present in the corresponding RCC subtypes. Both studies used data based on nephron-specific gene expression patterns and were able either to improve the prediction of patient outcome or identify gene expression networks defining the origin of RCC. However, as mentioned by Lindgren et al. [1], the transcriptional cues that determine segment-specific gene expression patterns are only partly understood. We have recently shown that the unique hypertonicity in the renal inner medulla regulates kidney and nephron-specific gene expression [4]. The group of Prof. Ian Frew showed that deletion of renal expression of the tumor suppressor von Hippel–Lindau (VHL) protein altered the urine concentration capability in mice [5]. They postulate that the mice cannot build up the hyperosmotic gradient in the kidneys that is necessary for urine concentration. The transcription factor nuclear factor of activated T-cells 5 (*NFAT5*) is the main transcription factor activated by the hyperosmotic environment, and induces the expression of several genes [6]. A recent study in that Special Issue of *Cancers* showed that microRNAs that mediate metabolic reprogramming in ccRCC also target *NFAT5* [7]. This was also associated with a reduced level of *NFAT5* target genes in the ccRCC samples compared to solid normal tissue.

In the present study, we analyzed if the hypertonicity-affected genes were also differentially expressed in ccRCC tumor samples and normal tissue, and if these genes were associated with the clinical outcome of the patients.

2. Results and Discussion

In contrast to our initial study, where we used microarrays, here we performed RNA-Seq using primary cultured inner medullary collecting duct (IMCD) cells cultivated at 300 or 900 mosmol/kg to identify differentially expressed transcripts affected by hypertonicity (for details see Table S1). We detected significant differences between the two conditions for 355 transcripts (false discovery rate FDR < 0.05; $\log_2$ fold change (FC) >3/<−3) and there were matching human transcripts for 284 of these (223 genes) (Figure 1A and Table S1). Hierarchical clustering of the TCGA Kidney Clear Cell Carcinoma (KIRC) samples based RNA-Seq data using the top 223 hypertonicity-affected genes clearly separated the normal non-tumor tissue samples ($n = 67$) from the tumor samples ($n = 449$; Figure 1B).

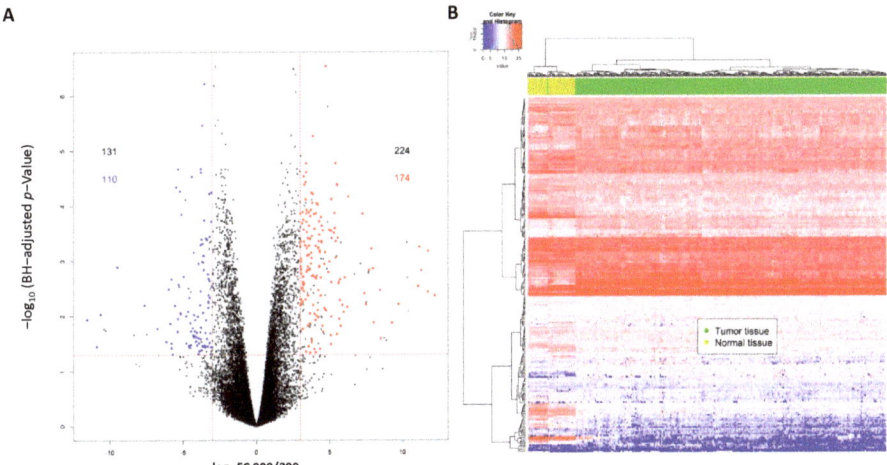

Figure 1. (**A**) Differentially expressed transcripts affected by hypertonicity in primary cultured inner medullary collecting duct (IMCD) cells either cultivated at 300 or 900 mosmol/kg. In total, 355 transcripts were differentially expressed (with a cut off log$_2$ fold change of >3 and <−3) and there were matched human transcripts for 284 of those. Of those, 110 transcripts were downregulated and 174 transcripts were upregulated by hypertonicity. (**B**) Hierarchical clustering of samples from The Cancer Genome Atlas (TCGA) Kidney Clear Cell Carcinoma (KIRC) cohort based on the hypertonicity-affected genes. The expression levels of the top 223 regulated genes were extracted from the TCGA KIRC cohort, and hierarchical clustering was performed. This set of genes was able to clearly separate clear cell renal cell carcinoma (ccRCC) samples (dark green) from the normal tissue samples (light green).

Part of the genes (41) showed a log$_2$ fold change of >3/<−3 between normal and tumor samples. Interestingly, several of the transcripts induced by hypertonicity were suppressed, and transcripts suppressed by hypertonicity were induced in the tumor samples compared to normal samples (Table S1).

The effect of hyper-osmolality on gene expression can be reverted by hypo osmotic switch [4]. For example one of the hypertonicity-induced transcripts (0 fragments per kilobase of transcript per million mapped reads (FPKM) at 300 vs. 75 FPKM at 900 mosmol/kg, see Table S1) was the E74-like ETS transcription factor 5 (*ELF5*). *ELF5* has been described as a tumor suppressor in RCC and is more or less absent in tumor samples (Table S1) [8]. Since *ELF5* has an important role as a tumor suppressor, we next asked whether it is possible to induce its expression in a ccRCC cell line by hyperosmolality. To test this, we used the established ccRCC cell line 786-0, and the same cell line that ectopically expresses WT-VHL (786-0-VHL). Both were cultivated either under isotonic (300 mosmol/kg) or for different periods of time under hyperosmotic (600 mosmol/kg) conditions. Indeed, the expression of *ELF5* could be induced by cultivation of 786-0 cells under hyperosmotic conditions as shown by PCR or qPCR analyses (Figure 2A,B). Interestingly, the induction of *ELF5* expression was higher in VHL+ cells than in VHL-deficient cells.

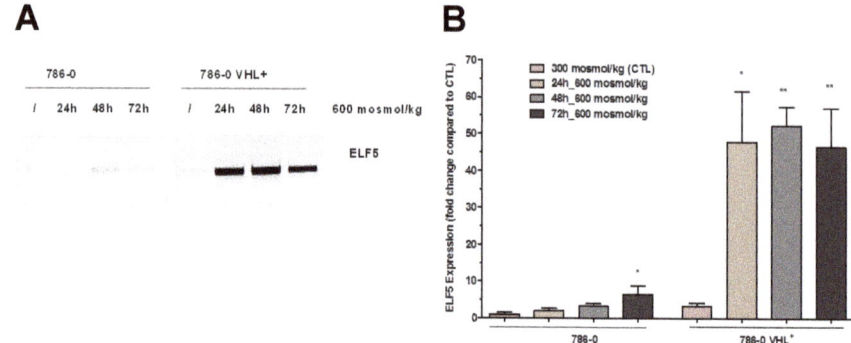

Figure 2. E74-like ETS transcription factor 5 (*ELF5*) expression in 786-0 cells is induced by environmental hypertonicity. von Hippel–Lindau (VHL)-deficient 786-0 and VHL-expressing (VHL+) 786-0 cells were cultivated either in normal medium (300) or for 24, 48, and 72 h in 600 mosmol/kg medium. (**A**) The expression of *ELF5* was analyzed by PCR. The osmolality was increased by the addition of 100 mM NaCl and 100 mM urea. The expression of *ELF5* was VHL dependent. (**B**) The expression of *ELF5* was quantified by real-time PCR in VHL-deficient 786-0 and VHL-expressing 786-0 VHL+ cells ($N > 3$, p-Value < 0.05 compared to control (CTL) using one-way ANOVA are marked by *, p-Value < 0.01 are marked by **). For more details about the PCR product of ELF5, please view the Supplementary Materials.

Our results clearly indicate that it is possible to induce the expression of the tumor suppressor ELF5 in RCC cells only by osmolality without any genetic manipulation. With the hyper-osmolality, we have identified a pathway that could be targeted for future intervention.

In the next step, we analyzed the predictive value of the hypertonicity-related genes for clinical outcome in ccRCC patients using the Cox proportional hazards model. Out of the 223 genes, 111 (49.8%) showed a significant effect (Table 1).

Table 1. Number of hypertonicity-affected genes and their impact on patient survival.

Effect on Cancer Specific Survival	Downregulated	Upregulated
hazardous	32	35
indifferent	46	66
favorable	9	35

Within the genes that had a significant impact on patients' survival, hypertonicity-downregulated genes tend to have a negative effect on survival (32 out of 41) while hypertonicity-upregulated genes have equal number of negative (35) and positive (35) effects. The corresponding data with the gene IDs and fold changes are provided in Table S1. This data suggests that the expression of hypertonicity-affected genes can be used to predict cancer-specific survival.

We next selected a minimum set of genes necessary for survival prediction using RNA-Seq data from the TCGA KIRC cohort. We identified 4 (*COL1A1*, *NDUFA4L2*, *S100A6*, *MT2A*) out of the 223 different genes that were regulated by hypertonicity in rats and subsequently defined our OSM score based on these four genes (Figure S1). Interestingly, all four genes have previously been associated with ccRCC tumorigenesis [9–12].

Our novel established OSM score based on these four genes was significantly associated with cancer-specific survival (Figure 3A; HR = 4.1; 95% CI: 2.78–6.07; $p = 4.39 \times 10^{-13}$; Cox proportional hazards regression model) in the TCGA cohort.

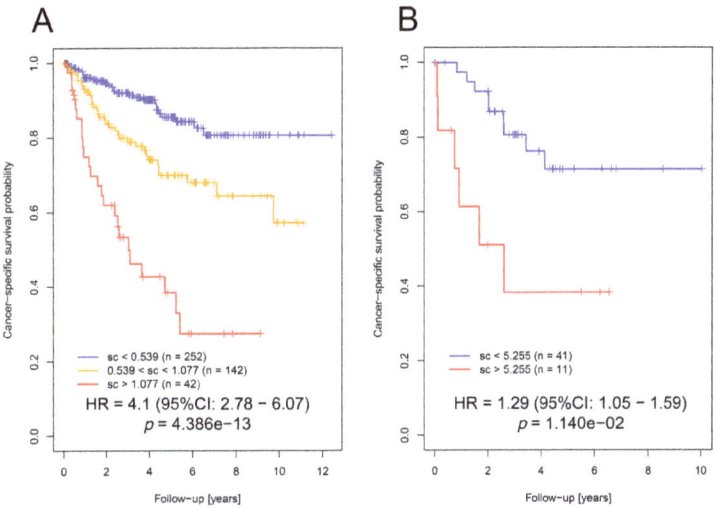

Figure 3. The OSM score could predict patient survival. (**A**) Kaplan–Meier plot indicating that hypertonicity-affected genes using the four selected genes (OSM score) can be applied for the prediction of patients' cancer-specific survival in the TCGA KIRC cohort. (**B**) Kaplan–Meier plot indicating that the OSM score can be applied for the prediction of patients' cancer-specific survival in the ccRCC validation cohort.

Multivariate analysis of the score together with clinicopathological parameters (T (primary tumor), N (regional lymph node), M (distant metastasis present at diagnosis), G (grading)) indicated that the score significantly predicted cancer-specific survival ($p = 2.3 \times 10^{-5}$, Table 2).

Table 2. Multivariate Cox regression for cancer-specific survival in the TCGA cohort ($n = 409$) and the validation cohort ($n = 51$).

Multivariate Analyses	Variable	Level	p-Value (Wald Test)	HR (95% CI)
Including T, N, M, G and OSM score (TCGA cohort)	OSM score		2.35×10^{-5}	2.6 (1.67–3.69)
	Primary tumor	T1/T2		1
		T3/T4	5.05×10^{-2}	1.7 (1–2.86)
	Lymph nodes	N0		1
		N1	6.15×10^{-2}	2.71 (0.95–7.72)
		NX	2.4×10^{-2}	0.6 (0.38–0.93)
	Distant metastasis	M0		1
		M1	1.55×10^{-12}	5.62 (3.48–9.07)
	Grade	G1/G2		1
		G3/G4	6.69×10^{-3}	2.35 (1.27–4.37)
Including T, N, M, G and OSM score (Validation cohort)	OSM score		1.58×10^{-2}	1.34 (1.06–1.7)
	Primary tumor	T1/T2		1
		T3/T4	2.54×10^{-1}	2.63 (0.5–13.9)
	Lymph nodes	N0		1
		N1/N2	1.27×10^{-1}	0.33 (0.08–1.36)
	Distant metastasis	M0		1
		M1	2.78×10^{-5}	41 (7.22–233.06)
	Fuhrman grade	G1/G2		1
		G3/G4	9.94×10^{-1}	1 (0.29–3.43)

Abbreviations: CI, confidence interval; HR, hazard ratio; Ref., reference level; T, primary tumor; N, regional lymph node; M, distant metastasis present at diagnosis; G, grading. Cases with grading information "GX" or metastasis status "MX" were excluded from multivariate analyses. OSM scores were determined based on gene expression data measured by RNA-Seq (TCGA) or microarray analyses (validation cohort).

The independent role for prediction in the multivariate model was proven by analysis of deviance ($p = 1.2 \times 10^{-4}$). To validate these results, the OSM score was calculated in an independent cohort of ccRCC patients ($n = 52$; for details see [13]) based on expression levels of the selected genes and their model coefficients. Notably, we showed that the OSM score was also significantly associated with cancer-specific survival (Figure 3B; HR = 1.29; 95% CI: 1.05–1.59; $p = 0.011$). Multivariate analysis confirmed its role in the prediction of cancer-specific survival ($p = 0.016$) in our validation cohort (Table 1; analysis of deviance $p = 0.0215$).

A link between loss of *VHL* and osmolality has also been shown using kidney-specific VHL knock-out mice [5]. The authors observed that the mice had increased diuresis. The same group developed a renal cancer mice model and investigated the gene expression profile in mouse ccRCCs and kidney cortices [14]. Using these gene expression data, we could demonstrate that the mouse ccRCCs and normal kidney cortices could be discriminated based on the osmolality-regulated genes (Figure S2). Our results indicate that *VHL* function is important for hyper-osmolality-induced gene expression, as seen for *ELF5*. In a recent manuscript that we have submitted to *Cancers* we were able to show that the deletion of *VHL* also reduced the expression of several other hyper-osmolality-induced genes. This implies that *VHL* is prominently involved in the regulation hyper-osmolality-induced pathways. Since up to 85% of RCC patients harbor loss of *VHL* function, it is mandatory to identify the underlying cellular and molecular mechanisms.

In summary, our in vitro and in vivo data demonstrate that osmolality is an interesting pathway for the future development of drugs or other interventions in ccRCC which has not been considered so far. Moreover, this is the first report that defines an expression pattern of genes that can not only be used to discriminate between normal vs. tumor tissue and is associated with cancer-specific survival in independent ccRCC cohorts, but have a common physiological mechanism regulating their expression. Thus, targeting osmolality represents a novel interesting option for ccRCC therapy development, and further studies are warranted to identify the functional relevance of hypertonicity-associated pathways in tumor development and proliferation.

3. Materials and Methods

3.1. Primary Renal Cell Culture and RNA-Seq

Experiments were approved by a governmental committee on animal welfare (Landesamt für Natur, Umwelt und Verbraucherschutz Nordrhein-Westfalen, Germany) and were performed in accordance with national animal protection guidelines (A 60/1993 and A 67/09).

Primary cultured IMCD cells were prepared as described before [4]. For each group, three biological replicates were used. The groups included cells which had been cultivated at 300 or 900 mosmol/kg for one week. Total RNA was isolated using the mirVana miRNA Isolation Kit (Thermo Scientific, Waltham, MA, USA); 500 ng of total RNA were depleted of ribosomal RNA using the RiboMinus kit (Thermo Fisher Scientific, Waltham, MA, USA) according to the manufacturer's instructions. Purified RNA was then fragmented by the addition of fragmentation buffer (200 mM Tris acetate, pH 8.2, 500 mM potassium acetate, and 150 mM magnesium acetate) and heating at 94 °C for 3 min in a thermocycler followed by ethanol precipitation with ammonium acetate and GlycoBlue (Thermo Fisher Scientific) as carrier. Fragmented RNA was then reverse transcribed using random hexamer and Superscript III (Thermo Fisher Scientific). The second strand was synthesized using the TargetAmp kit (Epicentre, Madison, WI, USA) according to the manufacturer's instructions. The final steps of library preparation (e.g., blunt end repair, adapter ligation, adapter fill-in, and amplification) were done according to Meyer and Kircher [15]. The barcoded libraries were purified and quantified using the Library Quantification Kit (Illumina/Universal; KAPA Biosystems, Wilmington, MA, USA) according to the manufacturer's instructions. A pool of up to 10 libraries was used for cluster generation at a concentration of 10 nM using an Illumina cBot. Sequencing of 2 × 100 bp was performed with an Illumina HiScanSQ sequencer at the sequencing core facility of the IZKF Leipzig (Faculty of Medicine, University Leipzig) using version 3 chemistry and flowcell according to the instructions of the manufacturer. Demultiplexing of raw reads, adapter trimming, and quality filtering were done according to Stokowy et al. [16] using TruSeq (Illumina) adapter sequences.

3.2. 786-0 Renal Cancer Cell Line and Real-Time PCR

The 786-0 and VHL-expressing 786-0-VHL were a kind gift of Prof. Barbara Seliger and were cultivated as described in [17]. For experimental setting, the cell culture medium was adjusted to 600 mosmol/kg by the addition of 100 mM NaCl and 100 mM urea. The cells were cultivated for different time points at 600 mosmol/kg. Total RNA isolation and cDNA synthesis were performed as described previously [4]. Real-time PCR was performed using the SYBR Green PCR Master Mix with the ABI PRISM 7900 Sequence Detection System. All instruments and reagents were purchased from Applied Biosystems (Darmstadt, Germany). Relative gene expression values were evaluated with the $2^{-\Delta\Delta Ct}$ method using *GAPDH* as reference gene [18]. The primer sequences for *ELF5* are *ELF5*-sense CGT GGA CTG ATC TGT TCA GCA ATG A, *ELF5*-antisense CAG GGT GGA CTG ATG TCC AGT ATG A and for *GAPDH GAPDH*-sense CAA GCT CAT TTC CTG GTA TGA C and *GAPDH*-antisense GTG TGG TGG GGG ACT GAG TGT GG.

3.3. Study Cohorts

Publicly available gene expression data from The Cancer Genome Atlas (TCGA) from a cohort of ccRCC patients (KIRC cohort, $n = 449$) were used to compare osmolality-induced genes expression between tumor and non-tumor samples. In this data set, 436 patients had both expression and CSS data and were used to develop the osmolality score. Expression data from tumor and non-tumor tissue were downloaded using the Bioconductor TCGAbiolinks package.

The validation cohort consisted of primary tumors with ccRCC histology ($n = 52$) of patients treated at the Department of Urology, University Hospital Tuebingen, Germany. Details of the study and tissue sample collection were described previously [13]. Transcriptome analyses was performed using the Human Transcriptome Array HTA 2.0 (Affymetrix/Thermo Fisher Scientific, Waltham, MA, USA), as described previously by Büttner et al. [13]. The accession number for genome-wide data at the European Genome-phenome Archive (EGA) (www.ebi.ac.uk/ega/home), which is hosted by the EBI and the CRG, is EGAS00001001176. Cancer-specific survival was used as endpoint in survival analyses of the development cohort (ccRCC KIRC) and the validation cohort, as described previously [13].

3.4. Statistical Analyses

RNA-Seq reads were aligned using bowtie2 and tophat2 to the rat reference genome (rnor6) according to Kim et al. [19]. Rat mRNA-Seq read counts were normalized and tested for differential expression using the Bioconductor edgeR package (v 3.24.3, [20]); 355 rat transcripts showed significant difference between two conditions: 900 and 300 mosmol/kg (Benjamini–Hochberg [21] adjusted p-Value < 0.05; $\log_2 FC >3/<-3$). Of these, 284 of them had matching human transcripts by gene symbol. For those 284 transcripts (223 genes), mRNA-Seq expression values (FPKM-UQ) of the TCGA-KIRC cohort (449 tumor samples with 67 matching tissue normal samples) were clustered (hierarchical clustering with agglomeration method ward. D2 and Euclidean distance). Clustering proved that selected transcripts expression clearly discriminated between tumor and normal samples. The potential impact of those genes' expression on TCGA-KIRC patients' ($n = 436$) cancer-specific survival (CSS) was tested by building a Cox proportional hazards model on each gene's expression separately (survival R package v 3.1-7, [21]). We found that 111 genes showed significant effect (Benjamini–Hochberg adjusted p-Value < 0.05). Later, we built a Cox proportional hazards model with lasso penalty based on the expression of the entire set of 223 genes (glmnet R package v 2.0-16, [22]). Four genes had non-zero coefficients according to the model, with minimal cross-validation error. Each TCGA-KIRC patient was assigned a survival score (termed the OSM score) calculated as the weighted sum of the expression of the four selected genes multiplied by the respective model coefficient. Analogously, the score was calculated for our independent RCC cohort ($n = 52$; [13]) based on selected genes expression (determined by microarray analyses) and the respective model coefficients. The value was multiplied by 100,000 times to avoid infinite hazards ratio. Patient cohorts were recursively partitioned based on the survival score using conditional inference trees [23] with the endpoint CSS. Multivariate survival analysis was performed using Cox proportional hazards regression models. Comparison of Cox models (with and without OSM score) was done using analysis of deviance [24].

4. Conclusions

Our study demonstrates that osmolality is an interesting pathway in ccRCC which has not yet been considered. The expression of hypertonicity-regulated genes is clearly associated with cancer-specific survival in ccRCC. We were also able to induce the expression of potentially tumor-suppressive genes by cultivating ccRCC cell lines under hyper-osmotic conditions.

Thus, targeting osmolality-associated pathways might represent a novel interesting therapeutic option for ccRCC.

Supplementary Materials: The following are available online at http://www.mdpi.com/2072-6694/12/1/6/s1, Figure S1: Selection of differentially expressed transcripts affected by hypertonicity for development of the novel OSM-score, Figure S2: Hierarchical clustering of samples from the normal kidney cortex and mouse ccRCCs based on the hypertonicity affected genes, Table S1: Differentially expressed transcripts affected by hypertonicity and expression differences of corresponding human transcripts in ccRCC tumor and non-tumor tissue of the TCGA KIRC cohort.

Author Contributions: S.K. performed research, analyzed data, and wrote the paper; K.K. analyzed data and wrote the paper; S.W. analyzed data and wrote the paper; J.L. performed research; J.B. contributed samples and wrote the paper; M.S. contributed samples and wrote the paper; E.S. designed research, analyzed data, and wrote the paper; B.E. designed research, performed research, analyzed data, and wrote the paper. All authors have read and agreed to the published version of the manuscript.

Funding: This work was supported by the Deutsche Forschungsgemeinschaft (DFG, German Research Foundation) ED 181/9-1, the Robert Bosch Stiftung (Stuttgart, Germany), the ICEPHA Graduate School Tuebingen-Stuttgart, The German Cancer Consortium (DKTK, Germany), and the Deutsche Forschungsgemeinschaft (DFG, German Research Foundation) under Germany's Excellence Strategy—EXC 2180-390900677.

Acknowledgments: We would like to thank Ian Frew, Clinic of Internal Medicine I, University Clinic Freiburg for his helpful discussion and interpretation of the data. The results shown here are partly based on data generated by the TCGA Research Network. We would like to thank The Cancer Genome Atlas initiative, all tissue donors, and investigators who contributed to the acquisition and analyses of the samples used in this study. Information about TCGA and the investigators and institutions who constitute the TCGA research network can be found at http://cancergenome.nih.gov/.

Conflicts of Interest: The authors declare no conflict of interest.

References

1. Lindgren, D.; Eriksson, P.; Krawczyk, K.; Nilsson, H.; Hansson, J.; Veerla, S.; Sjölund, J.; Höglund, M.; Johansson, M.E.; Axelson, H. Cell-Type-Specific Gene Programs of the Normal Human Nephron Define Kidney Cancer Subtypes. *Cell Rep.* **2017**, *20*, 1476–1489. [CrossRef]
2. Hsieh, J.J.; Purdue, M.P.; Signoretti, S.; Swanton, C.; Albiges, L.; Schmidinger, M.; Heng, D.Y.; Larkin, J.; Ficarra, V. Renal cell carcinoma. *Nat. Rev. Dis. Primers* **2017**, *3*, 17009. [CrossRef]
3. Büttner, F.; Winter, S.; Rausch, S.; Reustle, A.; Kruck, S.; Junker, K.; Stenzl, A.; Agaimy, A.; Hartmann, A.; Bedke, J.; et al. Survival Prediction of Clear Cell Renal Cell Carcinoma Based on Gene Expression Similarity to the Proximal Tubule of the Nephron. *Eur. Urol.* **2015**, *68*, 1016–1020. [CrossRef]
4. Schulze Blasum, B.; Schroter, R.; Neugebauer, U.; Hofschroer, V.; Pavenstadt, H.; Ciarimboli, G.; Schlatter, E.; Edemir, B. The kidney-specific expression of genes can be modulated by the extracellular osmolality. *FASEB J.* **2016**, *30*, 3588–3597. [CrossRef]
5. Schönenberger, D.; Rajski, M.; Harlander, S.; Frew, I.J. Vhl deletion in renal epithelia causes HIF-1α-dependent, HIF-2α-independent angiogenesis and constitutive diuresis. *Oncotarget* **2016**, *7*, 60971–60985. [CrossRef] [PubMed]

6. Jeon, U.S.; Kim, J.A.; Sheen, M.R.; Kwon, H.M. How tonicity regulates genes: Story of TonEBP transcriptional activator. *Acta Physiol.* **2006**, *187*, 241–247. [CrossRef] [PubMed]
7. Bogusławska, J.; Popławski, P.; Alseekh, S.; Koblowska, M.; Iwanicka-Nowicka, R.; Rybicka, B.; Kędzierska, H.; Głuchowska, K.; Hanusek, K.; Tański, Z.; et al. MicroRNA-Mediated Metabolic Reprograming in Renal Cancer. *Cancers* **2019**, *11*, 1825, confirmed.
8. Piggin, C.L.; Roden, D.L.; Gallego-Ortega, D.; Lee, H.J.; Oakes, S.R.; Ormandy, C.J. ELF5 isoform expression is tissue-specific and significantly altered in cancer. *Breast Cancer Res.* **2016**, *18*, 4. [CrossRef]
9. Ibanez de Caceres, I.; Dulaimi, E.; Hoffman, A.M.; Al-Saleem, T.; Uzzo, R.G.; Cairns, P. Identification of Novel Target Genes by an Epigenetic Reactivation Screen of Renal Cancer. *Cancer Res.* **2006**, *66*, 5021. [CrossRef] [PubMed]
10. Pal, D.; Sharma, U.; Singh, S.K.; Mandal, A.K.; Prasad, R. Metallothionein gene expression in renal cell carcinoma. *Indian J. Urol. IJU J. Urol. Soc. India* **2014**, *30*, 241–244.
11. Wang, L.; Peng, Z.; Wang, K.; Qi, Y.; Yang, Y.; Zhang, Y.; An, X.; Luo, S.; Zheng, J. NDUFA4L2 is associated with clear cell renal cell carcinoma malignancy and is regulated by ELK1. *PeerJ* **2017**, *5*, e4065. [CrossRef] [PubMed]
12. Lyu, X.-J.; Li, H.-Z.; Ma, X.; Li, X.-T.; Gao, Y.; Ni, D.; Shen, D.-L.; Gu, L.-Y.; Wang, B.-J.; Zhang, Y.; et al. Elevated S100A6 (Calcyclin) enhances tumorigenesis and suppresses CXCL14-induced apoptosis in clear cell renal cell carcinoma. *Oncotarget* **2015**, *6*, 6656–6669. [CrossRef] [PubMed]
13. Büttner, F.; Winter, S.; Rausch, S.; Hennenlotter, J.; Kruck, S.; Stenzl, A.; Scharpf, M.; Fend, F.; Agaimy, A.; Hartmann, A.; et al. Clinical utility of the S3-score for molecular prediction of outcome in non-metastatic and metastatic clear cell renal cell carcinoma. *BMC Med.* **2018**, *16*, 108. [CrossRef]
14. Harlander, S.; Schönenberger, D.; Toussaint, N.C.; Prummer, M.; Catalano, A.; Brandt, L.; Moch, H.; Wild, P.J.; Frew, I.J. Combined mutation in Vhl, Trp53 and Rb1 causes clear cell renal cell carcinoma in mice. *Nat. Med.* **2017**, *23*, 869–877. [CrossRef]
15. Meyer, M.; Kircher, M. Illumina Sequencing Library Preparation for Highly Multiplexed Target Capture and Sequencing. *Cold Spring Harb. Protoc.* **2010**, *2010*, pdb.prot5448. [CrossRef]
16. Stokowy, T.; Eszlinger, M.; Świerniak, M.; Fujarewicz, K.; Jarząb, B.; Paschke, R.; Krohn, K. Analysis options for high-throughput sequencing in miRNA expression profiling. *BMC Res. Notes* **2014**, *7*, 144. [CrossRef]
17. Leisz, S.; Schulz, K.; Erb, S.; Oefner, P.; Dettmer, K.; Mougiakakos, D.; Wang, E.; Marincola, F.M.; Stehle, F.; Seliger, B. Distinct von Hippel-Lindau gene and hypoxia-regulated alterations in gene and protein expression patterns of renal cell carcinoma and their effects on metabolism. *Oncotarget* **2015**, *6*, 11395–11406. [CrossRef] [PubMed]
18. Livak, K.J.; Schmittgen, T.D. Analysis of relative gene expression data using real-time quantitative PCR and the $2^{-\Delta\Delta Ct}$ Method. *Methods* **2001**, *25*, 402–408. [CrossRef]
19. Kim, D.; Pertea, G.; Trapnell, C.; Pimentel, H.; Kelley, R.; Salzberg, S.L. TopHat2: Accurate alignment of transcriptomes in the presence of insertions, deletions and gene fusions. *Genome Biol.* **2013**, *14*, R36. [CrossRef]
20. McCarthy, D.J.; Smyth, G.K.; Robinson, M.D. edgeR: A Bioconductor package for differential expression analysis of digital gene expression data. *Bioinformatics* **2009**, *26*, 139–140.
21. Benjamini, Y.; Hochberg, Y. Controlling the false discovery rate: A practical and powerful approach to multiple testing. *J. R. Stat. Soc. Ser. B* **1995**, *85*, 289–300. [CrossRef]
22. Friedman, J.; Hastie, T.; Tibshirani, R. Regularization Paths for Generalized Linear Models via Coordinate Descent. *J. Stat. Softw.* **2010**, *33*, 1–22. [CrossRef] [PubMed]
23. Hothorn, T.; Zeileis, A. Partykit: A Modular Toolkit for Recursive Partytioning in R. *J. Mach. Learn. Res.* **2015**, *16*, 3905–3909.
24. Therneau, T.M.; Grambsch, P.M. *Modeling Survival Data: Extending the Cox Model*; Springer: New York, NY, USA, 2000.

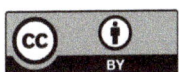

© 2019 by the authors. Licensee MDPI, Basel, Switzerland. This article is an open access article distributed under the terms and conditions of the Creative Commons Attribution (CC BY) license (http://creativecommons.org/licenses/by/4.0/).

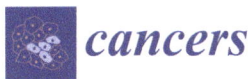

Commentary

Renal Cell Carcinoma with Sarcomatoid Features: Finally New Therapeutic Hope?

Renate Pichler [1],*, Eva Compérat [2], Tobias Klatte [3], Martin Pichler [4,5], Wolfgang Loidl [6], Lukas Lusuardi [7] and Manuela Schmidinger [8]

1. Department of Urology, Medical University Innsbruck, A-6020 Innsbruck, Austria
2. Department of Pathology, Hôspital Tenon, HUEP, Sorbonne University, 75005 Paris, France; eva.comperat@aphp.fr
3. Department of Urology, Royal Bournemouth Hospital, Bournemouth BH7 7DW, UK; Tobias.Klatte@gmx.de
4. Division of Clinical Oncology, Internal Medicine, Medical University of Graz, 8036 Graz, Austria; Martin.Pichler@medunigraz.at
5. Division of Cancer Medicine, MD Anderson Cancer Center, Houston, TX 77030, USA
6. Department of Urology, St Vincent's Hospital of Linz, 4010 Linz, Austria; Wolfgang.Loidl@ordensklinikum.at
7. Department of Urology & Andrology, Paracelsus Medical University Salzburg, 5020 Salzburg, Austria; l.lusuardi@salk.at
8. Clinical Division of Oncology, Department of Medicine I & Comprehensive Cancer Center, Medical University of Vienna, 1090 Vienna, Austria; Manuela.Schmidinger@meduniwien.ac.at
* Correspondence: Renate.Pichler@i-med.ac.at; Tel.: +43-0-512-504-24811; Fax: +43-0-512-504-28365

Received: 7 March 2019; Accepted: 22 March 2019; Published: 25 March 2019

Abstract: Renal cell carcinoma (RCC) with sarcomatoid differentiation belongs to the most aggressive clinicopathologic phenotypes of RCC. It is characterized by a high propensity for primary metastasis and limited therapeutic options due to its relative resistance to established systemic targeted therapy. Most trials report on a poor median overall survival of 5 to 12 months. Sarcomatoid RCC can show the typical features of epithelial-mesenchymal transition (EMT) and may contain epithelial and mesenchymal features on both the morphological and immunohistochemical level. On the molecular level, next-generation sequencing confirmed differences in driver mutations between sarcomatoid RCC and non-sarcomatoid RCC. In contrast, mutational profiles within the epithelial and sarcomatoid components of sarcomatoid RCC were shown to be identical, with TP53 being the most frequently altered gene. These data suggest that both epithelial and sarcomatoid components of RCC originate from the same progenitor cell, segregating primarily according to the underlying histologic epithelial subtype of RCC (clear cell, papillary or chromophobe). Current studies have shown that sarcomatoid RCC express programmed death 1 (PD-1) and its ligand (PD-L1) at a much higher level than non-sarcomatoid RCC, suggesting that blockade of the PD-1/PD-L1 axis may be an attractive new therapeutic strategy. Preliminary results of clinical trials evaluating checkpoint inhibitors in patients with sarcomatoid RCC showed encouraging survival data and objective response and complete response rates of up to 62% and 18%, respectively. These findings may establish a new standard of care in the management of patients with sarcomatoid RCC.

Keywords: sarcomatoid; RCC; immunotherapy; checkpoint inhibitors; survival; PD-L1

1. Introduction

Renal cell carcinoma (RCC) with sarcomatoid differentiation (sRCC) is a highly aggressive form of RCC. Histologically, sRCC shows loss of characteristic epithelial components and contains features such as spindle cells, high cellularity, and cellular atypia. These features are found in 5–8% of clear-cell RCC (ccRCC), 8–9% of chromophobe RCC, and 2–3% of papillary RCC [1–4]. About 75% of patients with sRCC present with metastatic disease [5,6] and outcomes are generally modest. Therapeutic strategies include vascular endothelial growth factor (VEGF)-targeted monotherapy [7], and combined strategies with sunitinib plus gemcitabine [8] or gemcitabine plus doxorubicin [9]. The majority of studies report on a poor median overall survival, ranging from 5 to 12 months [7–9].

2. The sRCC

The sRCC is not a distinct morphogenetic subtype of RCC [3,10]. It originates from epithelial-mesenchymal transition (EMT), and therefore contains both epithelial (carcinoma) and mesenchymal (sarcomatoid) features on both the morphological and immunhistochemical level [11], which is distinctive from primary sarcoma of the kidney [3,10]. The presence of even a small component of sarcomatoid differentiation was shown to independently predict poor survival compared to RCC without sarcomatoid features; thus, its description needs to be included in the surgical pathology report [3]. To which extent this would be necessary in tumors showing only 1% of sarcomatoid features is questionable, since pathology reports are extremely dependent on gross sampling.

Genomic profiling on paired epithelial and sarcomatoid areas of sRCC by next-generation sequencing confirmed different driver mutations between sRCC and ccRCC. However, the epithelial and sarcomatoid components of sRCC showed identical mutational profiles, with *TP53* (42%), *VHL* (35%), *CDKN2A* (27%), and *NF2* (19%) being the most frequently altered genes [12]. These findings have been confirmed by Wang et al. [13]: The epithelioid and sarcomatoid components of sRCC did not show differences in mutational load amongst cancer-related genes, whereas sRCC had a completely different molecular pathogenesis and distinctive mutational and transcriptional profiles compared to ccRCC. Indeed, the authors found fewer deletions at 3p21-25, a lower rate of two-hit loss of *VHL* and *PBRM1*, but more mutations in *TP53*, *PTEN*, and *RELN* [13]. Moreover, mutations in known cancer drivers, such as AT-rich interaction domain 1A (ARID1A) and BRCA1 associated protein 1 (BAP1), were significantly mutated in sarcomatoid patterns and mutually exclusive with TP53 and each other [14]. These data corroborate the hypothesis that both epithelial and sarcomatoid components of RCC may originate from the same progenitor cell, but clonal divergence occurs during tumor progression. This implicates that specific genes are involved in this process, leading to unique genetic alterations based on the observed EMT [1,15].

Induction of EMT may upregulate the expression of PD-L1 and other targetable immune checkpoint molecules in various cancer entities, such as claudin-low breast cancer [16], non-small cell lung cancer [17], or RCC [18] in vivo and in vitro. Interestingly, sRCC has been shown to express programmed death 1 (PD-1) and its ligand (PD-L1) at a much higher level than RCC without sarcomatoid elements [19], as seen in Figures 1 and 2. As higher tumoral PD-L1 expression seems to correlate with higher Fuhrmann grade [20], it is essential to compare the PD-L1 status between sRCC and grade 4 non-sarcomatoid ccRCC specifically [19]. Although sRCC is defined as grade 4 RCC, tumoral PD-L1 expression in the epithelioid component of sRCC was even higher than in non-sarcomatoid grade 4 ccRCC [19]. These results may suggest a biologic distinctiveness of sRCC compared to non-sarcomatoid ccRCC at the level of immune markers [19]. In this regard, tumoral PD-L1 and PD-1 expression was found in 54% and 96% of sRCC, compared to 17% and 62% of ccRCC specimens [21]. Moreover, the co-expression of both PD-L1 on tumor cells and PD-1 positive tumor-infiltrating lymphocytes was confirmed in 50% of all sRCC cases, compared to only one case (3%) with ccRCC [21]. These findings suggest that blockade of the PD-1/PD-L1 axis could be an attractive therapeutic approach in EMT-derived tumors, such as sRCC.

A small retrospective study by Ross et al., 2018, on response to checkpoint inhibitors in RCC patients with sarcomatoid differentiation presented as an abstract at American Society of Clinical Oncology (ASCO) Annual Meeting 2018 showed promising outcomes, with durable complete responses (CR) in up to 15% of patients, and an objective response rate (ORR) of 62% [22]. The genomic biomarker analyses of the phase III IMmotion151 study on bevacizumab plus atezolizumab versus sunitinib correlated angiogenesis and immune gene expression signatures with clinical outcomes from 832 RCC patients, focusing on sarcomatoid histology. Interestingly, the PD-L1 prevalence was higher in sRCC (63%), compared to non-sRCC (39%), whereas angiogenesis gene signature was lower in sRCC (34% vs. 65%) [23]. These results may explain why sRCC patients (n = 86) in the PD-L1+ study group showed the greatest therapeutic benefit with atezolizumab plus bevacizumab (progression-free survival: HR, 0.56 (95% CI: 0.38–0.83)) compared to sunitinib monotherapy [23,24]. In addition, the retrospective subgroup analysis of 112 sRCC intermediate or poor-risk patients from the CheckMate214 study [25] confirmed a higher rate of PD-L1 expression ($\geq$1%) in sRCC than in non-sRCC (47–53% vs. 26–29%). More importantly, immunotherapy with nivolumab plus ipilimumab achieved an unprecedently high ORR of 57%, with a CR rate of 18% and a median overall Survival (OS) of 31 months compared to vascular endothelial growth factor (VEGF)-targeted monotherapy with sunitinib (ORR, CR, median OS: 19%, 0% and 14 months) [26].

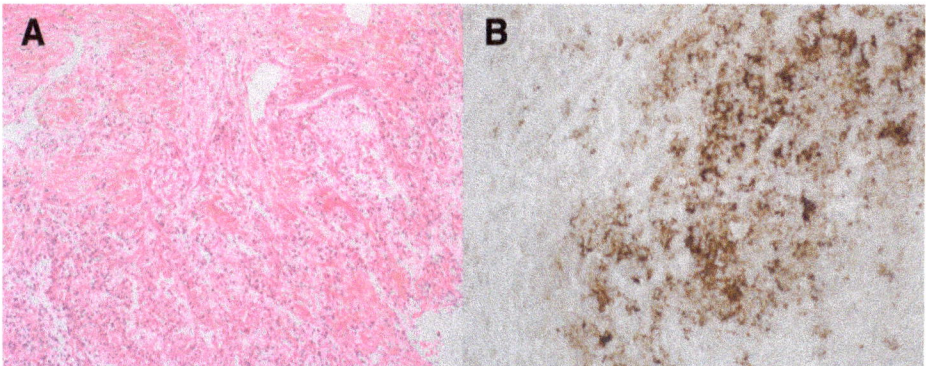

Figure 1. (**A**) Hematoxylin/eosin and phloxin staining for clear-cell RCC (ccRCC) with sarcomatoid features (50× magnification), considered as grade 4 according to the International Society of Urologic Pathologists (ISUP). (**B**) High PD-L1 (100× magnification) (E1L3N XP Rabbit mAB) cytoplasmatic staining of tumor cells in sRCC (>50% of tumor cells).

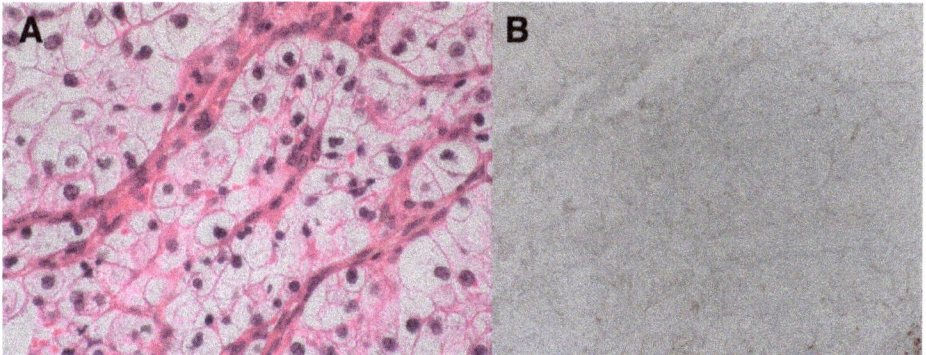

Figure 2. (**A**) Hematoxylin/eosin and phloxin staining for ccRCC without sarcomatoid features (400× magnification). (**B**) PD-L1 (E1L3N XP Rabbit mAB) cytoplasmatic staining of tumor cells, showing low PD-L1 expression (<5%), 100× magnification.

3. Conclusions

In summary, sRCC shows the typical features of EMT. On the molecular level, transcriptional data confirmed that sRCC is not a homogeneous RCC subtype and segregates primarily according to the underlying parental epithelial subtype (ccRCC, papillary or chromophobe RCC). Current biomarker studies have shown that sRCC tumors express PD-1/PD-L1 at a much higher level than non-sarcomatoid RCC. These findings will ultimately lead to a change in the treatment paradigm, shifting therapeutic decisions towards checkpoint inhibitors as first line treatment for sRCC.

Author Contributions: R.P. conceived and designed the work and was responsible for writing the draft. E.C. was responsible for pathological figures and PD-L1 staining. T.K., M.P., W.L., L.L., and M.S. critically revised the manuscript and were responsible for supervision.

Funding: This research received no external funding.

Conflicts of Interest: The authors declare no conflict of interest.

References

1. Jones, T.D.; Eble, J.N.; Wang, M.; Maclennan, G.T.; Jain, S.; Cheng, L. Clonal divergence and genetic heterogeneity in clear cell renal cell carcinomas with sarcomatoid transformation. *Cancer* **2005**, *104*, 1195–1203. [CrossRef] [PubMed]
2. Cheville, J.C.; Lohse, C.M.; Zincke, H.; Weaver, A.L.; Leibovich, B.C.; Frank, I.; Blute, M.L. Sarcomatoid renal cell carcinoma: An examination of underlying histologic subtype and an analysis of associations with patient outcome. *Am. J. Surg. Pathol.* **2004**, *28*, 435–441. [CrossRef]
3. De Peralta-Venturina, M.; Moch, H.; Amin, M.; Tamboli, P.; Hailemariam, S.; Mihatsch, M.; Javidan, J.; Stricker, H.; Ro, J.Y.; Amin, M.B. Sarcomatoid differentiation in renal cell carcinoma: A study of 101 cases. *Am. J. Surg. Pathol.* **2001**, *25*, 275–284. [CrossRef]
4. Amin, M.B.; Paner, G.P.; Alvarado-Cabrero, I.; Young, A.N.; Stricker, H.J.; Lyles, R.H.; Moch, H. Chromophobe renal cell carcinoma: Histomorphologic characteristics and evaluation of conventional pathologic prognostic parameters in 145 cases. *Am. J. Surg. Pathol.* **2008**, *32*, 1822–1834. [CrossRef] [PubMed]
5. Mian, B.M.; Bhadkamkar, N.; Slaton, J.W.; Pisters, P.W.; Daliani, D.; Swanson, D.A.; Pisters, L.L. Prognostic factors and survival of patients with sarcomatoid renal cell carcinoma. *J. Urol.* **2002**, *167*, 65–70. [CrossRef]
6. Merrill, M.M.; Wood, C.G.; Tannir, N.M.; Slack, R.S.; Babaian, K.N.; Jonasch, E.; Pagliaro, L.C.; Compton, Z.; Tamboli, P.; Sircar, K.; et al. Clinically nonmetastatic renal cell carcinoma with sarcomatoid dedifferentiation: Natural history and outcomes after surgical resection with curative intent. *Urol. Oncol.* **2015**, *33*, 166.e21-9. [CrossRef] [PubMed]
7. Golshayan, A.R.; George, S.; Heng, D.Y.; Elson, P.; Wood, L.S.; Mekhail, T.M.; Garcia, J.A.; Aydin, H.; Zhou, M.; Bukowski, R.M.; et al. Metastatic sarcomatoid renal cell carcinoma treated with vascular endothelial growth factor-targeted therapy. *J. Clin. Oncol.* **2009**, *27*, 235–241. [CrossRef] [PubMed]
8. Michaelson, M.D.; McKay, R.R.; Werner, L.; Atkins, M.B.; Van Allen, E.M.; Olivier, K.M.; Song, J.; Signoretti, S.; McDermott, D.F.; Choueiri, T.K. Phase 2 trial of sunitinib and gemcitabine in patients with sarcomatoid and/or poor-risk metastatic renal cell carcinoma. *Cancer* **2015**, *121*, 3435–3443. [CrossRef]
9. Roubaud, G.; Gross-Goupil, M.; Wallerand, H.; de Clermont, H.; Dilhuydy, M.S.; Ravaud, A. Combination of gemcitabine and doxorubicin in rapidly progressive metastatic renal cell carcinoma and/or sarcomatoid renal cell carcinoma. *Oncology* **2011**, *80*, 214–218. [CrossRef]
10. Delahunt, B.; Cheville, J.C.; Martignoni, G.; Humphrey, P.A.; Magi-Galluzzi, C.; McKenney, J.; Egevad, L.; Algaba, F.; Moch, H.; Grignon, D.J.; et al. The International Society of Urological Pathology (ISUP) grading system for renal cell carcinoma and other prognostic parameters. *Am. J. Surg. Pathol.* **2013**, *37*, 1490–1504. [CrossRef]
11. Mikami, S.; Katsube, K.; Oya, M.; Ishida, M.; Kosaka, T.; Mizuno, R.; Mukai, M.; Okada, Y. Expression of Snail and Slug in renal cell carcinoma: E-cadherin repressor Snail is associated with cancer invasion and prognosis. *Lab. Investig.* **2011**, *91*, 1443–1458. [CrossRef] [PubMed]
12. Malouf, G.G.; Ali, S.M.; Wang, K.; Balasubramanian, S.; Ross, J.S.; Miller, V.A.; Stephens, P.J.; Khayat, D.; Pal, S.K.; Su, X.; et al. Genomic Characterization of Renal Cell Carcinoma with Sarcomatoid Dedifferentiation Pinpoints Recurrent Genomic Alterations. *Eur. Urol.* **2016**, *70*, 348–357. [CrossRef] [PubMed]
13. Wang, Z.; Kim, T.B.; Peng, B.; Karam, J.; Creighton, C.; Joon, A.; Kawakami, F.; Trevisan, P.; Jonasch, E.; Chow, C.W.; et al. Sarcomatoid Renal Cell Carcinoma Has a Distinct Molecular Pathogenesis, Driver Mutation Profile, and Transcriptional Landscape. *Clin. Cancer Res.* **2017**, *23*, 6686–6696. [CrossRef]

14. Bi, M.; Zhao, S.; Said, J.W.; Merino, M.J.; Adeniran, A.J.; Xie, Z.; Nawaf, C.B.; Choi, J.; Belldegrun, A.S.; Pantuck, A.J.; et al. Genomic characterization of sarcomatoid transformation in clear cell renal cell carcinoma. *Proc. Natl. Acad. Sci. USA* **2016**, *113*, 2170–2175. [CrossRef] [PubMed]
15. Lebacle, C.; Pooli, A.; Bessede, T.; Irani, J.; Pantuck, A.J.; Drakaki, A. Epidemiology, biology and treatment of sarcomatoid RCC: Current state of the art. *World J. Urol.* **2019**, *37*, 115–123. [CrossRef] [PubMed]
16. Alsuliman, A.; Colak, D.; Al-Harazi, O.; Fitwi, H.; Tulbah, A.; Al-Tweigeri, T.; Al-Alwan, M.; Ghebeh, H. Bidirectional crosstalk between PD-L1 expression and epithelial to mesenchymal transition: Significance in claudin-low breast cancer cells. *Mol. Cancer* **2015**, *14*, 149. [CrossRef]
17. Lou, Y.; Diao, L.; Cuentas, E.R.; Denning, W.L.; Chen, L.; Fan, Y.H.; Byers, L.A.; Wang, J.; Papadimitrakopoulou, V.A.; Behrens, C.; et al. Epithelial-Mesenchymal Transition Is Associated with a Distinct Tumor Microenvironment Including Elevation of Inflammatory Signals and Multiple Immune Checkpoints in Lung Adenocarcinoma. *Clin. Cancer Res.* **2016**, *22*, 3630–3642. [CrossRef]
18. Wang, Y.; Wang, H.; Zhao, Q.; Xia, Y.; Hu, X.; Guo, J. PD-L1 induces epithelial-to-mesenchymal transition via activating SREBP-1c in renal cell carcinoma. *Med. Oncol.* **2015**, *32*, 212. [CrossRef]
19. Kawakami, F.; Sircar, K.; Rodriguez-Canales, J.; Fellman, B.M.; Urbauer, D.L.; Tamboli, P.; Tannir, N.M.; Jonasch, E.; Wistuba, I.I.; Wood, C.G.; et al. Programmed cell death ligand 1 and tumor-infiltrating lymphocyte status in patients with renal cell carcinoma and sarcomatoid dedifferentiation. *Cancer* **2017**, *123*, 4823–4831. [CrossRef] [PubMed]
20. Thompson, R.H.; Dong, H.; Kwon, E.D. Implications of B7-H1 expression in clear cell carcinoma of the kidney for prognostication and therapy. *Clin Cancer Res.* **2007**, *13*, 709s–715s. [CrossRef] [PubMed]
21. Joseph, R.W.; Millis, S.Z.; Carballido, E.M.; Bryant, D.; Gatalica, Z.; Reddy, S.; Bryce, A.H.; Vogelzang, N.J.; Stanton, M.L.; Castle, E.P.; et al. PD-1 and PD-L1 Expression in Renal Cell Carcinoma with Sarcomatoid Differentiation. *Cancer Immunol. Res.* **2015**, *3*, 1303–1307. [CrossRef] [PubMed]
22. Ross, J.A.; McCormick, B.Z.; Gao, J.; Msaouel, P.; Campbell, M.T.; Zurita, A.J.; Shah, A.Y.; Jonasch, E.; Matin, S.F.; Wood, C.G.; et al. Outcomes of patients (pts) with metastatic renal cell carcinoma (mRCC) and sarcomatoid dedifferentiation (sRCC) after treatment with immune checkpoint inhibitors (ICI): A single-institution retrospective study. *J Clin Oncol.* **2018**, *36*. [CrossRef]
23. Rini, B.I.; Huseni, M.; Atkins, M.B.; McDermott, M.F.; Powles, T.; Escudier, B.; Banchereau, R.; Liu, L.; Leng, N.; Fan, J.; et al. Molecular correlates differentiate response to atezolizumab (atezo) + bevacizumab (bev) vs sunitinib (sun): Results from a Phase III study (IMmotion151) in untreated metastatic renal cell carcinoma (mRCC). In Proceedings of the ESMO 2018, Munich, Germany, 19–23 October 2018.
24. Motzer, R.J.; Powles, T.; Atkins, M.B.; Escudier, B.; McDermott, D.F.; Suarez, C.; Bracarda, S.; Stadler, W.M.; Donskov, F.; Lee, J.L.; et al. IMmotion151: A Randomized Phase III Study of Atezolizumab Plus Bevacizumab vs Sunitinib in Untreated Metastatic Renal Cell Carcinoma (mRCC). *J. Clin. Oncol.* **2018**, *36*. [CrossRef]
25. Motzer, R.J.; Tannir, N.M.; McDermott, D.F.; Arén Frontera, O.; Melichar, B.; Choueiri, T.K.; Plimack, E.R.; Barthélémy, P.; Porta, C.; George, S.; et al. Nivolumab plus Ipilimumab versus Sunitinib in Advanced Renal-Cell Carcinoma. *N. Engl. J. Med.* **2018**, *378*, 1277–1290. [CrossRef] [PubMed]
26. McDermott, D.F.; Motzer, R.J.; Rini, B.I.; Aren Frontera, O.; George, S.; Powles, T.; Donskov, F.; Harrison, M.; Rodriguez-Cid, J.; Ishii, Y.; et al. ChechMate214 retrospective analyses of nivolumab plus ipilimumab or sunitinib in IMDC intermediate/poor-risk patients with previously untreated advanced renal cell carcinoma with sarcomatoid features. In Proceedings of the Seventeenth International Kidney Cancer Symposium, Miami, FL, USA, 2–3 November 2018.

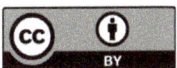

© 2019 by the authors. Licensee MDPI, Basel, Switzerland. This article is an open access article distributed under the terms and conditions of the Creative Commons Attribution (CC BY) license (http://creativecommons.org/licenses/by/4.0/).

MDPI
St. Alban-Anlage 66
4052 Basel
Switzerland
Tel. +41 61 683 77 34
Fax +41 61 302 89 18
www.mdpi.com

Cancers Editorial Office
E-mail: cancers@mdpi.com
www.mdpi.com/journal/cancers

www.ingramcontent.com/pod-product-compliance
Lightning Source LLC
LaVergne TN
LVHW070128100526
838202LV00016B/2245